Proteomics: Human Diseases and Advances

Proteomics: Human Diseases and Advances

Edited by **Steven Tiff**

hayle medical

New York

Published by Hayle Medical,
30 West, 37th Street, Suite 612,
New York, NY 10018, USA
www.haylemedical.com

Proteomics: Human Diseases and Advances
Edited by Steven Tiff

International Standard Book Number: 978-1-63241-331-4 (Hardback)

Printed in China.

Contents

Preface

Proteomics is a diverse field dealing in study of various proteins and their structure and functions. Biomedical research has reached the stage where a novel era of identifying a disease or a protein globally has emerged. During the post-genomic era, proteomics played an extremely significant role in analyzing molecular functions of proteins and determining biomarkers in diseases affecting human beings. Mass spectrometry, high-density antibody and protein collection, and 2D gel electrophoresis are few of the generally employed techniques in proteomics field. This book elucidates four significant and varied areas of present proteomic research: proteomic analysis of protein functions, organelles and secretome proteomics, proteomic discovery of disease biomarkers, and proteomic techniques for analyzing disease procedures. The use of these techniques in analyzing proteins in different diseases has now become a significant part of biomedical research across the globe. This book will serve as a useful source of reference for students, researchers as well as clinicians.

This book is the end result of constructive efforts and intensive research done by experts in this field. The aim of this book is to enlighten the readers with recent information in this area of research. The information provided in this profound book would serve as a valuable reference to students and researchers in this field.

At the end, I would like to thank all the authors for devoting their precious time and providing their valuable contribution to this book. I would also like to express my gratitude to my fellow colleagues who encouraged me throughout the process.

Editor

Part 1

Proteomic Discovery of Disease Biomarkers

1

Overview of Current Proteomic Approaches for Discovery of Vascular Biomarkers of Atherosclerosis

Lepedda Antonio Junior, Zinellu Elisabetta and Formato Marilena
University of Sassari/Dipartimento di Scienze Fisiologiche, Biochimiche e Cellulari
Italy

1. Introduction

Cardiovascular diseases are the leading cause of mortality and morbidity in developed countries being atherosclerosis the major contributor. Atherosclerosis is a form of chronic inflammation characterized by the accumulation of lipids and fibrous elements in medium and large arteries (Libby, 2002). The retention of apoB-100 containing lipoproteins (mainly LDL and Lp(a)) in the subendothelial space and their subsequent oxidation is thought to be the leading event in the development of atherosclerotic lesions (Williams & Tabas, 1995). The degree of inflammation, proteolysis, calcification and neovascularization affects the stability of advanced lesions. Plaque rupture and thrombosis are the most important clinical complications in the pathogenesis of stroke, coronary arteries and peripheral vascular diseases (Lutgens et al., 2003). So, the identification of early biomarkers of plaque presence and susceptibility to ulceration could be of primary importance in preventing such a life-threatening event. Disease aetiology is very complex and includes several important environmental and genetic risk factors such as hyperlipidemia, diabetes, and hypertension. In this regard elevated plasma levels of LDL cholesterol and low levels of HDL cholesterol have been long associated with the onset and development of atherosclerotic lesions. Although enormous efforts have been done to elucidate the molecular mechanisms underlying plaque formation and progression, they are not yet completely understood. In the last years, proteomic studies have been undertaken to both elucidate pathways of atherosclerotic degeneration and individuate new circulating markers to be utilized either as early diagnostic traits or as targets for new drug therapies.

This chapter will provide an overview of latest advances in proteomic studies on atherosclerosis and some related diseases, with particular emphasis on vascular tissue proteomics and lipoproteomics.

2. Application of proteomic technologies to the study of atherosclerosis

Atherosclerosis is a very complex pathology in terms of cell types involved, inflammatory mechanisms and multifactorial aetiology. Many efforts have been done to shed light on the mechanisms underlying atherogenesis and to identify new circulating biomarkers which, along with traditional risk factors, will help in early diagnosis and prevention as well as in monitoring the effects of pharmacological agents. To address these issues, proteomic studies have been focused on different matrices such as vascular cell/tissues, looking at both proteomes and secretomes, plasma/serum, urine, and purified plasma lipoprotein fractions (fig. 1).

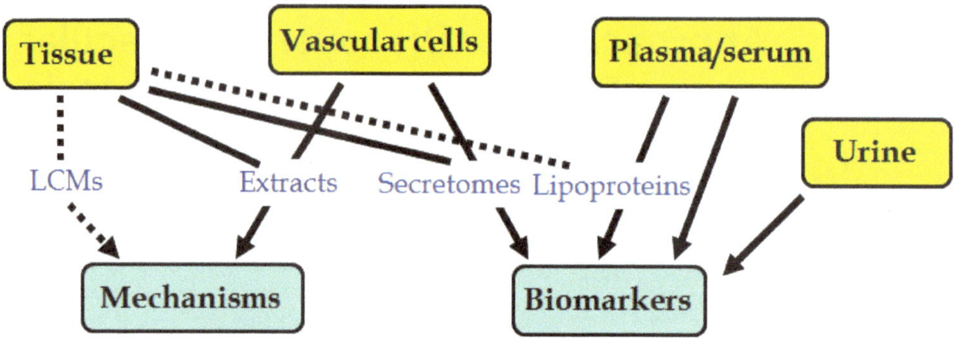

Fig. 1. Overview of the main targets of proteomic studies searching for both mechanisms of atherogenesis and biomarkers of atherosclerotic lesion presence and progression. Dotted lines represent almost unexplored paths. LCMs, laser-captured microdissections

To date, several proteomic approaches, such as 1D-2D electrophoresis (1DE-2DE) followed by mass spectrometry (MS) analyses, western arrays, protein arrays, and gel-free MS based proteomics, have been applied in the search of vascular biomarkers of atherosclerosis. Often, classical biochemical methods, mainly western blotting (WB), ELISA, and immunohistochemistry (IH) have been used to validate the proteomic results.

2.1 Vascular tissue proteomics

Even though tissue analyses frequently provide useful data, there are major drawbacks in analysing human atherosclerotic specimens. Atherosclerotic plaques are quite complex in terms of vascular cells and extracellular components. In this respect, besides vascular smooth muscle cells (VSMCs) and endothelial cells (ECs), they are composed of inflammatory cells, filtered plasma proteins, new-formed extracellular matrix, cellular debris and end-products of lipid and protein oxidation. Another critical point in the *in situ* analysis of protein expression within atherosclerotic plaques is the choice of the appropriate control. It would be desirable to utilize control specimens from the same vascular district of the same patient, in order to minimize intrinsic tissue differences, and from surgical endarterectomy rather than from post-mortem material, to avoid the occurrence of proteolytic modifications prior to analysis. Also the availability of a significant number of human specimens could be limiting. Because of the complexity of advanced lesions (Stary, 2000; Virmani et al., 2000) in terms of necrotic core dimension, fibrous cap thickness, inflammatory and proteolytic components, careful histochemical classification is needed. Moreover, results from different advanced lesion typologies are difficult to interpret because they could be either associated to the lesion development or merely a consequence of the advanced condition. In the latest years proteomic technologies have been applied to human diseased tissues to both characterize mechanisms of advanced atherosclerotic plaque development, mainly those responsible for its instability, and to identify markers useful in diagnosis and patients treatment. Compared to tissue specimens of human origin, animal models, mainly rodents, have been utilized to study the mechanisms underlying the early stages of lesion formation.

2.1.1 Studies on animal models

Apolipoprotein E-deficient mouse is the most popular murine model in cardiovascular research and has revealed important insights into mechanisms affecting atherogenesis. Mayr et al. analysed aortic lesions from apolipoprotein $E^{-}/^{-}$ and wild type mice classified as light, medium, and severe according to lesion-covered areas on the aortic surface (Mayr et al., 2005). As expected, authors found an increase of inflammatory cells, a decrease of VSMCs, and an accumulation of serum proteins associated to an impaired endothelial barrier function with lesion progression. Interestingly, immunoglobulins, that were barely detectable in apolipoprotein $E^{+}/^{+}$ mice, accumulated even in aortas of young apolipoprotein $E^{-}/^{-}$ mice. The authors identified 79 differentially expressed spots. Moreover, they suggested an increase in oxidative stress with lesion progression evaluating the ratio between the oxidized and the reduced forms of peroxiredoxin, the former resulting in a charge shift toward a more acidic isoelectric point. Overall, they found a linear relationship between the degree of peroxiredoxin-Cys oxidation and the extent of lesion formation in aortas of apolipoprotein E-deficient mice. Almofti et al. applied 2DE coupled to matrix-assisted laser desorption/ionization time of flight (MALDI TOF) MS analysis to a rat model of atherosclerosis. They induced atherosclerosis by a single dose of vitamin D3 associated with a high fat diet and identified 46 proteins differently expressed in diseased tissues. Among them, 18 proteins, including a group of oxidization-related enzymes, were found to be up-regulated, while 28 proteins were found down-regulated (Almofti et al., 2006). Vascular endothelium plays important physiological roles in vascular homeostasis, coagulation, inflammation, as well as tissue growth and repair. Impairment of the endothelial function is an early event in atherosclerotic lesion formation leading to overexpression of adhesion molecules as well as secretion of pro-inflammatory and chemotactic cytokines. An affinity-based proteomic approach was used by Wu et al. (Wu et al., 2007) to identify vascular endothelial surface proteins differentially expressed in aortic tissues of apolipoprotein E deficient mice. After *in situ* perfusion of vascular bed with a solution containing a biotin-derivative, biotinylated endothelial proteins were extracted, purified by affinity enrichment with streptavidin-agarose beads, and resolved by SDS-PAGE. The whole gel lanes were cut into slices that were subjected to tryptic digestion for nano liquid chromatography (LC) MS/MS analysis. In this way, 454 proteins, mainly extracellular or associated to cell membrane, were identified. Among them, there were cell adhesion molecules, accounting for the largest category, followed by proteins involved in signal transduction and transport. Interestingly, proteins associated with immune and inflammatory responses were more than doubled in atherosclerotic aorta (13%) in comparison to normal aorta (6%). On the other hand, proteins involved in lipid metabolism were decreased by 34% in atherosclerotic aorta. A rat model has been recently used for a proteomic study on the effects of blood shear stress on atherogenesis (Qi et al., 2008). It is well known that blood shear stress affects endothelial cell shape and orientation, as well as vascular wall permeability. Indeed, regions of arterial branching or curvature, where blood flow is not uniform, are preferential sites for lesion formation. By comparing homogenates of aortas kept under two levels of shear stress in a perfusion culture system for 24 hours, Qi et al. detected a reduced expression of protein Rho-GDP dissociation inhibitor alpha (Rho-GDIα) in low shear stress conditions and demonstrated, by siRNA technology, that this reduction enhances VSMC migration and apoptosis.

2.1.2 Studies on human tissues

As from 2003, 14 researches on human atherosclerotic plaque proteomics have been published; the diseased tissues used as matrices were coronary arteries (2/14), carotid arteries (11/14), and aortas (1/14).

Most of them were conducted by using two-dimensional electrophoresis coupled to mass spectrometry as analytical method (10/14). The sample source, the methodology applied, and the most relevant findings of these studies are summarized in table 1.

In 2003, You et al., by analysing 10 diseased (coronary artery disease, CAD) and 7 normal autoptic coronary arteries, reported about 2 fold increase of the ferritin light chain in the pathological specimens (You et al., 2003). Quantitative analysis by real-time PCR showed a decrease in ferritin light chain mRNA expression in diseased tissues suggesting that the increased expression of ferritin light chain in CAD coronary arteries may be related to increased protein stability. This result highlights the importance of protein expression analysis in studying disease-associated gene expression. Donners et al. analysed 5 stable plaques and 6 lesions with a thrombus from patients undergoing carotid endarterectomy, classified according to Virmani et al. (Donners et al., 2005). By 2DE analysis, they identified vinexin-β and α1-antitrypsin as differentially expressed. However, neither immunohistochemistry nor western blotting confirmed vinexin-β differential expression underlining the importance of validating proteomic results by other biochemical methods. Conversely, western blotting of 2D gels revealed, in lesions with a thrombus, the expression of six isoforms of the acute phase protein α1-antitrypsin, one of which was uniquely expressed in thrombus-containing plaques. Sung et al. analysed non-diseased and atherosclerotic specimens from 7 patients undergoing aorta bypass surgery. They identified a panel of 27 proteins differentially expressed in the atherosclerotic aorta involved in a number of biological processes, including calcium-mediated processes, migration of VSMCs, matrix metalloproteinase activation and regulation of pro-inflammatory cytokines (Sung et al., 2006). A different approach was adopted by Martin-Ventura et al. who analysed the protein secretion profiles obtained from 35 cultured atherosclerotic plaques (10 femoral, 25 carotids) and 36 control arteries (24 mammary, 12 radial) in the search of new biological markers potentially released by the arterial wall into the plasma (Duran et al., 2003; Martin-Ventura et al., 2004). In particular, they isolated and analysed the secretomes from non-complicated and ruptured/thrombosed areas of the same cultured carotid plaque so avoiding the variability of the control specimens. They showed that, compared to control arteries, heat shock protein 27 (HSP27) secretion into the culture medium was significantly lower in atherosclerotic plaques and barely detectable in complicated plaque supernatants, as confirmed by WB analysis. They also evidenced a 20-fold reduction in HSP27 levels in the plasma of patients with carotid stenosis respect to healthy controls so identifying HSP27 as a possible marker of atherosclerosis. The same research group evaluated the effects of incubation with atorvastatin, a 3-hydroxy-3-methylglutaryl CoenzymeA reductase inhibitor, on the secretomes of cultured atherosclerotic plaques (Durán et al., 2007). They identified 24 proteins that were increased and 20 proteins that were decreased in atherosclerotic plaque supernatants compared to controls. Interestingly, the presence of atorvastatin in culture medium reverted secretion of 66% proteins to control values. In this report, authors identified cathepsin D as a potential target for therapeutical treatment of atherosclerosis.

Human tissues (Methods)	Results	Known functions	Ref.
10 coronary arteries from CAD patients vs 7 normal autoptic coronary arteries (2DE of homogenates, LC-MS/MS, WB, rt-PCR)	↑ ferritin light chain ↓ ferritin light chain mRNA	modulation of oxidation	You et al., 2003
6 carotid plaques containing a thrombus vs 5 advanced stable lesions (2DE of homogenates, MALDI-TOF/TOF MS, LC-MS/MS, WB, IH)	↑ α1-antitrypsin	acute-phase protein	Donners et al., 2005
7 atherosclerotic aortic specimens vs biopsies of the normal tissue from the same patients (2DE of homogenates, MALDI-TOF MS, WB)	↑ 39 proteins (27 identified)	signal transduction angiogenesis MMP activation regulation of pro-inflammatory cytokines	Sung et al., 2006
35 atherosclerotic endarterectomies (10 femoral, 25 carotids) vs 36 control endarteries (24 mammary, 12 radial) (2DE of secretomes, MALDI-TOF MS, LC-MS/MS and IMAC combined with MALDI Q-TOF MS/MS, WB, ELISA, IH)	↓↓ HSP27 secretion ↓↓ HSP27 plasma levels	anti-inflammatory down-regulation of the apoptotic signaling pathway	Duran et al., 2003; Martin-Ventura et al., 2004
21 stenosing complicated carotid regions with/without atorvastatin treatement vs fibrous regions (ex vivo) (2DE of secretomes, MALDI-TOF MS, LC MS/MS, WB)	↑ 24 proteins ↓ 20 proteins Treatment reverts the differential protein secretion	modulation of oxidation and inflammation structural signaling pathway cholesterol metabolism	Durán et al., 2007
29 unstable carotid plaques vs 19 stable carotid plaques (2DE of extracts, MALDI-TOF MS, WB)	↑ ferritin light subunit ↑ superoxide dismutase 2 ↑ fibrinogen fragment D ↓ superoxide dismutase 3 ↓ glutathione S-transferase ↓ Rho GDP-dissociation inhibitor 1 ↓ annexin A10 ↓ HSP 20 ↓ HSP 27	modulation of inflammation and oxidative stress	Lepedda et al., 2009
10 complicated segments in the internal carotid artery (ICA) vs 10 stable segments in the common carotid artery (CCA) (2-D DIGE of homogenates, LC-MS/MS, IH)	↑ 6 proteins ↓ 11 proteins 2 proteins with isoform dependent distributions	signal transduction transport cell growth metabolism	Olson et al., 2010

Human tissues (Methods)	Results	Known functions	Ref.
10 carotid plaques vs reference synthetic gel (2DE of homogenates, LC-MS/MS)	Identification of proteins exclusive to plaque		Terzuoli et al., 2007; Porcelli et al., 2010)

IMAC, immobilized metal affinity chromatography. ↑, increase. ↓, decrease.

Table 1. 2DE coupled to MS studies on the human atherosclerotic plaque.

Since carotid plaque rupture and thrombosis are the most important clinical complications in the pathogenesis of cerebro-vascular diseases, many efforts have been done to elucidate mechanisms underlying plaque vulnerability and to identify reliable specific markers of plaques prone to rupture. In a previous study we provided evidence for a wide fragmentation of some apolipoproteins and arterial proteoglycans and for a pro-inflammatory microenvironment in unstable and much less in stable endarterectomy carotid plaques (Formato et al., 2004). Recently, we evaluated differential protein expression in a considerable number (n=48) of plaques obtained from carotid endarterectomy classified by immunohistochemistry in stable and unstable (Lepedda et al., 2009). Our study was carried out on the premise that plaque stability/instability is associated with distinct patterns of protein expression. We analysed extracts from finely minced tissues in order to allow enrichment in both topically expressed and filtered/retained proteins. A total of 57 distinct spots corresponding to 33 different proteins were identified in both stable and unstable plaques by peptide mass fingerprinting (PMF) analysis, most of which were of plasma origin (about 70%). This suggested the existence of an impaired endothelial barrier function independent from plaque typology. Compared to stable plaques, unstable ones showed reduced abundance of protective enzymes superoxide dismutase 3 and glutathione S-transferase, small HSP 27 and 20, annexin A10, and Rho GDP-dissociation inhibitor and a higher abundance of ferritin light subunit, superoxide dismutase 2 and fibrinogen fragment D. These proteins are described to play a role in either oxidative or inflammatory processes and in the formation and progression of the atherosclerotic plaque. Our proteomic approach, trying to differentiate unstable from stable human carotid plaques, identified, in the former, a panel of proteins with pro-oxidant and pro-inflammatory potentials according to our current understanding of the molecular basis of the atherosclerotic process.

To overcome inter-individual variations in protein expression, Olson et al. applied 2-D differential in gel electrophoresis (2D DIGE) in combination with MS/MS to compare protein distribution in 10 complicated segments located in the internal carotid artery (ICA) with that in 10 more stable segments in the common carotid artery (CCA) from the same patient (Olson et al., 2010). In this way, they identified 19 proteins with differential distribution between ICA and CCA segments. To overcome the problem of plaque heterogeneity, Terzuoli et al. proposed a method for selecting proteins exclusive to plaque by constructing a reference synthetic gel (Terzuoli et al., 2007; Porcelli et al., 2010). This gel, obtained by averaging the positions, shapes and optical densities of spots in 2DE maps from 10 carotid plaque samples was compared with an equivalent synthetic gel constructed using 10 plasma samples from the same carotid surgery patients. The comparison allowed discriminating between plasma and plaque proteins, the latter being potential markers of plaque vulnerability.

Some alternative proteomic approaches have been applied to date in the search of new biomarkers of the atherosclerotic process (table 2).

Human tissues (Methods)	Results	Known functions	Ref.
12 carotid endarterectomy specimens vs 7 non-atherosclerotic mammary arteries (Western array (823 Abs), WB, rt-PCR, IH)	↓↓ apoptosis-linked gene 2 ↑↑ Thrombospondin-2, Mn superoxide dismutase, apolipoprotein B-100, protein-tyrosine phosphatase 1C, apolipoprotein E ↓↓ glycogen synthase kinase-3β	mediator of apoptosis	Martinet et al., 2003
4 pooled unstable carotid plaques vs 4 pooled stable carotid plaques (protein microarray analysis of the expression of 512 proteins)	↑ 21 proteins ↓ 3 proteins	modulation of inflammatory, angiogenic, proliferative, and apoptotic pathways	Slevin et al., 2006
Histological sections from 35 coronary vessels in paraffin or frozen blocks (direct tissue proteomics AQUA methodology)	806 unique proteins identified with high confidence		Bagnato et al., 2007
Carotid plaques from 80 patients that had a secondary cardiovascular event vs 80 sex and age matched event-free patients (during a 3-year follow-up) (LC MS/MS)	Strong positive association between osteopontin and the occurrence of new vascular complications		de Kleijn et al., 2010

↑, increase. ↓, decrease.

Table 2. Alternative approaches in proteomics of the atherosclerotic plaque.

High-throughput western blot analysis, also called western array, was used to screen cell lysates from 12 carotid endarterectomy specimens and 7 non-atherosclerotic mammary arteries, obtained during bypass surgery, with 823 monoclonal antibodies mainly directed against signal-transducing proteins (Martinet et al., 2003). Western arrays showed a highly reproducible pattern of protein expression but also a high rate of false-positive signals (differential protein expression of only 7 of the 15 proteins detected by using this method was confirmed by standard immunoblot assay). A strong down regulation of apoptosis-linked gene 2 (ALG-2) was found, suggesting a novel mechanism inhibiting cell death in human advanced atherosclerotic plaques.

By using microarray technology, Slevin et al. compared the expression of 512 proteins associated with inflammatory, pro/anti-apoptotic, and angiogenesis pathways between 4 pooled fibrous stable carotid plaques and 4 pooled ulcerated, hemorrhagic unstable plaques (Slevin et al., 2006). In spite of the high sensitivity of protein microarrays, allowing detecting nanogram quantities, errors can occur because of weakly reacting or nonspecific antibodies, degraded proteins, and/or the efficiency of sample fluorescent labelling. However, western blotting analyses confirmed differential expression between stable and unstable plaque pools for all 11 proteins selected suggesting a high level of specificity of the array antibodies and the usefulness of this proteomic approach in the study of plaque pathogenesis.

Atherosclerotic tissue could also be laser-microdissected, which would allow one to compare different areas of the plaque such as necrotic core and shoulders/fibrous cap, providing valuable spatial information. Bagnato et al. applied the direct tissue proteomic (DTP) approach to paraffin or frozen blocks from 35 coronary atherosclerotic lesions classified by histopathological examination in early, intermediate, and advanced (Bagnato et al., 2007). In particular, different plaque regions were laser-microdissected (LCMs) from both paraffin and frozen sections and subjected to tryptic digestion followed by LC MS/MS to obtain area-specific proteomic information. Frozen sections were also homogenized and proteins resolved by SDS PAGE and analysed by LC MS/MS. Moreover, they used AQUA (absolute quantitation) methodology to quantify Stromal Cell-derived Factor 1 α (SDF1-α) and growth factors not detected by the above mentioned methods. These multiple approaches allowed them to identify 806 unique proteins with high confidence so obtaining a large scale protein profile of human atherosclerotic coronary arteries.

Recently, de Kleijn et al. analysed carotid endarterectomy specimens from 80 patients that had a secondary cardiovascular event in the 3-year follow-up and 80 sex and age matched event-free patients, by two HPLC fractionations coupled to MS (de Kleijn et al., 2010). They identified osteopontin as potential biomarker and validated data by assaying its level in a group of 574 patients that underwent carotid endarterectomy and a group of 151 patients that underwent femoral endarterectomy included in the follow-up. Osteopontin resulted highly predictive for secondary manifestations of cardiovascular events in other vascular territories.

Atherosclerosis is characterized by high oxidative and proteolytic activities. This process may lead to a pathological remodelling of aorta characterized by dilatation that can evolve toward vessel wall rupture (aortic aneurysm). Recently, Dejouvencel et al. focused their attention on intraluminal mural thrombus that develops in human abdominal aortic aneurysm (Dejouvencel et al., 2010). In particular, they analysed the protein released from three different aortic layers of the intramural thrombus (luminal, intermediate and abluminal), after 24 hours incubation on RPMI medium, by surface-enhanced laser desorption/ionization (SELDI) TOF MS profiling. They identified a peptide that was largely abundant in newly formed luminal layer respect to the other areas as hemorphin 7, a proteolytic fragment of the hemoglobin. The levels of this peptide were confirmed (by ELISA) to be higher in sera of abdominal aortic aneurysm patients respect to controls, and positively correlated with the volume of the thrombus. This peptide has been suggested as a potential marker of pathological vascular remodelling.

2.2 Vascular cell proteomics

As mentioned above, the study of atherosclerotic specimens are complicated by both the heterogeneous cellular composition and the inflammatory/proteolytic environment. In this respect, cell culture systems could represent a useful tool to partially overcome drawbacks of tissue analyses, allowing researchers to study single aspects of the atherosclerotic process in very controlled conditions. In the last years, studies on proteome (the intracellular proteins) and secretome (the proteins released into the cell culture medium) by 2DE and MS of ECs (Bruneel et al., 2003; Chen et al., 2007; Tunica et al., 2009), VSMCs (McGregor et al., 2001; Dupont et al., 2005; Lee et al., 2006), and monocytes/macrophages (Dupont et al., 2004; Fach et al., 2004; Slomianny et al., 2006; Zhang et al., 2007; Zhao et al., 2009) have been performed. Moreover, in the attempt to help in elucidating the mechanisms of atherogenesis, several proteomic studies have been carried out on vascular cells cultured in different experimental conditions (table 3). The most applied proteomic methodologies were 1DE-2DE coupled to MS analyses. Very few studies applied gel free proteomic approaches such as LC MS/MS (Fach et al., 2004; X.L. Wang et al., 2007; Zhao et al., 2009; Tunica et al., 2009; Zimman et al., 2010) and microarrays (Sukhanov et al., 2005).

2.3 Plasma/serum proteomics

Plasma is one of the most useful matrices to investigate for identifying new biomarkers. It carries resident proteins that represent the majority of plasma proteins, together with proteins released from vascular cells and other tissues. In this respect, variations in plasma proteome could reflect directly or indirectly a cardiovascular disease or other pathological conditions. Moreover, monitoring plasma proteome could be successful in patients follow up and in relation to drug therapies. Besides plasma, also serum is widely investigated, although its proteome is known to be drastically affected by blood coagulation. Plasma proteomic studies are challenging due to both the high dynamic range of protein concentrations and the number of low expressed proteins. Plasma is composed for up to 99% by 21 most abundant proteins and for the remaining 1% by about 50,000 low expressed protein variants, representing the so called "deep proteome" (Righetti et al., 2005). Plasma protein levels range from 40-50 mg/ml for albumin to less than 10 ng/ml for interleukins, chatepsins and peptide hormones. Therefore, differential proteomics of unfractionated plasma provides only limited information. In this regard, several pre-analytical depletion systems that imply affinity/immunoaffinity steps for simultaneous removal of the most represented plasma proteins have been set up. However, due to non-specific binding, many other proteins could be depleted. Besides depletion systems, also protein enrichment technology has been developed. This relies on solid-phase combinatorial ligand libraries, made of hexapeptides, to reduce the high dynamic range of protein concentration preventing the co-depletion of low-abundance proteins (Boschetti et al., 2007). Since variations in plasma protein expression can provide useful information on both physiological and pathological conditions of the different tissues in the body, many efforts have been made in characterizing the entire human plasma proteome. In this regard, during 2003-2005, 55 laboratories worldwide participating to the Human Plasma Proteome Project (HPPP) analysed reference specimens by using emerging technologies in the field of proteomics, and generated integrated databases for proteins detectable and identifiable in human serum and plasma (http://www.hupo.org/research/hppp/). They confidently identified 3020 proteins with a minimum of two high-scoring MS/MS spectra that have been searched for relevance to cardiovascular function and disease using PubMed search engine and specific keywords. On the basis of the current knowledge, the study individuated a subset of 345 proteins showing cardiovascular-related functions (markers of inflammation and/or cardiovascular disease, proteins implicated in coagulation, signalling, growth, differentiation, and vascular remodelling) (Berhane et al., 2005).

Experimental conditions	Endothelial cells	Smooth muscle cells	Monocytes/macrophages
Senescence	Kamino et al., 2003		
Shear stress	X.L. Wang et al., 2007; Huang et al., 2009	McGregor et al., 2004	
Pro-inflammatory conditions	Lomnytska et al., 2004; Pawlowska et al., 2005; González-Cabrero et al., 2007	Boccardi et al., 2007	
Oxidized/aggregated LDL	Chen et al., 2007	Sukhanov & Delafontaine, 2005; Padró et al., 2008	Fach et al., 2004; Conway & Kinter, 2005; Dupont et al., 2004; Kang et al., 2009; Burillo et al., 2009; Y.L. Yu et al., 2003a; Y.L.Yu et al., 2003b
Antioxidant/oxidant	Ha et al., 2005; Zimman et al., 2010	Jang et al., 2004; Lee et al., 2006	
Cholesterol loading	T. Wang et al., 2006		
HSP27 over-expression	Trott et al., 2009		
Drug treatment	M. Yu et al., 2004; Bieler et al., 2009; Millioni et al., 2010	Won et al., 2011	Barderas et al., 2009
PKCδ-/-		Mayr et al., 2004	
Hyperinsulinemia		Y. Wang et al., 2010	
Lipopolysaccharide or phorbol myristate			Gadgil et al., 2003; Sintiprungrat et al., 2010
ACS vs CAD			Barderas et al., 2007

ACS, acute coronary syndrome; CAD, coronary artery disease

Table 3. Literature overview of experimental conditions adopted in proteomic studies on ECs, VSMCs and monocytes/macrophages.

In the latest years, proteomics has been applied to plasma/serum to identify early diagnostic markers in relation to several cerebro-cardiovascular pathologies such as stroke (Allard et al., 2004; Kiga et al., 2008; Brea et al., 2009; Prentice et al., 2010), acute coronary syndrome (Mateos-Cáceres et al., 2004; Dardé et al., 2010), angiographic coronary disease (Donahue et al., 2006), acute myocardial infarction (AMI) (Distelmaier et al., 2009), coronary heart disease (CHD) (Prentice et al., 2010), coronary artery bypass grafting (CABG) (Banfi et al., 2010), aortic atherosclerotic plaque (Tabibiazar et al., 2006), and peripheral arterial disease (Wilson et al., 2007). Moreover, differential proteomic analysis has been addressed to elucidate effects on plasma proteome of different pharmacological treatments (Alonso-Orgaz et al., 2006; López-Farré et al., 2007). In this regard, the most applied proteomic methodologies were gel electrophoresis coupled to mass spectrometry analyses followed by gel free proteomic approaches such as LC MS/MS (Donahue et al., 2006; Wilson et al., 2007; Prentice et al., 2010) and microarrays (Tabibiazar et al., 2006). Almost all of these analytical approaches were preceded by one or more fractionation steps, mainly immunoaffinity depletion of the most abundant plasma protein species and ion exchange chromatography, to reduce the high complexity of plasma samples in terms of both number and dynamic range of protein species. Since many genetic and environmental factors affect atherosclerosis aetiology, one of the main drawbacks in differential analysis is the choice of a proper control group. In particular, results could be affected by coexisting pathological conditions such as dyslipidemia, hypertension and diabetes.

2.4 Urine proteomics

Urine is an easily accessible body fluid, stable against proteolytic degradation even after long storage times, and it represents a rich source of information. Urine protein and peptide composition results from glomerular filtration and proximal tubular absorption of circulating proteins (30%) and from the kidney and the urinary tract (70%) (Decramer et al., 2008). Urine proteomics is emerging as a powerful tool for identifying new biomarkers useful in diagnosis and monitoring of several human diseases. However, the urinary proteome analysis is not a simple task because the urine shows low protein concentration and high levels of salts or other interfering compounds. Moreover, urinary proteome is highly influenced by both inter-individual and intra-individual variability, the latter due to physical training, diet, drugs, caffeine consumption, etc. One of the priorities in this field during the coming years is to optimize sample preparation methods for urine proteomics (Thongboonkerd V., 2007). 2DE coupled with MS has represented for years the technique of choice for the analysis of urine proteins. Recently, Candiano et al. resolved 1118 spots in normal urine samples, 275 of which were characterized as isoforms of 82 proteins, 30 (108 spots) corresponding to typical plasma components (Candiano et al., 2010). However, the identity of most of the proteins found in normal urine by 2DE remains to be determined, the majority being low-molecular weight proteins (<30 kDa). By means of 1DE and HPLC as fractionation methods, and nano LC MS/MS and MS^3 as analytical methods, Adachi et al. identified 8041 peptides corresponding to 1543 proteins, probably representing the most advanced proteomic approach to urine characterization (Adachi et al., 2006).

The study of urinary proteome in relation to atherosclerosis is in its infancy but, in the last years, many efforts have been done. In particular, multiple urinary biomarkers of CAD have been described (Zimmerli et al., 2008; von Zur Muhlen et al., 2009; Delles et al., 2010) by means of capillary electrophoresis coupled online to micro time-of-flight mass spectrometry. A pattern of 238 CAD-specific polypeptides (49 of which have been sequenced) that identifies patients with high sensitivity and specificity has been defined.

2.5 Lipoproteomics

In 1995 Williams and Tabas published the "response-to-retention" hypothesis. According to this theory, early events in atherogenesis are related to a selective retention of LDL in the sub-endothelial space by means of specific interactions with some extracellular matrix components (Williams & Tabas, 1995). The molecular mechanisms underlying these processes are not completely understood, but knowledge of lipoprotein structure, apolipoprotein composition and their post-translational modifications could help in this respect. There are several types of lipoproteins differing for chemical compositions, physical properties and metabolic functions. They may be classified according to their densities in chylomicrons ($d < 0.95$ g/ml), very low density lipoproteins (VLDL, $d < 1.006$ g/ml), low density lipoproteins (LDL, $1.019 < d < 1.063$ g/ml), high density lipoproteins (HDL, $1.063 < d < 1.21$ g/ml) (Vance & Vance, 2008). A further class of lipoprotein particles is known as lipoprotein(a) (Lp(a)). Lp(a) is a LDL-like particle that carries, linked to apoB100 by a single disulfide bond, an heavily glycosylated multi-kringle protein named apolipoprotein(a). The physiological role of Lp(a) is unknown, although it is considered a risk factor for cardiovascular disease. Lipoproteins have attracted a great deal of interest because of their implication in the development of cardiovascular diseases, such as atherosclerosis. Although it is well known that high LDL-cholesterol and low HDL-cholesterol are positively correlated with the risk for the development of cardiovascular disease, clinical studies suggest that levels of apo B-100 and apo A-I may be better predictors (Walldius et al., 2001). Since the protein component of these particles is largely responsible for carrying out their various functions, detailed information about the apolipoprotein composition and structure may contribute to reveal their role in atherogenesis and to develop new therapeutic strategies for the treatment of lipoprotein-associated disorders. Applying proteomics to the study of lipoproteins seems to contribute significantly to the achievement of this goal. Indeed, recent proteomic studies have revealed that lipoproteins carry an array of proteins previously unsuspected. Among proteomic approaches, 2DE was applied to the study of lipoprotein particles for the first time in the 1970s (Emes et al., 1976) and allowed to reveal several protein isoforms (Zannis, 1986). With the improvement of 2DE technologies, due to the advent of immobilized pH gradient strips, in the last ten years several studies have been done in the attempt to elucidate the apolipoprotein cargo of the different lipoprotein species. In this respect, besides 2DE, several gel-free mass spectrometry based proteomics have been applied. So far, 31 proteomic studies on VLDL, LDL and HDL have been published, while no proteomic studies on chylomicrons or Lp(a) are present in literature. Among them, only 9 focused on lipoproteomics in relation to atherosclerosis in humans (table 4).

Before overviewing lipoproteomic studies, it is worth mentioning that the method used to isolate lipoproteins significantly affects the protein content of the resulting particles. Traditional methods, established in the 1950s (Havel et al., 1955), imply ultracentrifugation in high-salt media containing KBr or NaBr. Several lipoproteomic studies have been published using these procedures of lipoprotein isolation (Banfi et al., 2009; Davidson et al., 2009; Green et al., 2008; Heller et al., 2005, 2007; Hortin et al., 2006; Karlsson et al., 2005a, 2005b; Khovidhunkit et al., 2004; Mancone et al., 2007; Mazur et al., 2010; Rezaee et al., 2006; Vaisar et al., 2007, 2010; Alwaili et al, 2011). However, the high ionic strength and the high centrifugal field forces might cause either the dissociation of proteins or their exchange between different lipoprotein classes, altering the pattern of associated exchangeable apolipoproteins. Indeed, some of these studies reported a loss of proteins after a second step of ultracentrifugation (Banfi et al., 2009; Davidson et al., 2009; Mancone et al., 2007). Some others employed two ultracentrifuge procedures, using both salts and other compounds, such as sucrose and iodixanol (Bondarenko et al., 1999; Sun et al., 2010), reporting comparable results. By the way, Stahlman et al. reported that deuterium oxide (D_2O) is to be preferred over salts at least for LDL and HDL, since for VLDL isolation, the ionic strength of the solution is not so relevant (Ståhlman et al., 2008). Alternatively, lipoprotein can be isolated by means of

Subjects analysed	Purification methods Proteomic methods	Results	Ref.
VLDL			
1 hyperlipidemic subject vs 3 healthy subjects	ultracentrifugation in sucrose or in NaBr density gradient MALDI-TOF and ESI-TOF MS	↑ apo C-III	Bondarenko et al., 1999
LDL			
10 subjects with metabolic syndrome and subclinical carotid atherosclerosis vs 10 healthy controls 21 patients with type 2 diabetes and atherosclerosis vs 23 healthy controls.	ultracentrifugation in D_2O density gradient (small dense LDL) SELDI-TOF MS 1DE MALDI-TOF/TOF WB	Proteins differentially expressed in small dense LDL: ↑ apo C-III (3 isoforms), ↓ apo C-I (2isoforms), ↓ apo A-I, ↓ apo E	Davidsson et al., 2005
HDL			
20 control subjects for total HDL analysis 7 CAD subjects vs 6 control subjects for HDL_3 analysis	ultracentrifugation or affinity chromatography LC-ESI MS/MS	48 proteins identified in total HDL HDL_3 analysis: ↑apo C-IV, ↑PON1, ↑complement C3, ↑apo A-IV, ↑apo E	Vaisar et al., 2007
6 CAD subjects treated with niacin and atorvastatin for 12 months vs 6 non treated CAD subjects	sequential salt ultracentrifugation (HDL_3) LC–Fourier transform Ion Cyclotron Resonance –MS	↑PLTP, ↑apo F, ↑apo J, ↓apo E	Green et al., 2008
18 men with established CAD vs 20 apparently healthy men	sequential salt ultracentrifugation (HDL_2) MALDI-TOF MS and pattern recognition analysis LC-MALDI-TOF/TOF	↑apo C-III, ↓apo C-I ↑apo A-I peptides containing oxidized methionine	Vaisar et al., 2010
7 hypercholesterolemic subjects vs 9 normolipidemic subjects	ultracentrifugation in salt density gradient Shotgun LC-ESI MS/MS	↓apo A-I, ↑apo C-I, ↑apo C-III, ↑apo E	Heller et al., 2007
3 subjects having low HDL-cholesterol vs 3 subjects having high HDL-cholesterol	ultracentrifugation in salt density gradient (HDL_3) Top-down Differential Mass Spectrometry	380 peaks ↑ two forms of apo C-III	Mazur et al., 2010

Subjects analysed	Purification methods Proteomic methods	Results	Ref.
10 subjects having low HDL-cholesterol vs 10 subjects having high HDL cholesterol challenged with lipopolysaccharide (24 hours follow up)	apo A-I immunocapturing SELDI-TOF MS	profound changes in 21 markers in both groups	Levels et al., 2011
10 ACS subjects vs 10 stable CAD vs 10 healthy control subjects	KBr sequential ultracentrifugation 1D LC-MS/MS WB ELISA	67 proteins identified ↓ apo A-IV ↑SAA ↑complement C3	Alwaili et al., 2011

↑, increase. ↓, decrease.

Table 4. Overview of the lipoproteomic studies related to atherosclerosis in humans reviewed in the chapter.

immunopurification methods that rely on antibodies specific for the dominant protein of each class (Levels et al., 2007, 2011; Ogorzalek Loo et al., 2004; Rashid et al., 2002; Rezaee et al., 2006). Although this procedure does not lead to loss of weakly associated protein, it tends to nonspecifically co-purify associated proteins as serum contaminants and other lipoprotein fractions having the same antibody target (e.g. apolipoprotein A-I is the main HDL apolipoprotein but it is also present in both VLDL and LDL fractions). Other lipoprotein isolation methods that have been applied in lipoproteomic studies, involve electrophoretic techniques, specifically free solution isotachophoresis (Böttcher et al., 2000), and chromatographic techniques, such as fast protein liquid chromatography (Collins & Olivier, 2010; Richardson et al., 2009) and size exclusion/affinity chromatographies (Gordon et al., 2010).

2.5.1 VLDL

Both 2DE coupled to MS and gel-free MS approaches have been applied to the study of VLDL protein composition. Mancone et al., by using 2DE coupled to MALDI TOF/TOF MS analysis, provided a detailed map of VLDL, isolated by the classical ultracentrifugation method, from a plasma pool of 3 healthy volunteers. They identified two newly VLDL-associated proteins, namely apo L-I and prenylcysteine lyase that were known to be associated with HDL, and some post-translational modifications of Apo E (Thr^{212}glycosylations) and apo L-I (Ser^{296}phosphorylation) (Mancone et al., 2007). Sun et al. used two different analytical approaches to compare the protein content of VLDL and LDL isolated from pooled samples of healthy subjects by either NaBr or iodixanol gradient ultracentrifugation. By using a gel-free approach based on LC coupled to MS/MS analysis of tryptic digests labeled with iTRAQ (isobaric tag for relative and absolute quantitation) tags, they revealed 15 proteins differentially expressed in the two classes of lipoproteins. By using 2DE coupled with LC MS/MS, they further revealed 6 proteins differentially expressed as well. Moreover, the 5 apo A-I isoforms were found to be phosphorylated. This study, besides describing the VLDL and LDL lipoproteomes, provided insights into the metabolic changes, in terms of protein composition, during physiological VLDL to LDL transition (Sun et al., 2010). While the studies described above focused on the human lipoproteome of mature VLDL particles, other researches tried to shed light on VLDL assembly and maturation in animal models. For example, Rashid et al. immunopurified apo B from rat liver microsomes treated with chemical crosslinkers. Then, using LC MS/MS technology, they identified 99 unique proteins that co-immunoprecipitated with apo B, many of which were ribosomal proteins (Rashid et al., 2002).

Bondarenko et al. applied MALDI TOF and ESI TOF MS techniques to identify low molecular weight proteins constituting VLDL from 3 healthy subjects and 1 hyperlipidemic subject without previous tryptic digestion. By this approach they identified 15 apo C isoforms and 1 apo E isoform and observed higher level of apo C-III in the hyperlipidemic subject (Bondarenko et al., 1999).

2.5.2 LDL

LDL particles have been studied using different proteomic approaches. Karlsson et al. provided a 2DE map of LDL-associated proteins from a pooled plasma of 4 healthy subjects purified by KBr density gradient ultracentrifugation. Their results confirmed the presence of proteins known to be associated with LDL particles, showing that many of these were present in different isoforms. In particular, they detected three proteins not previously identified in LDL: serum amyloid A-IV, calgranulin A, and lysozyme C. To confirm that the proteins identified were truly associated with LDL rather than adsorbed during the isolation procedure, LDL was also purified by size-exclusion chromatography (Karlsson et al., 2005a). Moreover, they described three isoforms of apo M that were characterized for PTMs in a following work (Karlsson et al., 2006). Stahlman et al. applied 2DE coupled to MALDI TOF/TOF and SELDI TOF MS as well, to compare VLDL, LDL and HDL isolated from pooled plasma of 5 healthy donors by ultracentrifugation using either KBr or D_2O/sucrose to generate the gradient. VLDL profiles obtained with the two procedure of isolation were almost identical. Conversely, 2DE maps and SELDI TOF profiles of LDL and HDL were qualitatively similar, but differed in relative abundance of some protein species. Moreover, a reduced protein-lipids ratio was detected in LDL and HDL fractions purified by using KBr indicating that in the D_2O buffer the lipoproteins retained a higher content of exchangeable apoproteins (Ståhlman et al., 2008). LDL-associated proteins have also been studied using other proteomic approaches. Banfi et al. applied liquid-phase IEF and 1DE coupled with LC MS/MS to characterize the proteome of LDL isolated by density gradient ultracentrifugation from healthy subjects. They identified LDL-associated proteins not previously described, including prenylcysteine lyase (PCL1), orosomucoid, retinol-binding protein, and paraoxonase-1. The authors analysed PCL1 distribution in all the lipoprotein classes isolated by ultracentrifugation from 6 healthy subjects showing a decline from VLDL to LDL to HDL and its absence in lipoprotein-depleted plasma. Due to the oxidizing role of PCL1, they hypothesized that lipoproteins can themselves generate pro-oxidant species, thus suggesting a new role for lipoprotein in the development of atherosclerosis (Banfi et al., 2009). Bancells et al. analysed the proteome of LDL subfractions isolated by anion exchange chromatography after sequential ultracentrifugation of pooled healthy subjects plasma. Proteomic analysis, performed by LC MS/MS method, revealed the presence of 28 proteins most of which were involved in inflammation, coagulation and innate immunity, besides apolipoproteins involved in lipid metabolism. They observed that electronegative LDL, a minor subfraction of LDL fraction, has a higher content of minor proteins, especially apo F and apo J, compared to electropositive LDL (Bancells et al, 2010). Collins et al. performed a proteomic analysis, applying LC MS/MS, to compare the lipoprotein-associated proteins derived from plasma and serum samples. They isolated both HDL and LDL from healthy subjects by means of fast protein liquid chromatography-size exclusion chromatography (FPLC-SEC). 16 proteins, several of which were complement subcomponents, were found only in the LDL fraction. 65 proteins were identified to be unique to HDL, while another list of proteins was found to overlap between the two lipoprotein fractions. Regarding the differences between plasma- and serum-derived LDL and HDL particles, the authors reported that the most relevant differences regarded fibrinogen proteins which were depleted in serum. Therefore, they stated that, apart from significantly higher levels of apo B-100 in LDL purified from serum samples, comparative proteomic analysis of plasma and serum gives similar results (Collins & Olivier, 2010).

Up to date, only few studies on LDL proteomics and atherosclerosis have been reported. 2DE coupled with LC MS/MS and label-free quantitative MS (LFQMS) was applied by Richardson et al. to the analysis of LDL in the early stages of atherosclerosis in an animal model. LDL was isolated by fast protein LC (FPLC) from non-diabetic hyperlipidemic, diabetic dyslipidemic, diabetic dyslipidemic under exercise training, and healthy Yucatan pigs (Richardson et al., 2009). They identified 28 unique proteins and detected several differential expression patterns for apo E, A-I, C-III, fibrinogen, apo B, adiponectin, alpha-2-macroblobulin, complement C1q, ficolin, and apo J. Since LDL was isolated from pigs in the early stages of atherosclerosis, the alterations observed might be involved in the initiating stages of the disease. LDL-associated proteins have also been studied using other proteomic approaches. For example Davidsson et al. applied SELDI TOF technologies to compare LDL associated proteins from atherosclerotic patients (having either metabolic syndrome or diabetes) to that from healthy subjects. They focused on small dense LDL isolated by means of gradient ultracentrifugation using D_2O. The results showed that LDL from patients had lower content of apo A-I, apo C-I and apo E and higher content of apo C-III, the latter responsible for higher affinity for arterial proteoglycans that could facilitate LDL in situ oxidative modifications (Davidsson et al., 2005).

2.5.3 HDL

HDL is the most studied among lipoprotein particles, probably because of its anti-atherogenic functions. Proteomic studies in humans succeeded in identifying, besides the known apolipoproteins involved in the lipoprotein metabolism, other associated proteins such as acute-phase response proteins, proteinase inhibitors, and members of the complement activation. Therefore, characterizing the HDL proteome should help in the identification of novel anti-inflammatory and cardioprotective actions of HDL and could provide insights into lipid therapy. The most used among the several proteomic approaches that have been applied to characterize the HDL-associated proteins is 2DE coupled with MS. Böttcher et al. applied two-dimensional non-denaturing gradient gel electrophoresis (2D-GGE) and immunoblotting to analyse HDL subfractions isolated from healthy subjects. By means of free solution isotachophoresis (FS-ITP), they separated 3 HDL subfractions, namely fast (fHDL), intermediate (iHDL) and slow-migrating (sHDL). Proteomic analysis showed compositional differences in HDL subfractions. In particular, they observed that fHDL and iHDL contained the bulk of HDL and of apo A-I. Apolipoproteins other than apo A-I and apo A-II were not detectable in fHDL, while sHDL contained several minor apolipoproteins such as apo A-IV, apo D, apo E, apo J, and factor H. Apo C-III was found mainly in iHDL and sHDL with only little apo C-III in fHDL (Böttcher et al., 2000). A study performed by Ogorzalek Loo et al. suggests that a synergy between classical 2D gels and virtual 2D gels can be useful for studying HDL protein composition. Virtual 2DE is based on combining a first-dimensional isoelectric focusing (IEF) separation on polyacrylamide gels with MALDI MS surface scanning of the dried gel. In such a way, a virtual 2D gel can be created, generating an image in which mass spectrometry substitutes the second-dimension SDS-PAGE separation. By this approach the authors examined HDL isolated from human sera by selected-affinity immunosorption of apo A-I and revealed 42 unique masses for protein species with isoelectric points between pH 5.47–5.04 (Ogorzalek Loo et al., 2004). Heller et al. by using multiple proteomic approaches such as native or denaturing PAGE coupled with LC MS/MS, shotgun LC MS/MS and MALDI TOF MS profiling, analysed the protein complement of HDL_3, HDL_2, HDL_2/LDL and LDL/VLDL enriched fractions, isolated from a plasma pool of 10,000 healthy donors by density gradient ultracentrifugation. Therefore, they were able to characterize comprehensively the protein composition of the purified lipoprotein fractions (Heller et al., 2005). Karlsson et al. provided a detailed 2DE map of HDL_2 and HDL_3 isolated by salt gradient ultracentrifugation from pooled plasma of 4 healthy volunteers. Besides several isoforms of apolipoproteins already described to associate with HDL, they identified new proteins such as α-1-antitrypsin, two isoforms of salivary-α-amylase in HDL_2 and a glycosylated apoAII in HDL_3 (Karlsson et al., 2005b). By using 1DE and 2DE MALDI TOF MS and isotope-coded affinity tag (ICAT), Rezaee et al. detected many more proteins than Karlsson et al. in ultracentrifugally isolated HDL. This was the first study employing an ICAT method to identify lower abundance proteins. The overall identified proteins are known to be involved in different functions, such as lipid transport and metabolism, inflammation, immune system, hemostasis and thrombosis (Rezaee et al., 2006). The higher number of identified proteins could be ascribed to the use of ICAT method, that improve the sensitivity of the detection, as well as to the use of a single step of ultracentrifugation to isolate HDL. Khovidhunkit et al. investigated changes in proteins associated to HDL during inflammation by means of 2DE and LC MS/MS in an animal model. For this purpose, they analysed HDL isolated by salt gradient ultracentrifugation from sera of mice injected with normal saline or with endotoxin so detecting increased levels of SAA, apo E, apo A-IV and apo A-V and decreased levels of apo A-I and apo A-II in acute-phase HDL (Khovidhunkit et al., 2004).

Besides 2DE analyses, several groups have applied different gel-free proteomic approaches to characterize HDL proteome in healthy subjects. One of the first attempts was performed by Bondarenko et al. that used MALDI TOF MS and ESI TOF MS techniques to the analysis of intact protein of HDL isolated by density gradient ultracentrifugation in sucrose solution. They observed forty-nine peaks in the MALDI spectrum and 11 species in the ESI MS spectrum corresponding to the most abundant apolipoproteins, such as apo A-I, apo A-II, apo C-I, apo C-II, and apo C-III showing different isoforms due to post-translational modifications (Bondarenko et al., 2002). Applying immobilized pH gradient isoelectric focusing coupled with MALDI TOF MS, Farwig et al. were able to detect also SAA-IV in HDL isolated by ultracentrifugation in CsBiEDTA. They developed a successful method for recovering the apolipoproteins from immobilized pH gradient gels prior to MALDI analysis, demonstrating the analytical power of linking the IPG pI profile with MALDI TOF MS analysis (Farwig et al., 2003). Hortin et al. focused on HDL-associated low molecular weight peptides. By using HPLC and MALDI TOF MS or HPLC-ion trap mass spectrometry,

68 peptides in the 1-5 kDa size range were identified in ultracentrifugally isolated HDL. Among these, 19 were fragments derived from well-known HDL-associated protein while others were derived from non-lipoprotein plasma proteins as fibrinogen, α1-proteinase inhibitor, and transthyretin, suggesting that HDL particles may represent significant reservoirs of small peptides in the circulation (Hortin et al., 2006). Levels et al. applied SELDI TOF MS technologies to HDL isolated from normolipidemic individuals by means of immunocapturing directly on a SELDI protein chip covalently bound with anti-apo AI or anti apo-AII antibodies. In this way, 95 peaks in the 3–50 kDa molecular mass range and 27 more peaks between 50 and 160 kDa were detected (Levels et al., 2007). Gordon et al. applied MS-based proteomic approaches to the analysis of HDL purified from healthy subjects by means of gel filtration chromatography. To overcome problems related to nonspecific co-purification, they isolated only phospholipid-containing particles using calcium silicate hydrate (CSH), that were subjected to trypsin digestion while still bound to the CSH for identification by means of LC MS/MS. By this approach 47 proteins were identified. Among these, 14 were described as newly discovered HDL-associated proteins that support roles for HDL in complement regulation and protease inhibition (Gordon et al., 2010). To investigate the role of specific subspecies in the anti-atherogenic effects of HDL, Davidson et al. applied LC MS/MS to investigate the distribution of associated proteins across 5 subpopulations of HDL from healthy human volunteers. Subjecting one set of samples to sequential ultracentrifugation followed by salt gradient ultracentrifugation, and the other one to a single step of salt gradient ultracentrifugation they identified 22 and 28 proteins, respectively. Among them, the majority were apolipoproteins already known to be associated with ultracentrifugally-isolated HDL, while several complement factors and protease inhibitors already documented in other proteomic studies were not detected. By using peptide counts determined by MS, they monitored the relative abundance of a given protein across the HDL subfractions. Some proteins were found to associate preferentially to a specific subclass, while others were uniformly distributed across the subpopulations. This finding supports the proposal that HDL is composed of distinct subpopulations of particles that have discreet biological properties (Davidson et al., 2009).

A limited number of studies have focused on HDL proteomes in relation to atherosclerosis. Vaisar et al. used a shotgun LC MS/MS approach to identify proteins associated to total plasma HDL isolated from 20 healthy individuals. In this way, they described 48 proteins, 13 of which not yet known to associate to HDL. Moreover, they compared plasma HDL_3 fraction isolated from 6 healthy donors and 7 CAD patients. By means of Gene Ontology (GO) Consortium analysis, they were able to associate the array of HDL proteins to biological processes. Members of the complement pathway and endopeptidase inhibitors were found, suggesting that HDL plays also roles in regulating the complement system and protecting tissue from proteolysis. Thereafter, they found that some proteins associated to HDL_3 were upregulated in CAD patients, in particular apo C-IV, PON1, complement C3, apo A-IV, and apo E. Interestingly, they found three of these proteins also in HDL isolated from human carotid atherosclerotic tissues, being apo E the most abundant (Vaisar et al., 2007). In another study, they investigated whether combined statin and niacin therapy, which increase HDL cholesterol levels and reduce CAD risk, could reverse the changes in the protein composition observed in HDL_3. For this purpose HDL_3, isolated from 6 CAD patients before and 1 year after combined therapy, were subjected to LC–Fourier Transform Ion Cyclotron Resonance MS. By means of spectral counting and extracted ion chromatograms they found that treatment decreased apo E levels and increased apo J, apo F, and phospholipid transfer protein levels (Green et al., 2008). In a successive study, they investigated if protein composition was altered in HDL_2 isolated from CAD patients. Ultracentrifugally isolated HDL_2 was digested with trypsin and analysed by MALDI TOF MS and pattern recognition analysis. The most significant informative features were then subjected to LC MALDI MS/MS for identification. This analysis revealed that HDL_2 of CAD subjects carried a distinct protein cargo with increased levels of apo C-III and decreased levels of apo C-I, two apolipoproteins involved in the metabolism of HDL particles. Moreover, they found increased levels of apo A-I peptides containing oxidized methionine indicating the occurence of oxidative processes in CAD patients (Vaisar et al., 2010). Heller et al. used a shotgun LC MS/MS approach to characterize HDL protein composition of 7 hypercholesterolemic subjects and 9 normolipidemic ones. They used the peptide match score summation index, based on probabilistic peptide scores for absolute protein quantitation. By this approach, they found that in hypercholesterolemic subjects apo A-I levels were reduced while apo C-I, apo C-III, and apo E levels were increased, suggesting that HDL protein composition could be altered in lipemic disease (Heller et al., 2007). Mazur et al. applied differential top-down mass spectrometry to compare HDL_3 protein profiles between 3 subjects having low HDL cholesterol and 3 subjects having high HDL cholesterol. Differently from the so called "bottom up" proteomic methods that are based on the digestion of proteins into short peptides, "top-down" proteomic techniques characterize intact proteins. In this study HDL_3 samples were analysed by a reverse-phase nano-HPLC coupled to a linear trap quadrupole Fourier transform (LTQ-FT) hybrid mass spectrometer. The authors found 380 peaks that changed significantly in protein abundance between high HDL-c and low HDL-c subject groups demonstrating that this approach is suitable for the detection of quantitative differences in proteins and protein isoforms in human HDL samples (Mazur et al., 2010).

Very recently, Levels et al., applied SELDI TOF MS to HDL isolated, by apo A-I immunocapturing, from healthy subjects having low HDL-c and high HDL-c challenged with an endotoxin for 24 hours. Overall they observed profound changes in 21 markers in both study groups proteome irrespective of HDL cholesterol levels (Levels et al., 2011). Alwaili et al. applied 1D followed by LC-MS/MS to HDL isolated by sequential ultracentrifugation from male control, stable CAD, and ACS subjects (n=10/group). They identified 67 HDL-associated proteins involved in lipid binding, acute-phase response, immune response, and endopeptidase/protease inhibition. By means of spectral counting they found that nine proteins were differently abundant. Among them, apo A-IV was significantly reduced, whereas serum amyloid A and complement C3 were significantly increased in ACS patients compared to either controls or CAD subjects, as confirmed by western blotting and ELISA (Alwaili et al, 2011).

Recently, our research group started to study lipoproteomic profiles in relation to atherosclerosis (Formato et al., 2011). For this purpose we purified plasma VLDL, LDL, and HDL from patients undergoing carotid endarterectomy and from healthy normolipidemic donors by single isopycnic salt density gradient ultracentrifugation, followed by a second step of ultracentrifugation. Samples were subjected to 2DE followed by PMF analysis as reported in figure 2. In this way, we identified 21 spots corresponding to about 96% of 52 protein spots detected in VLDL, 22 spots corresponding to about 92% of 43 spots in LDL, and 20 spots corresponding to about 96% of 60 spots in HDL. The relative abundance of several identified lipoprotein-associated proteins differed between patients and healthy subjects (paper in preparation).

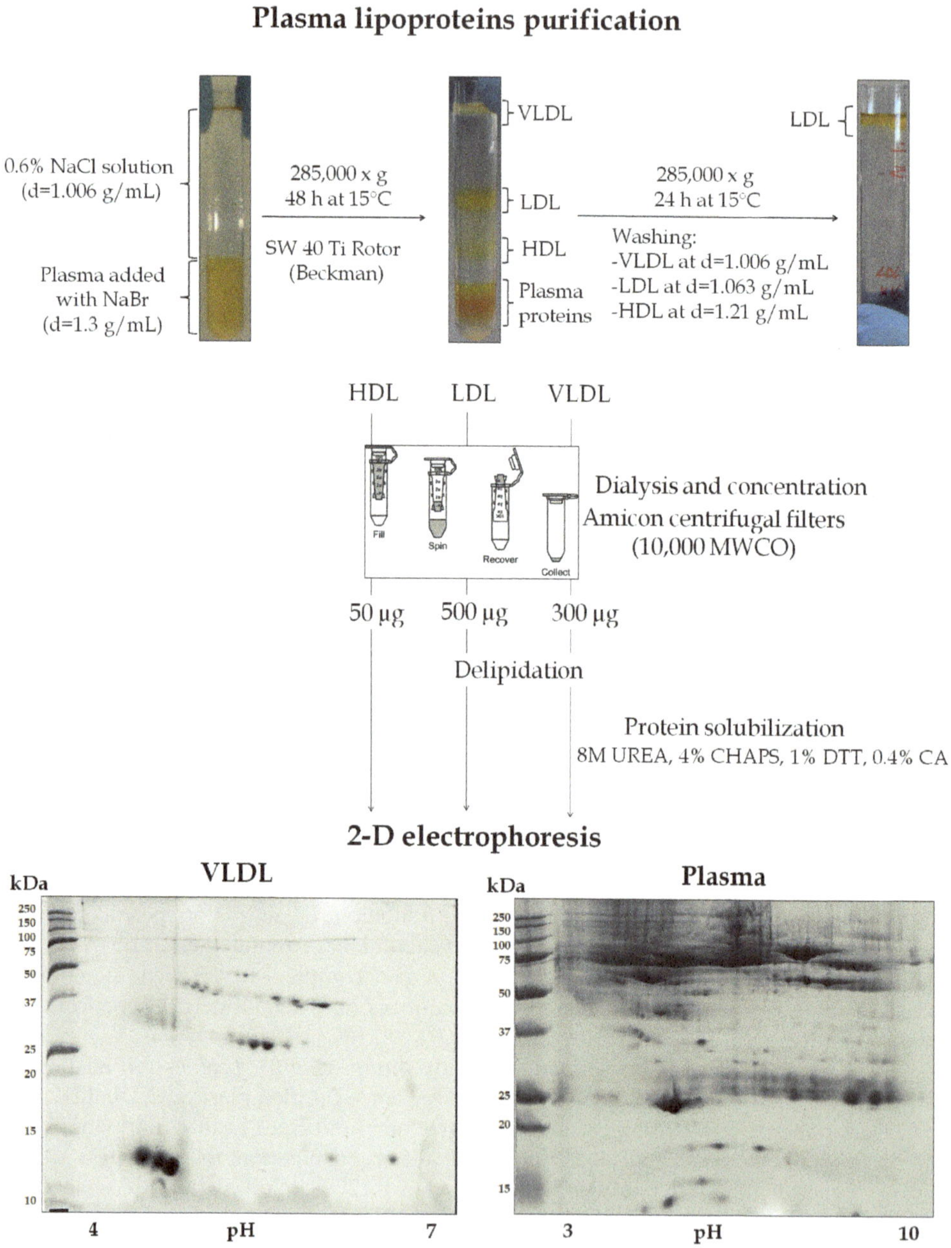

Fig. 2. Schematic workflow of the proteomic analysis of plasma lipoproteins adopted in our laboratory. Representative 2D maps of isolated VLDL and whole plasma are reported.

3. Conclusions

Plaque rupture and thrombosis are the most important clinical complications in the pathogenesis of vascular diseases. To date, many efforts have been done to elucidate mechanisms underlying plaque vulnerability and to identify reliable specific markers of plaques prone to rupture. In the last years, with the improvement of proteomic tools, large-scale technologies have been proved valuable in attempting to unravel pathways of complex diseases and biomarkers for early diagnosis and patients follow up. Collecting multiple biomarkers would be preferable over single markers in terms of higher sensitivity and specificity for the diagnosis of cardiovascular diseases. In this chapter, we have reviewed a great deal of information obtained by applying proteomics to the study of proteome/secretome from atherosclerotic tissues and plasma lipoproteins. In tissue proteomics, major drawbacks such as the plaque complexity, tissue sampling and availability, and the choice of the proper controls could affect the analysis. Even though results reported above seem to be quite promising, large-scale clinical studies are required to validate the usefulness of newly identified biomarkers. Moreover, there are several aspects of the atherosclerotic process that deserve further investigation. The analysis of laser captured microdissections by proteomics is still in its infancy but it could reveal valuable topological differences between specific areas of such a heterogeneous environment. Atherosclerotic plaques are characterized by the presence of an imbalance between oxidant and antioxidant species toward the former, leading to deep protein modifications. In this respect, recent advances in protein post-translational modifications analysis by mass spectrometry could be helpful. To date, many studies have been performed on proteome of purified plasma lipoproteins focusing mainly on HDL and LDL due to their association with atherosclerosis. As far as we know, no proteomic analyses have been performed on Lp(a). Since it is well known that elevated Lp(a) plasma levels are an important risk factor in atherogenesis, it would be of great interest to elucidate its apolipoprotein composition in relation to cardiovascular diseases. Another promising topic for future investigations is the characterization of proteomes of lipoproteins retained in atherosclerotic plaque. Finally, besides the great deal of work to be done in the future in both improving proteomic technologies and providing clues for the many aspects not yet investigated, it will also be necessary to put efforts on a comprehensive analysis of the huge quantity of data provided by the several proteomic studies.

4. Acknowledgments

This work has been supported by Fondazione Banco di Sardegna (Sassari, Italy) grant (Grant N° 536/2011.732).

5. References

Adachi, J.; Kumar, C.; Zhang, Y.; Olsen, J.V. & Mann, M. (2006). The human urinary proteome contains more than 1500 proteins, including a large proportion of membrane proteins, *Genome Biol*, Vol.7, No. 9, pp. R80

Allard, L.; Lescuyer, P.; Burgess, J.; Leung, K.Y.; Ward, M.; Walter, N.; Burkhard, P.R.; Corthals, G.; Hochstrasser, D.F. & Sanchez, J.C. (2004). ApoC-I and ApoC-III as potential plasmatic markers to distinguish between ischemic and hemorrhagic stroke, *Proteomics*, Vol.4, No. 8, pp. 2242-51

Almofti, M.R.; Huang, Z.; Yang, P.; Rui, Y. & Yang, P. (2006). Proteomic analysis of rat aorta during atherosclerosis induced by high cholesterol diet and injection of vitamin D3, *Clin Exp Pharmacol Physiol*, Vol.33, No. 4, pp. 305-9

Alonso-Orgaz, S.; Moreno, L.; Macaya, C.; Rico, L.; Mateos-Cáceres, P.J.; Sacristán, D.; Pérez-Vizcaíno, F.; Segura, A.; Tamargo, J. & López-Farré, A. (2006). Proteomic study of plasma from moderate hypercholesterolemic patients, *J Proteome Res*, Vol.5, No. 9, pp. 2301-8

Alwaili, K.; Bailey, D.; Awan, Z.; Bailey, S.D.; Ruel, I.; Hafiane, A.; Krimbou, L.; Laboissiere, S. & Genest, J. (2011). The HDL proteome in acute coronary syndromes shifts to an inflammatory profile, *Biochim Biophys Acta*, in press

Bagnato, C.; Thumar, J.; Mayya, V.; Hwang, S.I.; Zebroski, H.; Claffey, K.P.; Haudenschild, C.; Eng, J.K.; Lundgren, D.H. & Han, D.K. (2007). Proteomics analysis of human coronary atherosclerotic plaque: a feasibility study of direct tissue proteomics by liquid chromatography and tandem mass spectrometry, *Mol Cell Proteomics*, Vol.6, No. 6, pp. 1088-10

Bancells, C.; Canals, F.; Benítez, S.; Colomé, N.; Julve, J.; Ordóñez-Llanos, J. & Sánchez-Quesada, J.L. (2010). Proteomic analysis of electronegative low-density lipoprotein, *J Lipid Res*, Vol. 51, No.12, pp.3508-15

Banfi, C.; Brioschi, M.; Barcella, S.; Wait, R.; Begum, S.; Galli, S.; Rizzi, A. & Tremoli, E. (2009). Proteomic analysis of human low-density lipoprotein reveals the presence of prenylcysteine lyase, a hydrogen peroxide-generating enzyme, *Proteomics*. Vol.9, No.5, pp.1344-52

Banfi, C.; Parolari, A.; Brioschi, M.; Barcella, S.; Loardi, C.; Centenaro, C.; Alamanni, F.; Mussoni, L. & Tremoli, E. (2010). Proteomic analysis of plasma from patients undergoing coronary artery bypass grafting reveals a protease/antiprotease imbalance in favor of the serpin alpha1-antichymotrypsin, *J Proteome Res*, Vol.9, No. 5, pp. 2347-57

Barderas, M.G.; Tuñón, J.; Dardé, V.M.; De la Cuesta, F.; Durán, M.C.; Jiménez-Nácher, J.J.; Tarín, N.; López-Bescós, L.; Egido, J. & Vivanco, F. (2007). Circulating human monocytes in the acute coronary syndrome express a characteristic proteomic profile, *J Proteome Res*, Vol.6, No. 2, pp. 876-86

Barderas, M.G.; Tuñón, J.; Dardé, V.M.; De la Cuesta, F.; Jiménez-Nácher, J.J.; Tarín, N.; López-Bescós, L.; Egido, J. & Vivanco, F. (2009). Atorvastatin modifies the protein profile of circulating human monocytes after an acute coronary syndrome, *Proteomics*, Vol.9, No. 7, pp. 1982-93

Berhane, B.T.; Zong, C.; Liem, D.A.; Huang, A.; Le, S.; Edmondson, R.D.; Jones, R.C.; Qiao, X.; Whitelegge, J.P.; Ping, P. & Vondriska, T.M. (2005). Cardiovascular-related proteins identified in human plasma by the HUPO Plasma Proteome Project pilot phase, *Proteomics*, Vol.5, No. 13, pp. 3520-30

Bieler, S.; Meiners, S.; Stangl, V.; Pohl, T. & Stangl, K. (2009). Comprehensive proteomic and transcriptomic analysis reveals early induction of a protective anti-oxidative stress response by low-dose proteasome inhibition. *Proteomics*, Vol.9, No.12, pp.3257-67

Boccardi, C.; Cecchettini, A.; Caselli, A.; Camici, G.; Evangelista, M.; Mercatanti, A.; Rainaldi, G. & Citti, L. (2007). A proteomic approach to the investigation of early events involved in vascular smooth muscle cell activation, *Cell Tissue Res*, Vol.328, No. 1, pp. 185-95

Bondarenko, P.V.; Cockrill, S.L.; Watkins, L.K.; Cruzado, I.D. & Macfarlane, R.D. (1999). Mass spectral study of polymorphism of the apolipoproteins of very low density lipoprotein, *J Lipid Res*, Vol.40, No.3, pp.543-55

Bondarenko, P.V.; Farwig, Z.N.; McNeal, C.J. & Macfarlane, R.D. (2002). MALDI- and ESI-MS of the HDL apolipoproteins; new isoforms of apoA-I, II, *International Journal of Mass Spectrometry*, Vol.219, No.3, pp.671–80

Boschetti, E.; Lomas, L.; Citterio, A. & Righetti, P.G. (2007). Romancing the "hidden proteome", Anno Domini two zero zero seven, *J Chromatogr A*, Vol.1153, No. 1-2, pp. 277-90

Böttcher, A.; Schlosser, J.; Kronenberg, F.; Dieplinger, H.; Knipping, G.; Lackner, K.J. & Schmitz, G. (2000). Preparative free-solution isotachophoresis for separation of human plasma lipoproteins: apolipoprotein and lipid composition of HDL subfractions, *J Lipid Res.* Vol.41, No.6, pp.905-15

Brea, D.; Sobrino, T.; Blanco, M.; Fraga, M.; Agulla, J.; Rodríguez-Yáñez, M.; Rodríguez-González, R.; Pérez de la Ossa, N.; Leira, R.; Forteza, J.; Dávalos, A. & Castillo, J. (2009). Usefulness of haptoglobin and serum amyloid A proteins as biomarkers for atherothrombotic ischemic stroke diagnosis confirmation, *Atherosclerosis*, Vol.205, No. 2, pp. 561-7

Bruneel, A.; Labas, V.; Mailloux, A.; Sharma, S.; Vinh, J.; Vaubourdolle, M. & Baudin, B. (2003). Proteomic study of human umbilical vein endothelial cells in culture, *Proteomics*, Vol.3, No.5, pp.714-23

Burillo, E.; Recalde, D.; Jarauta, E.; Fiddyment, S.; Garcia-Otin, A.L.; Mateo-Gallego, R.; Cenarro, A. & Civeira, F. (2009). Proteomic study of macrophages exposed to oxLDL identifies a CAPG polymorphism associated with carotid atherosclerosis, *Atherosclerosis*, Vol.207, No. 1, pp. 32-7

Candiano, G.; Santucci, L.; Petretto, A.; Bruschi, M.; Dimuccio, V.; Urbani, A.; Bagnasco, S. & Ghiggeri, G.M. (2010). 2D-electrophoresis and the urine proteome map: where do we stand?, *J Proteomics*, Vol.73, No. 5, pp. 829-44

Chen, C.Y.; Lee, C.M.; Hsu, H.C.; Yang, C.Y.; Chow, L.P. & Lee, Y.T. (2007). Proteomic approach to study the effects of various oxidatively modified low-density lipoprotein on regulation of protein expression in human umbilical vein endothelial cell, *Life Sci*, Vol.80, No.26, pp.2469-80

Collins, L.A. & Olivier M. (2010). Quantitative comparison of lipoprotein fractions derived from human plasma and serum by liquid chromatography-tandem mass spectrometry, *Proteome Sci*, Vol.8, No. 42, pp.1-9

Conway, J.P. & Kinter, M. (2005). Proteomic and transcriptomic analyses of macrophages with an increased resistance to oxidized low density lipoprotein (oxLDL)-induced cytotoxicity generated by chronic exposure to oxLDL, *Mol Cell Proteomics*, Vol.4, No. 10, pp. 1522-40

Dardé, V.M.; de la Cuesta, F.; Dones, F.G.; Alvarez-Llamas, G.; Barderas, M.G. & Vivanco, F. (2010). Analysis of the plasma proteome associated with acute coronary syndrome: does a permanent protein signature exist in the plasma of ACS patients?, *J Proteome Res*, Vol.9, No. 9, pp. 4420-32

Davidson, W.S.; Silva, R.A.; Chantepie, S.; Lagor, W.R.; Chapman, M.J. & Kontush, A. (2009). Proteomic analysis of defined HDL subpopulations reveals particle-specific protein clusters: relevance to antioxidative function, *Arterioscler Thromb Vasc Biol*, Vol.29, No.6, pp.870-6

Davidsson, P.; Hulthe, J.; Fagerberg, B.; Olsson, B.M.; Hallberg, C.; Dahllöf, B. & Camejo, G. (2005) A proteomic study of the apolipoproteins in LDL subclasses in patients with the metabolic syndrome and type 2 diabetes, *J Lipid Res*, Vol.46, No.9, pp.1999-2006

de Kleijn, D.P.V.; Moll, F.L.; Hellings, W.E.; Ozsarlak-Sozer, G.; de Bruin, P.; Doevendans, P.A.; Vink, A.; Catanzariti, L.M.; Schoneveld, A.H.; Algra, A.; Daemen, M.J.; Biessen, E.A.; de Jager, W.; Zhang, H.; de Vries, J.; Falk, E.; Lim, S.K.; van der Spek, P.J.; Kwan Sze, S. & Pasterkamp, G. (2010). Local atherosclerotic plaques are a source of prognostic biomarkers for adverse cardiovascular events, *Arterioscler Thromb Vasc Biol*, Vol.30, pp. 612-19

Decramer, S.; Gonzalez de Peredo, A.; Breuil, B.; Mischak, H.; Monsarrat, B.; Bascands, J.L. & Schanstra, J.P. (2008). Urine in clinical proteomics, *Mol Cell Proteomics*, Vol.7, No. 10, pp. 1850-62

Dejouvencel, T.; Féron, D.; Rossignol, P.; Sapoval, M.; Kauffmann, C.; Piot, J.M.; Michel, J.B.; Fruitier-Arnaudin, I. & Meilhac, O. (2010). Hemorphin 7 reflects hemoglobin proteolysis in abdominal aortic aneurysm, *Arterioscler Thromb Vasc Biol*, Vol.30, No. 2, pp. 269-75

Delles, C.; Schiffer, E.; von Zur Muhlen, C.; Peter, K.; Rossing, P.; Parving, H.H.; Dymott, J.A.; Neisius, U.; Zimmerli, L.U.; Snell-Bergeon, J.K.; Maahs, D.M.; Schmieder, R.E.; Mischak, H. & Dominiczak, A.F. (2010). Urinary proteomic diagnosis of coronary artery disease: identification and clinical validation in 623 individuals, *J Hypertens*, Vol.28, No. 11, pp. 2316-22

Distelmaier, K.; Adlbrecht, C.; Jakowitsch, J.; Winkler, S.; Dunkler, D.; Gerner, C.; Wagner, O.; Lang, I.M. & Kubicek, M. (2009). Local complement activation triggers neutrophil recruitment to the site of thrombus formation in acute myocardial infarction, *Thromb Haemost*, Vol.102, No. 3, pp. 564-72

Donahue, M.P.; Rose, K.; Hochstrasser, D.; Vonderscher, J.; Grass, P.; Chibout, S.D.; Nelson, C.L.; Sinnaeve, P.; Goldschmidt-Clermont, P.J. & Granger, C.B. (2006). Discovery of proteins related to coronary artery disease using industrial-scale proteomics analysis of pooled plasma, *Am Heart J*, Vol.152, No. 3, pp. 478-85

Donners, M.M.; Verluyten, M.J.; Bouwman, F.G.; Mariman, E.C.; Devreese, B.; Vanrobaeys, F.; van Beeumen, J.; van den Akker, L.H.; Daemen, M.J. & Heeneman, S. (2005). Proteomic analysis of differential protein expression in human atherosclerotic plaque progression, *J Pathol*, Vol.206, No.1, pp. 39-45

Dupont, A.; Tokarski, C.; Dekeyzer, O.; Guihot, A.L.; Amouyel, P.; Rolando, C. & Pinet, F. (2004). Two-dimensional maps and databases of the human macrophage proteome and secretome, *Proteomics*, Vol.4, No. 6, pp. 1761-78

Dupont, A.; Corseaux, D.; Dekeyzer, O.; Drobecq, H.; Guihot, A.L.; Susen, S.; Vincentelli, A.; Amouyel, P.; Jude, B. & Pinet, F. (2005). The proteome and secretome of human arterial smooth muscle cells, *Proteomics*, Vol.5, No. 2, pp. 585-96

Duran, M.C.; Mas, S.; Martin-Ventura, J.L.; Meilhac, O.; Michel, J.B.; Gallego-Delgado, J.; Lázaro, A.; Tuñon, J.; Egido, J. & Vivanco, F. (2003). Proteomic analysis of human vessels: application to atherosclerotic plaques, *Proteomics*, Vol.3, No.6, pp. 973-8

Durán,M.C.; Martín-Ventura, J.L.; Mohammed, S.; Barderas, M.G.; Blanco-Colio, L.M.; Mas, S.; Moral, V.; Ortega, L.; Tuñón, J.; Jensen, O.N.; Vivanco, F. & Egido, J. (2007). Atorvastatin modulates the profile of proteins released by human atherosclerotic plaques, *Eur J Pharmacol*, Vol.562, No. 1-2, pp. 119-29

Emes, A.V.; Latner, A.L.; Rahbani-Nobar, M. & Tan, B.H. (1976). The separation of plasma lipoproteins using gel electrofocusing and polyacrylamide gradient gel electrophoresis, *Clin Chim Acta*, Vol.71, No.2, pp.293-301

Fach, E.M.; Garulacan, L.A.; Gao, J.; Xiao, Q.; Storm, S.M.; Dubaquie, Y.P.; Hefta, S.A. & Opiteck, G.J. (2004). In vitro biomarker discovery for atherosclerosis by proteomics, *Mol Cell Proteomics*, Vol.3, No. 12, pp. 1200-10

Farwig, Z.N.; Campbell, A.V. & Macfarlane, R.D. (2003). Analysis of high-density lipoprotein apolipoproteins recovered from specific immobilized pH gradient gel pI domains by matrix-assisted laser desorption/ionization time-of-flight mass spectrometry, *Anal. Chem*, Vol.75, pp.3823-30

Formato, M.; Farina, M.; Spirito, R.; Maggioni, M.; Guarino, A.; Cherchi, G.M.; Biglioli, P.; Edelstein, C. & Scanu, A.M. (2004). Evidence for a proinflammatory and proteolytic environment in plaques from endarterectomy segments of human carotid arteries, *Arterioscler Thromb Vasc Biol*, Vol.24, No. 1, pp. 129-35

Formato, M.; Lepedda, A.J.; Zinellu, E.; Cigliano, A.; Piredda, F.; Bacciu, P.P.; Guarino, A. & Spirito R. (2011). Apolipoprotein profiles in atherosclerotic disease, Proceedings of 79th European Atherosclerosis Society Congress, Goteborg, June, 2011

Gadgil, H.S.; Pabst, K.M.; Giorgianni, F.; Umstot, E.S.; Desiderio, D.M.; Beranova-Giorgianni, S.; Gerling, I.C. & Pabst, M.J. (2003). Proteome of monocytes primed with lipopolysaccharide: analysis of the abundant proteins, *Proteomics*, Vol.3, No. 9, pp. 1767-80

González-Cabrero, J.; Pozo, M.; Durán, M.C.; de Nicolás, R.; Egido, J. & Vivanco, F. (2007). The proteome of endothelial cells, *Methods Mol Biol*, Vol.357, pp.181-98

Gordon, S.M.; Deng, J.; Lu, L.J. & Davidson, W.S. (2010). Proteomic characterization of human plasma high density lipoprotein fractionated by gel filtration chromatography, *J Proteome Res*, Vol.9, No.10, pp.5239-49

Green, P.S.; Vaisar, T.; Pennathur, S.; Kulstad, J.J.; Moore, A.B.; Marcovina, S.; Brunzell, J.; Knopp, R.H.; Zhao, X.Q. & Heinecke, J.W. (2008) Combined statin and niacin therapy remodels the high-density lipoprotein proteome, *Circulation*, Vol.118, No12, pp.1259-67

Ha, M.K.; Chung, K.Y.; Bang, D.; Park, Y.K. & Lee, K.H. (2005). Proteomic analysis of the proteins expressed by hydrogen peroxide treated cultured human dermal microvascular endothelial cells, *Proteomics*, Vol.5, No.6, pp.1507-19

Havel, R. J.; Eder, H.A. & Bragdon, J.H. (1955). The distribution and chemical composition of ultracentrifugally separated lipoproteins in human serum, *J. Clin. Invest*, Vol.34, No.9, pp. 1345-53.

Heller, M.; Stalder, D.; Schlappritzi, E.; Hayn, G; Matter, U. & Haeberli, A. (2005). Mass spectrometry-based analytical tools for the molecular protein characterization of human plasma lipoproteins, *Proteomics*, Vol.5, No.10, pp. 2619-30

Heller, M.; Schlappritzi, E.; Stalder, D.; Nuoffer, J.M. & Haeberli, A. (2007) Compositional protein analysis of high density lipoproteins in hypercholesterolemia by shotgun LC-MS/MS and probabilistic peptide scoring, *Mol Cell Proteomics*, Vol.6, No.6, pp.1059-72

Hortin, G.L.; Shen, R.F.; Martin, B.M. & Remaley, A.T. (2006). Diverse range of small peptides associated with high-density lipoprotein, *Biochem Biophys Res Commun*, Vol. 340, No.3, pp.909-15

Huang, B.; Chen, S.C. & Wang, D.L. Shear flow increases S-nitrosylation of proteins in endothelial cells, (2009) *Cardiovasc Res*, Vol.83, No.3, pp.536-46

Jang, W.G.; Kim, H.S.; Park, K.G.; Park, Y.B.; Yoon, K.H.; Han, S.W.; Hur, S.H.; Park, K.S. & Lee, I.K. (2004). Analysis of proteome and transcriptome of tumor necrosis factor alpha stimulated vascular smooth muscle cells with or without alpha lipoic acid, *Proteomics*, Vol.4, No. 11, pp. 3383-93

Kamino, H.; Hiratsuka, M.; Toda, T.; Nishigaki, R.; Osaki, M.; Ito, H.; Inoue, T. & Oshimura, M. (2003). Searching for genes involved in arteriosclerosis: proteomic analysis of cultured human umbilical vein endothelial cells undergoing replicative senescence, *Cell Struct Funct*, Vol.28, No.6, pp.495-503

Kang, J.H.; Ryu, H.S.; Kim, H.T.; Lee, S.J.; Choi, U.K.; Park, Y.B.; Huh, T.L.; Choi, M.S.; Kang, T.C.; Choi, S.Y. & Kwon, O.S. (2009). Proteomic analysis of human macrophages exposed to hypochlorite-oxidized low-density lipoprotein, *Biochim Biophys Acta*, Vol.1794, No. 3, pp. 446-58

Karlsson, H.; Leanderson, P.; Tagesson, C. & Lindahl, M. (2005a). Lipoproteomics I: mapping of proteins in low-density lipoprotein using two-dimensional gel electrophoresis and mass spectrometry, *Proteomics*, Vol.5, No.2, pp. 551-65

Karlsson, H.; Leanderson, P.; Tagesson, C. & Lindahl, M. (2005b). Lipoproteomics II: mapping of proteins in high-density lipoprotein using two-dimensional gel electrophoresis and mass spectrometry, *Proteomics*. Vol.5, No.5, pp.1431-45

Karlsson, H.; Lindqvist, H.; Tagesson, C. & Lindahl, M. (2006). Characterization of apolipoprotein M isoforms in low-density lipoprotein, *J Proteome Res*, Vol.5, No.10, pp.2685-90

Khovidhunkit, W.; Duchateau, P.N.; Medzihradszky, K.F.; Moser, A.H.; Naya-Vigne, J.; Shigenaga, J.K.; Kane, J.P.; Grunfeld, C. & Feingold, K.R. (2004). Apolipoproteins A-IV and A-V are acute-phase proteins in mouse HDL, *Atherosclerosis*, Vol. 176, No.1, pp. 37-44

Kiga, C.; Sakurai, H.; Goto, H.; Hayashi, K.; Shimada, Y. & Saiki, I. (2008). Proteomic identification of haptoglobin as a stroke plasma biomarker in spontaneously hypertensive stroke-prone rats, *Life Sci*, Vol.83, No. 17-18, pp. 625-31

Lee, C.K.; Park H.J.; So, H.H.; Kim, H.J.; Lee, K.S.; Choi, W.S.; Lee, H.M.; Won, K.J.; Yoon, T.J.; Park, T.K. & Kim, B. (2006). Proteomic profiling and identification of cofilin responding to oxidative stress in vascular smooth muscle, *Proteomics*, Vol.6, No. 24, pp. 6455-75

Lepedda, A.J.; Cigliano, A.; Cherchi, G.M.; Spirito, R.; Maggioni, M.; Carta, F.; Turrini, F.; Edelstein, C.; Scanu, A.M. & Formato, M. (2009). A proteomic approach to differentiate histologically classified stable and unstable plaques from human carotid arteries, *Atherosclerosis*, Vol.203, No. 1, pp. 112-8

Levels, J.H.; Bleijlevens, B.; Rezaee, F.; Aerts, J.M. & Meijers, J.C. (2007). SELDI-TOF mass spectrometry of High-Density Lipoprotein, *Proteome Sci*, Vol. 6, pp.5-15

Levels, J.H.; Geurts, P.; Karlsson, H; Marée, R.; Ljunggren, S.; Fornander, L.; Wehenkel, L.; Lindahl, M.; Stroes, E.S.; Kuivenhoven, J.A. & Meijers, J.C. (2011). High-density lipoprotein proteome dynamics in human endotoxemia, *Proteome Sci*, Vol.9, No.34

Libby P. (2002). Inflammation in atherosclerosis, *Nature*, Vol.420, No.6917, pp. 868-74

Lomnytska, M.; Lukiyanchuk, V.; Hellman, U. & Souchelnytskyi, S. (2004). Transforming growth factor-beta1-regulated proteins in human endothelial cells identified by two-dimensional gel electrophoresis and mass spectrometry, *Proteomics*, Vol.4, No.4, pp.995-1006

López-Farré, A.J.; Mateos-Cáceres, P.J.; Sacristán, D.; Azcona, L.; Bernardo, E.; de Prada, T.P.; Alonso-Orgaz, S.; Fernández-Arquero, M.; Fernández-Ortiz, A. & Macaya, C. (2007).

Relationship between vitamin D binding protein and aspirin resistance in coronary ischemic patients: a proteomic study, *J Proteome Res*, Vol.6, No. 7, pp. 2481-7

Lutgens, E.; van Suylen, R.J.; Faber, B.C.; Gijbels, M.J.; Eurlings, P.M.; Bijnens, A.P.; Cleutjens, K.B.; Heeneman, S. & Daemen, M.J. (2003). Atherosclerotic plaque rupture: local or systemic process?, *Arterioscler Thromb Vasc Biol*, Vol.23, No.12, pp. 2123-30

Mancone, C.; Amicone, L.; Fimia, G.M.; Bravo, E.; Piacentini, M.; Tripodi, M. & Alonzi, T. (2007). Proteomic analysis of human very low-density lipoprotein by two-dimensional gel electrophoresis and MALDI-TOF/TOF, *Proteomics*, Vol.7, No.1, pp.143-54

Martinet, W.; Schrijvers, D.M.; De Meyer, G.R.; Herman, A.G. & Kockx, M.M. (2003). Western array analysis of human atherosclerotic plaques: downregulation of apoptosis-linked gene 2, *Cardiovasc Res*, Vol.60, No. 2, pp. 259-67

Martin-Ventura, J.L.; Duran, M.C.; Blanco-Colio, L.M.; Meilhac, O.; Leclercq, A.; Michel, J.B.; Jensen, O.N.; Hernandez-Merida, S.; Tuñón, J.; Vivanco, F. & Egido, J. (2004). Identification by a differential proteomic approach of heat shock protein 27 as a potential marker of atherosclerosis, *Circulation*, Vol.110, No.15, pp. 2216-9

Mateos-Cáceres, P.J.; García-Méndez, A.; López Farré, A.; Macaya, C.; Núñez, A.; Gómez, J.; Alonso-Orgaz, S.; Carrasco, C.; Burgos, M.E.; de Andrés, R.; Granizo, J.J.; Farré, J. & Rico, L.A. (2004). Proteomic analysis of plasma from patients during an acute coronary syndrome, *J Am Coll Cardiol*, Vol.44, No. 8, pp. 1578-83

Mayr, M.; Siow, R.; Chung, Y.L.; Mayr, U.; Griffiths, J.R. & Xu, Q. (2004). Proteomic and metabolomic analysis of vascular smooth muscle cells: role of PKCdelta, *Circ Res*, Vol.94, No. 10, pp. e87-96

Mayr, M.; Chung, Y.L.; Mayr, U.; Yin, X.; Ly, L.; Troy, H.; Fredericks, S.; Hu, Y.; Griffiths, J.R. & Xu, Q. (2005). Proteomic and metabolomic analyses of atherosclerotic vessels from apolipoprotein E-deficient mice reveal alterations in inflammation, oxidative stress, and energy metabolism, *Arterioscler Thromb Vasc Biol*, Vol.25, No. 10, pp. 2135-42

Mazur, M.T.; Cardasis, H.L.; Spellman, D.S.; Liaw, A.; Yates, N.A. & Hendrickson, R.C. (2010). Quantitative analysis of intact apolipoproteins in human HDL by top-down differential mass spectrometry. *Proc Natl Acad Sci U S A*. Vol.107, No.17, pp.7728-33

McGregor, E.; Kempster, L.; Wait, R.; Welson, S.Y.; Gosling, M.; Dunn, M.J. & Powel, J.T. (2001). Identification and mapping of human saphenous vein medial smooth muscle proteins by two-dimensional polyacrylamide gel electrophoresis, *Proteomics*, Vol.1, No. 11, pp. 1405-14

McGregor, E.; Kempster, L.; Wait, R.; Gosling, M.; Dunn, M.J. & Powell, J.T. (2004). F-actin capping (CapZ) and other contractile saphenous vein smooth muscle proteins are altered by hemodynamic stress: a proteonomic approach, *Mol Cell Proteomics*, Vol.3, No. 2, pp. 115-24

Millioni, R.; Puricelli, L.; Iori, E.; Arrigoni, G. & Tessari, P. (2010). The effects of rosiglitazone and high glucose on protein expression in endothelial cells, *J Proteome Res*, Vol.9, No.1, pp.578-84

Ogorzalek Loo, R.R.; Yam, L.; Loo, J.A. & Schumaker, V.N. (2004). Virtual two-dimensional gel electrophoresis of high-density lipoproteins, *Electrophoresis*. Vol. 25, No.14, pp.2384-91

Olson, F.J.; Sihlbom, C.; Davidsson, P.; Hulthe, J.; Fagerberg, B. & Bergström, G. (2010). Consistent differences in protein distribution along the longitudinal axis in symptomatic carotid atherosclerotic plaques, *Biochem Biophys Res Commun*, Vol.401, No. 4, pp. 574-80

Padró, T.; Peña, E.; García-Arguinzonis, M.; Llorente-Cortes, V. & Badimon, L. (2008). Low-density lipoproteins impair migration of human coronary vascular smooth muscle cells and induce changes in the proteomic profile of myosin light chain, *Cardiovasc Res*, Vol.77, No. 1, pp. 211-20

Pawlowska, Z.; Baranska, P.; Jerczynska, H.; Koziolkiewicz, W. & Cierniewski, C.S. (2005). Heat shock proteins and other components of cellular machinery for protein synthesis are up-regulated in vascular endothelial cell growth factor-activated human endothelial cells, *Proteomics*, Vol.5, No.5, pp.1217-27

Porcelli, B.; Ciari, I.; Felici, C.; Pagani, R.; Banfi, C.; Brioschi, M.; Giubbolini, M.; de Donato, G.; Setacci, C. & Terzuoli, L. (2010). Proteomic analysis of atherosclerotic plaque, *Biomed Pharmacother*, Vol.64, No. 5, pp. 369-72

Prentice, R.L.; Paczesny, S.; Aragaki, A.; Amon, L.M.; Chen, L.; Pitteri, S.J.; McIntosh, M.; Wang, P.; Buson Busald, T.; Hsia, J.; Jackson, R.D.; Rossouw, J.E.; Manson, J.E.; Johnson, K.; Eaton, C. & Hanash, S.M. (2010). Novel proteins associated with risk for coronary heart disease or stroke among postmenopausal women identified by in-depth plasma proteome profiling, *Genome Med*, Vol.2, No. 7, pp. 48

Qi, Y.X.; Qu, M.J.; Long, D.K.; Liu, B.; Yao, Q.P.; Chien, S. & Jiang, Z.L. (2008). Rho-GDP dissociation inhibitor alpha downregulated by low shear stress promotes vascular smooth muscle cell migration and apoptosis: a proteomic analysis, *Cardiovasc Res*, Vol.80, No. 1, pp. 114-22

Rashid, K.A.; Hevi, S.; Chen, Y.; Le Cahérec, F. & Chuck, S.L. (2002). A proteomic approach identifies proteins in hepatocytes that bind nascent apolipoprotein B, *J Biol Chem*, Vol. 277, No.24, pp.22010-7

Rezaee, F.; Casetta, B.; Levels, J.H.; Speijer, D. & Meijers, J.C. (2006). Proteomic analysis of high-density lipoprotein, *Proteomics*. Vol.6, No.2, pp.721-30

Richardson, M.R.; Lai, X.; Dixon, J.L.; Sturek, M. & Witzmann, F.A. (2009). Diabetic dyslipidemia and exercise alter the plasma low-density lipoproteome in Yucatan pigs, *Proteomics*, Vol.9, No.9, pp.2468-83

Righetti, P.G.; Castagna, A.; Antonucci, F.; Piubelli, C.; Cecconi, D.; Campostrini, N.; Rustichelli, C.; Antonioli, P.; Zanusso, G.; Monaco, S.; Lomas, L. & Boschetti, E. (2005). Proteome analysis in the clinical chemistry laboratory: myth or reality?, *Clin Chim Acta*, Vol.357, No. 2, pp. 123-39

Sintiprungrat, K.; Singhto, N.; Sinchaikul, S.; Chen, S.T. & Thongboonkerd, V. (2010). Alterations in cellular proteome and secretome upon differentiation from monocyte to macrophage by treatment with phorbol myristate acetate: insights into biological processes, *J Proteomics*, Vol.73, No. 3, pp. 602-18

Slevin, M.; Elasbali, A.B.; Miguel Turu, M.; Krupinski, J.; Badimon, L. & Gaffney, J. (2006). Identification of differential protein expression associated with development of unstable human carotid plaques, *Am J Pathol*, Vol.168, No. 3, pp. 1004-21

Slomianny M.C.; Dupont A.; Bouanou F.; Beseme O.; Guihot A.L.; Amouyel P.; Michalski J.C. & Pinet F. (2006). Profiling of membrane proteins from human macrophages: comparison of two approaches, *Proteomics*, Vol.6, No. 8, pp. 2365-75

Ståhlman, M.; Davidsson, P.; Kanmert, I.; Rosengren, B.; Borén, J.; Fagerberg, B. & Camejo, G. (2008). Proteomics and lipids of lipoproteins isolated at low salt concentrations in D2O/sucrose or in KBr, *J Lipid Res*, Vol. 49, No.2, pp.481-90

Stary, HC. (2000). Natural history and histological classification of atherosclerotic lesions: an update, *Arterioscler Thromb Vasc Biol*, Vol.20, No.5, pp. 1177-8

Sukhanov, S. & Delafontaine, P. (2005). Protein chip-based microarray profiling of oxidized low density lipoprotein-treated cells, *Proteomics*, Vol.5, No. 5, pp. 1274-80

Sun, H.Y.; Chen, S.F.; Lai, M.D.; Chang, T.T.; Chen, T.L.; Li, P.Y.; Shieh, D.B. & Young, K.C. (2010). Comparative proteomic profiling of plasma very-low-density and low-density lipoproteins, *Clin Chim Acta*, Vol.411, No.5-6, pp.336-44

Sung, H.J.; Ryang, Y.S.; Jang, S.W.; Lee, C.W.; Han, K.H. & Ko, J. (2006). Proteomic analysis of differential protein expression in atherosclerosis, *Biomarkers*, Vol.11, No.3, pp. 279-90

Tabibiazar, R.; Wagner, R.A.; Deng, A.; Tsao, P.S. & Quertermous, T. (2006). Proteomic profiles of serum inflammatory markers accurately predict atherosclerosis in mice, *Physiol Genomics*, Vol.25, No. 2, pp. 194-202

Terzuoli, L.; Felici, C.; Ciari, I.; Guerranti, R.; Pagani, R.; Marinello, E. & Porcelli, B. (2007). Synthetic gel of carotid artery plaque, *Int J Immunopathol Pharmacol*, Vol.20, No. 3, pp. 637-42

Thongboonkerd V. (2007). Practical points in urinary proteomics, *J Proteome Res*, Vol.6, No. 10, pp. 3881-90

Trott, D.; McManus, C.A.; Martin, J.L.; Brennan, B.; Dunn, M.J. & Rose, M.L. (2009). Effect of phosphorylated hsp27 on proliferation of human endothelial and smooth muscle cell, *Proteomics*, Vol.9, No.12, pp.3383-94

Tunica, D.G.; Yin, X.; Sidibe, A.; Stegemann, C.; Nissum, M.; Zeng, L.; Brunet, M. & Mayr, M. (2009) Proteomic analysis of the secretome of human umbilical vein endothelial cells using a combination of free-flow electrophoresis and nanoflow LC-MS/MS, *Proteomics*, Vol.9, No.21, pp.4991-6

Vaisar, T.; Pennathur, S.; Green, P.S.; Gharib, S.A.; Hoofnagle, A.N.; Cheung, M.C.; Byun, J.; Vuletic, S.; Kassim, S.; Singh, P.; Chea, H.; Knopp, R.H.; Brunzell, J.; Geary, R.; Chait, A.; Zhao, X.Q.; Elkon, K.; Marcovina, S.; Ridker, P.; Oram, J.F. & Heinecke, J.W. (2007). Shotgun proteomics implicates protease inhibition and complement activation in the antiinflammatory properties of HDL, *J Clin Invest*, Vol.117, No.3, pp.746-56

Vaisar, T.; Mayer, P.; Nilsson, E.; Zhao, X.Q.; Knopp, R. & Prazen, B.J. (2010) HDL in humans with cardiovascular disease exhibits a proteomic signature, *Clin Chim Acta.* Vol.411, No.13-14, pp.972-9

Vance, D.E. & Vance J.E. (2008). Biochemistry of lipids, lipoprotein and membranes (Fifth Edition), Elsevier B.V. ISBN: 978-0-444-53219-0

Virmani, R.; Kolodgie, F.D.; Burke, A.P.; Farb, A. & Schwartz, S.M. (2000). Lessons from sudden coronary death: a comprehensive morphological classification scheme for atherosclerotic lesions, *Arterioscler Thromb Vasc Biol*, Vol.20, No.5, pp. 1262-75

von Zur Muhlen, C.; Schiffer, E.; Zuerbig, P.; Kellmann, M.; Brasse, M.; Meert, N.; Vanholder, R.C.; Dominiczak, A.F.; Chen, Y.C.; Mischak, H.; Bode, C. & Peter, K. (2009). Evaluation of urine proteome pattern analysis for its potential to reflect coronary artery atherosclerosis in symptomatic patients, *J Proteome Res*, Vol.8, No. 1, pp. 335-45

Walldius, G.; Jungner, I.; Holme, I.; Aastveit, A.H.; Kolar, W. & Steiner, E. (2001). High apolipoprotein B, low apolipoprotein A-I, and improvement in the prediction of fatal myocardial infarction (AMORIS study): a prospective study, *Lancet*, Vol.358, No. 9298, pp. 2026-33

Wang, T.; Chen, Z.; Wang, X.; Shyy, J.Y. & Zhu Y. (2006). Cholesterol loading increases the translocation of ATP synthase beta chain into membrane caveolae in vascular endothelial cells, *Biochim Biophys Acta*, Vol.1761, No.10, pp.1182-90

Wang, X.L.; Fu, A.; Raghavakaimal, S. & Lee, H.C. (2007). Proteomic analysis of vascular endothelial cells in response to laminar shear stress, *Proteomics*, Vol.7, No.4, pp.588-96

Wang, Y.; Zhang, B.; Bai, Y.; Zeng, C. & Wang, X. (2010). Changes in proteomic features induced by insulin on vascular smooth muscle cells from spontaneous hypertensive rats in vitro, *Cell Biochem Biophys*, Vol.58, No. 2, pp. 97-106

Williams, K.J. & Tabas, I. (1995). The response-to-retention hypothesis of early atherogenesis, *Arterioscler Thromb Vasc Biol*, Vol.15, No.5, pp. 551-61

Wilson, A.M.; Kimura,E.; Harada, R.K.; Nair, N.; Narasimhan, B.; Meng, X.Y.; Zhang, F.; Beck, K.R.; Olin, J.W.; Fung, E.T. & Cooke, J.P. (2007). Beta2-microglobulin as a biomarker in peripheral arterial disease: proteomic profiling and clinical studies, *Circulation*, Vol.116, No. 12, pp. 1396-403

Won, K.J.; Lee, P.; Jung, S.H.; Jiang, X.; Lee, C.K.; Lin, H.Y.; Kang, H.; Lee, H.M.; Kim, J.; Toyokuni, S. & Kim, B. (2011). 3-morpholinosydnonimine participates in the attenuation of neointima formation via inhibition of annexin A2-mediated vascular smooth muscle cell migration, *Proteomics*, Vol.11, No. 2, pp. 193-201

Wu, J.; Liu, W.; Sousa, E.; Qiu, Y.; Pittman, D.D.; Maganti, V.; Feldman, J.; Gill, D.; Lu, Z.; Dorner, A.J.; Schaub, R. & Tan, X.Y. (2007). Proteomic identification of endothelial proteins isolated in situ from atherosclerotic aorta via systemic perfusion, *J Proteome Res*, Vol.6, No. 12, pp. 4728-36

You, S.A.; Archacki, S.R.; Angheloiu, G.; Moravec, C.S.; Rao, S.; Kinter, M.; Topol, E.J. & Wang, Q. (2003). Proteomic approach to coronary atherosclerosis shows ferritin light chain as a significant marker: evidence consistent with iron hypothesis in atherosclerosis, *Physiol Genomics*, Vol.13, No.1, pp. 25-30

Yu, M.; Chen, D.M.; Hu, G. & Wang, H. (2004). Proteomic response analysis of endothelial cells of human coronary artery to stimulation with carbachol, *Acta Pharmacol Sin*, Vol.25, No.9, pp.1124-30

Yu, Y.L.; Huang, Z.Y.; Yang, P.Y.; Rui, Y.C. & Yang, P.Y. (2003a). Proteomic studies of macrophage-derived foam cell from human U937 cell line using two-dimensional gel electrophoresis and tandem mass spectrometry, *J Cardiovasc Pharmacol*, Vol.42, No. 6, pp. 782-9

Yu, Y.L.; Yang, P.Y.; Fan, H.Z.; Huang, Z.Y.; Rui, Y.C. & Yang, P.Y. (2003b). Protein expressions in macrophage-derived foam cells: comparative analysis by two-dimensional gel electrophoresis, *Acta Pharmacol Sin*, Vol.24, No. 9, pp. 873-7

Zannis, V.I. (1986). Genetic polymorphism in human apolipoprotein E, *Methods Enzymol*, Vol.128, pp.823-51

Zhang, L.; Lun, Y.; Yan, D.; Yu, L.; Ma, W.; Du, B. & Zhu, X. (2007). Proteomic analysis of macrophages: a new way to identify novel cell-surface antigens, *J Immunol Methods*, Vol.321, No. 1-2, pp. 80-5

Zhao, C.; Zhang, H.; Wong, W.C.; Sem, X.; Han, H.; Ong, S.M.; Tan, Y.C.; Yeap, W.H.; Gan, C.S.; Ng, K.Q.; Koh, M.B.; Kourilsky, P.; Sze, S.K. & Wong, S.C. (2009). Identification of novel functional differences in monocyte subsets using proteomic and transcriptomic methods, *J Proteome Res*, Vol.8, No. 8, pp. 4028-38

Zimman, A.; Chen, S.S.; Komisopoulou, E.; Titz, B.; Martínez-Pinna, R.; Kafi, A.; Berliner, J.A. & Graeber, T.G. (2010). Activation of aortic endothelial cells by oxidized phospholipids: a phosphoproteomic analysis, *J Proteome Res*, Vol.9, No.6, pp.2812-24

Zimmerli, L.U.; Schiffer, E.; Zürbig, P.; Good, D.M.; Kellmann, M.; Mouls, L.; Pitt, A.R.; Coon, J.J.; Schmieder, R.E.; Peter, K.H.; Mischak, H.; Kolch, W.; Delles, C. & Dominiczak, A.F. (2008). Urinary proteomic biomarkers in coronary artery disease, *Mol Cell Proteomics*, Vol.7, No. 2, pp. 290-8

2

Urinary Exosomes for Protein Biomarker Research

Delfin Albert Amal Raj[1,2], Immacolata Fiume[1], Giovambattista Capasso[2] and Gabriella Pocsfalvi[1]
[1]*Mass Spectrometry and Proteomics, Institute of Protein Biochemistry – CNR, Naples*
[2]*Department of Internal Medicine, Chair of Nephrology, Faculty of Medicine, Second University of Naples, Naples*
Italy

1. Introduction

Exosomes represent a distinct class of membrane nanovesicles of endocytic origin that are released to the extracellular microenvironment from diverse cell types under both physiological and pathological conditions. Remarkable roles of exosomes have been revealed in intercellular communication, immune regulation, infection, aging and cancer. Exosomes carry and transfer proteins, nucleic acids and lipids, and are ubiquitous in most biofluids, such as urine, plasma, cerebrospinal fluid, etc. Membrane vesicles secreted by the epithelial cells of the urinary tract hold the promise to be an excellent source of disease relevant cargo proteins. In clinical proteomics urine is one of the most attractive biofluids as it can be obtained non-invasively, in large quantities and is relatively stable. Current isolation methods however are not sufficiently proficient to produce urinary exosomes (UEs) at a purity grade and with reproducibility suitable for downstream LC-MS based quantitative proteomics applications. Consequently urinary exosome based protein biomarker research today exclusively relies on targeted protein studies (Table 1).

This chapter describes the current state-of-the-art in exosome research in general and urinary exosomes in particular with a special focus on the potential of UEs in protein biomarker discovery. Recently we have developed an improved isolation/purification method based on double-cushion sucrose/D_2O ultracentrifugation (Raj et al., 2011b). The method relies on the solubilization of the major impurities associated with UEs in a carefully selected buffer solution. The new method separates exosomes from the heavier membrane fragments and/or vesicles more efficiently than current protocols and is compatible with LC-MS-based quantitative proteomics workflow.

2. Cell-derived exosomes: Biogenesis, composition and biological role

Cells rely on two basic mechanisms for active, vesicle-mediated macromolecular transport through the cellular plasma membrane: exocytosis and endocytosis (Figure 1). Both make use of membrane vesicles for the packaging and trafficking of molecules. While endocytosis is the process in which the extracellular substances enter into a cell without directly passing through the cell membrane, exocytosis is the primary means of cellular secretion. During both constitutive and regulated exocytosis the secretory-vesicles dock and/or fuse with the plasma membrane. Endocytic pathway (EP), which is primarily responsible for the uptake, trafficking and sorting of internalized proteins has a role in vesicle secretion too (Thery et al., 2002). In the EP, transmembrane proteins are sorted into lumenal vesicles of multivesicular bodies (MVBs). MVBs can have different destinies: they can fuse or mature with lysosomes where the degradation of their protein cargo takes place, or can fuse with the cell membrane to secrete the intraluminal vesicles (ILVs) into the extracellular space. These extracellularly released ILVs are called exosomes (Gruenberg et al., 2004, Keller et al., 2006). During this process, the second inward budding of the endosome membrane results in a positive orientation of the ILVs lipid membrane. Thus when the ILVs are released to the extracellular environment, they have the same orientation as the cell membrane and have been shown to display many of the surface markers from their cell of origin (Thery et al., 2002). The sorting process of membrane proteins during ILV formation is considered to be an active process and thus, exosomal surface proteins seem not to be a plain one-to-one representation of the surface markers for the cell of origin.

While the regulation of endocytic cargo sorting and its delivery to lysosomes have been extensively studied (Williams et al., 2007) relatively less is known about the factors which regulate the formation, the release and the cargo sorting into vesicles destined to be exosomes. The involvement of ubiquitinization and ESCRT (endosomal sorting complex required for transport) protein complexes have been shown by different groups (Gan et al., 2011, Shen et al., 2011). Though, ESCRT-independent mechanisms by means of ceramide-mediated budding of exosomes into ILVs within the MVBs have also been identified (Marsh et al., 2008, Trajkovic et al., 2008). Further evidence of ESCRT-independent pathway of ILV formation has come from studying the protein Pmel17, a main component of the c fibrils of pre-melanosomes, which is targeted to intraluminal vesicles of MVBs independently of ubiquitination, ESCRT0 and ESCRTI (Raposo et al., 2001). The most recent model on the formation of ILVs combines the lipid-driven membrane deformation theory with the ESCRT-regulated sorting mechanism (Babst, 2011).

Microvesicles (MVs) are generated by the outward budding and fission of membrane vesicles from the cell surface (Fig. 1) (Lee et al., 2011). MVs (100–1000 nm) are generally bigger in size than exosomes (30-100 nm). Yet due to the analytical difficulties in distinguishing between exosomes and MVs, which are also shed by normal and diseased cells, they are often grouped together.

Many mammalian cells like dendritic, mast, epithelial, neural, stem and hematopoietic cells, reticulocytes, astrocytes, adipocytes, and tumor cells have been reported to release exosomes (Denzer et al., 2000, van Niel et al., 2006). Exosomes purified from the cell culture supernatants are usually heterogeneous in size and contain functional mRNA translatable to proteins, mature microRNAs, lipids and proteins. Proteins of exosomes have been analyzed both by proteomics and targeted immunochemical methods, like Western-blot, FACS with immunolabeling, and immunoelectron microscopy. Protein composition analysis of exosomes shows a rather limited sub-cellular localization for the exosomal proteins. In fact, usually the preparations of exosomes are mostly enriched in cytosolic and membrane proteins and contain less proteins of nuclear, mitochondrial, endoplasmic-reticulum or Golgi-apparatus origin. Secondly, exosomes express a common set of proteins. These are structural components and proteins with a role in exosome biogenesis and trafficking. Cell type specific components which presumably reflect the biological function of the parent cell on

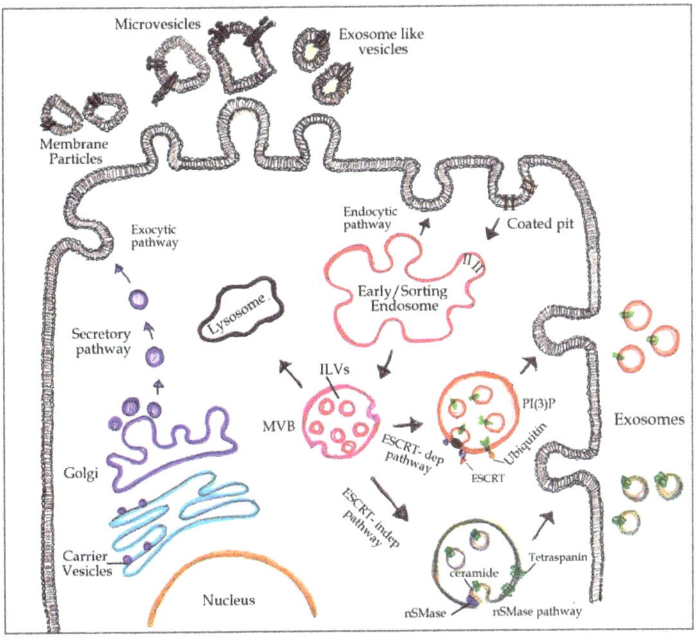

Fig. 1. Schematic representation of extracellular vesicles biogenesis. The formation, release and cargo sorting into vesicles destined to be exosomes may involve: i) ESCRT dependent pathway - involving the ubiquitination and ESCRT protein complexes and ii) ESCRT - independent pathway - like ceramide mediated budding. Microvesicles, membrane particles and exosome like vesicles are secreted by outward budding or fission from the cell surface.

the other hand could also be identified in exosome preparations (van Niel et al., 2006). Protein contents of exosomes from different cells have been mapped by proteomics and the most of the data obtained has been catalogued in Exocarta database (Mathivanan et al., 2009).

Despite their role in immune system modulation (Li et al., 2006), the biological role of exosome secretion remained largely elusive until recent years when Lötvall's group demonstrated that exosomes can transfer genetic information from one cell to another (Valadi et al., 2007, Taylor, 2010). Since then several mechanisms have been proposed to describe exosome-cell interactions: (i) cellular binding via conventional receptor–ligand interactions, similar to cell–cell communication. (ii) attaching/fusing with target cell membrane and (iii) internalization by recipient cells by endocytosis in a transcytotic manner. Besides the physiological roles of exosomes to remove the unwanted cellular debris, recent findings uncover an entirely new and exciting modes of cell–cell communication and paracrine signalling mediated by exosomes (Thery et al., 2002, Camussi et al., 2011). Emerging data shows their involvement in different diseases including inflammation, renal diseases, Alzheimer diseases, aging, bacterial and viral infections, allergies and cancer. Using different sources of tumor-derived exosomes, several groups claim that exosomes can prevent tumor development, induce tumor specific immunity, and provide a possible strategy for therapeutic tumor vaccination reviewed by van Niel et al. (van Niel et al., 2006).

3. Urinary exosomes

3.1 mRNA, miRNA and protein biomarkers in urinary exosomes

Urinary exosomes originate from those ILVs that are shed into the urinary space by the fusion of the outer membrane of MVBs with the apical plasma membrane of cells lining the urinary tract, including glomerular podocytes, renal tubule cells, and bladder. The number, and the physical, chemical and biological properties of UEs may change over time in association with disorders that affect the urinary system. Respect to the total urine sample, UEs result in a remarkable enrichment of low-abundance biomolecules with potentially high diagnostic value regarding the physiological and pathological state of the renal system. Therefore, it is not surprising that there is a great interest in the use of UEs as a novel biomarker source for early disease detection, classification, prediction severity, outcome and response to treatment. Since the first publication on proteomic profiling of UEs by the group of Knepper (Pisitkun et al., 2004), an increasing number of articles with keywords "exosome and urine" are to be found in the PubMed database. The principal aim of urinary exosome research today is to discover mRNA, microRNA and protein biomarkers.

Disease	Isolation method	Protein separation	Protein identification	Quantitation	Protein Biomarker candidate	Taxonomy	Ref
AKI	differential ultracentrifugation	2D-PAGE	MS Western blot	2D-PAGE	Fetuin-A	Rat Human	Zhou et al., 2006a
AKI	differential ultracentrifugation	SDS-PAGE	Western blot	Western blot	ATF3 WT-1	Rat Human	Zhou et al., 2008
FSGS	nanomembrane concentration	SDS-PAGE	MS Western blot	Western blot	Podocalyxin	Human	Cheruvanky et al., 2007
BC	differential ultracentrifugation	SDS-PAGE	MS	Spectral count	Resistin GTPase NRas EPS8L2 Mucin-4 EPS8L1 RAI3 GSA EHDP4 Galectin-3	Human	Smalley et al., 2008
PC	sucrose cushion ultracentrifugation	SDS-PAGE	Western blot	Western blot	PSA PSMA	Human	Mitchell et al., 2009
I/R	differential ultracentrifugation	SDS-PAGE	Western blot	Western blot	AQP1	Rat Human	Sonoda et al., 2009
GKD	sucrose gradient ultracentrifugation	SDS-PAGE	Western blot	Western blot	ADAM10	Human	Gutwein et al., 2010
NSCL	differential ultracentrifugation	SDS-PAGE	MS Western blot	Western blot	LRG1	Human	Li et al., 2011

AKI - acute kidney injury
FSGS - focal segmental glomerulosclerosis
BC - bladder cancer
PC - prostate cancer
I/R - renal ischemia/reperfusion
GKD - glomural kidney disease
NSCL – non-small cell lung cancer

Table 1. Different isolation/purification, protein separation, identification and quantitation methods used in urinary exosome related targeted protein biomarker studies.

mRNA transcripts encoding specific genes from various regions of the nephron, the collecting duct, the prostate and the bladder have been isolated from urinary exosome preparations (Miranda et al., 2010, Keller et al., 2011). Interestingly, RNA of UEs was found to be protected from RNase degradation which may suggest a functional role for the nucleic acids present in exosome (Keller et al., 2011). In the mRNA sample isolated from the urinary exosomes of prostate cancer patients PCA-3 and TMPRSS2:ERG, two known prostate cancer related biomarkers were detected (Nilsson et al., 2009). Urinary exosomes seem to be particularly rich in miRNAs too. The use of miRNA as diagnostic biomarkers in exosome research is an emerging field due to important potential advantages over standard mRNA (Li et al., 2010).

There are over a thousand proteins identified from UE preparations published in the Exocarta (Mathivanan et al., 2009) and the Urinary Exosome Protein Database (Pisitkun et al., 2004) including the six exosome markers commonly used in exosome research (Alix, Tsg101, CD63, CD9, CD81, HSP70). Proteins of UEs show a different profile from that of total urinary proteins but with a high degree of overlap. UEs are enriched in membrane and cytosolic cargo proteins from the different epithelial cells lining the urinary tract (Pisitkun et al., 2004, Gonzales et al., 2009). For clinical biomarker discovery, LC-MS based large-scale quantitative proteomic analysis would be the method of choice. However, at the urinary exosome level it is still a daunting task (Gonzales et al., 2008, Mitchell et al., 2009, Keller et al., 2011). Therefore, protein quantitation and expression analysis has mainly been performed by targeted studies like antibody-based Western blot analysis (Table 1). For this reason only a few protein biomarker candidates have so far been identified in UEs.

3.2 Isolation and purification

Protocols for collection, storage and processing of human urine for exosome isolation and protein characterization have recently been published (Zhou et al., 2006b). Concerning the isolation of UEs, current methods rely on ultracentrifugation or filtration, or the combination of these two. The majority of the studies use a two-step differential centrifugation protocol developed by Pisitkun et al (Pisitkun et al., 2004). The initial step is a low velocity sequential centrifugation which serves to remove cells and cellular debris (urinary sediment) from urine, leaving the exosomes in the supernatant. The second step is the ultracentrifugation for 1h to overnight of the supernatant at 100,000-200,000g velocity to sediment exosomes. The major short comings of this process are the high level of contamination from uromodulin (see later) and the lack of separation of exosomes from the other MVs and membrane particles.

To obtain higher purity grade UEs, the crude preparation obtained by the two-step differential centrifugation method can be further processed using the sucrose gradient or the sucrose cushion centrifugation. Sucrose gradient centrifugation can be performed on linear or step gradients typically using sucrose concentrations between 2.0 M - 0.25 M (Keller et al., 2007, Hogan et al., 2009, Simpson et al., 2009, Mathivanan et al., 2010). Instead of gradient, a small density cushion typically composed of 30% sucrose in deuterium oxide (D_2O), can also be employed for the purification of UEs (Mitchell et al., 2009, Simpson et al., 2009, Welton et al., 2010). In the sucrose cushion, formation of a mini density gradient takes place in the range of 1.10-1.18 g/cm^3. This range was shown to be suitable to enrich and purify exosomes preventing vesicle aggregation that pelleting could cause. Sucrose gradient and cushion centrifugations thus allow a better separation of exosomes from the vesicles of different densities respect to the differential centrifugation method, however it does not seem to eliminate the problem of the co-purifying uromodulin (Hogan et al., 2009).

Filtration-based protocols generally use polyether sulfone nano-membranes in a spin concentrator to isolate urinary exosomes (Cheruvanky et al., 2007). The method is simple, fast and is capable to isolate UEs from small volumes of urine (0.5–10 mL). Therefore it is very promising, especially for mRNA and miRNA based exosome biomarker research. Drawbacks of this method for protein biomarker research are the low yield and the high level of contamination caused by urinary proteins binding to the filter. To overcome this, recently a low protein binding membrane (hydrophilized polyvinylidene difluoride) has been used to isolate urinary exosomes (Merchant et al., 2010).

3.3 The uromodulin problem

Current methods are characterized by a high and variable level of uromodulin contamination (Hogan et al., 2009, Fernandez-Llama et al., 2010, Rood et al., 2010). Uromodulin, also referred to as Tamm–Horsfall glycoprotein, is a major glycoprotein produced by kidney cells. Uromodulin assembles into intracellular filaments in urine (Porter et al., 1955, Schaeffer et al., 2009). The filaments have an average width and length of 100 Å and 2.5 μm, respectively and tend to form a three-dimensional matrix with pores as shown by electron microscopy (Porter et al., 1955). This filament network traps exosomes and prevents their efficient isolation and purification by traditional methods. The uromodulin problem is one of the bottle neck of UE protein research because it considerably reduces sample yield and reproducibility (Fernandez-Llama et al., 2010). In order to facilitate the removal of high molecular weight aggregates recently, dithiothreitol (DTT) was applied to reduce the intermolecular disulfide bonds of uromodulin (Pisitkun et al., 2004, Fernandez-Llama et al., 2010). Treatment with DTT result in a higher yield of urinary exosomes. Notwithstanding it does not solve the problem efficiently. For this reason, urinary exosome samples prepared by the current methods are far from being ideal for quantitative proteomic analysis.

4. Interfacing urinary exosome isolation/purification and lysis with quantitative proteomics for protein biomarker research

Biomarkers support the diagnosis and medical management of various disorders. The remarkable progress made in proteomic technologies in the past decade have enabled researchers to consider designing studies to identify diagnostic and therapeutic biomarkers by analyzing complex proteome samples using unbiased mass spectrometry based methods. In urinary exosome research this has been hampered by the high and variable concentration of uromodulin causing low sample quantity, quality and low reproducibility. To meet the need of a global protein biomarker discovery platform we have set-up new protocols for the isolation/purification and also for the lysis and subsequent solubilization of membrane proteins. Paragraph 4.1 describes a novel urinary exosome preparation called double-cushion ultracentrifugation method and paragraph 4.2 shows its compatibility with downstream analysis.

We have employed a multiplex quantitative proteomics method, iTRAQ (isobaric Tagging for Relative and Absolute protein Quantification), in conjunction with multidimensional chromatography, followed by tandem mass spectrometry (MS/MS), to measure relative differences in the protein composition of urinary exosome samples (Figure 2). The aim of this work was to compare the protein content of UEs obtained by single- and double-

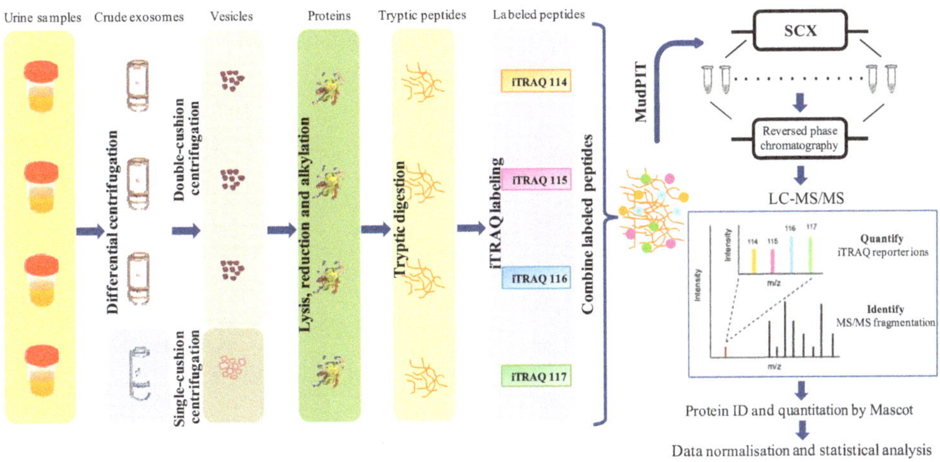

Fig. 2. Scheme of the MudPIT based 4-plex iTRAQ quantitative analysis comparing the double-cushion ultracentrifugation method with that of single-cushion.

cushion ultracentrifugation methods. Simultaneously, we compared samples obtained from a single person with a pool of healthy volunteers divided into two age groups (25-50 years and 50-70 years) in order to study feasibility of analysis of single patient versus pooled samples in the discovery phase of protein biomarker research.

4.1 A novel isolation/purification method based on uromodulin solubilization and double-cushion ultracentrifugation

The urinary exosome isolation/purification method which we have recently developed (Raj et al., 2011b) employs a double-cushion ultracentrifugation step performed in a carefully chosen buffer solution. Respect to other ultracentrifugation based methods which generally use a PBS buffer (150 mM NaCl at pH 7.2) the novel method employs a solubilising buffer composed of 20 mM Tris at pH 8.6. We have found that Tris buffer efficiently solubilizes uromodulin aggregates, keeps uromodulin in solution and does not lyses exosomes. This is in accordance with a previous in vitro study on uromodulin solubility which underlines the importance of alkaline pH, low sodium and calcium concentrations and sample dilution to prevent the formation of uromodulin aggregates (Kobayashi et al., 2001). After solubilizing the pellet obtained in the differential ultracentrifugation step, double-cushion ultracentrifugation is performed. The double-cushion is made of sucrose 1 M and sucrose 2 M prepared in 20 mM Tris pH 8.6 in D_2O and subsequently under layered below the sample in the centrifuge tube. This step was found to considerably improve the separation of exosomes from the heavier vesicles and/or membrane fragments.

4.2 Analysis of urinary vesicles at the various steps of isolation/purification

Exosomes were purified from pooled urine samples of ten healthy donors and separated on 4-12% gradient polyacrylamide gel then stained with colloidal Coomassie blue. SDS-PAGE analysis at the various phases of the isolation/purification process is shown in Figure 3.

Total urinary protein profiles before (Figure 3.A, Lane 1) and after exosome depletion (Figure 3.A, Lane 2) do not markedly differ from each other and show the typical pattern of

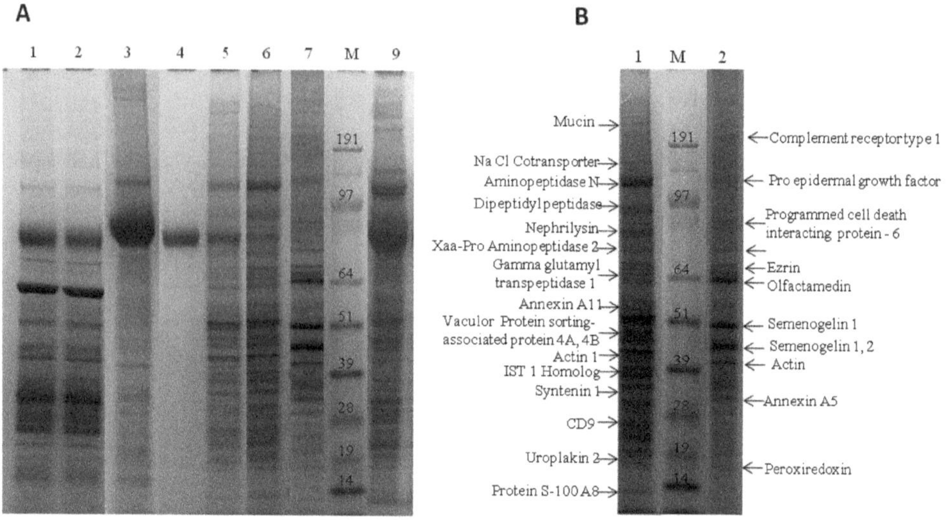

Fig. 3. SDS PAGE analyses A) at the different stages of urinary exosome isolation/purification through the double-cushion (lanes 1-7) and the single-cushion (lane 9) methods and, B) of the 1 M and 2 M sucrose fractions obtained after the double-cushion ultracentrifugation method (major proteins identified by *in-gel* digestion proteomics are indicated next to the band). Lanes in Figure A as follow: 1- Total urine; 2- Exosome depleted urine; 3- Crude exosome fraction after differential centrifugation; 4- 15,000g pellet; 5- 15,000g supernatant; 6- Purified exosomes (1 M sucrose fraction); 7- 2 M sucrose fraction; M- Protein molecular weight markers (kDa); 9- Urinary exosomes prepared by the single sucrose/D_2O cushion method. Lanes in Figure B are as follow: 1- 1 M sucrose fraction and 2- 2 M sucrose fraction and M- Protein molecular weight markers (kDa).

the major urinary proteins, like albumin, various IgG chains, uromodulin etc. After the two-step differential centrifugation the crude exosome pellet (Figure 3.A, lane 3) still contains a considerable amount of contaminating urinary proteins and in particular uromodulin at 85 kDa. These are in part removed after the solubilization step by low-speed centrifugation (Figure 3.A, lane 4-5) and, in part by the double-cushion ultracentrifugation. The later yields two fractions: the 1 M sucrose fraction which contains the exosome vesicles (Figure 3.A, lane 6) and the 2 M fraction which contains vesicles heavier than exosomes (Figure 3.A, lane 7). The efficiency of the uromodulin removal by the double-cushion sucrose ultracentrifugation methods can be appreciated by comparing the 1 M fraction (Figure 3.A, lane 6) with the crude exosome fraction (Figure 3.A, lane 3) and with the exosomes purified by the single-cushion method (Figure 3.A, lane 9). In Figure 3.B SDS-PAGE image of the two vesicle containing fractions, 1 M (lane 1) and 2 M (lane 2) are shown together with the major proteins identified in the gel bands. It is of note that not only the protein pattern but also the proteins identified in the major SDS-PAGE bands were found to be different, indicating the presence of two different types of vesicles in the two fractions. Semenogelin 1 and semenogelin 2 and olfactomedin for example have previously been identified in prostasomes, i.e. the secretory particles in human seminal fluid (Utleg et al., 2003). Therefore it is plausible to presume that the 2 M sucrose fraction contains heavier vesicles, like urinary secreted prostasomes.

Western blot analysis was performed to monitor the enrichment in exosomes and the reproducibility of sample preparation by the double-cushion ultracentrifugation. Exosomal proteins were separated on 4-12% gradient SDS-PAGE and electro blotted to PVDF membrane. Blots were probed with antibodies against two known exosome markers Alix and TSG101, together with NKCC2 a renal sodium transporter known to be present in urinary exosomes (Figure 4.). The enrichment of exosomes is excellent in the samples prepared by the double-cushion (Figure 4., lane 4-6) respect to the starting and exosome depleted urine samples (Figure 4., lane 2-3) and also to the sample prepared by the differential centrifugation method (Figure 4., lane 1). Importantly a very high degree of reproducibility was achieved in three independent urinary exosome preparations (Figure 4., lanes 4-6).

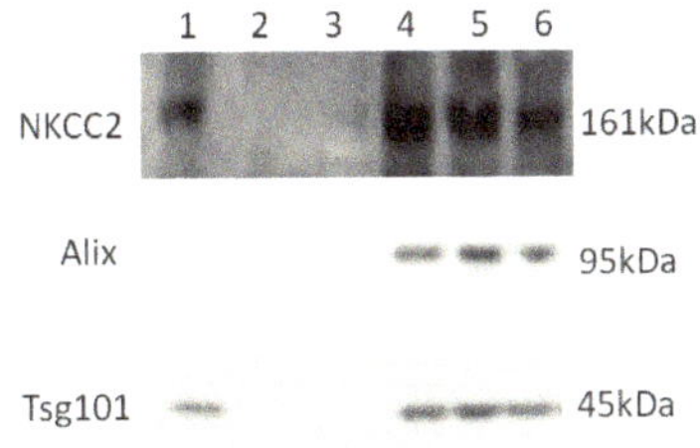

Fig. 4. Western blot analysis of urinary exosomes prepared by two different methods. Lane 1- Exosome purified by differential centrifugation; Lane 2- Total urine; Lane 3- Exosome depleted urine; Lane 4-6 – Exosomes purified in three independent experiments from pooled urine samples of ten healthy volunteers by the double-cushion method.

Exosome-like vesicles isolated from culture supernatant are limited by a lipid bilayer and in literature often described as saucer- or cup-shaped particles. Urinary exosomes isolated by the double-cushion ultracentrifugation method have a similar morphology as single cell line derived exosomes. The transmission electron microscopy (TEM) image shows (Figure 5) that diameters of the vesicles purified in the 1 M fraction are between 30 and 80 nm. Interestingly, the shape of the exosomes appeared to be nearly spherical with only a few elongated or cup-shaped specimens. After the double-cushion ultracentrifugation the sample is basically free from the long uromodulin filaments known to contaminate UEs prepared by traditional methods.

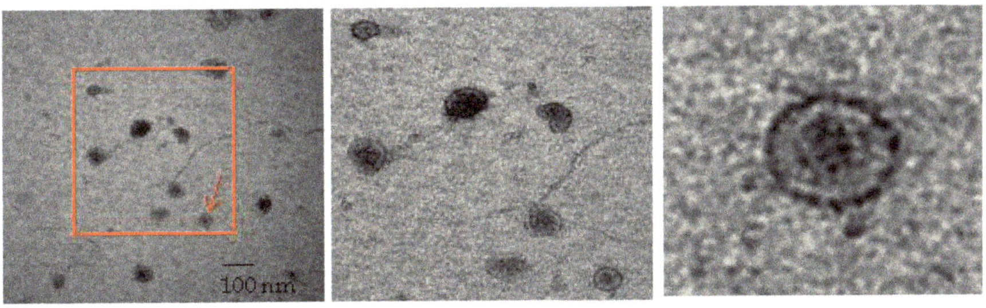

Fig. 5. Transmission electron microscopy image of urinary exosomes isolated and purified by the double-cushion ultracentrifugation method (1 M fraction). The image shows the typical morphology and size distribution of the vesicles. Frame shows the enlarged image (central) and the arrow shows a single vesicle enlarged on the right image.

5. Quantitative proteomics of urinary exosomes for protein biomarker discovery

Recently, we have developed protocols for lysis, protein extraction and *in-solution* digestion of UEs for MudPIT application to quantitative proteomics (Raj et al., 2011a). For the solubilization of exosomal membrane proteins the use of an acid cleavable detergent was found to be particularly useful. In a preliminary study four exosomal protein samples were prepared in parallel (Table 2) according to single- (sample 4) and double-cushion protocols (sample 1) from a pooled urine sample of 20 healthy donors (male, age group 25-45 years). Effects of age (sample 2) and sample pooling (sample 3) on the protein expression were also monitored in the same experiment.

Sample	Age (years)	Number of samples	Exosome preparation method	Label
1	25-45	20	Double-cushion	iTRAQ-114
2	50-70	20	Double-cushion	iTRAQ-115
3	43	1	Double-cushion	iTRAQ-116
4	25-45	20	Single-cushion	iTRAQ-117

Table 2. Samples analysed by *in-solution* digestion based MudPIT proteomics and iTRAQ labeling.

The 4-plex iTRAQ method (Ross et al., 2004) based on covalent labeling of the N-terminus and side-chain amines of peptides with four tags of varying mass was used for the protein quantitation (Figure 2.).

Protein samples were denatured, reduced, alkylated, enzymatically digested by trypsin and then labeled according to the manufacturer's protocol (iTRAQ reagent kit, Applied Biosystems). After iTRAQ labeling equal amounts of each sample (100 μg) were mixed, vacuum dried, detergent was acid cleaved and the resulting sample was desalted. The purified sample was then separated by two-dimensional HPLC. For strong cation-exchange (SCX) chromatography, in the first dimension, the following conditions were used: 95% solvent A (20% acetonitrile, 0.05% formic acid) and 5% solvent B (20% acetonitrile, 0.05% formic acid, 500mM KCl) for 3 min, solvent B ramped up to 90% in 40 min and maintained at 100% for 7 min. 47 fractions were collected between 0-55 min. Fractions were further separated in the second dimension on a reversed phase monolithic nano column using the following conditions: 95% solvent C (2% acetonitrile, 0.1% formic acid) and 5% solvent D (98% acetonitrile, 0.1% formic acid) for 5 min, ramp to 50% solvent D in 90 min and in 6 sec to 98% solvent D for 10 min. Eluting peptides were analyzed online by a QTOF type of tandem mass spectrometer (Qstar Elite) in an information dependent acquisition mode which facilitates both the protein identification and the multiplex quantitative analysis of the four samples. Tandem mass spectra were extracted and peak lists were generated by Analyst QS 2.0 software using the default parameters. Peak lists containing all acquired MS/MS spectra were searched against SwissProt 2010_09 (519348 sequences) database using Mascot Server (version 2.2) with trypsin specificity and allowing for up to one missed cleavage. iTRAQ at lysine residue and the N termini of the peptides and carbamidomethylation of cysteines were considered as fixed modifications whereas oxidations of methionine and iTRAQ at tyrosine residues were set as possible variable modifications. Mass tolerance was set to 50 ppm for precursor and to 0.1 Da for fragment ions, respectively. Low molecular mass reporter ions were used to relatively quantify the

peptides and the proteins from which they originate by Mascot iTRAQ 4-plex quantification method. Proteins which were quantified with a minimum of two unique peptides and $p<0.05$ significance threshold using MudPIT scoring have been considered.
More than hundred proteins were quantified in the iTRAQ analysis. Table 3. shows the weighted median ratios of the first 25 proteins ranked by Mascot protein score. Expression level of the major proteins isolated and purified by the double-cushion method are different from those purified with the single-cushion protocol (Table 3., ratio 117/114). In particular, cytoskeletal proteins (cubulin, megalin, actin, cofillin, moesin, tubulin, etc.) seem to be less abundant in the sample. They may be due to heterogeneous constituents of the cytoskeleton filaments present in urine which co-purify with the UEs in traditional methods. On the other hand a marked enrichment was observed in proteins which are related to the VPS4 complex of ESCRT machinery (IST1, VPS4A, and VPS4B), its associated proteins (CHM2A, CHMP5,

UniProt ID	Protein Name	Mascot score	115/114	116/114	117/114
AMPN_HUMAN	Aminopeptidase	1315	0.845	1.306	0.237
IST1_HUMAN	IST1 homolog	656	1.037	0.706	0.406
ACTB_HUMAN	Actin, cytoplasmic	430	1.408	1.631	0.733
DPEP1_HUMAN	Dipeptidase 1	370	0.857	0.700	0.430
VPS4A_HUMAN	Vacuolar protein sorting-associated protein 4A	350	1.150	0.742	0.473
CHM2A_HUMAN	Charged multivesicular body protein 2a	341	1.242	1.493	0.595
UROM_HUMAN	Uromodulin	282	0.958	0.578	22.450
CHMP5_HUMAN	Charged multivesicular body protein 5	279	1.082	0.569	0.161
RS27A_HUMAN	Ubiquitin-40S ribosomal protein S27a	275	1.051	0.764	0.445
GGT1_HUMAN	Gamma-glutamyltranspeptidase	267	0.840	1.045	0.342
NEP_HUMAN	Neprilysin	258	0.897	0.995	0.381
EZRI_HUMAN	Ezrin	254	1.245	1.093	0.776
ANX11_HUMAN	Annexin A11	252	1.393	0.435	0.601
PSCA_HUMAN	Prostate stem cell antigen	231	1.415	5.214	0.345
HSP7C_HUMAN	Heat shock cognate 71 kDa protein	208	1.186	0.990	0.428
PDC6I_HUMAN	Programmed cell death 6-interacting protein	231	1.093	0.684	0.500
CDC42_HUMAN	Cell division control protein 42 homolog	208	1.044	1.773	0.190
VPS4B_HUMAN	Vacuolar protein sorting-associated protein 4B	195	1.063	0.601	0.500
CHM4B_HUMAN	Charged multivesicular body protein 4b	181	1.308	0.923	0.559
POTEF_HUMAN	POTE ankyrin domain family member F	176	1.394	1.404	0.510
DPP4_HUMAN	Dipeptidyl peptidase 4	175	0.931	0.837	0.320
AQP1_HUMAN	Aquaporin-1	167	0.898	0.679	0.573
THY1_HUMAN	Thy-1 membrane glycoprotein	151	1.316	2.332	0.354
MUC1_HUMAN	Mucin-1	145	0.945	0.523	0.743
PROM1_HUMAN	Prominin-1	140	1.014	0.655	0.500

Table 3. The weighted median ratios of the 25 top-ranking proteins in the MudPIT based 4-plex iTRAQ experiment. 114, 115, 116 and 117 indicate sample-labeling by iTRAQ according to Table 2.

CHM4B) and proteins involved in the ubiquitination process (RS27A). The most abundant protein according to SDS-PAGE and MudPIT analyses is aminopeptidase (AMPN) known to reflect a periodicity in renal tubular function. Other proteins like AQP1, NEP, DPEP1 and DPP4 also related to renal function were identified among the most abundant proteins. Based on statistical analysis of the data, more than a 2-fold change was considered to be significant. Data obtained confirms that the double-cushion method efficiently removes the major urinary protein contamination characteristic of the current purification methods (more than a 20-fold change). In different single-cushion preparations (data not shown) the relative protein quantities vary considerably respect to that of uromodulin (i.e. mean of the fold changes of all quantified proteins unless uromodulin/uromodulin fold change). This can be explained by the poor reproducibility and it causes considerable complications in protein quantification and normalization. Comparing the two different age-groups we analysed, no significant difference in the expression was found in the 25 top-ranking exosomal proteins (Table 3., ratio 115/114). The individual sample, on the other hand shows few characteristic differences when compared with the pooled samples (116/114). In our study, the expression levels of PSCA and THY1 and ANX11 were found to be significantly altered respect to the age-matched control group. For a protein biomarker discovery platform which employs urinary exosomes as biomarker source, it is highly advisable to use a pooled control sample with a high number and clinically well defined individual samples.

6. Conclusions

Given the non-invasive nature of urine sample collection and the evolving biological significance of secreted membrane vesicles, unbiased quantitative analysis of biomolecules isolated from urinary exosomes is a step forward in clinical biomarker research. Recently we have set-up a multiplex quantitative approach for the analysis of protein contents of purified urinary exosomes (Figure 2.). This includes protocols for i.) the removal of major urinary exosome contaminations, ii.) the separation of urinary membrane vesicles of different sizes iii.) vesicle lysis and protein solubilization and, iv) the quantitative proteomics based urinary exosomal biomarker research. The novel isolation/purification procedure efficiently removes the major urinary exosomal contaminations and separates exosomes from other membrane vesicles. Thus it provides a good basis for the development of optimized methods for protein biomarker research. Quantitative MudPIT analysis performed on biological, analytical and technical replicates shows excellent reproducibility. No significant expression difference was found among normal healthy subjects grouped by age. Preliminary data suggests a superior performance in single sample biomarker analysis design over a pooling design. All together, these results suggest a prolific future of urinary exosomes in clinical proteomics of different diseases involving the renal and urinary tract.

7. Acknowledgment

The authors are grateful for the financial contribution of Italian Society of Nephrology granted by "Ricercando 2011" for the project entitled "Identification of reliable urinary biomarkers of Diabetic Nephropathy by means of powerful and complementary proteomic strategies". We also thank Rosarita Tatè and Michele Cermola (IGB, CNR) for the TEM analysis.

8. References

Babst, M. (2011). MVB vesicle formation: ESCRT-dependent, ESCRT-independent and everything in between. *Current Opinion in Cell Biology,* In Press, Corrected Proof.

Camussi, G., Deregibus, M. C., Bruno, S., Cantaluppi, V. & Biancone, L. (2011). Exosomes/microvesicles as a mechanism of cell-to-cell communication. *Kidney International,* 78 (9), 838-848.

Cheruvanky, A., Zhou, H., Pisitkun, T., Kopp, J. B., Knepper, M. A., Yuen, P. S. T. & Star, R. A. (2007). Rapid isolation of urinary exosomal biomarkers using a nanomembrane ultrafiltration concentrator. *American Journal of Physiololgy Renal Physiology,* 292 (5), F1657-1661.

Denzer, K., Kleijmeer, M. J., Heijnen, H. F., Stoorvogel, W. & Geuze, H. J. (2000). Exosome: from internal vesicle of the multivesicular body to intercellular signaling device. *Journal of Cell Science,* 113 (19), 3365-3374.

Fernandez-Llama, P., Khositseth, S., Gonzales, P. A., Star, R. A., Pisitkun, T. & Knepper, M. A. (2010). Tamm-Horsfall protein and urinary exosome isolation. *Kidney International,* 77 (8), 736-742.

Gan, X. & Gould, S. J. (2011). Identification of an inhibitory budding signal that blocks the release of HIV particles and exosome/microvesicle proteins. *Molecular Biology of the Cell,* 22 (6), 817-830.

Gonzales, P., Pisitkun, T. & Knepper, M. A. (2008). Urinary exosomes: is there a future? *Nephrology Dialysis Transplantation,* 23 (6), 1799-1801.

Gonzales, P. A., Pisitkun, T., Hoffert, J. D., Tchapyjnikov, D., Star, R. A., Kleta, R., Wang, N. S. & Knepper, M. A. (2009). Large-Scale Proteomics and Phosphoproteomics of Urinary Exosomes. *Journal of the American Society of Nephrology,* 20 (2), 363-379.

Gruenberg, J. & Stenmark, H. (2004). The biogenesis of multivesicular endosomes. *Nature Reviews Molecular Cell Biology,* 5 (4), 317-323.

Gutwein, P., Schramme, A., Abdel-Bakky, M., Doberstein, K., Hauser, I., Ludwig, A., Altevogt, P., Gauer, S., Hillmann, A., Weide, T., Jespersen, C., Eberhardt, W. & Pfeilschifter, J. (2010). ADAM10 is expressed in human podocytes and found in urinary vesicles of patients with glomerular kidney diseases. *Journal of Biomedical Science,* 17 (1), 3.

Hogan, M. C., Manganelli, L., Woollard, J. R., Masyuk, A. I., Masyuk, T. V., Tammachote, R., Huang, B. Q., Leontovich, A. A., Beito, T. G., Madden, B. J., Charlesworth, M. C., Torres, V. E., LaRusso, N. F., Harris, P. C. & Ward, C. J. (2009). Characterization of PKD Protein-Positive Exosome-Like Vesicles. *Journal of the American Society of Nephrology,* 20 (2), 278-288.

Keller, S., Ridinger, J., Rupp, A.-K., Janssen, J. & Altevogt, P. (2011). Body fluid derived exosomes as a novel template for clinical diagnostics. *Journal of Translational Medicine,* 9 (1), 86.

Keller, S., Rupp, C., Stoeck, A., Runz, S., Fogel, M., Lugert, S., Hager, H. D., Abdel-Bakky, M. S., Gutwein, P. & Altevogt, P. (2007). CD24 is a marker of exosomes secreted into urine and amniotic fluid. *Kidney International,* 72 (9), 1095-1102.

Keller, S., Sanderson, M. P., Stoeck, A. & Altevogt, P. (2006). Exosomes: From biogenesis and secretion to biological function. *Immunology Letters,* 107 (2), 102-108.

Kobayashi, K. & Fukuoka, S. (2001). Conditions for Solubilization of Tamm-Horsfall Protein/Uromodulin in Human Urine and Establishment of a Sensitive and

Accurate Enzyme-Linked Immunosorbent Assay (ELISA) Method. *Archives of Biochemistry and Biophysics,* 388 (1), 113-120.

Lee, T., D'Asti, E., Magnus, N., Al-Nedawi, K., Meehan, B. & Rak, J. (2011). Microvesicles as mediators of intercellular communication in cancer—the emerging science of cellular 'debris'. *Seminars in Immunopathology,* 1-13.

Li, J. Y., Yong, T. Y., Michael, M. Z. & Gleadle, J. M. (2010). Review: The role of microRNAs in kidney disease. *Nephrology,* 15 (6), 599-608.

Li, X.-B., Zhang, Z.-R., Schluesener, H. J. & Xu, S.-Q. (2006). Role of exosomes in immune regulation. *Journal of Cellular and Molecular Medicine,* 10 (2), 364-375.

Li, Y., Zhang, Y., Qiu, F. & Qiu, Z. (2011). Proteomic identification of exosomal LRG1: A potential urinary biomarker for detecting NSCLC. *Electrophoresis,* 32, 1-8.

Marsh, M. & van Meer, G. (2008). No ESCRTs for Exosomes. *Science,* 319 (5867), 1191-1192.

Mathivanan, S., Lim, J. W. E., Tauro, B. J., Ji, H., Moritz, R. L. & Simpson, R. J. (2010). Proteomics Analysis of A33 Immunoaffinity-purified Exosomes Released from the Human Colon Tumor Cell Line LIM1215 Reveals a Tissue-specific Protein Signature. *Molecular & Cellular Proteomics,* 9 (2), 197-208.

Mathivanan, S. & Simpson, R. J. (2009). ExoCarta: A compendium of exosomal proteins and RNA. *Proteomics,* 9 (21), 4997-5000.

Merchant, M. L., Powell, D. W., Wilkey, D. W., Cummins, T. D., Deegens, J. K., Rood, I. M., McAfee, K. J., Fleischer, C., Klein, E. & Klein, J. B. (2010). Microfiltration isolation of human urinary exosomes for characterization by MS. *Proteomics - Clinical Applications,* 4 (1), 84-96.

Miranda, K. C., Bond, D. T., McKee, M., Skog, J., Paunescu, T. G., Da Silva, N., Brown, D. & Russo, L. M. (2010). Nucleic acids within urinary exosomes/microvesicles are potential biomarkers for renal disease. *Kidney International,* 78 (2), 191-199.

Mitchell, P., Welton, J., Staffurth, J., Court, J., Mason, M., Tabi, Z. & Clayton, A. (2009). Can urinary exosomes act as treatment response markers in prostate cancer? *Journal of Translational Medicine,* 7 (1), 4.

Nilsson, J., Skog, J., Nordstrand, A., Baranov, V., Mincheva-Nilsson, L., Breakefield, X. O. & Widmark, A. (2009). Prostate cancer-derived urine exosomes: a novel approach to biomarkers for prostate cancer. *British Journal of Cancer,* 100 (10), 1603-1607.

Pisitkun, T., Shen, R.-F. & Knepper, M. A. (2004). Identification and proteomic profiling of exosomes in human urine. *Proceedings of the National Academy of Sciences of the United States of America,* 101 (36), 13368-13373.

Porter, K. R. & Tamm, I. (1955). Direct visualization of a mucoprotein component of urine. *Journal of Biological Chemistry,* 212 (1), 135-140.

Raj, D. A. A., Capasso, G., Fiume, I. & Pocsfalvi, G. (2011a). A multiplex quantitative proteomics strategy for protein biomarker studies in urinary exosomes *Kidney International,* accepted, manuscript ID: KI-09-11-1553.R1.

Raj, D. A. A., Capasso, G., Fiume, I. & Pocsfalvi, G. (2011b). Procedura di isolamento e di purificazione degli esosomi urinari per la ricerca di biomarcatori proteici. In U. I. B. M. patent deposited in 14 March 2011 (ed.), *Ufficio Italiano Brevetti e Marchi,* Italy.

Raposo, G. a., Tenza, D., Murphy, D. M., Berson, J. F. & Marks, M. S. (2001). Distinct Protein Sorting and Localization to Premelanosomes, Melanosomes, and Lysosomes in Pigmented Melanocytic Cells. *The Journal of Cell Biology,* 152 (4), 809-824.

Rood, I. M., Deegens, J. K. J., Merchant, M. L., Tamboer, W. P. M., Wilkey, D. W., Wetzels, J. F. M. & Klein, J. B. (2010). Comparison of three methods for isolation of urinary microvesicles to identify biomarkers of nephrotic syndrome. *Kidney Int*, 78 (8), 810-816.

Ross, P. L., Huang, Y. N., Marchese, J. N., Williamson, B., Parker, K., Hattan, S., Khainovski, N., Pillai, S., Dey, S., Daniels, S., Purkayastha, S., Juhasz, P., Martin, S., Bartlet-Jones, M., He, F., Jacobson, A. & Pappin, D. J. (2004). Multiplexed Protein Quantitation in Saccharomyces cerevisiae Using Amine-reactive Isobaric Tagging Reagents. *Molecular & Cellular Proteomics*, 3 (12), 1154-1169.

Schaeffer, C., Santambrogio, S., Perucca, S., Casari, G. & Rampoldi, L. (2009). Analysis of Uromodulin Polymerization Provides New Insights into the Mechanisms Regulating ZP Domain-mediated Protein Assembly. *Molecular Biology of the Cell*, 20 (2), 589-599.

Shen, B., Wu, N., Yang, J.-M. & Gould, S. J. (2011). Protein targeting to exosomes/microvesicles by plasma membrane anchors. *Journal of Biological Chemistry*.

Simpson, R. J., Lim, J. W. E., Moritz, R. L. & Mathivanan, S. (2009). Exosomes: proteomic insights and diagnostic potential. *Expert Review of Proteomics*, 6 (3), 267-283.

Smalley, D. M., Sheman, N. E., Nelson, K. & Theodorescu, D. (2008). Isolation and Identification of Potential Urinary Microparticle Biomarkers of Bladder Cancer. *Journal of Proteome Research*, 7 (5), 2088-2096.

Sonoda, H., Yokota-Ikeda, N., Oshikawa, S., Kanno, Y., Yoshinaga, K., Uchida, K., Ueda, Y., Kimiya, K., Uezono, S., Ueda, A., Ito, K. & Ikeda, M. (2009). Decreased abundance of urinary exosomal aquaporin-1 in renal ischemia-reperfusion injury. *American Journal of Physiology - Renal Physiology*, 297 (4), F1006-F1016.

Taylor, D. D. L., KY, US), Gercel-taylor, Cicek (Louisville, KY, US) (2010). Exosome-associated micro RNA as a dignostic marker. United States: University of Lousville ResearchFoundation Inc. (Louisville, KY, US).

Thery, C., Zitvogel, L. & Amigorena, S. (2002). Exosomes: composition, biogenesis and function. *Nature reviews*, 2, 569 - 579.

Trajkovic, K., Hsu, C., Chiantia, S., Rajendran, L., Wenzel, D., Wieland, F., Schwille, P., Brugger, B. & Simons, M. (2008). Ceramide Triggers Budding of Exosome Vesicles into Multivesicular Endosomes. *Science*, 319 (5867), 1244-1247.

Utleg, A. G., Yi, E. C., Xie, T., Shannon, P., White, J. T., Goodlett, D. R., Hood, L. & Lin, B. (2003). Proteomic analysis of human prostasomes. *The Prostate*, 56 (2), 150-161.

Valadi, H., Ekstrom, K., Bossios, A., Sjostrand, M., Lee, J. J. & Lotvall, J. O. (2007). Exosome-mediated transfer of mRNAs and microRNAs is a novel mechanism of genetic exchange between cells. *Nature Cell Biology*, 9 (6), 654-659.

van Niel, G., Porto-Carreiro, I., Simoes, S. & Raposo, G. (2006). Exosomes: A Common Pathway for a Specialized Function. *Journal of Biochemistry*, 140 (1), 13-21.

Welton, J. L., Khanna, S., Giles, P. J., Brennan, P., Brewis, I. A., Staffurth, J., Mason, M. D. & Clayton, A. (2010). Proteomic analysis of bladder cancer exosomes. *Molecular & Cellular Proteomics*.

Williams, R. L. & Urbe, S. (2007). The emerging shape of the ESCRT machinery. *Nature Reviwes Molecular Cell Biology*, 8 (5), 355-368.

Zhou, H., Cheruvanky, A., Hu, X., Matsumoto, T., Hiramatsu, N., Cho, M. E., Berger, A., Leelahavanichkul, A., Doi, K., Chawla, L. S., Illei, G. G., Kopp, J. B., Balow, J. E., Austin, H. A., III, Yuen, P. S. T. & Star, R. A. (2008). Urinary exosomal transcription factors, a new class of biomarkers for renal disease. *Kidney International,* 74 (5), 613-621.

Zhou, H., Pisitkun, T., Aponte, A., Yuen, P. S. T., Hoffert, J. D., Yasuda, H., Hu, X., Chawla, L., Shen, R. F., Knepper, M. A. & Star, R. A. (2006a). Exosomal Fetuin-A identified by proteomics: A novel urinary biomarker for detecting acute kidney injury. *Kidney International,* 70 (10), 1847-1857.

Zhou, H., Yuen, P. S. T., Pisitkun, T., Gonzales, P. A., Yasuda, H., Dear, J. W., Gross, P., Knepper, M. A. & Star, R. A. (2006b). Collection, storage, preservation, and normalization of human urinary exosomes for biomarker discovery. *Kidney International,* 69 (8), 1471-1476.

Exploring the Role of Biomarkers for the Diagnosis and Management of Traumatic Brain Injury Patients

Linda Papa
Graduate Medical Education, Orlando Health
Department of Emergency Medicine
University of Florida, College of Medicine
Florida State University, College of Medicine
University of Central Florida, College of Medicine
Orlando Regional Medical Center, Orlando, Florida
USA

1. Introduction

There are an estimated 10 million people affected annually by traumatic brain injury (TBI) across the globe.[1] In the United States, TBI is a major cause of death and disability[2] with about 52,000 annual deaths and 5.3 million Americans impaired by its effects. TBI is a contributing factor to over 30% of all injury-related deaths in the United States and it has been referred to as the silent epidemic of our time. [3, 4] European TBI prevalence data is not consistently reported by each country but it has been estimated that 1.6 million head-injured patients are hospitalized annually in Europe with an incidence rate of about 235 per 100,000. There is an average mortality rate of about 15 per 100,000 and a case fatality rate of about 11 per 100. The TBI severity ratio of hospitalized patients is about 22:1.5:1 for mild vs. moderate vs. severe cases, respectively.[5] According to the World Health Organization, TBI will surpass many diseases as the major cause of death and disability by the year 2020.[1]

Brain injuries can be focal, diffuse or a combination of focal and diffuse. The degree of brain injury depends on the primary mechanism/magnitude of injury, secondary insults and the patient's genetic and molecular response. Following the initial injury, cellular responses and neurochemical and metabolic cascades contribute to secondary injury.[6, 7] Focal brain injuries include contusions, brain lacerations, and hemorrhage leading to the formation of hematoma in the extradural, subarachnoid, subdural, or intracerebral compartments within the head. Traumatic brain injury represents a spectrum of injury severity. The number, types, and location of lesions as well as the magnitude of overlapping injuries across this spectrum of injury severity are still not clearly described and are challenging to classify.

There are two aspects to injury caused by TBI - the damage caused by the initial impact or insult, and that which may subsequently evolve over the ensuing hours and days referred to as secondary insults. Secondary insults can be mediated through physiologic events which decrease supply of oxygen and energy to the brain tissue or through a cascade of cytotoxic events. These events are mediated by many molecular and cellular processes.

2. The importance of mild and moderate TBI

Research in the field of TBI has long been dominated by research on severe brain injury. However, of the estimated 1.8 million people in the United States who sustain a TBI each year, over 90% will have either a "moderate" (GCS 9-12) or "mild" (GCS 13-15) injury; far outnumbering severe injuries.[2, 8, 9] Moderate TBI comprises over 10% of all TBI and mild TBI over 80%.[8] The majority of these patients will present to emergency departments (ED's) around the country for assessment and treatment.[10] The direct medical costs for treatment of TBI in the United States have been estimated at more than $4 billion annually.[11] If the costs of lost productivity that result from TBI are added to this then the overall estimated cost is closer to $56.3 billion. Moreover, mild TBI is significantly under-diagnosed and the likely societal burden is therefore even greater.[12] Mild and moderate TBI are often difficult to assess and distinguish clinically during the first hours after injury because neurological examinations are of restricted value. The distinction between mild, moderate and severe TBI is initially based on a GCS score and this may be influenced by factors such as perfusion and intoxication from drugs or alcohol, sedative medications, and other distracting injuries.

The term "mild TBI" is actually a misnomer. Individuals who incur a TBI and have an initial GCS score of 13-15 are acutely at risk for intracranial bleeding and diffuse axonal injury.[13] Additionally, a significant proportion is at risk for impairment of physical, cognitive, and psychosocial functioning.[14-18] Although some patients with mild TBI may be admitted to the hospital overnight, the vast majority are treated and released from emergency departments with basic discharge instructions. Most receive little guidance with respect to follow-up care. This group of TBI patients represents the greatest challenges to accurate diagnosis and outcome prediction. With perhaps no overt signs of acute head injury and a lack of clinical tools to detect the subtle cognitive deficits the patient is considered "unimpaired" and is discharged home and typically left to deal with persisting neurocognitive deficits on their own.[19] Accordingly, a significant minority has incomplete recoveries and has outcomes disproportionately worse than would have been predicted by the objective facts of the injury.[19, 20] The lack of clinical tools to detect the deficits that affect daily function leads to a state of frustration for patients and families that arises out of a failure to understand the nature of the difficulties encountered daily. Treatment protocols for mild TBI have only slowly begun to emerge and are still experimental. The injury is often seen as "not severe" and subsequently therapies have not been aggressively sought for these individuals. Unfortunately, despite the better understanding of the anatomical, cellular and molecular mechanisms of TBI, these advances have not yet yielded significant improvements in treatment. Among the potential barriers to treatment are the heterogeneity of traumatic brain injury, difficulty with stratification of patients by injury severity and lack of early markers of injury.[21-24]

3. The problem with current assessment of TBI

Prognostic tools for risk stratification of TBI patients are limited in the early stages of injury in the emergency setting for all severities of TBI. Unlike other organ-based diseases where rapid diagnosis employing biomarkers from blood tests are clinically essential to guide diagnosis and treatment, such as for myocardial ischemia or kidney and liver dysfunction, there are no rapid, definitive diagnostic tests for traumatic brain injury. Moreover, the reference standard for TBI is also more difficult to define than say cardiac ischemia. There is no early gold standard for stratification of patients by severity. Currently, diagnosis of TBI depends on a variety of measures including neurological examination and neuroimaging. Neuroimaging techniques such as CT scanning and MRI are used to provide objective information. However, CT scanning has low sensitivity to diffuse brain damage and confers exposure to radiation. MRI can provide information on the extent of diffuse injuries but its widespread application is restricted by cost, the limited availability of MRI in many centers, and the difficulty of performing it in physiologically unstable patients. Additionally, its role in the clinical management of TBI patients acutely has not been established.[25, 26]

While increasing CT use has reduced hospital admissions,[27] it has also raised concern over unnecessary exposure to ionizing radiation.[28-32] Although the calculation of projected cancer risk is still controversial, some studies suggest that CT scans of the head may be among the largest contributors to radiation exposure due to the frequency with which they are performed.[33] There is significant consensus that efforts should be made to prevent unnecessary radiation exposure while maintaining quality of care.[28, 29, 34, 35]

4. Challenges to the clinical application of biomarkers

There have been a number of cerebrospinal fluid (CSF) and serum biomarkers evaluated in TBI animal models and in humans. However, many of these candidate biomarkers have failed to exhibit adequate sensitivity and specificity for brain injury, and they have added minimal diagnostic and prognostic information. As a result many are skeptical about the potential of neurotrauma biomarkers to influence future clinical management and clinical trials. This reservation is based on a handful of biomarkers studied using compromised research designs and without the advantage of advancements made in the field of proteomics. Even though the application of proteomics in brain injury is still in its infancy[36, 37], neuroproteomics is penetrating the field of neurotrauma and brings great potential for improvements in research and patient care. As this technology advances and integrates other technologies such as bioinformatics and neuroimaging, characterization of CNS proteins will occur quickly and many more potential markers will be validated in a shorter timeframe.

Another important challenge in validating biomarkers for TBI will be that traditional outcome measures used to measure injury severity are, in and of themselves, limited. This is true for all severities of injury, and is particularly germane to the less severe injuries where neuroimaging, such as computed tomography (CT), may not demonstrate any obvious pathology. Traditionally, TBI has been separated into three very broad categories: mild, moderate and severe. Unfortunately, this classification scheme fails to capture the spectrum of TBI and the different types of injuries associated with it. The difficulty in classifying injury severity is one which has made clinical trials in the field of TBI challenging. Therapeutic clinical trials for TBI have met with negative results at a cost of over $200 million.[38, 39] These failures have been attributed to a multitude of factors but particularly to the heterogeneity of TBI which makes classification of the different injury types problematic. This heterogeneity, together with the lack of early definitive measures of severity opens the door for using biomarkers as early prognostic indicators. Potentially, biomarkers could provide early outcome measure for clinical trial obtainable much more reliably and economically than conventional neurological assessments, thereby significantly reducing the risks and costs of human clinical trials.

The release of substances and potential biomarkers after an injury is not a static process. Understanding the biokinetic properties of a biomarker will be essential to understanding the release pattern and "optimum" time for measurement. Clinicians and researchers will have to keep in mind that different injury types (for instance, mass lesions versus diffuse injuries) may demonstrate different kinetic parameters and, thus, may produce different quantities of a marker with different peaks and rates of decay. Moreover, secondary insults may also contribute to secondary elevations in a marker, altering its sensitivity and specificity at different time-points.

For markers measured in serum, the level of a biomarker may also reflect the extent of blood brain barrier disruption. Furthermore, extracranial sources of the biomarker may limit its specificity by creating false positives, thus compromising its clinical utility. For instance, the release of a potential CNS marker into the serum from other traumatized tissues or organs would hamper its clinical value in the setting of polytrauma. Another possible situation in which false positive marker values could occur is in the presence of a pre-existing disease state that may alter the metabolism or clearance of the marker, as with kidney or liver disease. Such factors need to be carefully assessed in rigorously designed clinical studies. Future studies should also ensure that adequate control groups are selected for comparison.

Ongoing studies by our group are currently being conducted to more fully elucidate the relationships between novel biomarkers and severity of injury and clinical outcomes in all severities of TBI patients. Before clinical application neurochemical markers will have to be rigorously evaluated and the above mentioned challenges taken into consideration.

5. Proteomic techniques in neurobiomarker discovery

Two dimensional gel electrophoresis (2D GE) and mass spectrometry has classically been the gold standard for protein identification. It is an excellent technique for discovering a multitude of proteins and is widely used. However, it requires specialized training and technical expertise. Some of the disadvantages include sample to sample variation, the inability to detect certain classes or sizes of proteins, and the need for many samples and controls.[40]

There are also non–gel-based mass spectrometry methods for identifying proteins that use high-resolution chromatography to separate complex mixtures of proteins prior to mass spectrometry. Typically the technique uses capillary chromatography for sensitivity and high-resolution mass spectrometry for identification of proteins. There is no need for two-dimensional gel electrophoresis for initial separation and it can analyze a wider range of proteins. However, the technique requires significant expertise and the cost of the materials and equipment to run this technique is much higher.[40]

Newer proteomic techniques are employing antibody-based methods such as high throughput immunoblotting and antibody panels and/or arrays (ELISA's). Antibodies are significantly more specific and selective than traditional techniques and allow the detection of proteins amid complex high-protein content biofluids such as serum or plasma.[41] Methods of amplifying the signal are under development so that only very small samples will be required for analysis. The drawback of this technique is its reliance on the sensitivity and specificity of the antibodies, and the inability to identify a wide range of proteins because the protein of interest must be pre-selected.

Examples of these techniques will be taken from studies conducted by our group. In two studies published in the Journal of Neurotrauma in 2007 by Pineda et al.[42] and in 2009 by

Brophy et al.[43] an immunoblotting technique employing sodium dodecyl sulfate-polyacrylamide gel electrophoresis (SDS-PAGE) was used to measure alpha-spectrin. Quantitative evaluation of intact αII-spectrin and its breakdown products (SBDP150, SBDP145 and SBDP120) was performed via computer-assisted densitometric scanning.
An example of the ELISA technique is taken from a study published in Critical Care Medicine in 2010 by Papa et al.[44] that measured Ubiquitin C-terminal hydrolase. In this study samples were measured using a standard UCH-L1 sandwich ELISA where reaction wells were coated with capture antibody and detection antibody was added to wells. The wells were developed with substrate solution and read with a spectrophotometer.

6. Status of biomarker research

Although there are a number of biochemical markers that have been investigated in TBI, our discussion will include the most current and widely studied ones. The most extensively studied among these are glial protein S-100 beta(β) [45-55], neuron-specific enolase (NSE)[56-63], and myelin basic protein (MBP)[41, 59, 64-66] Although some of these published studies suggest that these biomarkers correlate with degree of injury; conflicting results exist.[67-75]
S100β is the major low affinity calcium binding protein in astrocytes [76] and it is considered a marker of astrocyte injury or death. It can also be found in non-neural cells such as adipocytes, chondrocytes, and melanoma cells.[77] Elevated serum levels have been associated with increased incidence of post concussive syndrome and impaired cognition.[78, 79] Other studies have reported that serum levels of S-100β are associated with MRI abnormalities and with neuropsychological examination disturbances after mild TBI.[80, 81] A number of studies have found significant correlations between elevated serum levels of S-100β and CT abnormalities.[82-84] It has been suggested that adding the measurement of S-100B concentration to clinical decision tools for mild TBI patients could potentially reduce the number of CT scans by 30%.[84] Other investigators have failed to detect associations between S-100β with CT abnormalities.[67, 85, 86 87] The vast majority of these clinical studies have employed ELISA to measure levels of S100B. Although S-100β continues to be actively investigated and remains promising as an adjunctive marker, its utility as a biochemical diagnostic remains controversial. Some studies have observed high serum S-100β levels in trauma patients without head injuries suggesting that it lacks CNS specificity and is released from peripheral tissues.[88-90]
Neuron specific enolase is one of the five isozymes of the gycolytic enzyme enolase found in central and peripheral neurons and it has been shown be elevated following cell injury.[91] It has a molecular weight of 78 kDa and a biological half-life of 48 hours.[92] This protein is passively released into the extracellular space only under pathological conditions during cell destruction. Several reports on serum NSE measurements of mild TBI have been published.[59, 62, 91, 93] Most of these studies employed an enzyme immunoassay for NSE detection. Many of these studies either contained inadequate control groups or concluded that serum NSE had limited utility as a marker of neuronal damage. Early levels of NSE and MBP concentrations have been correlated with outcome in children, particularly those under 4 years of age.[64, 65, 94, 95] A limitation of NSE is the occurrence of false positive results in the setting of hemolysis.[96]
A supposedly cleaved form of tau, c-tau, has also been investigated as a potential biomarker of CNS injury. Tau is preferentially localized in the axon and tau lesions are apparently related to axonal disruption.[97, 98] CSF levels of c-tau were significantly elevated in TBI

patients compared to control patients and these levels correlated with clinical outcome.[99, 100] Though levels of c-tau were also elevated in plasma from patients with severe TBI, there was no correlation between plasma levels and clinical outcome.[101] A major limitation of all of these biomarkers is the lack of specificity for defining neuropathological cascades.

Alpha-II-spectrin (280 kDa) is the major structural component of the cortical membrane cytoskeleton and is particularly abundant in axons and presynaptic terminals.[102, 103] It is also a major substrate for both calpain and caspase-3 cysteine proteases.[104, 105] A hallmark feature of apoptosis and necrosis is an early cleavage of several cellular proteins by activated caspases and calpains. A signature of caspase-3 and calpain-2 activation is cleavage of several common proteins such as cytoskeletal αII-spectrin.[106] In a rat model, mean levels of both ipsilateral cortex (IC) and cerebral spinal fluid (CSF) spectrin breakdown products (SBDP) at 2, 6, and 24 h after two levels of controlled cortical impact (1.0 mm and 1.6 mm of cortical deformation) were significantly elevated by injury using immunoblotting.[107] Using the same proteomic Western blot technique, levels of spectrin breakdown products (SBDP's) have been reported in CSF from adults with severe TBI and they have shown a significant relationship with severity of injury and clinical outcome.[42, 108-113] Following a TBI the axonally enriched cytoskeletal protein α-II-spectrin is proteolyzed by calpain and caspase-3 to signature breakdown products (SBDPs). Calpain and caspase-3 mediated SBDP levels in CSF have shown to be significantly increased in TBI patients at several time points after injury, compared to control subjects. The time course of calpain mediated SBDP150 and SBDP145 (markers of necrosis) differs from that of caspase-3 mediated SBDP120 (marker of apoptosis). Average SBDP values measured early after injury correlated with severity of injury, CT scan findings and outcome at 6 months post injury.[43]

A promising candidate biomarker for TBI currently under investigation is Ubiquitin C-terminal Hydrolase-L1 (UCH-L1). UCH-L1 was previously used as a histological marker for neurons due to its high abundance and specific expression in neurons.[114] This protein is involved in the addition and removal of ubiquitin from proteins that are destined for metabolism.[115] It has an important role in the removal of excessive, oxidized or misfolded proteins during both normal and pathological conditions in neurons.[116] In initial studies, UCH-L1 was identified as a protein with a two-fold increase in abundance in the injured cortex 48 hours after controlled cortical impact in a rat model of TBI.[117] Subsequently, a UCH-L1 sandwich enzyme-linked immunosorbent assay quantitatively showed that CSF and serum UCH-L1 levels in rats were significantly elevated as early as 2 hours following both traumatic and ischemic injury.[118] Clinical studies in humans with severe TBI confirmed, using ELISA analysis, that the UCH-L1 protein was significantly elevated in human CSF[44, 119] and was detectable very early after injury and remained significantly elevated for 168 hours post-injury.[44] Further studies in severe TBI patients have revealed a very good correlation between CSF and serum levels.[120] Most recently, UCH-L1 was detected in the serum of mild and moderate TBI (MMTBI) patients within an hour of injury.[121] Serum levels of UCH-L1 discriminated MMTBI patients from uninjured and non-head injured trauma controls and were also able to distinguish mild TBI (concussion patients) from these controls. Most notable was that levels were significantly higher in those with intracranial lesions on CT than those without lesions.[121]

Glial Fibrillary Acidic Protein (GFAP) is a monomeric intermediate protein found in astroglial skeleton that was first isolated by Eng et al. in 1971.[122] GFAP is found in white and gray brain matter and is strongly upregulated during astrogliosis.[123] Current evidence indicates that serum GFAP might be a useful marker for various types of brain damage from neurodegenerative disorders[124, 125] and stroke[126] to severe traumatic brain injury.[127-131] Recently, Vos et al. described serum GFAP profile in severe and moderate TBI (GCS <12).[54] In a recent study by our group, GFAP was systematically assessed in human serum following mild and moderate TBI. We confirmed that the GFAP levels were significantly elevated in this population using ELISA analysis, including those with mild TBI. GFAP was able to discriminate TBI patients from uninjured controls. Additionally, serum levels were able to distinguish orthopedic and motor vehicle controls form TBI patients. GFAP was detectable in serum within a few hours of injury and was associated with measures of injury severity including the GCS score and CT lesions.[132, 133] The present work extends findings from studies in severe TBI to mild and moderate TBI.

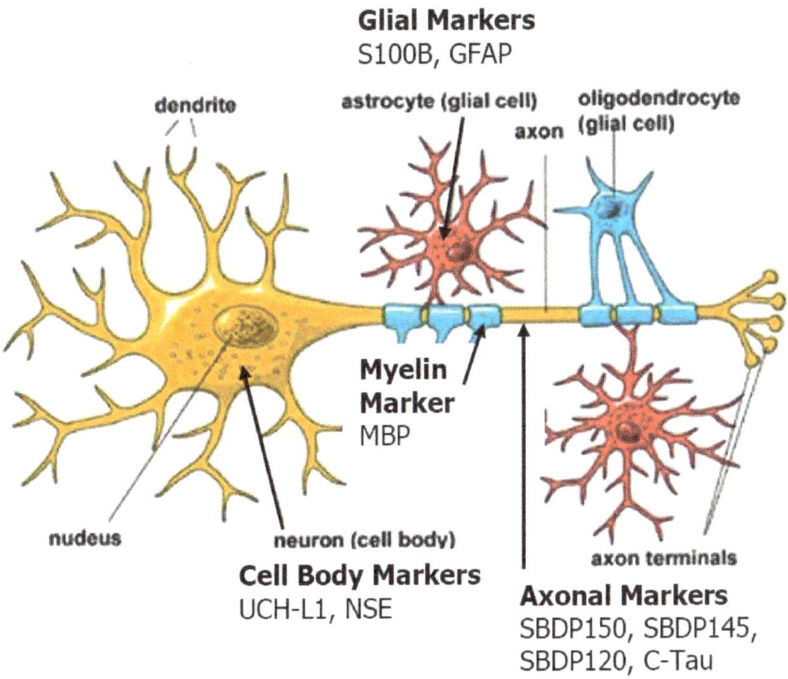

Fig. 1. The neuroanatomical locations of the above mentioned biomarkers.

7. Attributes of an ideal biomarker for TBI

Research in the field TBI biomarkers has increased exponentially over the last 20 years with most of the publications on the topic occurring in the last 10 years.[134] During the course of our work in the development of TBI biomarkers, it has become evident that there are a number of key features that a clinically useful biomarker should possess.[135] An "ideal biomarker" would: 1) demonstrate a high sensitivity and specificity for brain injury; 2) stratify patients by severity of injury; 3) have a rapid appearance in accessible biological fluid; 4) provide information on injury mechanisms; 5) have well defined biokinetc properties; 6) monitor progress of disease and response to treatment; 7) predict functional outcome; 8) be easily measured by widely available, simple techniques

Clinical researchers have developed methodological standards for developing clinical decision tools in order to ensure the validity of study results.[136, 137] As TBI biomarker research transitions from the bench to the bedside there are a number of important methodological issues that researchers will have to consider as they design their clinical protocols. Since TBI biomarkers are being designed for clinical management, the outcome or diagnosis being examined will need to be clearly defined and clinically important. In order to ensure external validity and the generalizability of the results, study patients will have to be selected without bias and represent a wide spectrum of clinical and demographic characteristics. When interpreting the data, clinical variables that potentially affect outcome will require careful consideration in the analysis. Multivariate statistical and bioinformatics models will also further improve classification of patients and help reduce systematic bias.[138] Another essential consideration will be the examination of biokinetic properties and temporal profiles of the biomarkers as well as systematic comparisons to controls.

8. The potential clinical role of biomarkers

Biochemical markers could help with clinical decision making by elucidating injury severity, injury mechanism(s), and monitoring progression of injury. Temporal profiles of changes in biomarkers could guide timing of diagnosis and treatment. Biomarkers could have a role in management decisions regarding patients at high risk of repeated injury. Accurate identification of these patients could facilitate development of guidelines for return to duty, work or sports activities and also provide opportunities for counseling of patients suffering from these deficits. Repeated mild TBI occurring within a short period (i.e. hours, days, or weeks) can be catastrophic or fatal, a phenomenon termed "second impact syndrome."[139, 140] Acute CT or MRI abnormalities are not usually found after these injuries, but levels of some neurotransmitters remain elevated, and a hypermetabolic state may persist in the brain for several days after the initial injury.[141] During this time the brain appears to be particularly vulnerable to additional TBI, which may result in severe sequelae, including greatly increased cerebral edema and even death.[139, 140]

Biomarkers could serve as prognostic indicators by providing information for patients and their families about the expected course of recovery. It opens the door to the initiation of early therapies. Identifying at-risk patients with less apparent TBI or differentiating injury pathology in those with more severe intracranial processes would be tremendously valuable in the management of these patients. For example, in a patient with a normal CT scan or MRI, a biomarker that could predict worsening neurological status or long-term disability would have great clinical utility.

There have been a large number of clinical trials studying potential therapies for traumatic brain injury (TBI) that have resulted in negative findings. Biomarkers measurable in blood would have important applications in clinical research of these injuries. Biomarkers could provide clinical trial outcome measures that are cost-effective and more readily available than conventional neurological assessments, thereby significantly reducing the risks and costs of human clinical trials. Biomarkers that represent highly sensitive and specific indicators of disease pathways have been used as substitutes for outcomes in clinical trials when evidence indicates that they predict clinical risk or benefit.

Lack of quickly accessible pathophysiologic information during the post-injury course has made pharmacologic intervention problematic. Biomarkers could provide more timely information on disease progression and the effects of interventions such as drugs and surgery. Biomarker measurements could potentially relate the effects of interventions on molecular and cellular pathways to clinical responses. In doing so, biomarkers would provide an avenue for researchers and clinicians to gain a mechanistic understanding of the differences in clinical response that may be influenced by uncontrolled variables.

Intoxicated, unconscious, sedated, or polytraumatized patients suspected of having a TBI pose a particular challenge to emergency and trauma physicians. Biomarkers could expedite the evaluation of such patients by providing information on the degree of brain injury prior to neuroimaging. Biomarkers in this setting could also help determine the need for early neurosurgical consultation or transfer to facilities with neurosurgical capabilities.

There are potential military applications as well. Serum biomarkers could help diagnose and/or triage brain injured military servicemen and women. TBI is a leading cause of combat casualty with an estimated 15-20% of all injuries sustained in 20th century conflicts being to the head.[142-144] America's armed forces are sustaining attacks by rocket-propelled grenades, improvised explosive devices, and land mines almost daily in the recent conflicts in Iraq and Afghanistan.[145] It has been suggested that over 50% of injuries sustained in combat are the result of such explosive munitions including bombs, grenades, land mines, missiles, and mortar/artillery shells. Neuroimaging techniques to diagnose brain injury acutely and other monitoring tools that assess secondary insults are not immediately available in combat zones and such casualties have to be evacuated. Triage and management of brain injured soldiers could be significantly improved if first responders had a quick and simple means of objectively assessing severity of brain injury and of monitoring secondary insults.

There is a unique opportunity to use the insight offered by biochemical markers to shed light on the complexities of the injury process. Accordingly, certain markers could be used as indicators of damage to a particular cell type or cellular process or may be indicative of a particular type of injury. Neuroanatomically, that could include evidence of, say, primary axonal damage versus glial damage. With such heterogeneity the solution may not lie with a single biomarker but more with a complementary panel of markers that may prove useful in distinguishing different pathoanatomic processes of injury.

9. Conclusion

The exploration and validation of biomarkers for TBI using advances in proteomics, neuroimaging, genomics, and bioinformatics must continue. Biomarkers of TBI measured through a simple blood test have the potential to significantly improve the management of TBI patients by providing timely information on the pathophysiology of injury; improving stratification of patients by injury severity; monitoring of secondary insults and injury progression; monitoring response to treatment; and predicting functional outcome. Biomarkers could provide major opportunities for the conduct of clinical research including confirmation of injury mechanism(s) and drug target identification. Ultimately the goal is improve outcome in patients suffering from these injuries.

10. References

[1] Hyder AA, Wunderlich CA, Puvanachandra P, Gururaj G, Kobusingye OC. The impact of traumatic brain injuries: a global perspective. *NeuroRehabilitation.* 2007;22(5):341-353.

[2] Consensus conference. Rehabilitation of persons with traumatic brain injury. NIH Consensus Development Panel on Rehabilitation of Persons With Traumatic Brain Injury. *Jama.* 1999;282(10):974-983.
[3] Faul M, Xu L, Wald MM, Coronado VG. Traumatic brain injury in the United States: emergency department visits, hospitalizations, and deaths. In: Services USDoHaH, ed. *Centers for Disease Control and Prevention, National Center for Injury Prevention and Control.* March 2010 ed. Atlanta, GA; 2010.
[4] Hoffman SW, Shesko K, Harrison CR. Enhanced neurorehabilitation techniques in the DVBIC Assisted Living Pilot Project. *NeuroRehabilitation.*26(3):257-269.
[5] Tagliaferri F, Compagnone C, Korsic M, Servadei F, Kraus J. A systematic review of brain injury epidemiology in Europe. *Acta Neurochir (Wien).* Mar 2006;148(3):255-268; discussion 268.
[6] Graham DI, Adams JH, Nicoll JA, Maxwell WL, Gennarelli TA. The nature, distribution and causes of traumatic brain injury. *Brain Pathol.* Oct 1995;5(4):397-406.
[7] Graham DI, Horsburgh K, Nicoll JA, Teasdale GM. Apolipoprotein E and the response of the brain to injury. *Acta Neurochir Suppl.* 1999;73:89-92.
[8] Yealy DM, Hogan DE. Imaging after head trauma. Who needs what? *Emerg Med Clin North Am.* Nov 1991;9(4):707-717.
[9] Vollmer DG, Dacey RG, Jr. The management of mild and moderate head injuries. *Neurosurg Clin N Am.* Apr 1991;2(2):437-455.
[10] Langlois JA, Rutland-Brown W, Thomas KE. *Traumatic Brain Injury in the United States: Emergency Department Visits, Hospitalizations, and Deaths.* Atlanta: Division of Injury and Disability Outcomes and Programs. National Center for Injury Prevention and Control. CDC; October 2004.
[11] TBI State Demonstration Grants. *J Head Trauma Rehabil.* Feb 2000;15(1):750-760.
[12] Thurman DJ. Epidemiology and Economics of Head Trauma. *Head Trauma: Basic Preclinical and Clinical Directions.* New York: Wiley-Liss; 2001:327-347.
[13] Stein SC, Fabbri A, Servadei F, Glick HA. A critical comparison of clinical decision instruments for computed tomographic scanning in mild closed traumatic brain injury in adolescents and adults. *Ann Emerg Med.* Feb 2009;53(2):180-188.
[14] Millis SR, Rosenthal M, Novack TA, et al. Long-term neuropsychological outcome after traumatic brain injury. *J Head Trauma Rehabil.* Aug 2001;16(4):343-355.
[15] Alves W, Macciocchi S, Barth JT. Postconcussive Symptoms After Uncomplicated Mild Head Injury. *J Head Trauma Rehabil.* 1993 1993;8(3):48-59.
[16] Rimel RW, Giordani B, Barth JT, Boll TJ, Jane JA. Disability caused by minor head injury. *Neurosurgery.* Sep 1981;9(3):221-228.
[17] Alexander MP. Mild traumatic brain injury: pathophysiology, natural history, and clinical management. *Neurology.* 1995;45(7):1253-1260.
[18] Barth JT, Macciocchi SN, Giordani B, Rimel R, Jane JA, Boll TJ. Neuropsychological sequelae of minor head injury. *Neurosurgery.* Nov 1983;13(5):529-533.
[19] Kennedy RE, Livingston L, Marwitz JH, Gueck S, Kreutzer JS, Sander AM. Complicated mild traumatic brain injury on the inpatient rehabilitation unit: a multicenter analysis. *J Head Trauma Rehabil.* May-Jun 2006;21(3):260-271.
[20] Kennedy JE, Lumpkin RJ, Grissom JR. A survey of mild traumatic brain injury treatment in the emergency room and primary care medical clinics. *Mil Med.* Jun 2006;171(6):516-521.

[21] Narayan RK, Michel ME, Ansell B, et al. Clinical trials in head injury. *J Neurotrauma.* May 2002;19(5):503-557.
[22] Saatman KE, Duhaime AC, Bullock R, Maas AI, Valadka A, Manley GT. Classification of traumatic brain injury for targeted therapies. *J Neurotrauma.* Jul 2008;25(7):719-738.
[23] Doppenberg EM, Choi SC, Bullock R. Clinical trials in traumatic brain injury: lessons for the future. *J Neurosurg Anesthesiol.* Jan 2004;16(1):87-94.
[24] Maas AI, Hukkelhoven CW, Marshall LF, Steyerberg EW. Prediction of outcome in traumatic brain injury with computed tomographic characteristics: a comparison between the computed tomographic classification and combinations of computed tomographic predictors. *Neurosurgery.* Dec 2005;57(6):1173-1182; discussion 1173-1182.
[25] Kesler ea. APECT, MR and quantitative MR imaging: correlates with neuropsycholgical. *Brain Injury.* 2000;14:851-857.
[26] Jagoda AS, Bazarian JJ, Bruns JJ, Jr., et al. Clinical policy: neuroimaging and decisionmaking in adult mild traumatic brain injury in the acute setting. *Ann Emerg Med.* Dec 2008;52(6):714-748.
[27] Wardlaw JM, Keir SL, Seymour J, et al. What is the best imaging strategy for acute stroke? *Health Technol Assess.* Jan 2004;8(1):iii, ix-x, 1-180.
[28] Brenner DJ, Hall EJ. Computed tomography--an increasing source of radiation exposure. *N Engl J Med.* Nov 29 2007;357(22):2277-2284.
[29] Fayngersh V, Passero M. Estimating radiation risk from computed tomography scanning. *Lung.* May-Jun 2009;187(3):143-148.
[30] Hall EJ, Brenner DJ. Cancer risks from diagnostic radiology. *Br J Radiol.* May 2008;81(965):362-378.
[31] Heilbrun ME, Chew FS, Tansavatdi KR, Tooze JA. The role of negative CT of the abdomen and pelvis in the decision to admit adults from the emergency department after blunt trauma. *J Am Coll Radiol.* Nov 2005;2(11):889-895.
[32] Livingston DH, Loder PA, Koziol J, Hunt CD. The use of CT scanning to triage patients requiring admission following minimal head injury. *J Trauma.* Apr 1991;31(4):483-487; discussion 487-489.
[33] Berrington de Gonzalez A, Mahesh M, Kim KP, et al. Projected cancer risks from computed tomographic scans performed in the United States in 2007. *Arch Intern Med.* Dec 14 2009;169(22):2071-2077.
[34] Schwartz DT. Counter-Point: Are We Really Ordering Too Many CT Scans? *West J Emerg Med.* May 2008;9(2):120-122.
[35] Stiell IG, Wells GA, Vandemheen K, et al. Variation in ED use of computed tomography for patients with minor head injury. *Ann Emerg Med.* Jul 1997;30(1):14-22.
[36] Choudhary J, Grant SG. Proteomics in postgenomic neuroscience: the end of the beginning. *Nat Neurosci.* May 2004;7(5):440-445.
[37] Collins MO, Yu L, Coba MP, et al. Proteomic analysis of in vivo phosphorylated synaptic proteins. *J Biol Chem.* Feb 18 2005;280(7):5972-5982.
[38] Choi SC, Bullock R. Design and statistical issues in multicenter trials of severe head injury. *Neurological Research.* 2001;Mar-Apr(23(2-3)):190-192.
[39] Doppenberg EM, Choi SC, Bullock R. Clinical trials in traumatic brain injury. What can we learn from previous studies? *Ann N Y Acad Sci.* Oct 15 1997;825:305-322.

[40] Denslow N, Michel ME, Temple MD, Hsu CY, Saatman K, Hayes RL. Application of proteomics technology to the field of neurotrauma. *J Neurotrauma.* May 2003;20(5):401-407.
[41] Wang KK, Ottens AK, Liu MC, et al. Proteomic identification of biomarkers of traumatic brain injury. *Expert Rev Proteomics.* Aug 2005;2(4):603-614.
[42] Pineda JA, Lewis SB, Valadka AB, et al. Clinical significance of alphaII-spectrin breakdown products in cerebrospinal fluid after severe traumatic brain injury. *J Neurotrauma.* Feb 2007;24(2):354-366.
[43] Brophy GM, Pineda JA, Papa L, et al. alphaII-Spectrin breakdown product cerebrospinal fluid exposure metrics suggest differences in cellular injury mechanisms after severe traumatic brain injury. *J Neurotrauma.* Apr 2009;26(4):471-479.
[44] Papa L, Akinyi L, Liu MC, et al. Ubiquitin C-terminal hydrolase is a novel biomarker in humans for severe traumatic brain injury. *Crit Care Med.* Jan 2010;38(1):138-144.
[45] MisslerU. S-100 protein and neuron-specific enolase concentrations in blood as indicators of infarction volume and prognosis in acute ischemic stroke. *Stroke.* 1997;28:1956-1960.
[46] Ytrebo LM NG, Korvald C, et al. Renal elimination of protein S-100beta in picgs with acute encephalopathy. *Scand J Clin Lab Invest.* 2001;61:217-225.
[47] Jonsson H JP, Hoglund P, Alling C, Blomquist S. The elimination of S-100b and renal function after cardiac surgery. *J Cardiothorac Vasc Aneth.* 2000;14:698-701.
[48] Usui A KK, Abe T, Murase M, Tanaka M, Takeuchi E. S-100ao protein in blood and urine during open-heart surgery. *Clin Chem.* 1989;35:1942-1944.
[49] Raabe A, Grolms C, Seifert V. Serum markers of brain damage and outcome prediction in patients after severe head injury. *Br J Neurosurg.* 1999;13(1):56-59.
[50] Haimoto HH, S; Kato, K. Differential distribution of immunoreactive S100-a and S100-b proteins in normal nonnervous human tissues. *Lab Invest.* 1987;57:489-498.
[51] Woertgen C, Rothoerl RD, Holzschuh M, Metz C, Brawanski A. Comparison of serial S-100 and NSE serum measurements after severe head injury. *Acta Neurochir (Wien).* 1997;139(12):1161-1164; discussion 1165.
[52] Romner B, Ingebrigtsen T, Kongstad P, Borgesen SE. Traumatic brain damage: serum S-100 protein measurements related to neuroradiological findings. *J Neurotrauma.* Aug 2000;17(8):641-647.
[53] Korfias S, Stranjalis G, Boviatsis E, et al. Serum S-100B protein monitoring in patients with severe traumatic brain injury. *Intensive Care Med.* Feb 2007;33(2):255-260.
[54] Vos PE, Jacobs B, Andriessen TM, et al. GFAP and S100B are biomarkers of traumatic brain injury: an observational cohort study. *Neurology.* Nov 16 2010;75(20):1786-1793.
[55] Berger RP, Pierce MC, Wisniewski SR, Adelson PD, Kochanek PM. Serum S100B concentrations are increased after closed head injury in children: a preliminary study. *J Neurotrauma.* Nov 2002;19(11):1405-1409.
[56] BW M. A soluble protein characteristic of the nervous system. *Biochem Biophys Res Commun.* 1965;19:739-744.
[57] Donato R. Functional roles of S100 proteins, calcium-binding proteins of the EF-hand type. *Biochim Biophys Acta.* 1999;1450:191-231.
[58] Cooper E. Neuron-specific enolase. *Int J Biol Markers.* 1994(4):205-210.

[59] Yamazaki Y, Yada K, Morii S, Kitahara T, Ohwada T. Diagnostic significance of serum neuron-specific enolase and myelin basic protein assay in patients with acute head injury. *Surg Neurol.* Mar 1995;43(3):267-270; discussion 270-261.
[60] de Kruijk JR, Leffers P, Menheere PP, Meerhoff S, Twijnstra A. S-100B and neuron-specific enolase in serum of mild traumatic brain injury patients. A comparison with health controls. *Acta Neurol Scand.* Mar 2001;103(3):175-179.
[61] Raabe A, Grolms C, Seifert V. Serum markers of brain damage and outcome prediction in patients after severe head injury. *Br J Neurosurg.* Feb 1999;13(1):56-59.
[62] Ross SA, Cunningham RT, Johnston CF, Rowlands BJ. Neuron-specific enolase as an aid to outcome prediction in head injury. *Br J Neurosurg.* Oct 1996;10(5):471-476.
[63] Naeimi ZS, Weinhofer A, Sarahrudi K, Heinz T, Vecsei V. Predictive value of S-100B protein and neuron specific-enolase as markers of traumatic brain damage in clinical use. *Brain Inj.* May 2006;20(5):463-468.
[64] Berger RP, Adelson PD, Pierce MC, Dulani T, Cassidy LD, Kochanek PM. Serum neuron-specific enolase, S100B, and myelin basic protein concentrations after inflicted and noninflicted traumatic brain injury in children. *J Neurosurg.* Jul 2005;103(1 Suppl):61-68.
[65] Berger RP, Beers SR, Richichi R, Wiesman D, Adelson PD. Serum biomarker concentrations and outcome after pediatric traumatic brain injury. *J Neurotrauma.* Dec 2007;24(12):1793-1801.
[66] Beers SR, Berger RP, Adelson PD. Neurocognitive outcome and serum biomarkers in inflicted versus non-inflicted traumatic brain injury in young children. *J Neurotrauma.* Jan 2007;24(1):97-105.
[67] Piazza O, Storti MP, Cotena S, et al. S100B is not a reliable prognostic index in paediatric TBI. *Pediatr Neurosurg.* 2007;43(4):258-264.
[68] Martens P. Serum neuron-specific enolase as a prognostic marker for irreversible brain damage in comatose cardiac arrest surviviors. *Acad Emerg Med.* 1996;3:126-131.
[69] Rainey T, Lesko M, Sacho R, Lecky F, Childs C. Predicting outcome after severe traumatic brain injury using the serum S100B biomarker: results using a single (24h) time-point. *Resuscitation.* Mar 2009;80(3):341-345.
[70] Bazarian JJ, Zemlan FP, Mookerjee S, Stigbrand T. Serum S-100B and cleaved-tau are poor predictors of long-term outcome after mild traumatic brain injury. *Brain Inj.* Jun 2006;20(7):759-765.
[71] Watt SE, Shores EA, Baguley IJ, Dorsch N, Fearnside MR. Protein S-100 and neuropsychological functioning following severe traumatic brain injury. *Brain Inj.* Sep 2006;20(10):1007-1017.
[72] Morochovic R, Racz O, Kitka M, et al. Serum S100B protein in early management of patients after mild traumatic brain injury. *Eur J Neurol.* Oct 2009;16(10):1112-1117.
[73] Dirnagl U CI, and Moskowitz MA. Pathology of ischaemic stroke: an integrated view. *TINS.* 1999;22(9):391-397.
[74] Laskowitz ea. Serum Markers of Cerebral Ischemia. *Journal of Stroke and Cerebrovascular Diseases.* 1998;7(4 (July-August)):234-241.
[75] Roine ea. Neurological outcome after out-of-hospital cardiac arrest. Prediction by cerebrospinal fluid enzyme analysis. *Arch Neurol.* 1989;46:753-756.

[76] Xiong H, Liang WL, Wu XR. [Pathophysiological alterations in cultured astrocytes exposed to hypoxia/reoxygenation]. *Sheng Li Ke Xue Jin Zhan.* Jul 2000;31(3):217-221.

[77] Zimmer DB, Cornwall EH, Landar A, Song W. The S100 protein family: history, function, and expression. *Brain Res Bull.* 1995;37(4):417-429.

[78] Ingebrigtsen T, Romner B. Management of minor head injuries in hospitals in Norway. *Acta Neurol Scand.* Jan 1997;95(1):51-55.

[79] Waterloo K, Ingebrigtsen T, Romner B. Neuropsychological function in patients with increased serum levels of protein S-100 after minor head injury. *Acta Neurochir (Wien).* 1997;139(1):26-31; discussion 31-22.

[80] Ingebrigtsen T, Romner B. Serial S-100 protein serum measurements related to early magnetic resonance imaging after minor head injury. Case report. *J Neurosurg.* Nov 1996;85(5):945-948.

[81] Ingebrigtsen T, Waterloo K, Jacobsen EA, Langbakk B, Romner B. Traumatic brain damage in minor head injury: relation of serum S-100 protein measurements to magnetic resonance imaging and neurobehavioral outcome. *Neurosurgery.* Sep 1999;45(3):468-475; discussion 475-466.

[82] Ingebrigtsen T, Romner B, Marup-Jensen S, et al. The clinical value of serum S-100 protein measurements in minor head injury: a Scandinavian multicentre study. *Brain Inj.* Dec 2000;14(12):1047-1055.

[83] Muller K, Townend W, Biasca N, et al. S100B serum level predicts computed tomography findings after minor head injury. *J Trauma.* Jun 2007;62(6):1452-1456.

[84] Biberthaler P, Linsenmeier U, Pfeifer KJ, et al. Serum S-100B concentration provides additional information fot the indication of computed tomography in patients after minor head injury: a prospective multicenter study. *Shock.* May 2006;25(5):446-453.

[85] Phillips JP, Jones HM, Hitchcock R, Adama N, Thompson RJ. Radioimmunoassay of serum creatine kinase BB as index of brain damage after head injury. *Br Med J.* Sep 20 1980;281(6243):777-779.

[86] Rothoerl RD, Woertgen C, Holzschuh M, Metz C, Brawanski A. S-100 serum levels after minor and major head injury. *J Trauma.* Oct 1998;45(4):765-767.

[87] Bechtel K, Frasure S, Marshall C, Dziura J, Simpson C. Relationship of serum S100B levels and intracranial injury in children with closed head trauma. *Pediatrics.* Oct 2009;124(4):e697-704.

[88] Rothoerl RD, Woertgen C. High serum S100B levels for trauma patients without head injuries. *Neurosurgery.* Dec 2001;49(6):1490-1491; author reply 1492-1493.

[89] Romner B, Ingebrigtsen T. High serum S100B levels for trauma patients without head injuries. *Neurosurgery.* Dec 2001;49(6):1490; author reply 1492-1493.

[90] Anderson RE, Hansson LO, Nilsson O, Dijlai-Merzoug R, Settergen G. High serum S100B levels for trauma patients without head injuries. *Neurosurgery.* 2001;49(5):1272-1273.

[91] Skogseid IM, Nordby HK, Urdal P, Paus E, Lilleaas F. Increased serum creatine kinase BB and neuron specific enolase following head injury indicates brain damage. *Acta Neurochir (Wien).* 1992;115(3-4):106-111.

[92] Schmechel D, Marangos PJ, Brightman M. Neurone-specific enolase is a molecular marker for peripheral and central neuroendocrine cells. *Nature.* Dec 21-28 1978;276(5690):834-836.

[93] Ergun R, Bostanci U, Akdemir G, et al. Prognostic value of serum neuron-specific enolase levels after head injury. *Neurol Res.* Jul 1998;20(5):418-420.
[94] Varma S, Janesko KL, Wisniewski SR, et al. F2-isoprostane and neuron-specific enolase in cerebrospinal fluid after severe traumatic brain injury in infants and children. *J Neurotrauma.* Aug 2003;20(8):781-786.
[95] Bandyopadhyay S, Hennes H, Gorelick MH, Wells RG, Walsh-Kelly CM. Serum neuron-specific enolase as a predictor of short-term outcome in children with closed traumatic brain injury. *Acad Emerg Med.* Aug 2005;12(8):732-738.
[96] Johnsson P, Blomquist S, Luhrs C, et al. Neuron-specific enolase increases in plasma during and immediately after extracorporeal circulation. *Ann Thorac Surg.* Mar 2000;69(3):750-754.
[97] Kosik KS, Finch EA. MAP2 and tau segregate into dendritic and axonal domains after the elaboration of morphologically distinct neurites: an immunocytochemical study of cultured rat cerebrum. *J Neurosci.* Oct 1987;7(10):3142-3153.
[98] Higuchi M, Lee VM, Trojanowski JQ. Tau and axonopathy in neurodegenerative disorders. *Neuromolecular Med.* 2002;2(2):131-150.
[99] Shaw GJ, Jauch EC, Zemlan FP. Serum cleaved tau protein levels and clinical outcome in adult patients with closed head injury. *Ann Emerg Med.* Mar 2002;39(3):254-257.
[100] Zemlan FP, Jauch EC, Mulchahey JJ, et al. C-tau biomarker of neuronal damage in severe brain injured patients: association with elevated intracranial pressure and clinical outcome. *Brain Res.* Aug 23 2002;947(1):131-139.
[101] Chatfield DA, Zemlan FP, Day DJ, Menon DK. Discordant temporal patterns of S100beta and cleaved tau protein elevation after head injury: a pilot study. *Br J Neurosurg.* Oct 2002;16(5):471-476.
[102] Goodman SR, Zimmer WE, Clark MB, Zagon IS, Barker JE, Bloom ML. Brain spectrin: of mice and men. *Brain Res Bull.* 1995;36(6):593-606.
[103] Riederer BM, Zagon IS, Goodman SR. Brain spectrin(240/235) and brain spectrin(240/235E): two distinct spectrin subtypes with different locations within mammalian neural cells. *J Cell Biol.* Jun 1986;102(6):2088-2097.
[104] Wang KK, Posmantur R, Nath R, et al. Simultaneous degradation of alphaII- and betaII-spectrin by caspase 3 (CPP32) in apoptotic cells. *J Biol Chem.* Aug 28 1998;273(35):22490-22497.
[105] McGinn MJ, Kelley BJ, Akinyi L, et al. Biochemical, structural, and biomarker evidence for calpain-mediated cytoskeletal change after diffuse brain injury uncomplicated by contusion. *J Neuropathol Exp Neurol.* Mar 2009;68(3):241-249.
[106] Pike BR, Flint J, Dave JR, et al. Accumulation of calpain and caspase-3 proteolytic fragments of brain-derived alphaII-spectrin in cerebral spinal fluid after middle cerebral artery occlusion in rats. *J Cereb Blood Flow Metab.* Jan 2004;24(1):98-106.
[107] Ringger NC, O'Steen BE, Brabham JG, et al. A novel marker for traumatic brain injury: CSF alphaII-spectrin breakdown product levels. *J Neurotrauma.* Oct 2004;21(10):1443-1456.
[108] Cardali S, Maugeri R. Detection of alphaII-spectrin and breakdown products in humans after severe traumatic brain injury. *J Neurosurg Sci.* Jun 2006;50(2):25-31.
[109] Papa L, D'Avella D, Aguennouz M, et al. Detection of Alpha-II Spectrin And Breakdown Products In Humans After Severe Traumatic Brain Injury [abstract]. *Acad Emerg Med.* May 2004;11(5).

[110] Papa L, Lewis SB, Heaton S, et al. Predicting Early Outcome Using Alpha-II Spectrin Breakdown Products In Human CSF After Severe Traumatic Brain Injury [abstract]. *Acad Emerg Med.* May 2006;13(5 (Suppl 1)).

[111] Papa L, Pineda J, Wang KKW, et al. Levels of Alpha-II Spectrin Breakdown Products in Human CSF and Outcome After Severe Traumatic Brain Injury [abstract]. *Acad Emerg Med.* May 2005;12(5 (Suppl 1)).

[112] Farkas O, Polgar B, Szekeres-Bartho J, Doczi T, Povlishock JT, Buki A. Spectrin breakdown products in the cerebrospinal fluid in severe head injury--preliminary observations. *Acta Neurochir (Wien).* Aug 2005;147(8):855-861.

[113] Mondello S, Robicsek SA, Gabrielli A, et al. alphaII-spectrin breakdown products (SBDPs): diagnosis and outcome in severe traumatic brain injury patients. *J Neurotrauma.* Jul 2010;27(7):1203-1213.

[114] Jackson P, Thompson RJ. The demonstration of new human brain-specific proteins by high-resolution two-dimensional polyacrylamide gel electrophoresis. *J Neurol Sci.* Mar 1981;49(3):429-438.

[115] Tongaonkar P, Chen L, Lambertson D, Ko B, Madura K. Evidence for an interaction between ubiquitin-conjugating enzymes and the 26S proteasome. *Mol Cell Biol.* Jul 2000;20(13):4691-4698.

[116] Gong B, Leznik E. The role of ubiquitin C-terminal hydrolase L1 in neurodegenerative disorders. *Drug News Perspect.* Jul-Aug 2007;20(6):365-370.

[117] Kobeissy FH, Ottens AK, Zhang Z, et al. Novel differential neuroproteomics analysis of traumatic brain injury in rats. *Mol Cell Proteomics.* Oct 2006;5(10):1887-1898.

[118] Liu MC, Akinyi L, Scharf D, et al. Ubiquitin C-terminal hydrolase-L1 as a biomarker for ischemic and traumatic brain injury in rats. *Eur J Neurosci.* Feb 2010;31(4):722-732.

[119] Siman R, Toraskar N, Dang A, et al. A panel of neuron-enriched proteins as markers for traumatic brain injury in humans. *J Neurotrauma.* Nov 2009;26(11):1867-1877.

[120] Brophy G, Mondello S, Papa L, et al. Biokinetic Analysis of Ubiquitin C-Terminal Hydrolase-L1 (Uch-L1) in Severe Traumatic Brain Injury Patient Biofluids. *J Neurotrauma.* Feb 10.

[121] Papa L, Lewis LM, Falk JL, et al. Serum levels of UCH-L1 distinguishes mild and moderate traumatic brain injury from trauma controls and is associated with lesions on computed tomography [abstract]. *J Neurotrauma.* 2011;28(July):A1-A134.

[122] Eng LF, Vanderhaeghen JJ, Bignami A, Gerstl B. An acidic protein isolated from fibrous astrocytes. *Brain Res.* May 7 1971;28(2):351-354.

[123] Duchen LW. General pathology of neurons and neuroglia. In: Adams JA, Corsellis JAN, Duchen LW, eds. *Greenfield's Neuropathology.* London: Edward Arnold; 1984:1-52.

[124] Baydas G, Nedzvetskii VS, Tuzcu M, Yasar A, Kirichenko SV. Increase of glial fibrillary acidic protein and S-100B in hippocampus and cortex of diabetic rats: effects of vitamin E. *Eur J Pharmacol.* Feb 21 2003;462(1-3):67-71.

[125] Mouser PE, Head E, Ha KH, Rohn TT. Caspase-mediated cleavage of glial fibrillary acidic protein within degenerating astrocytes of the Alzheimer's disease brain. *Am J Pathol.* Mar 2006;168(3):936-946.

[126] Herrmann M, Vos P, Wunderlich MT, de Bruijn CH, Lamers KJ. Release of glial tissue-specific proteins after acute stroke: A comparative analysis of serum concentrations

of protein S-100B and glial fibrillary acidic protein. *Stroke.* Nov 2000;31(11):2670-2677.
[127] Missler U, Wiesmann M, Wittmann G, Magerkurth O, Hagenstrom H. Measurement of glial fibrillary acidic protein in human blood: analytical method and preliminary clinical results. *Clin Chem.* Jan 1999;45(1):138-141.
[128] Pelinka LE, Kroepfl A, Leixnering M, Buchinger W, Raabe A, Redl H. GFAP versus S100B in serum after traumatic brain injury: relationship to brain damage and outcome. *J Neurotrauma.* Nov 2004;21(11):1553-1561.
[129] Pelinka LE, Kroepfl A, Schmidhammer R, et al. Glial fibrillary acidic protein in serum after traumatic brain injury and multiple trauma. *J Trauma.* Nov 2004;57(5):1006-1012.
[130] van Geel WJ, de Reus HP, Nijzing H, Verbeek MM, Vos PE, Lamers KJ. Measurement of glial fibrillary acidic protein in blood: an analytical method. *Clin Chim Acta.* Dec 2002;326(1-2):151-154.
[131] Nylen K, Ost M, Csajbok LZ, et al. Increased serum-GFAP in patients with severe traumatic brain injury is related to outcome. *J Neurol Sci.* Jan 15 2006;240(1-2):85-91.
[132] Papa L, Akinyi L, Demery J, et al. Levels of Serum GFAP Are Associated With Severity Of Injury In Patients With Mild And Moderate Traumatic Brain Injury [abstract]. *Acad Emerg Med.* May 2008;15(5):Suppl.
[133] Papa L, Lewis LM, Falk JL, et al. Elevated Levels of Serum Glial Fibrillary Acidic Protein Breakdown Products in Mild and Moderate Traumatic Brain Injury Are Associated With Intracranial Lesions and Neurosurgical Intervention. *Ann Emerg Med.* Nov 7 2011.
[134] Kochanek PM, Berger RP, Bayr H, Wagner AK, Jenkins LW, Clark RS. Biomarkers of primary and evolving damage in traumatic and ischemic brain injury: diagnosis, prognosis, probing mechanisms, and therapeutic decision making. *Curr Opin Crit Care.* Apr 2008;14(2):135-141.
[135] Papa L, Robinson G, Oli M, et al. Use of Biomarkers for Diagnosis and Management of Traumatic Brain Injury Patients. *Expert Opinion on Medical Diagnostics.* 2008;2(8):937-945.
[136] Stiell IG, Wells GA. Methodologic standards for the development of clinical decision rules in emergency medicine. *Ann Emerg Med.* Apr 1999;33(4):437-447.
[137] Laupacis A, Sekar N, Stiell IG. Clinical prediction rules. A review and suggested modifications of methodological standards. *Jama.* Feb 12 1997;277(6):488-494.
[138] Maas AI, Marmarou A, Murray GD, Teasdale SG, Steyerberg EW. Prognosis and clinical trial design in traumatic brain injury: the IMPACT study. *J Neurotrauma.* Feb 2007;24(2):232-238.
[139] Cantu RC. Return to play guidelines after a head injury. *Clin Sports Med.* Jan 1998;17(1):45-60.
[140] Erlanger DM, Kutner KC, Barth JT, Barnes R. Neuropsychology of sports-related head injury: Dementia Pugilistica to Post Concussion Syndrome. *Clin Neuropsychol.* May 1999;13(2):193-209.
[141] McCrory PR, Berkovic SF. Second impact syndrome. *Neurology.* Mar 1998;50(3):677-683.
[142] Carey ME. Analysis of wounds incurred by U.S. Army Seventh Corps personnel treated in Corps hospitals during Operation Desert Storm, February 20 to March 10, 1991. *J Trauma.* Mar 1996;40(3 Suppl):S165-169.

[143] Sapsford W. Penetrating brain injury in military conflict: does it merit more research? *J R Army Med Corps.* Mar 2003;149(1):5-14.

[144] Okie S. Traumatic brain injury in the war zone. *N Engl J Med.* May 19 2005;352(20):2043-2047.

[145] Warden D. Blast Injury. http://www.dvbic.org/cms.php?p=Blast_injury]. Accessed April 9, 2008.

4

Circadian Proteomics and Its Unique Advantage for Discovery of Biomarkers of Heart Disease

Peter S. Podobed, Gordon M. Kirby and Tami A. Martino
Cardiovascular Research Group, Biomedical Sciences, University of Guelph, Ontario Canada

1. Introduction

Current statistics from the World Health Organization, Heart and Stroke Foundation of Canada, and the American Heart Association show that cardiovascular disease remains a leading cause of death (Heart and Stroke Foundation of Canada [HSFO], 2011; Roger et al., 2011; World Health Organization [WHO], 2011). Innovative and integrative approaches aimed at understanding and treating heart disease are needed. In this chapter we introduce a novel field of investigation called cardiovascular circadian proteomics. This approach is based on the application of high throughput proteomic technologies for discovery of molecular processes in cardiovascular tissues over the 24-hour day/night cycles. Time is a crucial but frequently overlooked factor affecting our physiology in health and disease. Circadian cardiovascular proteomics offers considerable promise to advance our understanding of heart disease (indeed disease in general), and opens new avenues for treatment of patients clinically.

2. The circadian system and its importance to cardiovascular physiology

Life on earth is subject to a 24-hour day/night (circadian or diurnal) cycle. Circadian systems have evolved to allow physiological and behavioural processes to be synchronous with this cycle - mammals are adapted to sleep either during the day or at night. Circadian clocks allow us to entrain to environmental cues and hence anticipate the differing physiologic and behavioural demands of daily events. In mammals, the system is organized as a hierarchy with multiple oscillators, as has been well reviewed (Hastings et al., 2003; Rajaratnam & Arendt, 2001; Reppert & Weaver, 2001, 2002). At the top is the hypothalamic suprachiasmatic nucleus (SCN), a brain region functioning as a master rhythmic regulator (Figure 1A). The SCN integrates light information received from the eyes to coordinate clocks throughout the body. There are additional circadian regulatory systems such as the food entrainable clock (Storch & Weitz, 2009) which we are just now beginning to understand, but are beyond the scope of this review. We observe the output of the entrained clocks as daily physiologic rhythms, many of which are crucial to the cardiovascular system, such as the cyclic variation in heart rate (HR) and blood pressure (BP). Daily HR and BP follow the diurnal variation of our autonomic nervous system and increase around wake-time to help sustain cardiac output, then decrease during the period of vagal dominance at night and in the early morning (Guo & Stein, 2003; Imai et al., 1990).

Circadian rhythms also underlie the timing of onset of adverse cardiovascular events. The incidence of myocardial infarction in humans peaks in the morning (~6:00A.M.-12:00 noon) (Cohen et al., 1997; Goldberg et al., 1990; Muller et al., 1985). A similar pattern is observed in the incidences of sudden cardiac death (Muller et al., 1989; Willich et al., 1987), ventricular tachyarrhythmia (Eksik et al., 2007; Tofler et al., 1995), and rupture of aortic aneurysms (Manfredini et al., 2004; Mehta et al., 2002; Sumiyoshi et al., 2002). Precursor risk factors such as vasomotor tone, platelet aggregability, and other factors involved in thrombosis or thrombolysis also exhibit daily rhythms (Andrews et al., 1996; Angleton et al., 1989; Decousus et al., 1985; Maemura et al., 2000; Otto et al., 2004). Recent studies link timing of onset of adverse cardiac events with a circadian clock mechanism, reviewed in (Durgan & Young, 2010; Martino & Sole, 2009; Sole & Martino, 2009).

Proteins involved in the molecular clock mechanism have been identified in the last 10+ years, and daily oscillations of this mechanism in peripheral tissues, including the myocardium, are believed to be primarily combination of self-sustaining cycling along with neural/hormonal cues from the SCN. It is illustrated in Figure 1B and described in many excellent reviews (Hastings et al., 2003; Reddy et al., 2005; Roenneberg & Merrow, 2005). Though we focus here on protein cycling, it is important to note that there are post-translational rhythms as well, such as phosphorylation. Though beyond the scope of this review the reader is directed to several examples (Akashi et al., 2002; Lowrey et al., 2000; Iitaka et al., 2005; Yin et al., 2006).

In the following sections, we describe how application of the circadian concepts, in combination with state-of-the-art proteomics, provides significant new opportunities for understanding disease physiology, for biomarker discovery, and helping patients clinically.

3. Discovery of the circadian heart proteome

Our laboratory is focussed on discovering the circadian heart proteome both in normal tissue and in disease. Initial studies are done using murine models of cardiovascular disease, and later are translated clinically. Here we describe the circadian proteome in normal C57Bl/6 mouse heart, and in our well-established murine model of heart disease termed pressure-overload induced cardiac hypertrophy by Transverse Aortic Constriction (TAC). To induce heart disease, eight week old male mice were entrained to a 12:12 light (L): dark (D) cycle and administered TAC surgery where a ligature was placed distal to the third bifurcation of aorta (Figure 2A). In sham operated animals the surgical procedure was identical, but the ligature was not tightened. (Figure 2A). For proteomic studies, heart tissues were collected one week later (as the heart remodels), at six time-points 4 hours apart over the 24-hour L:D cycle (Figure 2B). The proteome was analyzed by two-dimensional difference in gel electrophoresis (2D-DIGE) and mass spectrometry (MS). Figure 2B illustrates the experimental workflow design. The technical details are described below.

3.1 Protein purification and labelling

The cytoplasmic soluble proteome was purified from either TAC or sham left ventricular heart tissue. Cardiac tissue was immersed in 600 μl ice-cold cell lysis buffer (10 mM Tris pH 8, 8 M Urea, 4% w/v 3-[(3-cholamidopropyl)dimethylammonio]-1-propanesulfonate (CHAPS), and protease inhibitors). The lysis buffer helps to solubilize, denature, and

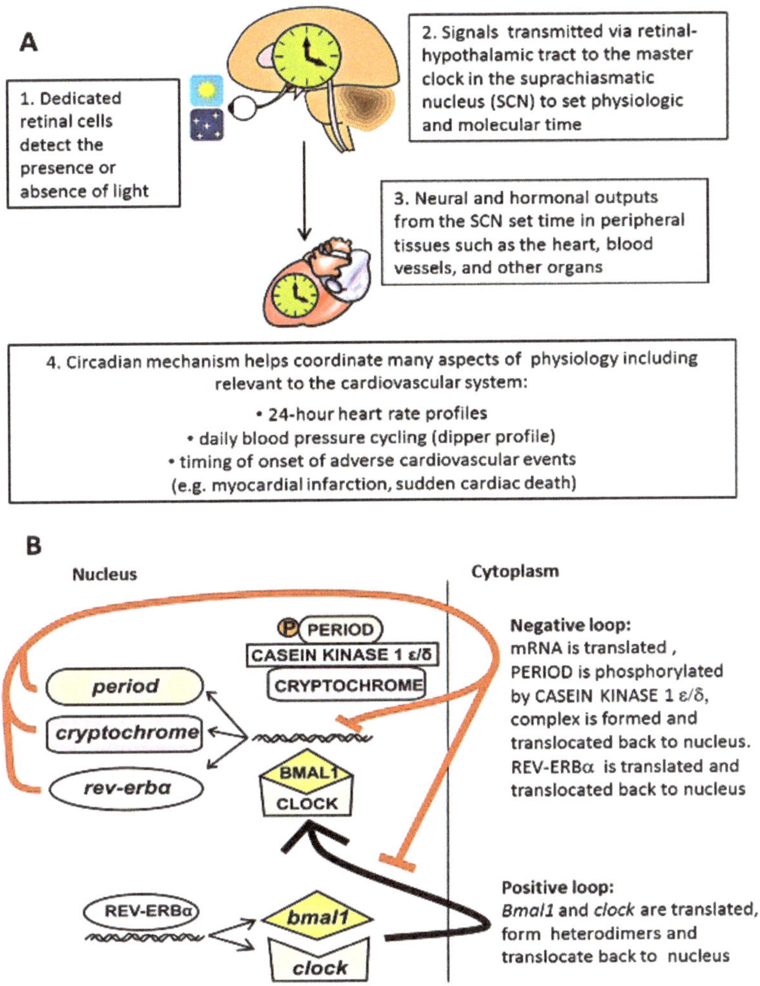

A) Light activates dedicated retinal receptors and signals the hypothalamic suprachiasmatic nucleus (SCN). The SCN is a master body clock, and orchestrates physiologic and molecular rhythms in peripheral organs including the heart. Rhythms relevant to the heart include the daily cycling of heart rate and blood pressure, also timing of onset of acute cardiac events such as myocardial infarction.
B) The molecular clock mechanism is dependent upon oscillating levels of proteins that interact via a 24-hour autoregulatory feedback. On the positive arm BMAL1 and CLOCK combine as heterodimers and bind to E-box elements upstream in the coding regions of other core clock elements, PERIOD and CRYPTOCHROME. These are phosphorylated by CASEIN KINASE 1 EPSILON (or DELTA), form heterodimers, then translocate to the nucleus. There, they bind to the same E-box elements thus negatively regulating their own expression. The positive loop also initiates production of RETINOIC ACID-RELATED ORPHAN NUCLEAR RECEPTOR ALPHA resulting in its inhibition, and completion of the 24-hour cycle. CAPITAL=Proteins; *italic*=mRNA.

Fig. 1. The Circadian System.

disaggregate proteins. Cell disruption was carried out using a Potter-Elvehjem tissue grinder. Following centrifugation the supernatant was collected and proteins were quantified by Bradford assay.

Prior to protein separation, 50 μg of each sample was labelled with CyDyes (Cy3/Cy5), and an internal control was pooled from both lysates and labelled with Cy2 (Figure 2B). To account for any bias due to preferential binding of CyDyes, a dye swap approach was also done in a separate experiment, so that the samples were alternatively labelled with the reciprocal dye. CyDyes form a covalent bond between their NHS ester reactive group and epsilon amino group of protein's lysine residues. The labelling reaction does not cause a significant change in isolectric point because lysine carries an intrinsic +1 charge at neutral or acidic pH, which is replaced by CyDye's +1 charge. CyDyes were added so that there was a stoichiometric excess of proteins and thus only 1-5% of lysines were labelled. The reaction was carried out for 30 minutes in the dark, and then quenched with 10 mM lysine.

3.2 First dimension isoelectric focussing

Proteins were separated in the first dimension by isoelectric focusing (IEF) based on our standard operating protocol (Hobson et al., 2007). In the experiment shown here (Figure 3) we used nonlinear 13 cm immobilized pH gradient (IPG) strips pH 3 - 10 (GE Healthcare). The CyDye labelled samples were combined and mixed with rehydration buffer (8 M urea, 2% w/v CHAPS, Dithiothreitol (DTT), 0.5% v/v carrier pharmalytes). Then, samples in rehydration buffer were applied at the bottom of the IPG strip holder. The strip was put on top of the sample solution and covered with paraffin oil to prevent crystallization of urea, water loss and carbon dioxide dissolving at the alkaline end of the strip. IEF was done using an Ettan IPGphore unit. The initial step was active rehydration, allowing proteins to slowly enter the strip along its whole length under the influence of a small current (30 V for 10 h). The next series of steps were 500 V step and hold for 2 h, 1000 V gradient for 1 h, 8000 V gradient for 2.5 h, 8000 V step and hold for 16000 V h, 500 V step and hold for 2 h. The result was that proteins migrated to a position in accordance with their isoelectric point.

3.3 Second dimension electrophoresis

For the second dimension, the sample containing IPG strips were equilibrated with sodium dodecyl sulfate (SDS) running buffer (75 mM Tris (pH 8.8), 6 M Urea, 30% v/v Glycerol and 2% w/v SDS). DTT was added to reduce disulfide bonds, and iodoacetamide (IAA) to alkylate thiol groups what prevented disulfide bonds from reforming. After equilibration the IPG strip was applied directly on top of a large format 16 X 14 cm 12% acrylamide gel. Agarose was poured on top of the strip to prevent air from getting underneath and to hold strip in place. Molecular markers were applied 4 cm from the positive end of the strip. The proteins were then separated vertically according to their molecular weight by SDS-polyacrylamide gel electrophoresis (PAGE) on a DALT 6 electrophoresis unit at 20 ^{0}C, 6 W/ gel for 18 h.

3.4 Protein detection and bioinformatics analysis

After 2D-DIGE, the relative abundance of proteins from the TAC heart disease versus sham protein lysates was detected using a high resolution fluorescent scanner Typhoon 9410 (GE Healthcare). The excitation/emission wavelengths for the CyDyes were as follows: Cy2, 480 nm/530 nm (blue), Cy3, 540 nm/590 nm (green) and Cy5, 620 nm/680 nm (red). Images

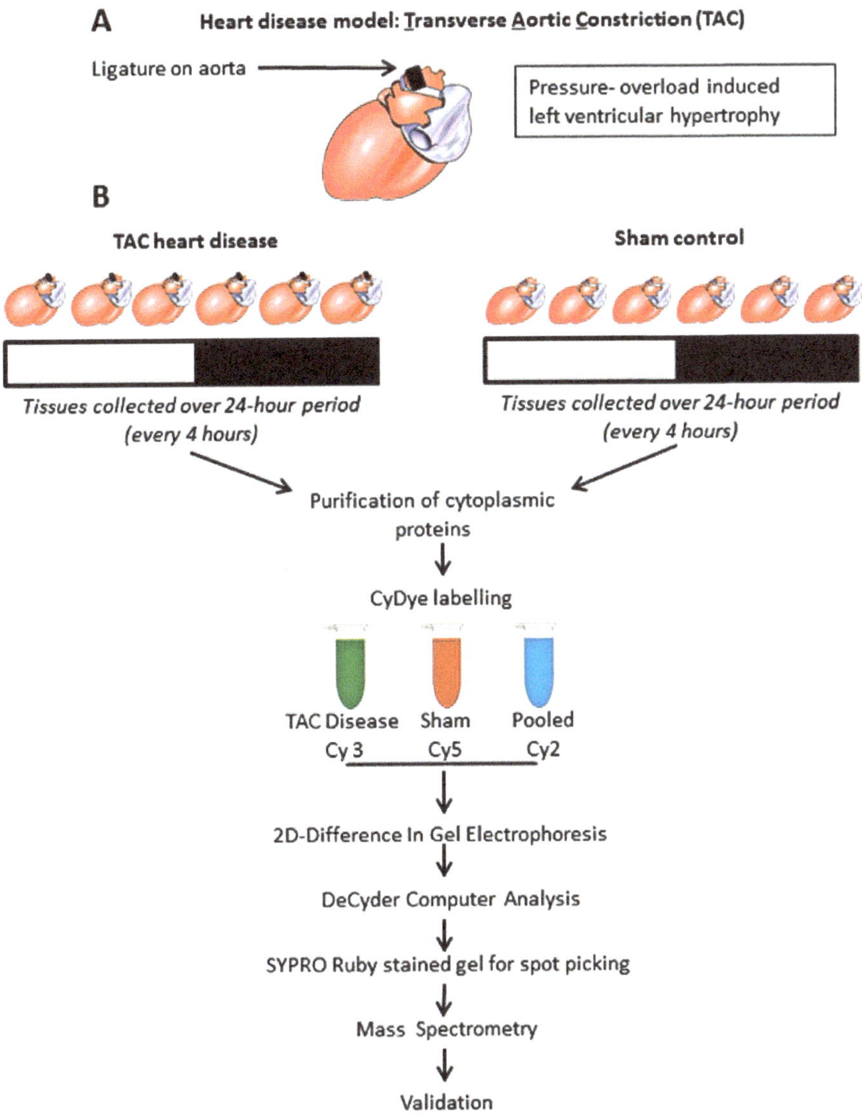

A) Heart disease model. Pressure overload cardiac hypertrophy is induced by transverse aortic constriction (TAC). A ligature is placed distal to the third bifurcation of aorta. Sham animals undergo the same procedure except the ligature is not tightened. B) Two-dimensional difference in gel electrophoresis (2D-DIGE) and mass spectrometry (MS) approach to characterize the circadian cardiovascular proteome in health and disease. Heart tissue is collected from TAC disease and sham control animals at 6 timepoints over the 24-hour light/dark cycle. The cytoplasmic proteome from TAC vs. sham hearts is labelled with Cy3 and Cy5 dye, respectively. An internal control consists of pooled samples labelled with Cy2. After 2D-DIGE protein expression is analyzed with DeCyder. SYPRO Ruby gel for picking spots of interest is created. Proteins are excised and identified by MS. Results are validated by Western blot.

Fig. 2. Experimental design.

were visualized with Image Quant TL software. An overlay image of Cy3 and Cy5 scans is illustrated in Figure 3A. Proteins that had higher abundance in TAC heart disease vs. sham appeared as a red spot. Lower levels in TAC heart disease vs. sham appeared green. Equal amounts of protein in TAC heart disease vs. sham were yellow.

Statistical analysis and quantification of protein expression was achieved by DeCyder software (GE Healthcare). In the first step of DeCyder workflow, difference in gel analysis (DIA) used a codetection algorithm to detect and match differently labelled samples (Cy2, Cy3 and Cy5) within the same gel. It was necessary to define a specific area of interest within a gel and then manually confirm that the program detected all the spots within that area. Spot intensity corresponding to protein abundance was quantified after background subtraction and normalization. The second step termed biological variance analysis (BVA) simultaneously analyzed multiple DIGE gels by matching all the spots to a master gel, defined by user. Protein expression was compared between gels and statistically verified. Based on spot intensity, DeCyder constructed 3D views of relative protein abundance. The standardized volume of the peaks was used to calculate fold change.

In this study, and as shown in Figure 3B, we found three spots (# 596, 615, and 1012) that were upregulated in TAC heart disease compared to sham at our sleep-wake transition timepoint (ZT23). Spot # 596 had a 1.18 fold change, spot # 615 had a 1.48 fold change, and spot # 1012 had 1.77 fold change. To identify the proteins of interest, a pick gel was created containing 300 μg of unlabelled protein. Glass plates were treated with Bind-Silane (γ-methacryloxypropyltrimethoxysilane) so that the gel was covalently attached to the surface. After electrophoresis, proteins were fixed in 10% methanol and 7% acetic acid solution for 2 hours, then stained with SYPRO Ruby for 18 hours and destained in 40% methanol/10% acetic acid solution for 2 hours. The gel was scanned with a Typhoon 9410 scanner at 532 nm (670 BP 30 emission filter). Images were uploaded to DeCyder and matched to the previous DIGE gel. Unique coordinates for each spot were created using position markers. After manual confirmation, an Ettan Spot picker (GE Healthcare) was used to excise proteins from the gel.

3.5 Trypsin digestion and mass spectrometry

To determine the identification of the proteins in gel spots # 596, 615 and 1012, we used an In-Gel Tryptic Digestion Kit (Thermo Scientific) followed by mass spectrometry (MS). Trypsin is a serine protease that cleaves the peptide bonds at the carboxyl side of lysine and arginine amino acids. Following digestion, tryptic peptide fragments were separated by nano-LC which consisted of a trap column (300μm ID) and an analytical column (75 μm ID) packed with 5μm, 300Å Zorbax SB C18 beads. A linear binary gradient was used where solvent A was 98% H_2O:2% CH_3CN and 0.1% (v/v) formic acid and solvent B was 2% H_2O : 98% CH_3CN and 0.1% (v/v) formic acid. Peptides were eluted over a 2 - 95% solvent B gradient for 100 min at a rate of 300 nL/min. The eluant from the nano-LC was coupled to a hybrid triple/quadrupole linear ion trap mass spectrometer (QTRAP 4000, ABSciex) through a nano-spray ionization source equipped with a 15 μm ID emittor tip. Our preferred database for searching was Mascot (http://www.matrixscience.com). This database contains information on more than 10 million proteins, with inherent redundancies built in since peptides can correspond to more than one protein. Each of the spots generated a list of possible protein candidates, and Mascot score and E value helped identify the correct match. The molecular weight and pI of the identified protein was comparable to the expected molecular weight and pI of the corresponding spot from the 2-DE gel.

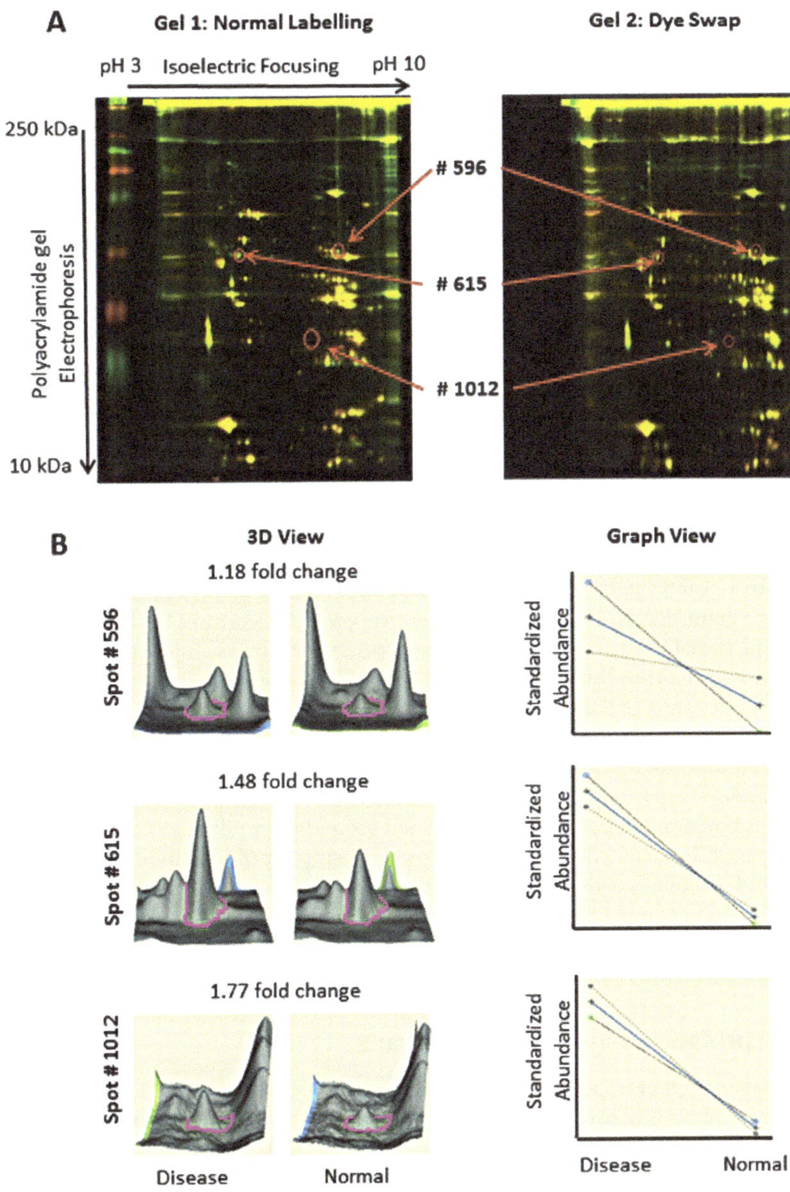

A) 2D-DIGE image. The gel on the left had proteins purified from TAC (heart disease) labelled with Cy3 and those from sham heart labelled with Cy5. Gel on the right shows alternatively labelled samples, where TAC proteins are labelled with Cy5 and sham with Cy3. Location of the proteins of interest is shown with arrows. B) DeCyder computer analysis of three identified protein spots # 596, 615 and 1012. Based on standardized abundance these protein spots increased in TAC vs. sham. Expression changes are shown by 3D and Graph views.

Fig. 3. Circadian Cardiovascular Proteomics.

3.6 Role of proteins identified in TAC heart disease

Our laboratory is interested in circadian cardiovascular proteomics to better understand molecular processes underlying heart disease and clinical treatments. The TAC upregulated spots 519, 615 and 1012 were identified by MS as Succinyl-CoA:3-ketoacid-coenzyme A transferase 1, mitochondrial (SCOT), Desmin (DESM), and PDZ and LIM domain protein 1 (PDLIM1) respectively. Three examples from ZT23 (one hour before lights on, murine sleep-time) were shown here; other proteins were identified from different times of day or night. Figure 4 shows a representative mass spectrum for one of the identified proteins, SCOT (spot #519), as well as the number and list of tryptic hits, Mascot score, E-value, and protein sequence. Functionally, SCOT is a mitochondrial matrix protein and is the key rate limiting enzyme for ketone body metabolism (Fukao et al., 2004; Orii et al., 2008). That it exhibits increased expression around sleep time suggests that it plays a role in changing cardiac energy sources. The second identified protein, DESMIN (spot # 615) is crucial for muscle structure and function, as reviewed in (Paulin & Li, 2004). The third protein, PDLIM1 (spot #1012) is a cytoskeletal protein involved in cardiac contractility and cardioprotection, as reviewed in (Arias-Loza et al., 2008; Johnsen et al., 2009).

3.7 Validation: Western blotting

Candidate circadian biomarkers identified by 2D-DIGE and MS are validated by Western blot protein expression analyses using an independent set of cytoplasmic soluble proteins from TAC and sham hearts. Proteins (20 μg) are separated according to their mass by 12% SDS-PAGE and transferred to polyvinylidene fluoride membrane (Bio-Rad) using a semi-dry transfer apparatus (Bio-Rad). Membranes are blocked for 2 hours at room temperature with 5% non-fat dry milk in TBS-T 0.05 % (20 mM Tris Base, 137mM NaCl, 0.05 % Tween 20, pH 7.6) and incubated overnight at 4 ^{0}C with primary antibodies against SCOT, DESM or PDLIM1. The antibodies are diluted according to the manufacturer's instructions. Anti-actin antibody (1:40000, Milipore) is used as a loading control. Immunoreactive protein bands are visualized with horseradish peroxidise-conjugated secondary antibodies (1:5000, Sigma) and ECLplus reagent (GE Healthcare). Blots are scanned using Storm 860 molecular imager (GE Healthcare) and protein expression is quantified by Image J software (NIH). Expression levels of SCOT, DESM and PDLIM1 in TAC samples at ZT23 are compared to sham, thus independently validating 2D-DIGE approach. Validating the candidate proteins/biomarkers in human samples will increase their significance and is key to translational applications.

4. Circadian proteomes in other body organs

Our time-of-day circadian approach led to discovery of SCOT, DESMIN, and PDLIM which were upregulated in TAC cardiac hypertrophy at sleep time. Other groups have also met with success investigating circadian proteomics in different tissues and clinical paradigms. A summary of identified circadian proteomes is shown in Table 1. The first identification of a circadian proteome was reported by Reddy and colleagues (Reddy et al., 2006), using a 2D-DIGE/MS approach to study murine liver. Mice were entrained to 12:12 L:D cycles, then placed in constant darkness (12:12 D:D) and sacrificed at 6 consecutive time-points 4 hours apart. It was observed that 135 (21%) out of 642 detected protein spots rhythmically cycled over the 24-hour period. Many of the newly identified circadian proteins were key rate limiting enzymes including ketohexokinase, succinate dehydrogenase 1, aldolase 2, enolase 1/aconitase 2, carbamoyl phosphate synthetase 1, CPS1, arginosuccinate synthetase 1, and arginase 1.

Tissue	Methods	Proteins with circadian expression pattern	Function	Reference
Liver CD1 mice	Mice were entrained under 12:12 L:D and then transferred to 12:12 D:D (constant darkness). Liver tissue was collected every 4-h over 24-h starting at CT 0 (n = 3/ time point) 2D-DIGE MALDI-TOF MS LC MS/MS	Arginosuccinate synthetase 1 (ASS1)	Urea cycle	(Reddy et al., 2006)
		Carbamoyl phosphate synthetase 1 (CPS1)	Urea cycle	
		Arginase 1 (ARG1)		
		Ketohexokinase (KHK)	Fructose metabolism	
		Succinate dehydrogenase 1 (SDH1)		
		Aldolase 2 (ALDO2)	Glycolysis	
		Enolase 1 (ENO1)		
		Aconitase 2 (ACO2)	Kreb's cycle	
Pineal gland Wistar rats	Rats were entrained under 12:12 L:D. Pineal glands were collected at ZT6 (6 hours after lights on) and ZT18 (6 hours after lights off) (n = 8/ time point) 2D-PAGE MALDI-TOF MS	**Dark period (rodent wake time)**		(Moller, Sparre et al. 2007)
		Alpha enolase	Glycolysis pathway	
		Gamma enolase		
		Vimentin	Morphogenesis	
		Creatine kinase, B chain	Energy transduction	
		Guanine deaminase	Purine catabolism	
		Peptidyl-prolyl cis-trans isomerase A	Protein folding	
		Annexin A2 and A5	Ca^{2+}-regulated membrane-binding	
		Light period (rodent sleep time)		
		Malate Dehydrogenase	Krebs cycle	
		Citrate synthase		
		Triosephosphate Isomerise		
		Ubiquinolcytochrome c reductase core protein I	Mitochondrial electron transport	
		RNA recognition motif	Processing of pre-mRNAs	
		Chaperonin containing TCP1	Chaperone, signal transduction	
		ER protein ERp29 precursor(Erp31)		
		Transitional endoplasmic reticulum ATPase	Vesicle budding from the endoplasmic reticulum	
		Complement C3 Precursor	Activation of the complement system	
		Phosphoserine phosphatise	Biosynthesis of serine from carbohydrates	
		Contrapsin-like protease inhibitor 1 and 3 precursor	Protein metabolism	

Tissue	Methods	Proteins with circadian expression pattern	Function	Reference
Retina C57BL/6 mice	Mice were entrained under 12:12 L:D and transferred to 12:12 D:D. Retinal tissue was collected every 6-h over 24-h starting at CT 2 (n = 5/ time point) 2D-PAGE MALDI-TOF MS	N-ethylmaleimide-sensitive fusion protein	Vesicle transport	(Tsuji, Hirota et al. 2007)
		Charged Multivesicular body protein 4b		
		Reticulocalbin-2 precursor	Calcium binding	
		Calbindin D28	Photoreceptor adaptation, gating of photic input	
		Heterogeneous ribonucleoprotein A/B	RNA-binding	
		T-complex 1 subunit delta	Protein folding, phototransduction, morphological changes	
		Leukotriene A4 hydrolase	Metabolism	
		Proteasome subunit alpha type 1	Protein degradation	
SCN releasate Long-Evans/BluGill rats	Rats were entrained under 12:12 L:D and transferred to 12:12 D:D. Samples were taken every 4-h over 24-h starting at CT 0 LC MALDI-TOF MS LC MS/MS	Angiotensin I		(Hatcher et al., 2008)
		Arginine vasopressin[b]		
		Proenkephalin 219–229		
		Galanin		
		Neurokinin-B		
		Neurotensin		
		POMC, melanotropin α		
		PEN		
		Big LEN		
		Little SAAS		
		Somatostatin-14[b]		
		proSomatostatin 89-100		
		Substance P		
		Thymosin β-4		
Urine *Tau* mutant hamsters	Hamsters entrained under 14:10 L:D cycle. SDS-PAGE LC MS/MS	Cytochrome C (CYCS)	Apoptosis	(Martino et al., 2008)
Blood C57Bl/6	Mice entrained to 12:12 L:D cycle SELDI	Fingerprinting assay	Proof of concept that de-novo proteins cycle in the blood, and that the daily rhythmic variation changes in heart disease	Ref Martino same one as below
Blood C57BL/6 mice	Mice entrained under 12:12 L:D cycle. Samples collected every 4 hours, starting at ZT 23 (n = 3/ time point) SDS-PAGE LC MS/MS	Transthyretin	Transports thyroxin (T4) and retinol (vitamin A)	(Martino, Tata et al. 2007)
		Apolipoprotein A1 precursor	Lipid and cholesterol regulation	
		Apolipoprotein E precursor		
		Apolipoprotein J		
		Plasminogen	Plasmin formation	
		Complement C3 precursor	Activation of compliment system	

Tissue	Methods	Proteins with circadian expression pattern	Function	Reference
Blood metabolome C57BL/6 and CBA/N mice	Mice entrained under 12:12 L:D cycles, then transferred to either 12:12L:D or 12:12 D:D. Blood collected in fasting animals over 24-h starting at ZT 4 or CT 4 LC-MS CE-MS	Trimethylamine N-oxide		(Minami et al., 2009)
		Glutamine 2-Aminobutyrate		
		Cytidine		
		Sarcosine		
		Carnitine		
		Valine		
		Tryptophan		
		4-Guanidinobutyrate		
		Isoleucine		
		3-Methylhistidine		
		Leucine		
		Proline		
		Guanidoacetate		
		1-Methylnicotinamide		
		Citrulline		
		Creatinine		
		Glycine		
		Methionine sulfoxide		
		a-Aminoadipate		
		Methionine		
		Phenylalanine		
		N,N-Dimethylglycine		
		Thr 13C		
		Threonine		
		Ornithine		
		Hydroxyproline		
		Creatine		
		Corticosterone		
		lysophosphatidylcoline		

Table 1. Circadian proteomes.

The circadian proteome in the rat pineal gland was identified using 2D-PAGE, silver stain and tandem mass spectrometry (MS/MS) (Moller et al., 2007). In this study, rats were entrained to 12:12 L:D cycle. Pineal glands were collected at two timepoints: ZT06 which is 6 hours after lights on (light phase, rats asleep) and ZT18 which is 6 hours after lights off (dark phase, rats awake). A total of 1737 pineal gland proteins were detected, 35 showed greater abundance during sleep time and 25 during wake time. Proteins upregulated during wake time were involved in glycolysis (alpha- and gamma-enolase), morphogenesis (vimentin), energy transduction (Creatine kinase), purine catabolism (guanine deaminase), protein folding (peptidyl-prolyl cis–trans isomerase A), and Ca^{2+}-dependent membrane binding (annexin A2, annexin A5). Proteins with increased abundance during sleep mapped to the Krebs cycle (malate dehydrogenase, citrate synthase, triosephosphate isomerise), mitochondrial electron transport (ubiquinol-cytochrome c reductase core protein 1), RNA binding and processing (RNA recognition motif), protein folding (chaperone-containing TCP1, ER protein ERp29 precursor), cell transport (transitional ER ATPase), complement (C3 precursor), and metabolism (phosphoserine phosphotase, contrapsin-like protease inhibitor 1 and 3 precursors).

The circadian proteome of the mouse retina was characterized by 2D-PAGE and Coomassie Brilliant stain (Tsuji et al., 2007). C57Bl/6 mice were entrained at 12:12 L:D cycle, then placed in constant darkness (12:12 D:D) and sacrificed on the fourth day at 4 timepoints: CT2, CT8, CT14, and CT20. CT2 corresponded to subjective dawn and CT12 to subjective dusk. A total of 415 protein spots were detected and 11 exhibited circadian rhythms. The cycling proteins were important in vesicular transport (N-ethylmaleimide-sensitive fusion protein, charged multivesicular body protein 4b), calcium-binding (calbindin D28, reticulocalbin-2 precursor), RNA-binding (heterogeneous ribonucleoprotein A/B), protein folding (T-complex 1 delta), metabolism (leukotriene A4 hydrolase), and protein degradation (proteasome subunit alpha1).

The circadian peptidome released from rat hypothalamic SCN was characterized using a gel-free approach (Hatcher et al., 2008). Long-Evans/BluGill rats were entrained to 12:12 L:D and then transferred to constant darkness. Animals were sacrificed during subjective day-time (CT 0-12) and brain slices containing SCN and optic nerve were prepared. SCN releasates were obtained from extracellular fluid with pipettes containing solid-phase extraction material or from the SCN itself with micrometer-sized beads with solid-phase extraction material. Samples of releasate were collected at the beginning and end of CT 0–4, 4–8, 8–12, 12–16, 16–20, and 20–24 intervals and analyzed with MALDI TOF MS. Identified peptides were independently verified with LC-MS/MS. Arginine vasopressin showed a robust circadian rhythm with a peak during sleep time. Other identified peptides were angiotensin I, arginine vasopressin[b], proenkephalin, galanin, neurokinin-B, neurotensin, melanotropin α, PEN, big LEN, little SAAS, somatostatin-14b, proSomatostatin, substance P and thymosin β-4. Interestingly, this study also detected previously unknown peptides, which prompted further investigation of their biological role.

5. The circadian proteome helps to understand disease and identify new biomarkers

Disturbances of the circadian rhythm, such as might occur in humans in shift work or sleep disorders, can affect many physiologic processes (e.g. circadian rhythms of heart rate, body temperature, sympathetic nervous activity, chemical, inflammatory, and metabolic processes). The proteome should characteristically change as well, revealing de novo biomarkers. We investigated this using a +/tau hamster model bearing a mutation in the core circadian clockwork protein casein kinase 1 epsilon (Martino et al., 2008). The circadian rhythm disruption in these animals etiologically caused heart and kidney disease. The animals exhibited profound proteinuria. To detect proteomic changes, urine samples collected from +/tau vs. controls were analyzed on 10-20% tricine gels stained with Coomassie dye. Bands were excised from the gel, trypsin digested, subjected to MS/MS on a LCQ DECA XP ion trap, and analyzed using Sequest. Protein identification was validated by Western blot. As shown in Table 1, a ~15 kDa protein band, appearing only in the urine of the +/tau animals, was identified by MS as cytochrome c, a biomarker of cellular apoptosis. Apoptosis was confirmed in the renal tissues of +/tau mutants by terminal uridine deoxynucleotidyl transferase dUTP nick end labelling (TUNEL) staining. Thus by using circadian approaches, a novel biomarker of renal disease was discovered. This was a particularly exciting discovery as there are notably very few biomarkers of developing renal disease. For example, a usual biomarker for kidney disease is creatinine, however, this represents just chemical waste generated from muscle metabolism and is only an indirect marker of renal function. Here we identified a direct indicator of early and ongoing tissue damage, by investigating circadian proteome expression. This marker is easily obtained by collecting urine samples, thus making it potentially ideal for point-of-care or routine diagnostics. Additional examples of circadian-based biomarkers, including many fundamental to human health and disease, are described below.

6. Circadian biomarkers in blood

Circadian proteomics can be used for discovery of de-novo blood biomarkers of heart disease. Established cardiovascular factors (e.g. hypertension, smoking, diabetes) do not fully explain the risk for heart disease, and there is substantial interest in the development of new biomarkers to identify persons at risk and who may be targeted for preventative measures. In those with heart disease, biomarkers are in demand to help track disease progression and aid physicians in better treating their patients. Although a number of strategies are currently used to identify biomarkers, there have been very few clinical advances, and thus new approaches such as circadian proteomics are warranted.

As an example, we recently investigated diurnal proteome cycling in murine blood (Martino et al., 2007). Blood was the preferred tissue for biomedical investigation because of its ease of accessibility and minimal invasiveness for sampling. As shown in Table 1, the first approach was proof of concept and used surface-enhanced laser desorption ionization (SELDI) MS. Only proteins retained on ion exchange solid phase chromatographic surfaces (or chips) were examined; substances with other biochemical properties remain open to future investigation. Expression profiles were collected over a wide mass range; those of lower molecular weight (1-10 kDa range) classically contained bioactive peptides, while those in the midrange (10-50 kDa) and larger (>50 kDa) reflected peptides/proteins involved in cell structural and functional processes. With SELDI MS we essentially created a fingerprint of blood protein expression over the 24-hour time, from which one could then quantify, statistically analyze and graph data to visualize daily protein rhythms.

Since one of the drawbacks of SELDI MS was a relative inability to further identify the fingerprint proteins, the diurnal blood proteome was also characterized following prefractionation on column chromatography with an ion exchange resin (Martino et al., 2007). As shown in Table 1, proteins comprising effluent, salt elution, and bead retentive fractions were visualized by SDS-PAGE and silver stain. Protein bands that exhibited cyclic variation over 24 hours were excised, trypsin digested, and then injected by electro spray ionization (ESI) into a LCQ DECA XP ion trap. Proteins were identified by comparison searching molecular mass against murine databases. Many of the identified blood proteins with diurnal expression linked to cycles in physiology were those released from liver, such as transthyretin, apolipoprotein A1 precursor, apolipoprotein E precursor, apolipoprotein J, plasminogen and complement C3 precursor. Ultimately, comparing daily rhythms in sera from healthy individuals vs. heart disease patients would allow for the creation of new biomarker profiles and discovery platforms.

Another study examining diurnal biomarkers in blood measured 24-hour profiles of small chemical substances (peptides, amino acids, hormones) (Minami et al., 2009). As shown in Table 1, blood was drawn every 4 hours over the 24-hour period from CBA mice maintained

SCOT: Succinyl-CoA:3-ketoacid-coenzyme A transferase 1, mitochondrial

A

Peptide: GGHVNLTMLGAMQVSK, 2^+

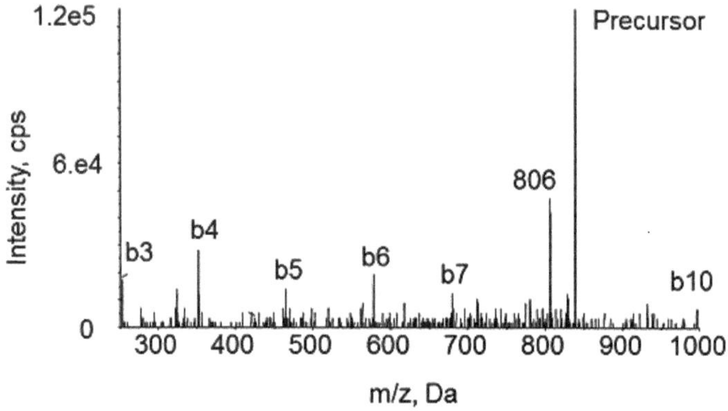

B

Peptides

KGNAHKI
KLLSSGLRL
KCTLPLTGKQ
KGVFDVDKKN
RNFNLPMCKA
KDGSVAIASKPRE
KFYTDPVEAVKD
KYGDLANWMIPGKM
KGMGGAMDLVSSSKTKV
RMISSYVGENAEFERQ
RGGHVNLTMLGAMQVSKY
RQFLSGELEVELTPQGTLAERI
RAGGAGVPAFYTSTGYGTLVQEGGSPIKY

Total number of peptides sequenced: 24
Mascot score: 150
E-value: 4.0 ×10^{-21}

C

Protein sequence and peptide coverage

*MAAL***KLLSSGLRL***GASARSSRGALHKGCVCYFSV*
*STRHHT***KFYTDPVEAVKD***IPNGATLLVGGFGLC*
GIPENLIGALLKTGVKDLTAVSNNAGVDNFGLGLL
*LRSKQIK***RMISSYVGENAEFERQFLSGELEVEL**
TPQGTLAERIRAGGAGVPAFYTSTGYGTLVQ
EGGSPIKYNKDGSVAIASKPRE*VREFNGQHFIL*
*EEAITGDFALVKAWKADRAGNVIFRKSA***RNFNLP**
MCKA*AGTTVVEVEEIVDIGSFAPEDIHIPKIYVHRL*
IKGEKYEKRIERLSLRKEGDGKGKSGKPGGDVRERI
IKRAALEFEDGMYANLGIGIPLLASNFISPNMTVH
LQSENGVLGLGPYPLKDEADADLINAGKETVTVLP
*GASFFSSDESFAMI***RGGHVNLTMLGAMQVSK**
YGDLANWMIPGKMVKGMGGAMDLVSSSK
TKV*VVTMEHSA***KGNAHK***IMEKCTLPLTGKQCV*
*NRIITE***KGVFDVDKKN***GLTLIELWEGLTVDDIKKST*
GCDFAVSPNLMPMQQIST

A) Representative mass spectrum of the SCOT peptide: RGGHVNLTMLGAMQVSKY. B) A total of 24 peptides were identified, corresponding to 13 unique sequences. The Mascot score is 150, E-value is 4.0 ×10^{-21}. C) Identified peptides and their corresponding match to the SCOT protein sequence.

Fig. 4. MS based identification of Succinyl-CoA:3-ketoacid-coenzyme A transferase 1, mitochondrial (SCOT).

under L:D or D:D conditions and LC-MS analysis was performed that led to the detection of 176 negative and 142 positive ion peaks. Importantly, in transgenic murine model of clock disruption (Cry1-/- and Cry2-/-), expression of these metabolites was altered, suggesting that they were controlled by the clock mechanism. The authors demonstrated that their metabolite timetable could be used to accurately determine body time in mice with different genetic background, age, sex and feeding regime. The overall purpose of doing this was to create maps of body time, which could be applied clinically to optimize understanding of disease or determine the best times for administering drugs and therapies.

7. Circadian rhythms in neuro/hormone biomarkers

Long before protein cycling was even discovered, it was already known that some key neuroendocrine hormones important to the heart had daily rhythmic patterns of expression. Cycling of many of these hormones drives the protein rhythms we observe in normal heart and other tissues, and the changes that occur in disease. Further details are described below and in Figure 5 and Table 2.

7.1 Sleep-time hormones

The first example is melatonin, and its expression in humans is elevated in the dark but suppressed by light (thus it is sometimes called the "hormone of darkness") (Brzezinski, 1997). It has a cardioprotective effect through antioxidant and anti-inflammatory activity, reviewed by (Tengattini et al., 2008). It is a useful circadian biomarker of heart disease. Nocturnal melatonin levels were low in patients with acute myocardial infarction (MI) vs. healthy controls within the first 24 hours after hospital admission (Dominguez-Rodriguez et al., 2002). Also, patients with ST-segment MI who developed adverse events during follow-up had significantly lower nocturnal melatonin levels than patients without the events (Dominguez-Rodriguez et al., 2006). In another study it was revealed that nocturnal melatonin levels were reduced in patients with cardiac syndrome X vs. controls (Altun et al., 2002). Second, the renin-angiotensin-aldosterone system (RAAS) also exhibits circadian rhythm. Aldosterone produced by the adrenal cortex regulates Na^+ and K^+ homeostasis. Aldosterone plasma levels peak during sleep time (11:00 P.M. - 7:00 A.M.) (Charloux et al., 1999). As a biomarker of heart disease, it has been reported that while normal subjects showed an 81% decrease during the wake period, there was only a 40% decrease in low renin hypertensive patients (Grim et al., 1974). Similarly, plasma renin activity (PRA) cycles in healthy subjects with peak activity during sleep (Charloux et al., 1999). Patients with hypertensive heart disease exhibited a greater increase in PRA during sleep-time as compared to normotensive patients (Tuck et al., 1985).

Finally, growth hormone secretion by the anterior pituitary gland is pulsatile and has a circadian rhythm with the highest peak occurring at midnight (Surya et al., 2006). Growth hormone is involved in regulation of cardiac metabolism and contractility, reviewed by (Volterrani et al., 2000). In some heart failure patients (New York Heart Association classes I-III) there is a loss of circadian rhythm and overall reduction of growth hormone secretion (Duncan et al., 2003).

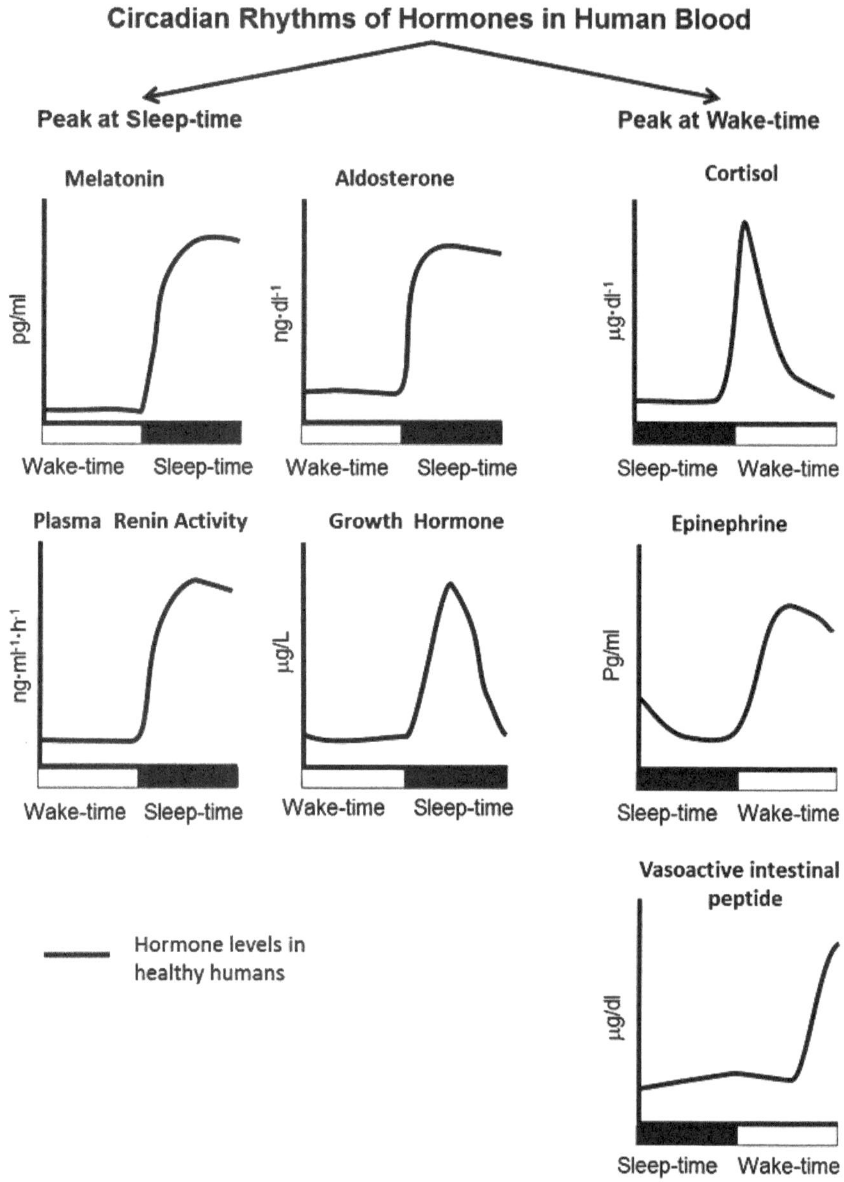

Left; Melatonin, aldosterone, plasma renin activity, growth hormone peak during sleep time. Right; cortisol, epinephrine, vasoactive intestinal peptide peak during wake time. X-axis: white bar = light period, black bar = dark. Rhythms illustrated here are based on the references listed in Table 2.

Fig. 5. Dirunal cycling of hormones in blood.

Hormone	Selective function(s) relevant to the cardiovascular system	Hormone Cycling		References
		In healthy humans	Altered cycling in specified cardiovascular disease	* Used in Figure 5 § Heart disease # Additional references
Melatonin	Antioxidant, circadian entrainment	Nocturnal peak in blood (in the dark) Secretion is suppressed by light and activated in the dark	Nocturnal decrease observed within the first 24h period in patients with myocardial infarct (MI) Low levels of melatonin correlate with adverse events during follow up in ST-segment MI patients Nocturnal decrease in patients with cardiac syndrome X vs. healthy controls	* (Brzezinski, 1997) # (Claustrat et al., 1986) # (Follenius et al., 1995) § (Dominguez-Rodriguez et al., 2006) § (Dominguez-Rodriguez et al., 2002) § (Altun et al., 2002)
Aldosterone	Regulates Na^+/K^+ homeostasis, blood pressure	Peak serum levels during sleep time	Does not decrease normally during the day in low renin hypertensive patients vs. healthy controls	* (Charloux et al., 1999) # (Katz et al., 1975) # (Lightman et al., 1981) § (Grim et al., 1974)
Plasma Renin Activity	Regulates blood pressure	Significantly higher plasma activity during sleep time	Significantly upregulated only at night in some patients with essential hypertension	* (Charloux et al., 1999) # (Katz et al., 1975) § (Tuck et al., 1985)
Growth Hormone	Affects metabolism and contractility	Nocturnal plasma peak Exhibits pulsatile expression	Overall decrease and loss of circadian rhythm in some patients with chronic heart failure (NY Heart Association classes I-III)	* (Surya et al., 2006) # (Takahashi et al., 1968) # (Hartman et al., 1991) § (Duncan et al., 2003)

Hormone	Selective function(s) relevant to the cardiovascular system	Hormone Cycling		References
		In healthy humans	Altered cycling in specified cardiovascular disease	* Used in Figure 5 § Heart disease # Additional references
Cortisol	Regulates blood sugar levels, increases blood pressure	Serum levels peak around wake-time	Peaks at 4:00 A.M. in some low renin hypertensive patients	* (Charloux et al., 1999) * (Lightman et al., 1981) # (Lockinger et al., 2004) # (Cugini et al., 1991) § (Grim et al., 1974)
Epinephrine	Increases heart rate and blood pressure Mediates sympathetic response	Plasma levels peak during wake time	Nocturnal increase in some patients with obstructive sleep apnea vs. healthy controls	* (Linsell et al., 1985) # (Scheer et al., 2009) # (Akerstedt & Froberg, 1979) § (Alonso-Fernandez et al., 2005)
Vasoactive intestinal peptide	Regulates vasodilation, heart rate, force of contraction	Plasma peak before sleep (20:00), trough at night (0:00)	Circadian rhythm is lost in patients with orthotopic heart transplant	* (Cugini et al., 1991) # (Cugini et al., 1992) § (Cugini et al., 1993)

Table 2. Circadian rhythms in neuro/hormones in humans

7.2 Wake time hormones

Cortisol exhibits diurnal variation with serum levels peaking early in the morning around wake time and troughing late in the evening (Charloux et al., 1999; Lightman et al., 1981). It may also be a useful biomarker or mediator of disease as plasma cortisol peaks earlier at 4:00 A.M. in some low renin hypertensive patients, as compared to 8:00 A.M. in normal controls (Grim et al., 1974). Epinephrine stimulates sympathetic activity including in the cardiovascular system. It exhibits a robust endogenous circadian rhythm that peaks during wake time (Linsell et al., 1985), and this expression changes in obstructive sleep apnea heart failure patients, in which there is increased nocturnal sympathetic tone (Alonso-Fernandez et al., 2005; Bradley & Floras, 2009). Lastly, vasoactive intestinal peptide affects vasodilation, heart rate and force of contraction, reviewed by (Henning & Sawmiller, 2001). It has a circadian rhythm with a peak before sleep time (20:00) and a trough later at night (0:00) (Cugini et al., 1991). The rhythm of this peptide is lost in patients with orthotopic heart transplant (Cugini et al., 1993).

8. Clinical translation

Discovery of the circadian cardiovascular proteome and it's endogenous drivers provides a new understanding of cardiovascular health and disease, where time is a new paradigm of functional significance. Proteomic biomarkers can be easily implemented with ELISA-type point-of-care diagnostic platforms that could be routinely applied in physician offices, or even potentially in the consumer's home. One of the practical applications of cardiovascular circadian proteomics is chronotherapy, which requires easily accessible markers of body time for optimizing the timing of drug treatments. For example, we recently demonstrated that the efficacy of treatment with the angiotensin converting enzyme inhibitor (ACEi) captopril exhibits a diurnal pattern, consistent with the diurnal variation in ACE expression (Martino et al., 2011). ACEi are common medications given to cardiovascular patients with hypertension, after a myocardial infarction or with heart failure. We found that drug administration at sleep-time improved heart function, but wake-time did not differ from placebo. This approach can be used in other diseases such as cancer (Hrushesky & Bjarnason, 1993; Innominato et al., 2010) and neuroendocrine disorders (Chung et al., 2011) as well.

9. Conclusion

Circadian cardiovascular proteomics is an important new area of research that provides an excellent opportunity to elucidate molecular processes that underlie our health and disease across the 24-hour light/dark period. At this early stage, temporal analysis of the proteome in cardiovascular tissues (i.e. heart or blood) of experimental animal models reveals remarkable 24-hour variations in protein abundances. Diurnal protein profiles differ remarkably between health and disease. Characterization of these proteins is the key to understanding normal body physiology as well as providing new diagnostic capabilities, and new approaches to treatment by aiding in the design of personalized therapeutics.

10. Acknowledgments

Supported by a Grant from the Heart and Stroke Foundation (NA6466 to T.A. Martino).

11. References

Akashi, M., Tsuchiya, Y., Yoshino, T., & Nishida, E. (2002). Control of intracellular dynamics of mammalian period proteins by casein kinase I epsilon (CKIepsilon) and CKIdelta in cultured cells. *Mol Cell Biol*, Vol. 22, No. 6, pp. 1693-703, issn 0270-7306

Akerstedt, T., & Froberg, J. E. (1979). Sleep and stressor exposure in relation to circadian rhythms in catecholamine excretion. *Biol Psychol*, Vol. 8, No. 1, pp. 69-80, issn 0301-0511

Alonso-Fernandez, A., Garcia-Rio, F., Racionero, M. A., Pino, J. M., Ortuno, F., Martinez, I., & Villamor, J. (2005). Cardiac rhythm disturbances and ST-segment depression episodes in patients with obstructive sleep apnea-hypopnea syndrome and its mechanisms. *Chest*, Vol. 127, No. 1, pp. 15-22, issn 0012-3692

Altun, A., Yaprak, M., Aktoz, M., Vardar, A., Betul, U. A., & Ozbay, G. (2002). Impaired nocturnal synthesis of melatonin in patients with cardiac syndrome X. *Neurosci Lett,* Vol. 327, No. 2, pp. 143-5, issn 0304-3940

Andrews, N. P., Gralnick, H. R., Merryman, P., Vail, M., & Quyyumi, A. A. (1996). Mechanisms underlying the morning increase in platelet aggregation: a flow cytometry study. *J Am Coll Cardiol,* Vol. 28, No. 7, pp. 1789-95, issn 0735-1097

Angleton, P., Chandler, W. L., & Schmer, G. (1989). Diurnal variation of tissue-type plasminogen activator and its rapid inhibitor (PAI-1). *Circulation,* Vol. 79, No. 1, pp. 101-6, issn 0009-7322

Antos, C. L., McKinsey, T. A., Frey, N., Kutschke, W., McAnally, J., Shelton, J. M., Richardson, J. A., *et al.* (2002). Activated glycogen synthase-3 beta suppresses cardiac hypertrophy in vivo. *Proc Natl Acad Sci U S A,* Vol. 99, No. 2, pp. 907-12, issn 0027-8424

Arias-Loza, P. A., Jazbutyte, V., & Pelzer, T. (2008). Genetic and pharmacologic strategies to determine the function of estrogen receptor alpha and estrogen receptor beta in cardiovascular system. *Gend Med,* Vol. 5 Suppl A, pp. S34-45, issn 1550-8579

Bradley, T. D., & Floras, J. S. (2009). Obstructive sleep apnoea and its cardiovascular consequences. *Lancet,* Vol. 373, No. 9657, pp. 82-93, issn 1474-547X

Brzezinski, A. (1997). Melatonin in humans. *N Engl J Med,* Vol. 336, No. 3, pp. 186-95

Charloux, A., Gronfier, C., Lonsdorfer-Wolf, E., Piquard, F., & Brandenberger, G. (1999). Aldosterone release during the sleep-wake cycle in humans. *Am J Physiol,* Vol. 276, No. 1 Pt 1, pp. E43-9, issn 0002-9513

Chung, S., Son, G. H., & Kim, K. (2011). Circadian rhythm of adrenal glucocorticoid: its regulation and clinical implications. *Biochim Biophys Acta,* Vol. 1812, No. 5, pp. 581-91, issn 0006-3002

Claustrat, B., Brun, J., Garry, P., Roussel, B., & Sassolas, G. (1986). A once-repeated study of nocturnal plasma melatonin patterns and sleep recordings in six normal young men. *J Pineal Res,* Vol. 3, No. 4, pp. 301-10, issn 0742-3098

Cohen, M. C., Rohtla, K. M., Lavery, C. E., Muller, J. E., & Mittleman, M. A. (1997). Meta-analysis of the morning excess of acute myocardial infarction and sudden cardiac death. *Am J Cardiol,* Vol. 79, No. 11, pp. 1512-6, issn 0002-9149

Cugini, P., Lucia, P., Di Palma, L., Re, M., Canova, R., Gasbarrone, L., & Cianetti, A. (1992). The circadian rhythm of atrial natriuretic peptide, vasoactive intestinal peptide, beta-endorphin and cortisol in healthy young and elderly subjects. *Clin Auton Res,* Vol. 2, No. 2, pp. 113-8, issn 0959-9851

Cugini, P., Lucia, P., Di Palma, L., Re, M., Leone, G., Battisti, P., Canova, R., *et al.* (1991). Vasoactive intestinal peptide fluctuates in human blood with a circadian rhythm. *Regul Pept,* Vol. 34, No. 3, pp. 141-8, issn 0167-0115

Cugini, P., Lucia, P., Scibilia, G., Di Palma, L., Cioli, A. R., Cianetti, A., Gasbarrone, L., *et al.* (1993). Lack of circadian rhythm of plasma concentrations of vasoactive intestinal peptide in patients with orthotopic heart transplants. *Br Heart J,* Vol. 70, No. 4, pp. 363-5, issn 0007-0769

Decousus, H. A., Croze, M., Levi, F. A., Jaubert, J. G., Perpoint, B. M., De Bonadona, J. F., Reinberg, A., *et al.* (1985). Circadian changes in anticoagulant effect of heparin infused at a constant rate. *Br Med J (Clin Res Ed),* Vol. 290, No. 6465, pp. 341-4, issn 0267-0623

Dominguez-Rodriguez, A., Abreu-Gonzalez, P., Garcia-Gonzalez, M., & Reiter, R. J. (2006). Prognostic value of nocturnal melatonin levels as a novel marker in patients with ST-segment elevation myocardial infarction. *Am J Cardiol,* Vol. 97, No. 8, pp. 1162-4, issn 0002-9149

Dominguez-Rodriguez, A., Abreu-Gonzalez, P., Garcia, M. J., Sanchez, J., Marrero, F., & de Armas-Trujillo, D. (2002). Decreased nocturnal melatonin levels during acute myocardial infarction. *J Pineal Res,* Vol. 33, No. 4, pp. 248-52, issn 0742-3098

Duncan, B., Moyna, N. M., Heller, G. V., McGill, C., Katten, D., Finta, L., Velusamy, M., *et al.* (2003). A 24-hour comparison of serum growth hormone concentrations in patients with heart failure versus healthy controls. *Pharmacotherapy,* Vol. 23, No. 2, pp. 147-52, issn 0277-0008

Durgan, D. J., & Young, M. E. (2010). The cardiomyocyte circadian clock: emerging roles in health and disease. *Circ Res,* Vol. 106, No. 4, pp. 647-58, issn 1524-4571

Eksik, A., Akyol, A., Norgaz, T., Aksu, H., Erdinler, I., Cakmak, N., Alper, A. T., *et al.* (2007). Circadian pattern of spontaneous ventricular tachyarrhythmias in patients with implantable cardioverter defibrillators. *Med Sci Monit,* Vol. 13, No. 9, pp. CR412-416, issn 1234-1010

Follenius, M., Weibel, L., & Brandenberger, G. (1995). Distinct modes of melatonin secretion in normal men. *J Pineal Res,* Vol. 18, No. 3, pp. 135-40, issn 0742-3098

Fukao, T., Lopaschuk, G. D., & Mitchell, G. A. (2004). Pathways and control of ketone body metabolism: on the fringe of lipid biochemistry. *Prostaglandins Leukot Essent Fatty Acids,* Vol. 70, No. 3, pp. 243-51, issn 0952-3278

Goldberg, R. J., Brady, P., Muller, J. E., Chen, Z. Y., de Groot, M., Zonneveld, P., & Dalen, J. E. (1990). Time of onset of symptoms of acute myocardial infarction. *Am J Cardiol,* Vol. 66, No. 2, pp. 140-4, issn 0002-9149

Grim, C., Winnacker, J., Peters, T., & Gilbert, G. (1974). Low renin, "normal" aldosterone and hypertension: circadian rhythm of renin, aldosterone, cortisol and growth hormone. *J Clin Endocrinol Metab,* Vol. 39, No. 2, pp. 247-56, issn 0021-972X

Guo, Y. F., & Stein, P. K. (2003). Circadian rhythm in the cardiovascular system: chronocardiology. *Am Heart J,* Vol. 145, No. 5, pp. 779-86, issn 1097-6744

Hartman, M. L., Faria, A. C., Vance, M. L., Johnson, M. L., Thorner, M. O., & Veldhuis, J. D. (1991). Temporal structure of in vivo growth hormone secretory events in humans. *Am J Physiol,* Vol. 260, No. 1 Pt 1, pp. E101-10, issn 0002-9513

Hastings, M. H., Reddy, A. B., & Maywood, E. S. (2003). A clockwork web: circadian timing in brain and periphery, in health and disease. *Nat Rev Neurosci,* Vol. 4, No. 8, pp. 649-61, issn 1471-003X

Hatcher, N. G., Atkins, N., Jr., Annangudi, S. P., Forbes, A. J., Kelleher, N. L., Gillette, M. U., & Sweedler, J. V. (2008). Mass spectrometry-based discovery of circadian peptides. *Proc Natl Acad Sci U S A,* Vol. 105, No. 34, pp. 12527-32, issn 1091-6490

Henning, R. J., & Sawmiller, D. R. (2001). Vasoactive intestinal peptide: cardiovascular effects. *Cardiovasc Res,* Vol. 49, No. 1, pp. 27-37, issn 0008-6363

Hobson, D. J., Rupa, P., Diaz, G. J., Zhang, H., Yang, M., Mine, Y., Turner, P. V., *et al.* (2007). Proteomic analysis of ovomucoid hypersensitivity in mice by two-dimensional difference gel electrophoresis (2D-DIGE). *Food Chem Toxicol,* Vol. 45, No. 12, pp. 2372-80, issn 0278-6915

Hrushesky, W. J., & Bjarnason, G. A. (1993). Circadian cancer therapy. *J Clin Oncol,* Vol. 11, No. 7, pp. 1403-17, issn 0732-183X

Heart and Stroke Foundation of Canada [HSFO]. Heart disease statistics. 7.27 2011, Available from: <http://www.heartandstroke.com/site/c.ikIQLcMWJtE/b.3483991/k.34A8/Statistics.htm#heartdisease>

Iitaka, C., Miyazaki, K., Akaike, T., & Ishida, N. (2005). A role for glycogen synthase kinase-3beta in the mammalian circadian clock. *J Biol Chem,* Vol. 280, No. 33, pp. 29397-402, issn 0021-9258

Imai, Y., Abe, K., Munakata, M., Sakuma, H., Hashimoto, J., Imai, K., Sekino, H., *et al.* (1990). Circadian blood pressure variations under different pathophysiological conditions. *J Hypertens Suppl,* Vol. 8, No. 7, pp. S125-32, issn 0952-1178

Innominato, P. F., Levi, F. A., & Bjarnason, G. A. (2010). Chronotherapy and the molecular clock: Clinical implications in oncology. *Adv Drug Deliv Rev,* Vol. 62, No. 9-10, pp. 979-1001, issn 1872-8294

Johnsen, S. A., Gungor, C., Prenzel, T., Riethdorf, S., Riethdorf, L., Taniguchi-Ishigaki, N., Rau, T., *et al.* (2009). Regulation of estrogen-dependent transcription by the LIM cofactors CLIM and RLIM in breast cancer. *Cancer Res,* Vol. 69, No. 1, pp. 128-36

Katz, F. H., Romfh, P., & Smith, J. A. (1975). Diurnal variation of plasma aldosterone, cortisol and renin activity in supine man. *J Clin Endocrinol Metab,* Vol. 40, No. 1, pp. 125-34

Lightman, S. L., James, V. H., Linsell, C., Mullen, P. E., Peart, W. S., & Sever, P. S. (1981). Studies of diurnal changes in plasma renin activity, and plasma noradrenaline, aldosterone and cortisol concentrations in man. *Clin Endocrinol (Oxf),* Vol. 14, No. 3, pp. 213-23, issn 0300-0664

Linsell, C. R., Lightman, S. L., Mullen, P. E., Brown, M. J., & Causon, R. C. (1985). Circadian rhythms of epinephrine and norepinephrine in man. *J Clin Endocrinol Metab,* Vol. 60, No. 6, pp. 1210-5, issn 0021-972X

Lockinger, A., Koberle, D., Konig, P. S., Saria, A., Herold, M., Cornelissen, G., & Halberg, F. (2004). Neuropeptide chronomics in clinically healthy young adults: circaoctohoran and circadian patterns. *Peptides,* Vol. 25, No. 4, pp. 533-42, issn 0196-9781

Lowrey, P. L., Shimomura, K., Antoch, M. P., Yamazaki, S., Zemenides, P. D., Ralph, M. R., Menaker, M., *et al.* (2000). Positional syntenic cloning and functional characterization of the mammalian circadian mutation tau. *Science,* Vol. 288, No. 5465, pp. 483-92, issn 0036-8075

Maemura, K., de la Monte, S. M., Chin, M. T., Layne, M. D., Hsieh, C. M., Yet, S. F., Perrella, M. A., *et al.* (2000). CLIF, a novel cycle-like factor, regulates the circadian oscillation of plasminogen activator inhibitor-1 gene expression. *J Biol Chem,* Vol. 275, No. 47, pp. 36847-51, issn 0021-9258

Manfredini, R., Boari, B., Gallerani, M., Salmi, R., Bossone, E., Distante, A., Eagle, K. A., *et al.* (2004). Chronobiology of rupture and dissection of aortic aneurysms. *J Vasc Surg,* Vol. 40, No. 2, pp. 382-8, issn 0741-5214

Martino, T. A., & Sole, M. J. (2009). Molecular time: an often overlooked dimension to cardiovascular disease. *Circ Res,* Vol. 105, No. 11, pp. 1047-61, issn 1524-4571

Martino, T. A., Tata, N., Bjarnason, G. A., Straume, M., & Sole, M. J. (2007). Diurnal protein expression in blood revealed by high throughput mass spectrometry proteomics and implications for translational medicine and body time of day. *Am J Physiol Regul Integr Comp Physiol,* Vol. 293, No. 3, pp. R1430-7, issn 0363-6119

Martino, T. A., Oudit, G. Y., Herzenberg, A. M., Tata, N., Koletar, M. M., Kabir, G. M., Belsham, D. D., *et al.* (2008). Circadian rhythm disorganization produces profound cardiovascular and renal disease in hamsters. *Am J Physiol Regul Integr Comp Physiol,* Vol. 294, No. 5, pp. R1675-83, issn 0363-6119

Martino, T. A., Tata, N., Simpson, J. A., Vanderlaan, R., Dawood, F., Kabir, M. G., Khaper, N., *et al.* (2011). The primary benefits of angiotensin-converting enzyme inhibition on cardiac remodeling occur during sleep time in murine pressure overload hypertrophy. *J Am Coll Cardiol,* Vol. 57, No. 20, pp. 2020-8, issn 1558-3597

Mehta, R. H., Manfredini, R., Hassan, F., Sechtem, U., Bossone, E., Oh, J. K., Cooper, J. V., *et al.* (2002). Chronobiological patterns of acute aortic dissection. *Circulation,* Vol. 106, No. 9, pp. 1110-5, issn 1524-4539

Minami, Y., Kasukawa, T., Kakazu, Y., Iigo, M., Sugimoto, M., Ikeda, S., Yasui, A., *et al.* (2009). Measurement of internal body time by blood metabolomics. *Proc Natl Acad Sci U S A,* Vol. 106, No. 24, pp. 9890-5, issn 1091-6490

Moller, M., Sparre, T., Bache, N., Roepstorff, P., & Vorum, H. (2007). Proteomic analysis of day-night variations in protein levels in the rat pineal gland. *Proteomics,* Vol. 7, No. 12, pp. 2009-18, issn 1615-9853

Muller, J. E., Tofler, G. H., & Stone, P. H. (1989). Circadian variation and triggers of onset of acute cardiovascular disease. *Circulation,* Vol. 79, No. 4, pp. 733-43, issn 0009-7322

Muller, J. E., Stone, P. H., Turi, Z. G., Rutherford, J. D., Czeisler, C. A., Parker, C., Poole, W. K., *et al.* (1985). Circadian variation in the frequency of onset of acute myocardial infarction. *N Engl J Med,* Vol. 313, No. 21, pp. 1315-22, issn 0028-4793

Orii, K. E., Fukao, T., Song, X. Q., Mitchell, G. A., & Kondo, N. (2008). Liver-specific silencing of the human gene encoding succinyl-CoA: 3-ketoacid CoA transferase. *Tohoku J Exp Med,* Vol. 215, No. 3, pp. 227-36, issn 1349-3329

Otto, M. E., Svatikova, A., Barretto, R. B., Santos, S., Hoffmann, M., Khandheria, B., & Somers, V. (2004). Early morning attenuation of endothelial function in healthy humans. *Circulation,* Vol. 109, No. 21, pp. 2507-10,

Paulin, D., & Li, Z. (2004). Desmin: a major intermediate filament protein essential for the structural integrity and function of muscle. *Exp Cell Res,* Vol. 301, No. 1, pp. 1-7,

Rajaratnam, S. M., & Arendt, J. (2001). Health in a 24-h society. *Lancet,* Vol. 358, No. 9286, pp. 999-1005, issn 0140-6736

Ralph, M. R., & Menaker, M. (1988). A mutation of the circadian system in golden hamsters. *Science,* Vol. 241, No. 4870, pp. 1225-7, issn 0036-8075

Reddy, A. B., Wong, G. K., O'Neill, J., Maywood, E. S., & Hastings, M. H. (2005). Circadian clocks: neural and peripheral pacemakers that impact upon the cell division cycle. *Mutat Res,* Vol. 574, No. 1-2, pp. 76-91, issn 0027-5107

Reddy, A. B., Karp, N. A., Maywood, E. S., Sage, E. A., Deery, M., O'Neill, J. S., Wong, G. K., *et al.* (2006). Circadian orchestration of the hepatic proteome. *Curr Biol,* Vol. 16, No. 11, pp. 1107-15, issn 0960-9822

Reppert, S. M., & Weaver, D. R. (2001). Molecular analysis of mammalian circadian rhythms. *Annu Rev Physiol,* Vol. 63, pp. 647-76, issn 0066-4278

Reppert, S. M., & Weaver, D. R. (2002). Coordination of circadian timing in mammals. *Nature,* Vol. 418, No. 6901, pp. 935-41, issn 0028-0836

Roenneberg, T., & Merrow, M. (2005). Circadian clocks - the fall and rise of physiology. *Nat Rev Mol Cell Biol,* Vol. 6, No. 12, pp. 965-71, issn 1471-0072

Roger, V. L., Go, A. S., Lloyd-Jones, D. M., Adams, R. J., Berry, J. D., Brown, T. M., Carnethon, M. R., *et al.* (2011). Heart disease and stroke statistics--2011 update: a report from the American Heart Association. *Circulation,* Vol. 123, No. 4, pp. e18-e209, issn 1524-4539

Scheer, F. A., Hilton, M. F., Mantzoros, C. S., & Shea, S. A. (2009). Adverse metabolic and cardiovascular consequences of circadian misalignment. *Proc Natl Acad Sci U S A,* Vol. 106, No. 11, pp. 4453-8, issn 1091-6490

Sole, M. J., & Martino, T. A. (2009). Diurnal physiology: core principles with application to the pathogenesis, diagnosis, prevention, and treatment of myocardial hypertrophy and failure. *J Appl Physiol,* Vol. 107, No. 4, pp. 1318-27, issn 1522-1601

Storch, K. F., & Weitz, C. J. (2009). Daily rhythms of food-anticipatory behavioral activity do not require the known circadian clock. *Proc Natl Acad Sci U S A,* Vol. 106, No. 16, pp. 6808-13, issn 1091-6490

Sumiyoshi, M., Kojima, S., Arima, M., Suwa, S., Nakazato, Y., Sakurai, H., Kanoh, T., *et al.* (2002). Circadian, weekly, and seasonal variation at the onset of acute aortic dissection. *Am J Cardiol,* Vol. 89, No. 5, pp. 619-23, issn 0002-9149

Surya, S., Symons, K., Rothman, E., & Barkan, A. L. (2006). Complex rhythmicity of growth hormone secretion in humans. *Pituitary,* Vol. 9, No. 2, pp. 121-5, issn 1386-341X

Takahashi, Y., Kipnis, D. M., & Daughaday, W. H. (1968). Growth hormone secretion during sleep. *J Clin Invest,* Vol. 47, No. 9, pp. 2079-90, issn 0021-9738

Tengattini, S., Reiter, R. J., Tan, D. X., Terron, M. P., Rodella, L. F., & Rezzani, R. (2008). Cardiovascular diseases: protective effects of melatonin. *J Pineal Res,* Vol. 44, No. 1, pp. 16-25, issn 0742-3098

Tofler, G. H., Gebara, O. C., Mittleman, M. A., Taylor, P., Siegel, W., Venditti, F. J., Jr., Rasmussen, C. A., *et al.* (1995). Morning peak in ventricular tachyarrhythmias detected by time of implantable cardioverter/defibrillator therapy. The CPI Investigators. *Circulation,* Vol. 92, No. 5, pp. 1203-8, issn 0009-7322

Tsuji, T., Hirota, T., Takemori, N., Komori, N., Yoshitane, H., Fukuda, M., Matsumoto, H., *et al.* (2007). Circadian proteomics of the mouse retina. *Proteomics,* Vol. 7, No. 19, pp. 3500-8, issn 1615-9853

Tuck, M. L., Stern, N., & Sowers, J. R. (1985). Enhanced 24-hour norepinephrine and renin secretion in young patients with essential hypertension: relation with the circadian pattern of arterial blood pressure. *Am J Cardiol,* Vol. 55, No. 1, pp. 112-5, issn 2-9149

Volterrani, M., Manelli, F., Cicoira, M., Lorusso, R., & Giustina, A. (2000). Role of growth hormone in chronic heart failure. Therapeutic implications. *Drugs,* Vol. 60, No. 4, pp. 711-9, issn 0012-6667

World Health Organization [WHO]. 2011. Cardiovascular Diseases. 7.27 2011, Available from: <http://www.who.int/cardiovascular_diseases/en/>

Willich, S. N., Levy, D., Rocco, M. B., Tofler, G. H., Stone, P. H., & Muller, J. E. (1987). Circadian variation in the incidence of sudden cardiac death in the Framingham Heart Study population. *Am J Cardiol,* Vol. 60, No. 10, pp. 801-6, issn 0002-9149

Yin, L., Wang, J., Klein, P. S., & Lazar, M. A. (2006). Nuclear receptor Rev-erbalpha is a critical lithium-sensitive component of the circadian clock. *Science,* Vol. 311, No. 5763, pp. 1002-5, issn 1095-9203

5

From Biomarker Discovery to Clinical Evaluation for Early Diagnosis of Lung Surgery-Induced Injury

Mei-Ling Tsai, Shu-Hui Chen,
Chih-Ching Chang and Ming-Ho Wu
*National Cheng Kung University,
Taiwan, Republic of China*

1. Introduction

Lung cancer is one of the most common cancers in the world (Chiang et al., 2010; Landis et al., 1998). Surgical removal of the tumor mass offers the best chance for a cure in patients with non-small-cell lung cancer. A tumor in stages I (confined to the lung without nodal or distant metastasis), II (involvement of only lymph nodes within the lung), and IIIA (involvement of nodes on the same side as the tumor) is considered potentially resectable for cure (Martini et al., 1995).

Based on tumor size and location, lung surgery is mainly divided into three types: wedge resection (removal of a small area in one lobe of either right or left lung), lobectomy (removal of one lobe from a right or left lung), and pneumonectomy (removal of an entire right or left lung). The mortality rate is much higher after pneumonectomy (61%) than lobectomy (35%) (Gunluoglu et al., 2011). Among the post-surgical factors, aberrant local inflammation and abnormal fluid drainage are the most common for inducing pulmonary edema. Excessive accumulation of fluid in the alveoli causes lung injury and hinders functional recovery. A severe form of acute lung injury results in acute respiratory distress syndrome. Sudden and life-threatening lung failure is the most detrimental factor in post-surgical mortality (Jordan et al., 2000).

With the progression from lung injury to acute respiratory distress syndrome, proinflammatory cytokines are increased, such as interleukin-1β (Donnelly et al., 1996; Geiser et al., 2001) and tumor necrosis factor-α (Tremblay et al., 2002). However, the production of vascular endothelial growth factor is reduced in the early stage but not altered in the late stage (Medfor & Millar, 2006). Interleukin-1β and tumor necrosis factor-α are further elevated in the sustained phase (Bhatia & Moochhala, 2004). The increases in proinflammatory cytokines are not correlated with injury-induced mortality (Donnelly et al., 1996). Corticosteroid which alters host inflammatory responses do not show beneficial effects in the early stage of acute respiratory distress syndrome (Kollef et al., 1995). Current reviews suggest that activation of inflammation-independent pathways in the early stage and inflammation-dependent pathways in the late stage contribute to the development of acute respiratory distress syndrome (Spragg et al., 2010; Bhatia & Moochhala, 2004).

To effectively reduce post-surgical mortality, early detection of acute respiratory distress syndrome may provide in-depth information for the design of management plans, including non-pharmacological therapies (Villar et al., 2011).

2. Proteomic analysis of bronchoalveolar lavage fluid in biomarker studies

To effectively identify the biomarkers of various lung diseases, bronchoalveolar lavage fluid from the lower airways and alveoli is collected for genomic or cytological analysis of cellular components (Meyer, 2007). This lung-specific fluid can be used for protein analysis. Identification of the non-cellular components in bronchoalveolar lavage fluid may provide valuable data for the early detection of acute lung injury.

2.1 Current advances in proteomic analysis of bronchoalveolar lavage fluid

In the past decades, over 100 human proteins or protein isoforms have been identified in bronchoalveolar lavage fluid from patients with various lung diseases (Wattiez et al., 1999; Lenz et al., 1993; Sadaghdar et al., 1992; Sabounchi-Schütt et al., 2001; Vesterberg et al., 2001). The major challenge today is to identify the lead proteins and validate the potential biomarkers (Turtoi et al., 2011a). To overcome this difficulty, integration of clinical studies with proteomic analysis of bronchoalveolar fluid is a potential solution (Turtoi et al., 2011b).

2.2 Sampling concern in proteomic analysis of bronchoalveolar lavage fluid

In clinical proteomics, the most difficult challenge before sample analysis is patient selection and sample collection (Apweiler et al., 2009). In the case of lung cancer patients, the major concern is to collect bronchoalveolar lavage fluid from those who may develop post-surgical lung edema. Although both bronchoalveolar lavage fluid and bronchial washings are collected using similar procedures, the former is collected from terminal alveoli after instilling more than 140 ml of sterile saline and the latter is collected from major airways after instilling less than 140 ml of saline. Because of the concern that excessive fluid accumulation may cause the complication of lung edema, bronchial washing is a better choice for conducting clinical proteomics.

2.3 Technical limitations in proteomic analysis of bronchoalveolar lavage fluid

In conventional proteomic analysis, two-dimensional gel electrophoresis provides good protein separation. However, it restricts the discovery of proteins with extreme biochemical properties such as size, isoelectric point, and solubility (Rabilloud, 2002). In comparison, one-dimensional gel electrophoresis provides easy comparison of banding patterns in protein profiling but is less efficient in protein separation. Moreover, the high salt concentration in the bronchoalveolar lavage fluid interferes with the resolution of protein separation to a lesser extent in one-dimensional gel electrophoresis (Plymoth, 2003).

2.4 Application of 1D gel with liquid chromatography and MS/MS in biomarker discovery

The rapid development of LC/MS/MS offers a better solution to one-dimensional gel electrophoresis (Schirle et al., 2003). A similar approach has been used to discover proteins with molecular weight greater than 100 kDa (such as α2-macroglobulin). The discovery of hundreds of proteins in bronchoalveolar lavage fluid demonstrates its feasibility in biomarker identification (Wu et al., 2005; Chang et al., 2007).

2.5 Sensitivity and specificity of the lead proteins after proteomic analysis

To accelerate the translation of biomarker discovery from bench to bedside, the development of techniques has been divided into 5 stages (Pepe et al., 2001). In Phase 1, potential biomarkers are discovered by various approaches, such as proteomic analysis. After the leads are identified by biochemical studies, measurable classifiers or outcomes are developed in Phase 2. Based on the analysis of their specificity and sensitivity, the cutoff point of the measurable outcome is determined and used in Phase 3. Based on patient history and clinical data, the number and nature of clinical cases is well defined in Phase 3. Suitable criteria for a clinical trial are determined in Phase 4. Phase 5 is a randomized trial to compare the specificity and sensitivity of the leads with those of current biomarkers in the market.

Today, the importance of sensitivity and specificity in biomarker selection has shifted proteomic studies from large-scale analysis to clinically-relevant validation. In addition to large-scale analysis in protein or metabolite identification (Mou et al., 2011; Huang et al., 2011), the leads are selected based on their sensitivity and specificity.

3. Translational study from protein identification to clinical application

The purpose of this study was to discover potential biomarkers for the early detection of acute respiratory distress syndrome. To avoid sampling-induced complications, bronchial washings from lung cancer patients before and after surgical therapy (lobectomy) were collected. To reduce population heterogeneity, cancer stage, hormonal variation, and tumor location were well-defined. Only patients older than 60 years, had right lung cancer at stages IA and IB, and agreed to receive right lung lobectomy were recruited.

Those patients who met the inclusion and exclusion criteria were selected as controls. The inclusion criteria were: defined cancer in any lobe of the right lung, non-smoker, age ≥60 years, elective operation, operation period <210 min, forced expiratory volume in 1 s (FEV1) >80%, and no prior major lung resection or thoracic irradiation. Exclusion criteria were: age <60 years, operation period >210 min, FEV1 <60%, emergency or urgent operation, and prior major lung resection or distant thoracic irradiation. Based on our criteria, 7 patients (5 females and 2 males with ages ranging between 61 and 77 years) were included as controls. A review was conducted from the medical records and prospective database. The study protocol was approved by the Human Medical Studies Committee at National Cheng Kung University Medical College Hospital. Informed consent was given by all participants or their legal guardians .

Prior to a large-scale analysis of proteins in bronchial washings, the protein profiles of washings from different compartments of the lungs before and after lobectomy were compared. In the right lung where tumor tissues were identified, no clear bands at molecular weights >75 kDa were found in washings collected before or after lobectomy. In the left lung, no clear bands at molecular weights >75 kDa were found in the washings collected before lobectomy. After lobectomy, more bands at molecular weights >75 kDa were found. The intensity of each band was much greater (Fig. 1). Similar patterns were found in all samples studied.

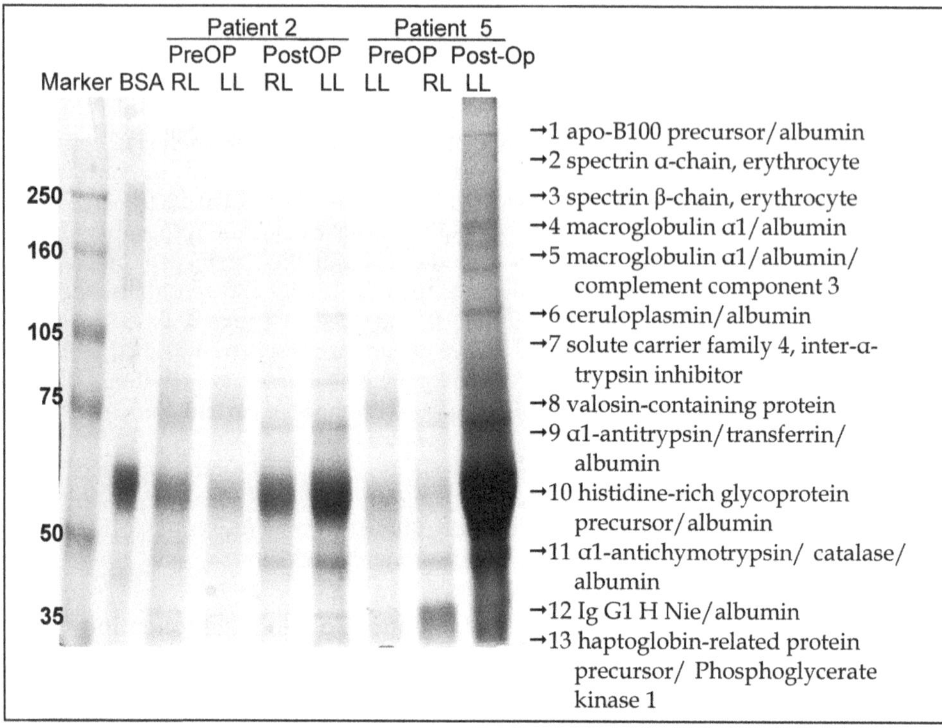

Fig. 1. Protein profiling of bronchial washes from right (RL) and left lungs (LL) from patients before (Pre-Op) and after (Post-Op) right lung lobectomy. Bovine serum albumin (BSA) was used a positive control because albumin was identified in various bands.

The banding pattern allowed us to hypothesize that the proteins at molecular weights >75 kDa are exuded into alveoli after surgery. One-dimensional gel electrophoresis coupled with LC/MS/MS allowed us to identify the proteins in 13 major bands. As listed in Table 1, 8 proteins had molecular weights >100 kDa, including α2-macroglobulin.

To test our hypothesis that protein exudation is surgery-dependent, the relative abundance of α1-antitrypsin (47 kDa) and α2-macroglobulin (162 kDa) in bronchial washings was measured by Western blot analysis. α1-antitrypsin was found in washings collected before and after lobectomy (data not shown) but α2-macroglobulin was only found after lobectomy (Fig. 2).

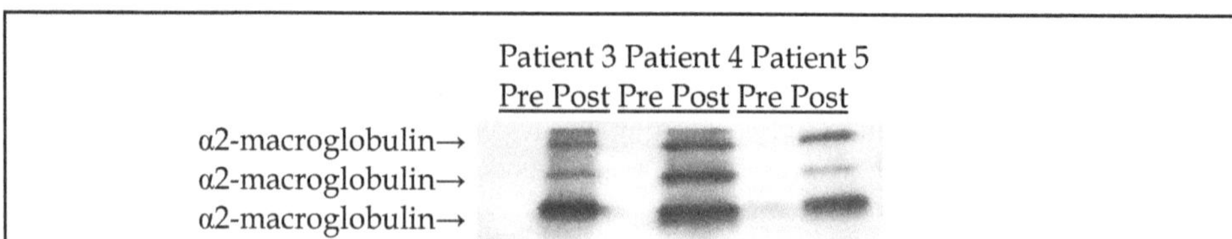

Fig. 2. Relative abundance of α2-macroglobulin in bronchial washings before (Pre) and after (Post) lobectomy.

No	GI number	Protein name	MW (kDa)	No. of matched peptides	Sequence coverage	Score
1	28780	apo-B100 precursor	516.384	6	2%	285
2	1174412	spectrin α chain, erythrocyte	280.904	5	3%	257
3	134798	spectrin β chain, erythrocyte	247.040	7	4%	291
4	179674	complement component C4A	194.365	5	4%	216
5	4557385	complement component 3 precursor	188.612	8	7%	451
6	224053	α2-macroglobulin	162.096	2	1%	86
7	4557485	ceruloplasmin (ferroxidase)	122.998	2	2%	91
8	1483187	inter-α-trypsin inhibitor family heavy chain-related protein (IHRP)	103.553	2	2%	82
9	4507021	solute carrier family 4, anion exchanger, member 1	102.017	3	4%	213
10	6005942	valosin-containing protein	89.962	4	9%	130
11	28592	serum albumin	71.351	12	19%	615
12	3287489	hsp89-α-δ-N	63.850	2	5%	85
13	4504489	histidine-rich glycoprotein precursor	60.527	2	4%	69
14	553788	transferrin	55.233	4	10%	177
15	69990	α1-glycoprotein	52.488	2	6%	84
16	386789	hemopexin precursor	52.266	2	2%	81
17	38408	immunoglobulin M heavy chain	50.135	3	9%	112
18	229601	Ig G1 H Nie	49.812	3	12%	127
19	177827	α1-antitrypsin	46.790	2	7%	67
20	10334547	immunoglobulin heavy chain	42.319	2	8%	57
21	123510	haptoglobin-related protein precursor	39.505	2	6%	114
22	121039	Ig gamma-1 chain C region	36.605	3	14%	118
23	121043	Ig gamma-2 chain C region	36.500	2	11%	55
24	183817	β-globin	19.209	4	33%	221
25	442753	Chain D, Hemoglobin Ypsilanti	16.021	5	50%	206

Table 1. Proteins identified in bronchial washings from the left lung of a patient receiving right lung lobectomy.

3.1 Vascular endothelial growth factor and lobectomy-induced inflammation

Since vascular endothelial growth factor is a potent inducer of vascular permeability (Lee, 2005) and its expression is positively correlated with inflammation-induced protein exudation and leukocyte infiltration (Chang et al., 2005), it is plausible to suggest that an increase in vascular endothelial growth factor is associated with surgery-induced protein exudation and leukocyte infiltration.

As shown in Table 2, the vascular endothelial growth factor level was positively correlated with total protein concentration ($y = 0.0025x + 1.0755$, $R^2 = 0.7359$, $P < 0.05$) and cell count ($y = 0.0696x - 0.6441$, $R^2 = 0.8463$, $P < 0.05$) but not with operation duration or PaO_2/FiO_2. The correlation analysis supported the hypothesis that the induction of vascular endothelial growth factor after surgery contributes to leukocyte infiltration and protein exudation.

Patient No	Operation duration (min)	PaO_2/FiO_2	Cell count (10^4 cells/ml)	Protein conc. (μg/ml)	VEGF (pg/ml)
1	152	270.167	2.5	0.641	162.80
2	191	202.500	67.0	3.412	613.68
3	234	435.000	100.0	4.826	1517.40
4	160	220.800	22.5	1.737	89.95
5	196	336.000	3.5	2.462	99.79
6	140	338.333	0.5	0.660	109.64
7	221	505.600	5.0	1.302	359.69

PaO_2: arterial partial pressure of oxygen; FiO_2: inspired oxygen fraction; PaO_2/FiO_2: oxygenation index

Table 2. Clinical data of 7 patients who received right lung lobectomy without complications

3.2 α2-macroglobulin and α1- antitrypsin in lobectomy-induced inflammation

The relative expression of α2-macroglobulin at bands 2, 4, and 5 from bronchial washings was correlated with protein concentration, leukocyte number, and the level of vascular endothelial growth factor (Fig. 3).

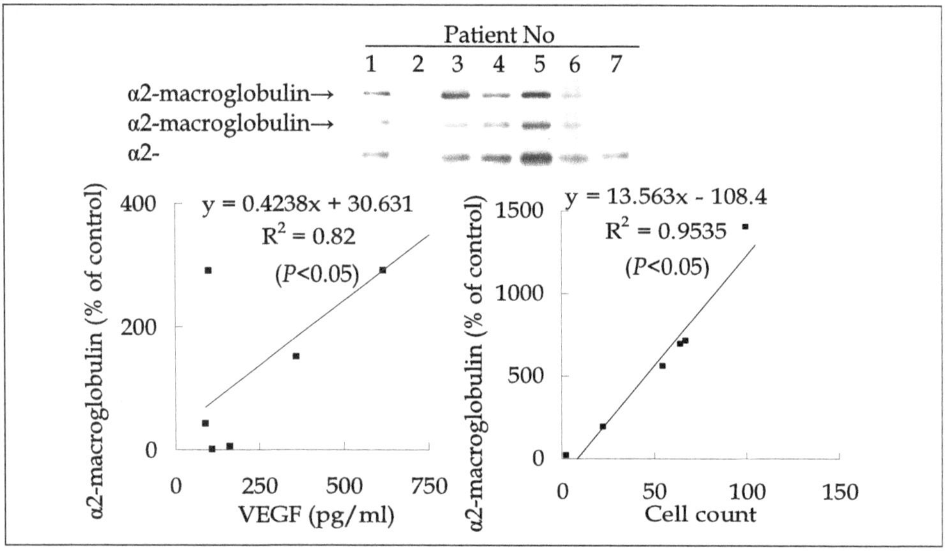

Fig. 3. Correlation analysis of α2-macroglobulin and VEGF/total cells in bronchial washings.

Likewise, the relative expression of α1-antitrypsin at bands 5, 7, and 8 from bronchial washing was positively correlated with protein concentration, leukocyte number, and the level of vascular endothelial growth factor (data not shown). These data supported our hypothesis that the increase of vascular endothelial growth factor after surgery facilitates leukocyte infiltration and the exudation of acute-phase proteins (such as α1-antitrypsin and α2-macroglobulin) into alveoli.

3.3 Characterization of α2-macroglobulin and α1-antitrypsin in lobectomized patients with acute respiratory distress syndrome

Based on the report of the joint American–European Consensus Conference, the acute respiratory distress syndrome is well defined as follows: bilateral infiltrates on frontal chest radiography, the absence of left atrial hypertension (pulmonary capillary wedge pressure <18 mmHg or no clinical signs of left ventricular failure), and severe hypoxemia with a PaO_2/FiO_2 ratio <200 mmHg (Bernard et al., 1994). Five patients who received lung surgery and met these criteria were studied.

3.3.1 Characterization of patients with acute respiratory distress syndrome

The group with lobectomy free of complications had levels of total protein and total leukocyte numbers in their bronchial washings similar to those who developed acute respiratory distress syndrome (P >0.05, Fig. 4). These data indicate that lung surgery induces inflammation (leukocyte infiltration and protein exudation) in the groups with and without the complication of acute respiratory distress syndrome. So, factors other than inflammation contribute to the development of this syndrome.

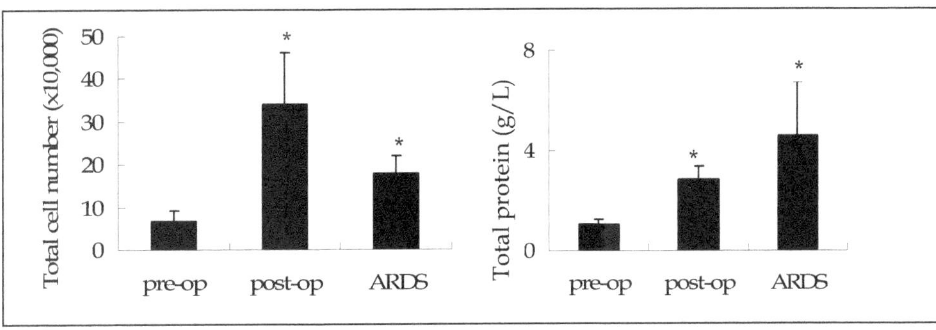

*Significant difference from pre-op.

Fig. 4. Total leukocyte number and protein concentration in patients before (pre-op) and after lobectomy (post-op) with no complication and those with acute respiratory distress syndrome (ARDS).

In lung cancer patients, an increase of vascular endothelial growth factor is positively associated with poor prognosis (P = 0.018; Han et al., 2001) but not with a worse postoperative year-survival rate (P = 0.0643; Liao et al., 2001). These reports are also consistent with our finding that the increase of vascular endothelial growth factor after lung surgery does not contribute to surgery-induced acute respiratory distress syndrome.

3.3.2 Protein profiling of bronchial washings from lobectomized patients with acute respiratory distress syndrome

Unlike patients with no complications, those with acute respiratory distress syndrome showed white or gray patches on the chest X-ray. In one-dimensional gel electrophoresis, the protein profiling of bronchial washings from patients without complications showed a much clearer banding pattern than those from patients with acute respiratory distress syndrome (Fig. 5). Eight bands from each gel were cut and subjected to LC/MS/MS for protein identification. No protein was identified in Lane 1. The most significant difference was that albumin appeared in almost every band of the samples from patients without complications but not in those with acute respiratory distress syndrome. In contrast, α1-antitrypsin was identified only in bands 6 and 7 from the group without complications but was found in bands 2, 3, 4, 5, 6, and 7 in the group with the complication (Fig. 5).

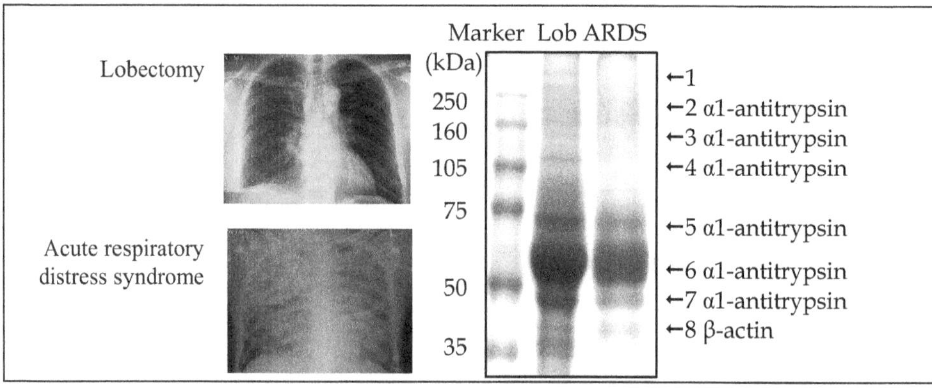

Fig. 5. Comparison of chest X-rays and protein profiling of bronchial washings in lobectomized patients with no complications (lobectomy, Lob) and those with acute respiratory distress syndrome (ARDS).

3.3.3 α2-macroglobulin and α1-antitrypsin in bronchial washings from lobectomized patients with acute respiratory distress syndrome

As shown in Fig. 6, both α2-macroglobulin and α1-antitrypsin were detected in bronchial washings after surgery.

After quantification, the total amounts of α2-macroglobulin at bands 2, 4, and 5 and α1-antitrypsin at bands 5, 7, and 8 did not show any statistical difference between the groups with and without complications. The most important finding was lower levels of α1-antytrypsin at bands 7 and 8 in the group without complications than the acute respiratory distress syndrome group (Fig. 6). It is likely that α1-antitrypsin variants at bands 5, 7, and 8 can be used as biomarkers for the early detection of acute respiratory distress syndrome.

In bronchial washings collected from the patients with acute respiratory distress syndrome, leukocyte number was not correlated with the total amounts of α2-macroglobulin or α1-antitrypsin. Our analyses again supported the notion that surgery-induced inflammation is not an important indicator in the early phase of acute respiratory distress syndrome.

It has been reported that α1-antitrypsin can be produced by lung epithelial cells (Venember et al., 1994) but α2-macroglobulin cannot. Our preliminary data confirmed the expression of

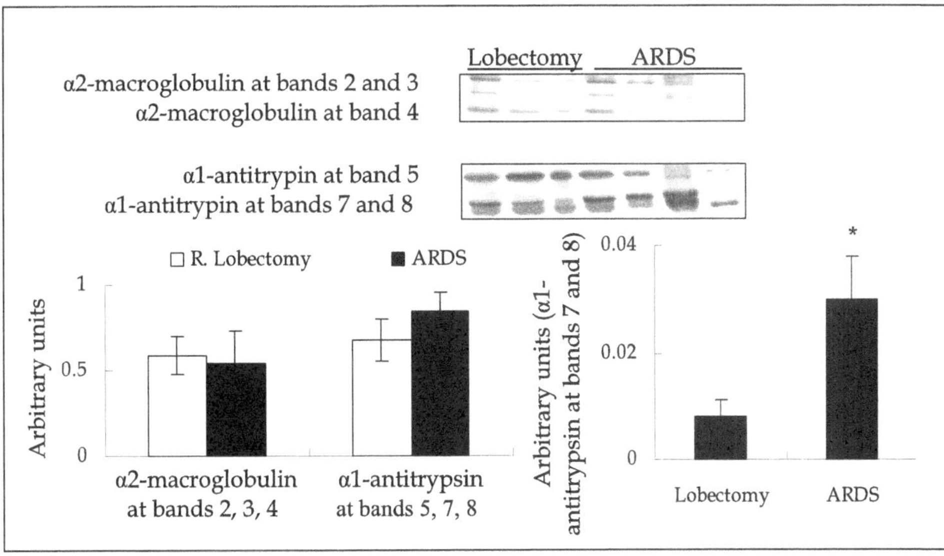

Fig. 6. Relative expression of α1-antitrypsin and α2-macroglobulin (macroglobulin) in the lobectomized group without complications (lobectomy) and in the group with acute respiratory distress syndrome (ARDS).

α1-antitrypsin in A549, a lung epithelial cell line. The changes in α1-antitrypsin variants could be due to functional changes in lung epithelial cells.

3.4 Specificity and sensitivity of α1-antitrypsin variants as potential biomarkers for acute respiratory distress syndrome

It is of importance to turn the relative expression of α1-antitrypsin in bronchial washings into a measurable outcome because only the measurable outcome is used to determine the cutoff value. Based on the cutoff value, sensitivity (the proportion of subjects who test positive among those with the condition) and specificity (the proportion of subjects who test negative among those without the condition) can be calculated.

As shown in Fig. 6, α1-antitrypsin variants at bands 7 (47 kDa) and 8 (40 kDa) had a lower abundance in the group without complications than the group with acute respiratory syndrome. To avoid variations in sample loading and the intensity in each calculation, the ratio of the expression of α1-antitrypsin at band 5 (70 kDa) to that at bands 7 and 8 was used as the measurable outcome. Based on this calculation, the cutoff value was 0.5. A ratio <0.5 was considered an indication of acute respiratory distress syndrome.

Table 3 shows the ratio for each patient from the complication-free group. Four out of 7 patients had a ratio <0.5. The specificity of α1-antitrypsin for true negative patients was 0.43 (3/7).

Table 4 shows the ratio for each patient from the complication group. Three out of 5 patients had a ratio <0.5. The sensitivity of α1-antitrypsin for true positive patients was 0.6 (3/5).

Patient No	Ratio of expression of α1-antitrypsin at band 5 to that at bands 7 and 8	Cutoff value = 0.5
1	0.000: 0.027	<0.5
2	0.043: 0.099	<0.5
3	0.019: 0.024	>0.5
4	0.017: 0.023	>0.5
5	0.018: 0.087	<0.5
6	0.000: 0.006	<0.5
7	0.042: 0.053	>0.5

Table 3. Ratio of the expression of α1-antitrypsin at band 5 to that at bands 7 and 8 in the lobectomized patients without acute respiratory distress syndrome.

Patient No	Ratio of expression of α1-antitrypsin at band 5 to that at bands 7 and 8	Cutoff value = 0.5
A	0.081: 0.177	<0.5
B	0.043: 0.199	<0.5
C	0.081: 0.086	>0.5
D	0.015: 0.040	<0.5
E	0.025: 0.048	>0.5

Table 4. Ratio of the expression of α1-antitrypsin at band 5 to that at bands 7 and 8 in lobectomized patients with acute respiratory distress syndrome.

3.5 Further improvement of specificity and sensitivity for detecting acute respiratory distress syndrome using dual biomarkers

As shown in Tables 3 and 4, the sensitivity of α1-antitrypsin variants for detecting acute respiratory distress syndrome (0.6) was better than the specificity (0.43). The major concern is how to optimize the cutoff value and improve the specificity. In table 3, patients 1 and 6 with ratios <0.5 showed the lowest values in cell counts and protein concentration. Meanwhile, the expression of α2-macroglobulin was almost undetectable, which indicates minor inflammation in the patients. The lower ratio of relative expression of α1-antitrypsin at band 5 to that at bands 7 and 8 was false-positive.

α1-antitrypsin was found in the lungs before and after surgery; α2-macroglobulin only occurred in the lungs after surgery. To avoid the lower levels of α1-antitrypsin variants which may create a false-positive result, α2-macroglobulin can be recruited as a second biomarker. The ratio of α1-antitrypsin variants was considered as a true result only when the sample expressed detectable α2-macroglobulin in bronchial washings. Accordingly, the specificity for true negative patients changed to 0.71 (5/7). The prediction for true negatives was improved.

4. From identification of leads to further validation using α2-macroglobulin and α1-antitrypsin variants as an example

After the discovery of potential biomarkers by proteomic analysis in this study, the first challenge was to identify the leads from the proteins discovered after developing a quick screening test. After Phase 1, the second challenge was to provide clear justification to optimize the cutoff values.

4.1 Contribution of this study to the discovery of biomarkers for detecting acute respiratory distress syndrome

Ideally, quantitative proteomic analysis should be used to reveal lobectomy-induced changes of all proteins in bronchial washings. However, the unique compartment of the lung allowed us to analyze exudate components which may not exist before surgery, such as α2-macroglobulin. Based on the important mechanism of surgery-induced inflammation in the early phase of lung injury, one-dimensional gel electrophoresis in this study was an easy and suitable tool to identify α2-macroglobulin as an indicator of vascular endothelial growth factor-mediated permeability.

The second contribution of this study was to take advantage of one-dimensional gel electrophoresis with pattern analysis to reveal the pattern changes of α1-antitrypsin between the groups with and without post-surgical complications. The difference found allowed us to identify α1-antytripsin variants as biomarkers for the early detection of acute respiratory distress syndrome.

4.2 Limitations of this study

In this study, α1-antitrypsin variants were considered as biomarkers for acute respiratory distress. No mechanistic data are provided to explain why and how the formation of α1-antitrypsin variants are related to the progression from surgery-induced inflammation to acute respiratory distress syndrome.

The association between α1-antitrypsin variants and infection was first reported in 2010 (Zhang et al., 2010). The decrease of the α1-antitrypsin variant at 130 kDa and the increase of the variant at 40 kDa is associated with human immunodeficiency virus-induced infection. Glycoproteomic analysis shows that changes in α1-antitrypsin variants may be due to a shift of glycosylation. In future, glycoproteomic analysis of α1-antitrypsin variants should be further explored.

Although the analysis of their specificity and sensitivity, the cutoff point of the measurable outcome, and criteria for patient selection are clearly and easily determined, the small number of clinical cases in this study limits the generalization of α2-macroglobulin and α1-antitrypsin as markers for acute respiratory distress syndrome. To use them as measurable biomarkers in Phase 3, it is necessary to increase the number and the complexity of clinical cases for further validation on whether the cutoff points determined are suitable for early diagnosis of acute respiratory distress syndrome.

One-dimensional gel electrophoresis does not offer a good way for protein separation. Comparative proteomic analysis only compares the intensity of each spot. These two approaches may our discovery of new proteins. The technology of stable isotope dimethyl labeling coupled with LC/MS/MS permits further quantification of specific peptides of each protein and provides a better quantification tool after one-dimensional electrophoresis (Huang et al., 2006). This approach then compensates for the limitation of one-dimensional gel electrophoresis.

5. Conclusion

Both inflammation -dependent and -independent mechanisms contribute to the progression from lung injury to acute respiratory distress syndrome. Stage-dependent changes in biomarkers allow us to monitor the progression of the diseases and develop new treatments in a stage-dependent manner.

In this study, α2-macroglobulin and α1-antitrypsin were positively correlated with vascular endothelial growth factor, clearly showing lobectomy-induced inflammation. The total amount of α1-macroglobulin can be used as a biomarker of increased vascular permeability in the lung. The severity of lobectomy-induced inflammation is similar to that of inflammation in acute respiratory distress syndrome but respiratory function becomes much worse in patients with the syndrome. Concomitantly, the patients with acute respiratory distress syndrome had lower levels of α1-antitrypsin at higher molecular weights and higher levels of α1-antitrypsin at lower molecular weights. Similarly, human immunodeficiency virus-induced infection is associated with the decreased abundance of α1-antitrypsin at higher molecular weights and the increased abundance of α1-antitrypsin at lower molecular weights (Zhang et al., 2010). Because α1-antitrypsin exists in lung epithelial cells (Venember et al., 1994), the changes of α1-antitrypsin variants in the patients with acute respiratory distress may reflect lung epithelial damage.

6. Acknowledgment

The authors appreciate the technical support of Shih-Hsin Ho, Hong-Da Wang, and Yan-Jie Chen, clinical sample collections by Drs. Jia-Ming Chang and Chang-Wen Chen, and grant support from the National Science Council, Taiwan (NSC-95-2314-B-006-125-MY2 and NSC-95-2323-B-006-004).

7. References

Apweilerm, R., Aslanidis, C., Deufel, T., Gerstner, A., Hansen, J., Hochstrasser, D., Kellner, R., Kubicek, M., Lottspeich, F., Maser, E., Mewes, HW., Meyer, HE., Müllner, S., Mutter, W., Neumaier, M., Nollau, P., Nothwang, HG., Ponten, F., Radbruch, A., Reinert, K., Rothe, G., Stockinger, H., Tárnok, A., Taussig, MJ., Thiel, A., Thiery, J., Ueffing, M., Valet, G., Vandekerckhove, J., Wagener, C., Wagner, O., & Schmitz, G. (2009). Approaching clinical proteomics: current state and future fields of application in cellular proteomics. *Cytometry A*, Vol.75, No.10, (October 2009), pp. 816-32, ISSN 1552-4930

Bernard, GR., Artigas, A., Brigham, KL., Carlet, J., Falke, K., Hudson, L., Lamy, M., Legall, JR., Morris, A., & Spragg, R. (1994). The American-European Consensus Conference on ARDS. Definitions, mechanisms, relevant outcomes, and clinical trial coordination. *American Journal of Respiratory and Critical Care Medicine*, Vol.149, No. 3 Pt 1, (March 1994), pp. 818-24, ISSN 1073-449X

Bhatia, M., & Moochhala, S. (2004). Role of inflammatory mediators in the pathophysiology of acute respiratory distress syndrome. *Journal of Patholog*, Vol.202, No.2, (February 2004), pp. 145-56, ISSN 1096-9896

Chang, CC., Chiu, HF., Wu, YS., Li, YC., Tsai, ML., Shen, CK., & Yang, CY. (2005). The induction of vascular endothelial growth factor by ultrafine carbon black contributes to the increase of alveolar-capillary permeability. *Environmental Health Perspectives*, Vol.113, No.4, (April 2005), pp.454-60, ISSN 0091-6765

Chang, CC., Chen, SH., Ho, SH., Yang, CY., Wang, HD., & Tsai, ML. (2007). Proteomic analysis of proteins from bronchoalveolar lavage fluid reveals the action mechanism of ultrafine carbon black-induced lung injury in mice. *Proteomics*, Vol.7, No.23, (December 2007), pp.4388-97, ISSN 1615-9861

Chiang, CJ., Chen, YC., Chen, CJ., You, SL., & Lai, MS. (2010). Cancer trends in Taiwan. Taiwan Cancer Registry Task Force. *Japanese Journal of Clinical Oncology*, Vol.40, No.10, (October 2010), pp.897-904, ISSN 0368-2811

Donnelly, SC., Strieter, RM., Reid, PT., Kunkel, SL., Burdick, MD., Armstrong, I., Mackenzie, A., & Haslett, C. (1996). The association between mortality rates and decreased concentrations of interleukin-10 and interleukin-1 receptor antagonist in the lung fluids of patients with the adult respiratory distress syndrome. *Annals of Internal Medicine*, Vol.125, No.3, (August 1996), pp.191–6, ISSN 1539-3704

Geiser, T., Atabai, K., Jarreau, PH., Ware, LB., Pugin, J., & Matthay, MA. (2001). Pulmonary edema fluid from patients with acute lung injury augments in vitro alveolar epithelial repair by an IL-1beta-dependent mechanism. *American Journal of Respiratory and Critical Care Medicine*, Vol.163, No.6, (May 2001), pp.1384–8, ISSN 1073-449X

Gunluoglu, MZ., Demir, A., Turna, A., Sansar, D., Melek, H., Dincer, SI., & Gurses, A. (2011). Extent of lung resection in non-small lung cancer with interlobar lymph node involvement. *Annals of Thoracic and Cardiovascular Surgery*, Vol.17, No.3, (June 2011), pp.229-35, ISSN 1341-1098

Han, H., Silverman, JF., Santucci, TS., Macherey, RS., d'Amato, TA., Tung, MY., Weyant, RJ., & Landreneau, RJ. (2001). Vascular endothelial growth factor expression in stage I non-small cell lung cancer correlates with neoangiogenesis and a poor prognosis. *Annals of Surgical Oncology*, Vol.8, No.1, (January-February 2001), pp.72-9, ISSN 1068-9265

Huang, SY., Tsai, ML., Tsai, CJ., Wu, JL., Hsu, JL., Ho, SH., & Chen SH. (2006). Quantitation of protein phosphorylation in pregnant rat uteri using stable isotope dimethyl labeling coupled with IMAC. *Proteomics*, Vol.6, No.6, (March 2006), pp.1-12, ISSN 1615-9861

Huang, Z., Lin, L., Gao, Y., Chen, Y., Yan, X., Xing, J., & Hang, W. (2011). Bladder cancer determination via two urinary metabolites: a biomarker pattern approach. (in press). *Molecular & Cellular Proteomics*, ISSN 1535-9484

Jordan, S., Mitchell, JA., Quinlan, GJ., Goldstraw, P., & Evans, TW. (2000). The pathogenesis of lung injury following pulmonary resection. *European Respiratory Journal,* Vol.15, No.4, (April 2000), pp.790-9, ISSN 1399-3003

Kollef, MH., & Schuster, DP. (1998). The acute respiratory distress syndrome. *The New England Journal of Medicine,* Vol.332, No.1, (January 1995), pp.27-37, ISSN 1533-4406

Landis, SH., Murray, T., Bolden, S., & Wingo, PA. (1998). Cancer statistics, *CA-a Cancer Journal for Clinicians.* Vol.48, No.1, (January-February 1998), pp.6-29, ISSN 1542-4863

Lee, YC. (2005). The involvement of VEGF in endothelial permeability: a target for anti-inflammatory therapy. *Current Opinion in Investigational Drugs,* Vol.6, No.11, (November 2005), pp.1124-30, ISSN 1472-4472

Lenz, AG, Meyer, B., Costabel, U., & Maier, K. (1993). Bronchoalveolar lavage fluid proteins in human lung disease: analysis by two-dimensional electrophoresis. *Electrophoresis,* Vol.14, No. 3, (March 1993), pp. 242-4, ISSN 1522-2683

Liao, M., Wang, H., Lin, Z., Feng, J., & Zhu, D. (2001). Vascular endothelial growth factor and other biological predictors related to the postoperative survival rate on non-small cell lung cancer. *Lung Cancer,* Vol.33, No.2-3, (August-September 2001), pp.125-32, ISSN 0169-5002

Martini, N., Bains, MS., Burt, ME., Zakowski, MF., McCormack, P., Rusch, VW., & Ginsberg, RJ. (1995). Incidence of local recurrence and second primary tumors in resected stage I lung cancer. *The Journal of Thoracic and Cardiovascular Surgery,* Vol.109, No.1, (January 1995), pp.120-9, ISSN 0022-5223

Medford, AR., & Millar, AB. (2006). Vascular endothelial growth factor (VEGF) in acute lung injury (ALI) and acute respiratory distress syndrome (ARDS): paradox or paradigm? *Thorax,* Vol.61, No.7, (July 2006), pp.621-6, ISSN 1468-3296

Meyer, KC. (2007). Bronchoalveolar lavage as a diagnostic tool. *Seminars in Respiratory and Critical Care Medicine,* Vol.28, No.5, (October 2007), pp.546-60, ISSN 1069-3424

Mou, Y., Xing, R., & Liu, C. (2011). Diagnosis of Gallbladder Cancer Using Matrix-Assisted Laser Desorption/Ionization Time-of-Flight Profiling. (in press). *The American Journal of the Medical Sciences,* ISSN 1538-2990

Pepe, MS., Etzioni, R., Feng, Z., Potter, JD., Thompson, M., Thornquist, M., Winget, M., & Yasui, Y. (2001). Phases of biomarker development for early detection of cancer. *Journal of the National Cancer Institute.* Vol.93, No.14, (July 2001), pp.1054–61. ISSN 1460-2105

Plymoth, A., Löfdahl, CG., Ekberg-Jansson, A., Dahlbäck, M., Lindberg, H., Fehniger, TE., & Marko-Varga, G. (2003). Human bronchoalveolar lavage: biofluid analysis with special emphasis on sample preparation. *Proteomics,* Vol.3, No.6, (June 2003), pp.962-72 ISSN 1615-9861

Rabilloud, T. (2002). Two-dimensional gel electrophoresis in proteomics: old, old fashioned, but it still climbs up the mountains. *Proteomics,* Vol.2, No.1, (January 2002), pp.3–10, ISSN 1615-9861

Sabounchi-Schütt, F., Aström, J., Eklund, A., Grunewald, J., & Bjellqvist, B. (2001). Detection and identification of human bronchoalveolar lavage proteins using narrow-range immobilized pH gradient DryStrip and the paper bridge sample application method. *Electrophoresis*, Vol.22, No.9, (May 2001), pp.1851–60, ISSN 1522-2683

Sadaghdar, H., Huang, ZB., & Eden, E. (1992). Correlation of bronchoalveolar lavage findings to severity of Pneumocystis carinii pneumonia in AIDS. Evidence for the development of high-permeability pulmonary edema. *Chest* Vol.*102*, No.1, (July 1992), pp.63-9. ISSN 1931-3543

Schirle, M., Heurtier, MA., & Kuster, B. (2003). Profiling core proteomes of human cell lines by one-dimensional PAGE and liquid chromatography-tandem mass spectrometry. *Molecular & Cellular Proteomics,* Vol.2, No.12, (December 2003), pp.1297-305, ISSN 1535-9484

Spragg, RG., Bernard, GR., Checkley, W., Curtis, JR., Gajic, O., Guyatt, G., Hall, J., Israel, E., Jain, M., Needham, DM., Randolph, AG., Rubenfeld, GD., Schoenfeld, D., Thompson, BT., Ware, LB., Young, D., & Harabin, AL. (2010). Beyond mortality: future clinical research in acute lung injury. *American Journal of Respiratory and Critical Care Medicine*, Vol.181, No.10, (May 2010), pp.1121-7, ISSN 1073-449X

Tremblay, LN., Miatto, D., Hamid, Q., Govindarajan, A., & Slutsky, AS. (2002). Injurious ventilation induces widespread pulmonary epithelial expression of tumor necrosis factor-alpha and interleukin-6 messenger RNA. *Critical Care Medicine,* Vol.30, No.8, (August 2002), pp.1693–1700, ISSN 1530-0293

Turtoi, A., De Pauw, E., & Castronovo, V. (2011a). Innovative proteomics for the discovery of systemically accessible cancer biomarkers suitable for imaging and targeted therapies. *American Journal of Pathology,* Vol.178, No.1, (January 2011), pp.12-8 ISSN 0002-9440

Turtoi, A., Dumont, B., Greffe, Y., Blomme, A., Mazzucchelli, G., Delvenne, P., Mutijima, EN., Lifrange, E., De Pauw, E., & Castronovo, V. (2011b). Novel Comprehensive Approach for Accessible Biomarker Identification and Absolute Quantification from Precious Human Tissues. *Journal of Proteome Research,* Vol.10, No.7, (July 2011), pp.3160-82, ISSN 1535-3907

Venembre, P., Boutten, A., Seta, N., Dehoux, MS., Crestani, B., Aubier, M., & Durand, G. Secretion of alpha 1-antitrypsin by alveolar epithelial cells. FEBS Letters, Vol.346, No.2-3, (June 1994), pp.171-4. ISSN 0014-5793

Vesterberg, O., Palmberg, L., & Larsson, K. (2001). Albumin, transferrin and alpha2-macroglobulin in bronchoalveolar lavage fluid following exposure to organic dust in healthy subjects. *International Archives of Occupational and Environmental Health,* Vol.74, No.4, (May 2001), pp.249-54, ISSN 1432-1246

Villar, J., Blanco, J., Zhang, H., & Slutsky, AS. (2011). Ventilator-induced lung injury and sepsis: two sides of the same coin? *Minerva Anestesiologica,* Vol.77, No.6, (June 2011), pp.647-53, ISSN 1827-1596

Wattiez, R., Hermans, C., Bernard, A., Lesur, O., & Falmagne, P. (1999). Human bronchoalveolar lavage fluid: two-dimensional gel electrophoresis, amino acid microsequencing and identification of major proteins. *Electrophoresis,* Vol.20, No.7, (June 1999), pp.1634-45, ISSN 1522-2683

Wu, J., Kobayashi, M., Sousa, EA., Liu, W., Cai, J., Goldman, SJ., Dorner, AJ., Projan, SJ., Kavuru, MS., Qiu, Y., & Thomassen, MJ. (2005). Differential proteomic analysis of bronchoalveolar lavage fluid in asthmatics following segmental antigen challenge. *Molecular & Cellular Proteomics,* Vol.4, No.9, (September 2005), pp.1251-64, ISSN 1535-9484

Zhang, L., Jia, X., Zhang, X., Cao, J., Yang, P., Qiu, C., Shen, Y., Ma, F., Liu, L., Sun, J., Shen, F., Yin, L., Liu, L., Yao, Y., & Lu, H. (2010). Alpha-1 antitrypsin variants in plasma from HIV-infected patients revealed by proteomic and glycoproteomic analysis. *Electrophoresis,* Vol.31, No.20, (October 2010), pp.3437-45, ISSN 1522-2683

Part 2

Proteomic Analysis of Protein Functions

6

Proteomic Approaches to Unraveling the RB/E2F Regulatory Pathway

Jone Mitxelena[1], Nerea Osinalde[2], Jesus M. Arizmendi[2], Asier Fullaondo[1] and Ana M. Zubiaga[1]
[1]*Dept. Genetics, Physical Anthropology and Animal Physiology*
University of the Basque Country, UPV/EHU, Bilbao
[2]*Dept. Biochemistry and Molecular Biology,*
University of the Basque Country, UPV/EHU, Bilbao
Spain

1. Introduction

Correct entry into and progression through the cell cycle require an intact RB/E2F pathway, and its deregulation is now considered a general hallmark of cancer (Nevins 2001). Pioneer work in the early 90's showed that E2F activity is controlled through the temporal association of E2F factors with Retinoblastoma (RB) tumor suppressor proteins (pRB, p107 and p130), also called pocket proteins (Bandara & La Thangue 1991; Chellappan et al. 1991). The additional finding that RB activity is regulated through phosphorylations by cyclin dependent kinases (CDKs) provided the groundwork for the current model of cell cycle control (Weinberg 1995). According to this model, non-phosphorylated RB binds to E2F in G0/G1, leading to the repression of E2F target genes. Subsequent phosphorylation of RB by CDKs in mid-to late G1 disrupts its association with E2F. As a result, free E2F triggers the expression of target genes necessary for entry into and progression through the cell cycle (Burkhart & Sage 2008). This pathway is thought to be disrupted in most human cancers, either by activation of positively acting components such as G1 cyclins and CDKs, or the inactivation of negatively acting components such as RB and cyclin kinase inhibitors (Nevins 2001). The predicted consequence of deficient RB-mediated regulation is that E2F activity is constantly unleashed from the inhibitory effects of RB (DeGregori & Johnson 2006; Dimova & Dyson 2005; Iaquinta & Lees 2007).
Mammalian E2F is a family of related factors (E2F1-8), originally discovered for their pivotal role in transcriptional regulation of genes associated with DNA replication and G1/S progression (Attwooll et al. 2004; Trimarchi & Lees 2002). More recently, microarray expression profiling analyses and ChIP-chip analyses (chromatin immunoprecipitation coupled to microarray technology) in cells overexpressing individual E2Fs have revealed that the transactivation function of these factors exceeds beyond G1/S transition regulation. In fact, E2Fs regulate a wide spectrum of genes with diverse biological functions, including regulation of apoptosis, autophagy, mitosis, chromosome organization, macromolecule metabolism, or differentiation (Ma et al. 2002; Muller et al. 2001; Polager et al. 2008; Ren et al. 2002; Weinmann et al. 2002; Young et al. 2003). Thus, the role of E2F transcription factors in cellular physiology is probably more complex than it was originally thought to be.

Traditionally, the mammalian E2F family has been divided into "activators" (E2F1-3) and "repressors" (E2F4-8). However, recent *in vivo* data have questioned this oversimplified classification. Indeed, accumulating evidence suggests that most E2Fs can function both as activators as well as repressors, depending on the cellular context (Balciunaite et al. 2005; Iglesias et al. 2004; Infante et al. 2008; Lang et al. 2001; Lee et al. 2011; Ma et al. 2002; Morris et al. 2000; Muller et al. 2001; Polager et al. 2008; Young et al. 2003). Likewise, both oncogenic and tumor suppressor properties have been assigned to these factors (DeGregori & Johnson 2006; Johnson & DeGregori 2006). The mechanisms underlying this bimodal impact of individual E2Fs, and their implication in human cancer development remain to be elucidated. This is a particularly relevant point that needs to be addressed, since strategies based on E2F biology are being devised for the development of anticancer therapies (Kaelin, Jr. 2003). An additional level of complexity in the understanding of E2F function *in vivo* derives from the considerable functional overlap existing among several E2F members (Chen et al. 2009a; DeGregori & Johnson 2006). Nonetheless, the characterization of mouse models lacking individual E2Fs has revealed that these factors play unique roles in development, tissue homeostasis and tumor formation (Chen et al. 2009a; DeGregori & Johnson 2006; Trimarchi & Lees 2002).
Functional specificity of individual E2F factors is thought to be established through the regulation of distinct sets of target genes. In fact, there is growing evidence that this specificity is achieved by interaction of E2Fs with other proteins or by post-translational modifications (PTMs) on E2Fs or E2F-containing complexes. Much of this evidence has been gathered through proteomic approaches such as yeast two-hybrid screening, two-dimensional electrophoresis (2-DE) followed by mass spectrometry (MS) or shotgun proteomics (Figure 1). In this review, the application of proteomics in the study of RB/E2F regulatory pathway is summarized. Results derived from these experiments are expanding our current understanding of the RB/E2F biology in several important ways. They are piecing together the interactions within macromolecular complexes that regulate transcription of E2F target genes. Furthermore, they are helping define the mechanisms underlying RB/E2F-dependent control of cellular physiology and pathology.

2. Identification of proteins that interact with E2Fs

It has long been recognized that E2F activity is regulated through the association of E2F factors with specific protein partners. In fact, E2F1, the founder member of the family, was first identified as a sequence-specific DNA-binding activity that co-precipitated with RB (Chittenden et al. 1991). Recent development of non-hypothesis driven proteomic approaches has allowed a more extensive analysis of protein-protein interactions in the E2F field. Several methods have been successfully applied in the identification of RB/E2F interacting partners, in particular, yeast two-hybrid screenings and affinity purification coupled to MS.

2.1 Genome-wide yeast two-hybrid interaction screening

The yeast two-hybrid method is one of the most widely used methods for mapping protein-protein interactions. In this method, the "bait" protein is typically expressed in yeast as a chimeric protein fused to the DNA-binding domain of a known transcription factor (usually *Gal4*). All other "target" proteins that the bait protein is going to be screened against are expressed within the cell fused to the activation domain of this same transcription factor.

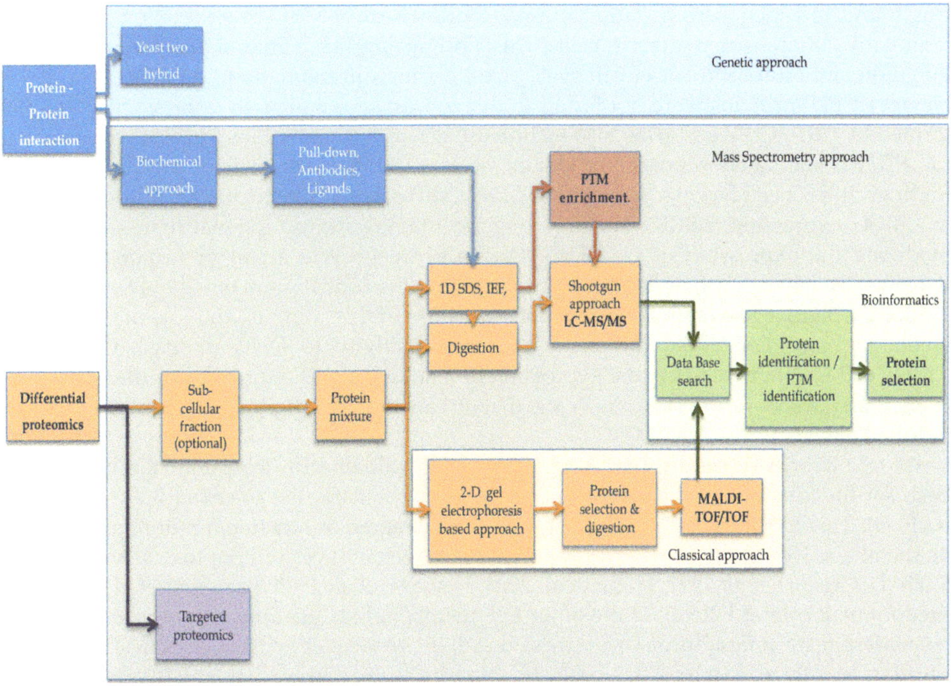

Fig. 1. A schematic diagram showing proteomic approaches to analyzing regulatory signaling pathways.

The interaction between the bait and target proteins brings into close proximity the DNA binding and activation domains of the transcription factor, resulting in the activation of a reporter gene (Fields & Song 1989). Given that the conditions applied in this methodology are not physiological, some of the detected interactions may not represent true interactions. Consequently, this experimental system is thought to yield a high false positive rate. Consequently, interactions detected by this system need to be further validated in an appropriate physiological system. Despite the mentioned drawbacks, it is also true that the yeast two-hybrid interaction screening provides a method to scrutinize protein-protein interactions within living cells, whereas other approaches measure protein interactions after the complexes have been removed from the cellular environment.

Interaction proteomics has been helpful in exploring the intricate macromolecular interactions established by RB and E2F for the regulation of gene expression. Work from many laboratories has shown that RB mediates transcriptional repression through the recruitment of a large number of co-repressors, resulting in an alteration of chromatin conformation that hinders transcription. Most RB/E2F co-repressors, including histone deacetylases (HDAC1-3), nucleosome remodeling proteins (BRG1), DNA methyl transferases (DNMT1) or RBP1 have been identified through hypothesis-driven classical biochemical approaches (Brehm et al. 1998; Luo et al. 1998; Magnaghi-Jaulin et al. 1998). Interestingly, HBP1 and CtIP/CtBP co-repressors were discovered by yeast two-hybrid screening analyses using the pocket protein p130 as the bait (Meloni et al. 1999a; Tevosian et al. 1997). HBP1, a tumor suppressor member of the HMG family of transcription factors, was found to function as a transcriptional repressor of N-MYC in association with RB in terminally differentiated muscle cells. This finding implies a role of this complex in the initiation and establishment of cell cycle arrest during differentiation (Tevosian et al. 1997). However, E2F proteins were not found in this repressor complex. By contrast, the complex formed by CtIP/CtBP and p130 also included E2F1, and provided an additional mechanism for RB/E2F-mediated repression (Meloni et al. 1999b). In agreement with the original findings, it has been recently shown that CtIP/CtBP plays a transcriptional co-repressor role in ZBRK1 expression. ZBRK1 is a zinc finger-containing transcriptional repressor that can modulate the expression of GADD45A to induce cell cycle arrest in response to DNA damage (Liao et al. 2010). It has been proposed that the contribution of RB to DNA damage-induced growth arrest may depend on the formation of this complex and loss of CtIP/CtBP–mediated repression could affect the cellular sensitivity to DNA damage. Conversely, CtIP/CtBP is able to activate the expression of a subset of E2F-target genes after its release from RB-imposed repression, implying that it can also function as an activator in other cellular contexts (Liu & Lee 2006).

Yeast two-hybrid screening has been particularly valuable to delve into the mechanistic basis for the functional specificity of E2F factors, particularly the so-called E2F "activators" (E2F1-3). This E2F subfamily exhibits a significant degree of functional redundancy among its members. However, E2F1 appears to be a stronger inducer of apoptosis than E2F2 and E2F3 (DeGregori et al. 1997; Hong et al. 2008; Kowalik et al. 1998; Lazzerini et al. 2005). The predominant role of E2F1 over the other E2F members in triggering apoptosis is thought to be conferred by unique protein partners that E2F1 associates with. The critical domain to specifically induce apoptosis has been shown to lie in the marked box of E2F1 (Hallstrom & Nevins 2003). Taking advantage of this knowledge, the E2F1 marked box has been used by Hallstrom and Nevins as the bait to screen for protein partners that could mediate E2F1-dependent apoptosis. JAB1 (c-JUN activating-binding protein) was identified as an E2F1-specific binding protein that functions synergistically with E2F1 to induce apoptosis coincident with an induction of p53 protein accumulation (Hallstrom & Nevins 2006). Interestingly, JAB1 association appears to regulate exclusively the apoptotic role of E2F1, as cell cycle entry is not affected by this E2F protein partner. In addition to JAB1, several more E2F1-interacting proteins were detected in this screen (Table 1), although their functional relevance in E2F1 function remains to be determined.

Remarkably, the E2F marked box has emerged as an important domain for mediating protein interactions that could dictate specificity of promoter recognition. For example, E2F2 and E2F3, but not E2F1 or E2F4, have been shown to interact specifically with RYBP (Ring-1 and YY1-binding protein) through their marked box. RYBP recruits these E2Fs to target promoters containing YY1 binding sites such as the CDC6 promoter. It has been proposed that the formation of an E2F2/3-RYBP-YY1 complex would facilitate the timely activation of CDC6 (Schlisio et al. 2002). An independent yeast two-hybrid screen with E2F3 as the bait discovered TFE3 (an E-box binding factor) as a protein that specifically interacts with E2F3. This association, which is dependent on the marked box of E2F3, facilitates transcriptional activation of the p68 subunit gene of DNA Polα (Giangrande et al. 2003). Furthermore, this screen also yielded several more proteins that bound specifically the marked box of E2F3 (Table 1). Some of these proteins, such as CBP, RYBP or MGA had previously been shown to interact with E2Fs (Morris et al. 2000; Ogawa et al. 2002; Schlisio et al. 2002; Trouche et al. 1996), providing a strong validation of the screen. By contrast, E2F1, E2F2 and E2F4 are unable to bind TFE3 or to activate transcription of p68. Based on the characterization of all

E2F member	Interacting Protein	Function	Reference
E2F1	JAB1	Promotes apoptosis	Hallstron & Nevins 2006
	EAPP	Activates transcription of TK and represses transcription of p14^{ARF}. Promotes proliferation	Novy et al. 2005
	SKIP, CBP, TEF-5, B-MYB, MGA	n.d.	Giangrande et al. 2003
	MCRS1, E1F1, FHOD1, FLNA, SUI1, A-FABP, MX1, RNF2, PRMT3, RANBP9	n.d.	Hallstron & Nevins 2006
E2F2	RYBP	Activates transcription of CDC6	Schlisio et al. 2002
	B-MYB	n.d.	Giangrande et al. 2003
	ALIEN	n.d.	Escher et al. 2007
	EAPP	n.d.	Novy et al. 2005
E2F3	RYBP	Activates transcription of CDC6	Schlisio et al. 2002
	TFE3	Activates the p68 subunit gene of DNA Polα	Giangrande et al. 2003
	RXR-BP, WNK1, PKI-B, SKIP, RYBP, CBP, TEF-5, B-MYB, MGA, SPIB	n.d.	Giangrande et al. 2003
	HSP86, A-FABP, MX1, RNF2, PRMT3, RANBP9	n.d.	Hallstron & Nevins 2006
	ALIEN	n.d.	Escher et al. 2007
	EAPP	n.d.	Novy et al. 2005
E2F4	ALIEN	n.d.	Escher et al. 2007
	MGA	n.d.	Giangrande et al. 2003
E2F5	ALIEN	n.d.	Escher et al. 2007
E2F6	ALIEN	n.d.	Escher et al. 2007

Table 1. E2F-specific binding partners identified through proteomic approaches. n.d.: not determined

these interactions it has been proposed that transcriptional regulation of specific E2F target genes can only be achieved when relevant interacting proteins act jointly forming a functional complex on the promoter (Freedman et al. 2009). Therefore, the unique marked box of each individual E2F factor appears to play a pivotal role in determining the specificity of interaction.

Other proteins exhibit E2F-binding activity independently of the marked box, allowing the mapping of distinct functional domains within the E2Fs. A yeast two-hybrid interaction screen with the amino-terminal region of E2F1 comprising the NLS but lacking the marked box led to the cloning of EAPP (E2F-associated phosphoprotein) (Novy et al. 2005). EAPP appears to potentiate the proliferative functions of E2F1 in several ways. It enhances the transcription of growth-correlated E2F-target genes like thymidine kinase whereas it represses the expression of the tumor suppressor p14^{ARF}, an E2F1-target gene that can mediate E2F-induced apoptosis. Of note, EAPP can also interact with E2F2 and E2F3a through their amino-terminal regions (Novy et al. 2005). Consequently, EAPP could mediate proliferation related redundant functions of the E2F "activators" through binding to their well-conserved N-terminal region.

E2F6 together with E2F7 and E2F8 have features that set them apart from other members of the E2F family. These factors lack RB-binding and transactivation domains, and pocket proteins are thought not to complex with E2F6-8 (Cartwright et al. 1998; Gaubatz et al. 1998; Trimarchi et al. 1998). Thus, there is a particular interest in identifying the proteins that interact with these non-classical E2F members and determining their mechanism for transcriptional regulation of target genes. Two independent yeast two-hybrid analyses have described distinct interactions between E2F6 and components of the Polycomb Group (PcG), known mammalian transcriptional repressors (Bunker & Kingston 1994). In the first study, E2F6 was shown to associate with members of the PRC1 complex, including some PcG proteins (RING1, MEL-18, MPH1, and BMI1) as well as RYBP (Trimarchi et al. 2001). The second screening identified the PcG protein EPC1 as a novel E2F6-binding protein, in complex with EZH2 and SIN3B (Attwooll et al. 2005). In both cases, the association of E2F6 with PcG proteins could account for an RB-independent mechanism for the recruitment of repressive complexes to E2F6 target promoters and the consequent transcriptional repression (Trimarchi et al. 2001). It should be mentioned that this work did not detect an interaction between RYBP and E2F2 or E2F3, as shown by Schlisio and co-workers (Schlisio et al. 2002). The basis for this discrepancy is not clear, but could reflect methodological differences. However, the common ability of E2F2, E2F3 and E2F6 to interact with RYBP, suggests that E2F2 and E2F3 may be able to repress a subset of target genes by RB-independent mechanisms.

2.2 Affinity purification coupled to mass spectrometry

Identification of protein-protein interactions is becoming increasingly easier since the extraordinary advances that have taken place in recent years in mass spectrometry (MS). Affinity purification coupled to mass spectrometry is currently the preferred method for screening protein-protein interactions, owing to the sensitivity, specificity and reliability of this approach (Gavin et al. 2002; Ho et al, 2002; Krogan et al. 2006; Sellers et al. 1998). In contrast to classical biochemical methods, MS-based proteomics is a discovery or explorative non-hypothesis driven science. However, it should be noted that the identification of protein complexes remains a significant challenge. This is because many interactions are transient and can be easily lost during sample preparation. Additionally, many proteins are expressed at low levels, and it remains difficult to purify them. In fact, isolating the protein complex is the most critical step in determining the success of a proteomic analysis. The most widely used method for protein complex isolation is antibody-based immunoprecitation (IP), although MS is also compatible with other affinity purification methods used to map protein-protein interactions, such as oligoprecipitation and tagged protein precipitation by affinity ("protein pull-down")(Gavin et al. 2002; Meng et al. 2006).

A wide range of RB/E2F partners have been identified to date by MS. Remarkably, the discovered proteins are mainly involved in transcriptional repression, which highlights the critical role of the RB/E2F network in the timely suppression of target gene expression. Combining immunological methods with an uncommon mass spectrometric technique named SELDI (surface-enhanced laser desorption/ionization)(Lehmann et al. 2005), co-repressor ALIEN was identified in E2F1 containing endogenous protein complexes (Escher et al. 2007). Additional co-immunoprecipitation experiments revealed specific interactions of ALIEN with E2F2 through E2F6. ALIEN is able to repress E2F1 transcriptional activity when tethered to target promoters containing E2F binding sites (Tenbaum et al. 2007). The mechanism for this repressive activity remains undetermined. An RB-dependent process has been proposed, based on the finding that ALIEN interacts with pRB/p107 and HDAC (Escher et al. 2007). However, ALIEN-mediated co-repression is also evident in cells lacking functional RB (Tenbaum et al. 2007).

Affinity purification coupled to MS analysis has been particularly useful in the identification of native RB/E2F transcriptional repressor complexes (Table 2). They were firstly characterized in *Drosophila melanogaster* (Korenjak et al. 2004). Subsequently, homologous complexes were identified in other animal species, including *Caenorhabditis elegans* and human (Harrison et al. 2006; Litovchick et al. 2007), emphasizing the importance of this pathway. Before the application of proteomic methods, a wide assortment of chromatin-modifying and binding complexes had been implicated in RB-mediated repression (Frolov & Dyson 2004). However, it is unclear which of the many reported interactions are biologically meaningful, due to the non-physiological methods employed for the screening. In an effort to characterize native RB/E2F repressor complexes in *Drosophila*, Brehm´s group took advantage of the relative simplicity of the *Drosophila* dRB/E2F network, consisting of two pocket proteins, RBF1 and RBF2, and two E2F proteins, dE2F1 and dE2F2 that heterodimerize with a common partner, dDP. By classical chromatography followed by MS analysis of the resulting fractions, they isolated an RBF multisubunit complex, termed dREAM (Korenjak et al. 2004), which contains RBF1/2, dE2F2, dDP, dMyb and dMyb-interacting proteins (Mip/TWIT, CAF1p55, Mip40 and Mip120). Interestingly, an independent analysis of Myb-associated proteins, involving affinity chromatography and DALPC mass spectrometry analysis (direct analysis of large protein complexes) resulted in the identification of a similar complex in *Drosophila* that was called Myb–MuvB complex (Lewis et al. 2004).

In agreement with a role in transcriptional repression, the identified complexes localize to transcriptionally silent sites on polytene chromosomes and mediate stable repression of a specific set of E2F targets that have sex- and differentiation-specific expression patterns. The mechanism by which these repressive complexes mediate the silencing of their target genes has been controversial, and enzymatic and non-enzymatic modes of repression have been suggested (Korenjak et al. 2004; Lewis et al. 2004). The finding that dREAM only binds deacetylated histone H4, characteristic of repressed chromatin, suggests that dREAM complexes perform their repressive function through binding unmodified nucleosomes and therefore protecting them from activating modifications (Korenjak et al. 2004). This hypothesis was further supported by the identification of histone deacetylase Rpd3, the HDAC1 homolog in *Drosophila*, associated with the repressor complex (Lewis et al. 2004). Strikingly, at least seven, and possibly all dREAM subunits are related to *C. elegans* synMuv class B genes (Fay & Han 2000). These proteins encompass the DRM complex, genetically resolved by Harrison and collaborators, which controls vulval differentiation in the worm (Harrison et al. 2006). The similarity between the worm DRM and the fly dREAM and Myb–

E2F member	Complex	Function	Reference
Drosophila E2F2	dREAM: RBF1/2, dDP,dMyb, Mip/TWIT,CAF1p55, Mip40 , Mip120, Rpd3	Transcriptional repression of developmentally regulated genes	Korenjak et al. 2004
	Myb-MuvB: RBF1/2, dDP,dMyb, Mip40, Caf1p55, Mip130 , Mip120, dLin52, Rpd3, L(3)MBT	Transcriptional repression of developmentally regulated genes	Lewis et al. 2004
E2F1	CtIP/CtBP, p130	Repression of ZBRK1. RB-dependent growth arrest after DNA damage	Meloni et al. 1999 Liao Ching-Chun, 2010
	ALIEN, pRB/p107, CDK2	Repression of E2F1 expression and cellular proliferation	Escher et al. 2007 Tenbaum et al. 2007
E2F4/5	DREAM: p130, LIN9, LIN37, LIN52, LIN54 LIN53/RBBP4	Transcriptional repression of cell cycle genes in G0	Litovchick et al. 2007
E2F6	Complex: RYBP, RING1, MEL-18, MPH1, BMI1	not determined	Trimarchi et al. 2001
	Complex: EPC1, EZH2, SIN3B	Target gene repression in proliferating cells	Attwoll et al. 2005
	Complex: MGA, MAX RING1/2, MBLR, h-l(3)MBT-like, YAF2, HP1γ	Target gene repression in quiescent cells	Ogawa et al. 2002

Table 2. Multiprotein complexes encompassing E2F factors identified by proteomic approaches.

MuvB complexes indicates that the DRM complex likely acts in transcriptional repression of E2F targets, and implies a remarkable conservation in the mechanism of pocket protein function across species.

An integration of proteomic, genomic, and bioinformatic approaches has allowed DeCaprio's group the identification and functional characterization of human DREAM, the homolog of the fly dREAM (Litovchick et al. 2007). To determine the composition of this complex the authors purified p130-associated proteins and applied a multidimensional protein identification method (MudPIT). This method couples biphasic and triphasic microcapillary columns to high performance liquid chromatography followed by tandem mass spectrometry analysis (Florens & Washburn 2006). The core components of the identified complex include p130, E2F4/5, DP1/2 and mammalian orthologs of synMuvB proteins LIN9, LIN37, LIN52, LIN54, and LIN53/RBBP4 (also known as LIN complex). Interestingly, the human DREAM repressor complex differs from the fly complex in that it lacks MYB. In fact, MYB immunoprecipitates with LIN9, LIN37, and LIN54, but not with E2F or p130 in human cells, indicating the existence of two distinct transcriptional complexes incorporating either p130 or MYB. Indeed, several reports have demonstrated that the complex composition is dynamic and cell cycle phase-dependent. In quiescent cells LIN complex proteins associate with p130 and E2F4, and the complex binds to its target genes. In late G1/S phase, E2F4 and p130 dissociate and the LIN complex associates with MYB (Litovchick et al. 2007; Schmit et al. 2007), forming a new complex that is required for activation of G2/M genes. The dynamic interaction of the LIN complex with different DNA-binding proteins (E2F4 *vs.* MYB) supports a model in which DREAM is bound in G0 to E2F-regulated promoters via E2F4/p130 and in S-phase to G2/M promoters via MYB. Another finding that distinguishes the human complex from its fly and worm orthologs is that human DREAM does not appear to regulate target genes involved in development (Litovchick et al. 2007).

Mass spectrometry has also been applied to elucidate the mechanism by which E2F6 regulates transcriptional repression in quiescent cells. E2F6 was shown to interact directly with MGA and MAX (Ogawa et al. 2002). These proteins are known to bind as heterodimers to E boxes such as the MYC binding elements, and to antagonize MYC function (Hurlin et al. 1999). Given that MYC and E2F share common functions such as mitotic responses, cell cycle stimulation and induction of apoptosis, it has been proposed that E2F- and MYC-responsive genes could be co-regulated by E2F6 (Ogawa et al. 2002). In the complex containing E2F6-MGA-MAX, several Polycomb group proteins (RING1/2, MBLR, h-l(3)MBT-like protein, and YAF2) are also present, together with HP1γ, a methyltransferase related to gene silencing in euchromatic loci (Horsley et al. 1996). The recruitment of E2F6 to its target genes could form a "platform" that is required for nucleating PcG proteins. Subsequent recruitment of HP1γ to this platform would propagate chromatin inactivation, leading to entire repressed regions (Ogawa et al. 2002). It is remarkable that as many as three types of E2F6 repressor complexes containing different PcG proteins have been identified by proteomic methods (Table 2). The biological relevance for such diversity has not been clarified, although there is evidence that these complexes could be formed at different phases throughout the cell cycle. MAX and HP1γ were found associated with E2F target promoters in G0, but not following re-entry into the cell cycle, suggesting a role for this complex in gene repression in quiescent cells (Ogawa et al. 2002). By contrast, the PcG protein EZH2 only forms complexes with E2F6-EPC1 in proliferating cells, suggesting that this complex regulates genes required for cell cycle progression (Attwooll et al. 2005).

Deciphering the protein interactome of upstream components of the RB/E2F pathway has also led to the characterization of new functions of the pathway. This is the case of a recently work published by Sicinski´s group in which cyclin D1 protein partners were characterized by immunoaffinity purification coupled to MS analysis (Jirawatnotai et al. 2011). Identification of cyclin D1 interactors revealed a network of DNA repair proteins, including RAD51, a key DNA recombinase that drives the homologous recombination process in response to DNA damage (Baumann & West 1998). Remarkably, the finding that Cyclin D1´s function in DNA repair appears to be independent of its kinase activity could have clinical applications. For instance, a large pool of RB-negative cancers, which do not require D-cyclins for proliferation, may still be benefited by therapeutic interventions targeting cyclin D1 in combination with radiation treatment. This work clearly shows how interacting-proteomics can fundamentally change our understanding of signaling networks and how combining multiple approaches is possible to unveil novel therapeutic strategies to different disorders such as oncogenic malignancies.

3. Post-translational modifications on E2F transcription factors

Post-translational modifications (PTMs) are gene non-template chemical modifications occurring at distinct amino acid side chains of proteins. PTMs can change the size, charge-state, structure or conformation of proteins. As a result, PTMs influence several aspects that directly or indirectly affect protein function. Sub-cellular localization (Mueller et al. 2009), protein half-life (Min et al. 2010) or binding affinity to other molecules such as nucleic acids, lipids or other proteins (Takasaki et al. 1999) are usually conditioned by these modifications. Consequently, PTMs play a key role in functional proteomics and are involved in the modulation of almost every single cellular process. Not surprisingly, malfunctions on these critical cellular processes have usually been related to several diseases (Ko et al. 2010; Song et al. 2010). More than 300 types of PTMs have been described to date and the number and variety of identified modifications is continuously increasing (Zhao & Jensen 2009). Some modifications such as phosphorylation, acetylation, glycosylation and methylation are very common and are found in almost every protein while others, for example biotinylation, are very rare. Given the high abundance, dynamism and diversity of PTMs, they likely constitute one of the most complex regulatory mechanisms in eukaryotic cells.

The E2F transcription factors are not an exception to such modifications, as they are known to be regulated by a variety of PTMs. In the mid 90's *in vitro* assays showed that ubiquitination occurring at the C-terminal end of E2F1 is determinant in mediating cell cycle-dependent degradation of this transcription factor by the ubiquitin/proteasome pathway (Hofmann et al. 1996). Additionally, two independent studies concluded that E2F1-3 but not E2F4-6 can be acetylated by p300/CBP acetyltransferases. Further *in vitro* acetylation assays using deletion mutants of E2F1, restricted the site of acetylation to three conserved lysine residues located at the N-terminal region of its DNA binding domain. This modification could be reversed by HDAC1, and was found to influence the DNA-binding ability of E2F1 and consequently its transcriptional activity (Martinez-Balbas et al. 2000; Marzio et al. 2000). More recently, Set9 methyltransferase and LSD1 demethylase have been shown to regulate E2F1-mediated p53-independent cell death (Kontaki & Talianidis 2010; Xie et al. 2011). Interestingly, a complex cross-talk between different PTMs was found on E2F1. Precisely, Set9-catalyzed methylation at Lys185 inhibits acetylation and phosphorylation events involved in the stabilization of E2F1, while ubiquitination, known to favor protein degradation, is stimulated (Kontaki & Talianidis 2010). Although these diverse PTMs have been described to affect the biological functions of E2Fs, phosphorylation has been the most studied modification.

3.1 Biochemical analysis of phosphorylations

Phosphorylation of proteins is a highly dynamic process involved in the regulation of several essential cellular functions such as cell cycle regulation, differentiation and signal transduction. Given its biological relevance, the identification and kinetic studies of protein phosphorylation have become a major challenge in molecular biology. Pioneer works describing phosphorylation events on E2F were mainly based on results obtained from electrophoretic mobility shift assays (Peeper et al. 1995) and *in vitro* kinase assays (Lin et al. 2001; Vandel & Kouzarides 1999). A major common feature of these studies is that they were hypothesis-driven, that is, the identification of the PTMs was, to an extent, a targeted approach. Moreover, each work was focused on individual proteins where a single or a few modifications were described at a time. Consequently, the information about PTMs affecting the biological function of E2Fs has been considerably limited. Indeed, these classical approaches have led to the identification and characterization of merely 7 phosphorylations on E2F1 over a period of 10 years, all of which are registered in the Phosphosite database (Hornbeck et al. 2004). Phosphorylation of E2F1 at Ser332 and Ser337 disrupts its interaction with RB to become transcriptionally active (Fagan et al. 1994). By contrast, phosphorylation at Ser375 increases its ability to interact with RB and, consequently, decreases its DNA binding capacity (Peeper et al. 1995). Phosphorylation of E2F1 residues Ser403 and Thr433 by TFIIH kinase in S-phase triggers rapid degradation of the transcription factor (Vandel & Kouzarides 1999). Finally, two residues on E2F1, Ser31 and Ser364, can be phosphorylated in response to DNA damage by ATM/ATR and Chk1 kinases, respectively. Both phosphorylations are involved in E2F1-mediated apoptosis (Lin et al. 2001; Stevens et al. 2003). Phosphorylation of E2F3a at Ser124 and its role in DNA-damage induced apoptosis has also been described by classical biochemical approaches (Martinez et al. 2010).

3.2 MS-based identification of phosphorylations

Recent advances in mass spectrometry have largely overcome the disadvantages faced by classical biochemical approaches allowing the large-scale identification of phosphorylated peptides and the more challenging localization of them within the peptide sequence. In order to decipher the biological meaning of site-specific phosphorylation events in the regulation of cellular processes, quantitative phosphoproteomics studies have produced a considerable body of work during the last 5 years. As a result, thousands of new phosphorylations have been identified (Huttlin et al. 2010; Monetti et al. 2011), some of them corresponding to E2F family members.

Due to the low stoichiometry of site-specific phosphorylation, refinement of phosphopeptide enrichment methodologies has been crucial for the fruitful characterization of this type of PTM by MS. Currently, there are several phosphopeptide enrichment methods available, such as strong cation exchange chromatography (SCX) (Beausoleil et al. 2004), hydrophilic interaction chromatography (HILIC) (Boersema et al. 2007), immobilized metal affinity chromatography (IMAC) (Li & Dass 1999) and titanium dioxide enrichment method (TiO_2) (Larsen et al. 2005; Pinkse et al. 2004). They all manage to separate phosphorylated peptides from non-phosphorylated ones taking advantage of the properties that the negative charge of the phosphate groups confer to phosphopeptides. Antibody-based enrichment approaches have also been demonstrated to be very efficient and useful for phosphoprotein/phosphopeptide enrichment (Choudhary et al. 2009). For optimal analysis of the phosphoproteome these methods are usually combined in multi-stage enrichment strategies (Thingholm et al. 2008). In addition, implementation of quantitation methods has opened new perspectives in studies of complex and dynamic biological signaling networks. In the past decade, highly accurate techniques based on stable isotope labeling for protein quantitation by MS have been developed. Stable isotope labeling of amino acids in cell culture (SILAC) (Ong et al. 2002) and iTRAQ (Ross et al. 2004) are currently the most frequently used techniques in quantitative MS-based phosphoproteomics.

The first global *in vivo* SILAC-based quantitative phosphoproteomic study to be reported was performed by Mann's group. It combined SCX and TiO_2 enrichment of phosphopeptides followed by LC-MS/MS analysis to quantify changes in phosphopeptide levels in response to EGF treatment (Olsen et al. 2006). From the 6,600 phosphosites corresponding to 2,244 proteins that were detected in this study, the previously described E2F1 phosphoserine-375 (pSer375) (Peeper et al. 1995) was identified. This large-scale analysis showed that the phosphorylation state of E2F1 Ser375 is independent of EGF treatment, since the amount of phosphopeptide remained constant over time after the addition of the stimulus (Olsen et al. 2006).

Similar studies carried out by Dephoure and colleagues combined SILAC-based quantitation with SCX followed by TiO_2 and IMAC to assess the quantitative atlas of mitotic phosphorylation on HeLa cells. MS analysis of enriched phosphopeptides revealed the presence of E2F1 pSer375 in G1 phase cell lysates. In addition, two new phosphorylations were identified on E2F2 and a single one on E2F7. E2F2 residues Ser133 and Tyr130 were shown to be phosphorylated during the M phase of the cell cycle while E2F7 Ser410 was found to be phosphorylated in G1 phase (Dephoure et al. 2008).

Additional quantitative phosphoproteomic studies have reported the identification of a large number of phosphoresidues on various members of the E2F family, some of which had not been reported before (Figure 2). To decipher the phosphorylation dynamics occurring during early differentiation of human embryonic stem cells, a SILAC-based quantitation combined with SCX and TiO_2 followed by MS analysis was performed (Van et al. 2009). Of the 5,222 identified proteins, 1,399 were phosphorylated in 3,067 residues. Two phosphorylated residues, pSer16 and pThr14 precisely, corresponded to E2F4 and were first described in this work. Quantitative phosphoproteomic analysis of T cell receptor signaling revealed the existence of 2 new phosphorylations on E2F family members. Apart from the phosphorylations at Ser375 and Ser332, previously described to affect E2F1 binding affinity for RB (Fagan et al., 1994; Peeper et al., 1995), a new phosphorylated serine at position 340 was detected on E2F1. Moreover, phosphorylation on E2F2 Ser117 was also observed in this analysis (Mayya et al. 2009).

A quantitative phosphoproteomic analysis focused on dissecting the rapamycin-dependent activation of oncogenic cascades also identified several new phosphorylation sites on E2Fs (Chen et al. 2009b). Differentially SILAC labeled cells were cultured in the presence or absence of rapamycin, and stimulated with EGF. Both protein lysates were combined, digested and phosphopeptides were subjected to double IMAC purification followed by MudPIT LC-MS/MS analysis. Of the 6,175 phosphosites identified in this screening, 3 corresponded to E2F8. For the first time, E2F8 Ser355, Ser357 and Ser358 were found phosphorylated. Quantitative phosphoproteomics was also applied in mouse cells to unravel the signaling cascade initiated in response to the oncogenic mutant receptor tyrosine kinase FIt3. This kinase has been involved in the development of several hematopoietic malignancies (Stirewalt & Radich 2003). A total of 14,700 phosphosites were identified, of which 1 corresponded to E2F7 (pTyr416) and 5 to E2F8 (pSer20, pSer71, pSer102, pSer358 and pSer429) (Choudhary et al. 2009). The Tyr416 residue of mouse E2F7 is not conserved in humans. By contrast, 4 of the 5 novel murine E2F8 phosphosites identified in this screening are conserved in humans, suggesting that they may be biologically relevant (Choudhary et al. 2009). In fact, pSer71 of E2F8 has recently been detected in the phosphoproteome of human embryonic stem cells undergoing differentiation (Rigbolt et al. 2011). In this report, an additional phosphosite on E2F8, pSer316, was described. Recently, in an attempt to elucidate the mechanism that regulates the switch of the MuvB core from B-MYB to DREAM, phosphorylation of E2F4 at Ser384 was detected. This phosphorylation could contribute to entry of cells into quiescence (Litovchick et al. 2007).

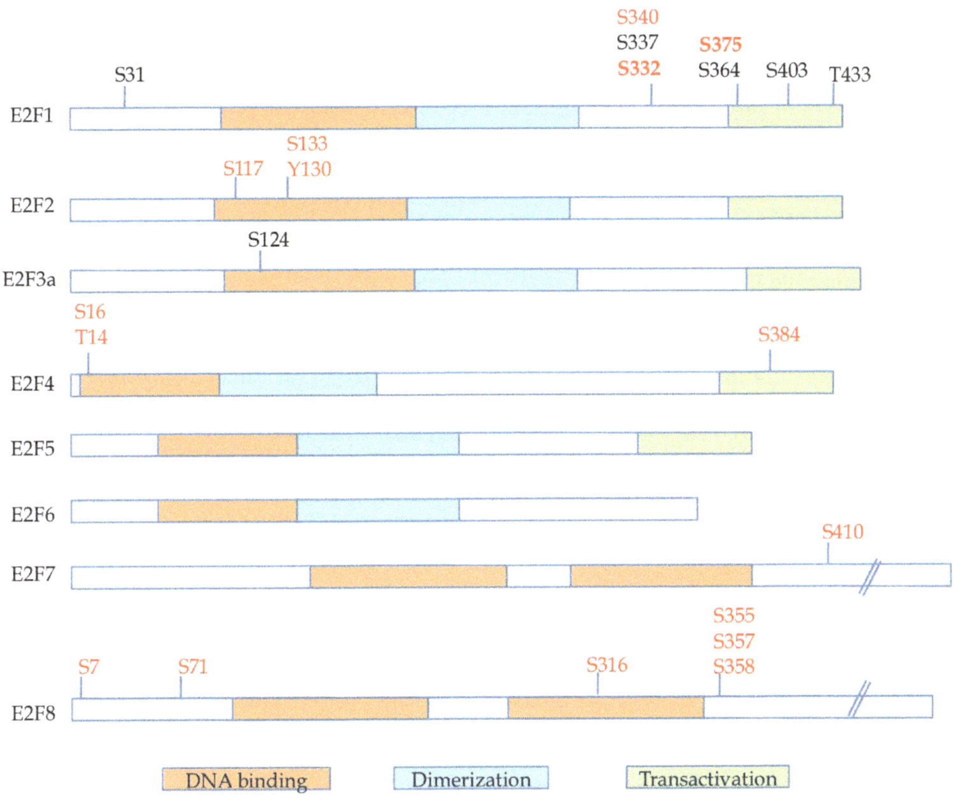

Fig. 2. Phosphorylations detected in human E2F family members. In black phosphorylations detected by classical biochemical methods; in red, phosphorylations detected by MS; in bold red, phosphorylations detected by both methods. S: Serine; T: Threonine; Y: Tyrosine.

Novel methodological approaches in SILAC-based quantitative phosphoproteomics include a double phosphopeptide enrichment using IMAC followed by HILIC. This kind of strategy has allowed the identification of pSer7 on E2F8 (Yao et al. 2011). Furthermore, quantitative data indicated that protein SUMOylation influences phosphorylation detected at residue Ser7, since inhibition of SUMOylation was found to increase the amount of pSer7. This new evidence of cross-talk between different PTMs underscores once more the complexity of PTMs and the relevance of the combinatorial PTM patterns.

4. Protein profiling to elucidate E2F function

A large number of potential E2F targets have been discovered recently through the application of high throughput transcriptomic analyses. However, mRNA abundance poorly correlates with protein levels. This discrepancy can in part be explained by several post-transcriptional mechanisms such as alternative splicing of pre-mRNAs, microRNA mediated regulation, or selective degradation and post-translational modifications of proteins. Therefore, protein expression analyses should be carried out in addition to mRNA expression analyses to achieve a full picture of E2F regulated pathways.

Two-dimensional gel electrophoresis (2-DE) combined with protein identification by MS has been the most popular method in expression proteomics. In this global protein profiling approach, 2-DE is used to separate proteins within a complex mixture based on their pI and molecular weight. Subsequent staining and image analysis can detect differences in spot intensities, rendering a list of proteins that are differentially expressed between the conditions under comparison. The resulting spots are then excised and analyzed by MS (Görg et al. 2004). Global protein expression analyses of cells that either overexpress or are deficient for individual E2Fs have emerged as a useful methodology to elucidate the spectrum of E2F activity. Pützer's group analyzed protein expression in p53-deficient osteosarcoma cells (Saos-2) expressing E2F1 fused to the murine estrogen receptor ligand-binding domain (ER). This construction permitted conditional activation of E2F1 after addition of 4-hydroxytamoxifen (4-OHT) to the cultures (Stanelle et al. 2002). 2-DE analysis of E2F1 induced and non-induced Saos-2 cells' proteome led to the identification of 33 novel differentially regulated E2F1 target proteins by MALDI-MS (Li et al. 2006b), 15 upregulated and 18 dowregulated. Only eight of these differentially regulated proteins harbor E2F-consensus sites in their promoter (Rabinovich et al. 2008): SRSF1, TUBB, GDI2, H2B.1, TCP1γ, HNRNPA2/B1, HNRNPK and MATR3. Nevertheless, since E2F1 overexpression was the only stimulus applied to the culture, most of the identified target genes are probably E2F1 targets. Functional analysis of E2F1-regulated target genes suggests that E2F1 plays predominantly a negative role in Saos-2 cellular proliferation. By altering the balance between anti- and pro-apoptotic Bcl-2 family members, E2F1 would render cells susceptible to both mitochondrial apoptosis and ER-stress related death signals (Li et al. 2006b). These results are consistent with the findings described by several groups, including ours, in mouse models lacking E2F1, and favor the hypothesis that E2F1 plays anti-proliferative and pro-apoptotic roles *in vivo* (Field et al. 1996; Garcia et al. 2000; Yamasaki et al. 1996).

A similar pro-apoptotic role has been attributed to E2F1 in proteomic analyses involving p53-wild-type osteosarcoma cells (U2OS) carrying an inducible E2F1 transgene. 2-DE followed by MS led to the identification of 76 proteins, 53 overexpressed and 23 suppressed after E2F1 induction (Liontos et al. 2009). Many of them appear to be potentially novel E2F1-regulated targets. As many as 63% and 77% of the overexpressed and suppressed proteins, respectively, harbor E2F1 responsive elements in their promoters. The spectrum of identified E2F1-regulated proteins included chaperones, metabolic enzymes, proteins associated with RNA processing, components of the protein degradation/turnover machinery, cytoskeletal and motor/contractile related proteins, regulatory and cell signaling molecules, transport carriers and channels, as well as putative oncogenes. A significant number of the identified E2F1 downstream targets are part of pro-apoptotic signaling cascades regulating ATM and/or p53. In agreement with an oncosuppressor function for E2F1 *in vivo*, the authors reported a positive correlation between E2F1 expression and DNA damage response and apoptosis in primary osteosarcoma tumors with wild-type p53. This picture is contrary to the general view that the increased levels of E2F activators, such as those observed in many cancer types, are mediating uncontrolled proliferation (Chen et al. 2009a). Whether deregulated expression of E2F proteins promotes or limits cancer progression has not been unequivocally established. Other factors, such as RB or p53 status may determine the final outcome of E2F-dependent activity in each particular context.

Protein profiling analyses performed by our group are also helping to unveil the physiological role of E2F2. A repressor function for E2F2 is emerging from these studies, in agreement with DNA microarray and functional data. When quiescent E2F2$^{-/-}$ and wild-type T lymphocyte expression profiles were gathered by 2-DE followed by MS, we identified a set of deregulated proteins involved in TCR-mediated signaling, cell survival and stress responses (Azkargorta et al. 2006). The aberrant expression of these proteins was linked to the hyperproliferative phenotype that characterizes E2F2-deficient cells (Iglesias et al. 2004; Infante et al. 2008; Murga et al. 2001; Zhu et al. 2001). Interestingly, comparative proteomics has also revealed novel pathways regulated by E2F2. We have recently found that mediators of the Aryl-hydrocarbon receptor (AHR) are aberrantly expressed in the proteome of proliferating E2F2$^{-/-}$ lymphocytes relative to wild-type counterparts (Azkargorta et al. 2010). Consequently, E2F2$^{-/-}$ cells exhibit an increase in their sensitivity to dioxin-triggered apoptosis. These results suggest that E2F2 modulates cellular sensitivity to xenobiotic signals through the negative regulation of the AHR pathway.

Remarkably, a comparison of proteome and transcriptome profiling results derived from the same cellular systems has shown a clear discrepancy in individual targets regulated by E2Fs (Azkargorta et al. 2006; Azkargorta et al. 2010; Infante et al. 2008; Li et al. 2006a; Liontos et al. 2009; Muller et al. 2001). These discrepancies may be explained by the different methods of assay/sample preparation, different detection sensitivity, alternative splicing, post-transcriptional regulation, PTMs, selective degradation of proteins, and the time discrepancy between mRNA and protein expression. Thus, proteomics and DNA-based technologies should be considered as complementary approaches.

4.1 The RB/E2F pathway in cancer protein profiling

Transcriptomic analyses have demonstrated a commonly conserved RB/E2F-dependent "proliferation signature" in cancer cells, supporting a role for this pathway in regulation of cellular proliferation in normal as well as tumor cells (Whitfield et al. 2006). Given the prevalence of this signature in cancer, a similar finding would be expected at the protein level. However, most 2-DE/MS-based proteomic analyses of tumor cells performed to date have not displayed this pathway unequivocally, probably due to the limitations of the technology. An important drawback of traditional 2-DE-based proteomic methods is that they can only reveal the presence of highly abundant proteins within the cells, whereas proteins that function at low levels, such as certain transcription factors and checkpoint/regulatory proteins, are not easily identified if no pre-enrichment and/or pre-fractionation steps are applied (Gygi et al. 2000). In general, the number of proteins identified in these experiments is quite low, in the range of 100-300 proteins per experiment. This number is several orders of magnitude lower than the thousands of genes that can be interrogated by DNA microarray analyses. Consequently, cancer proteome profiles gathered to date with this technology should, in general, be considered as preliminary.

An RB/E2F dependent signature was appreciable in the proteome of cervical cancer cells with high-risk HPV infection analyzed by 2-DE and MS. Differentially expressed proteins in cervical cancer cells were identified and functionally classified as proteins involved in the regulation of the cell cycle, general genomic stability, telomerase activation and cell immortalization (Choi et al. 2005). A significant proportion of these genes (30%), particularly those present in the nuclear fraction, are well-known E2F transcriptional targets (PCNA, CDC25A, MCM3,4,8, CHRAC-1), most of which were upregulated. As exceptions, XRCC2 involved in DNA repair and CASP-2 involved in apoptosis induction, which were downregulated. These results are consistent with a model in which functional inactivation of RB by HPV oncoprotein E7 unleashes E2F and triggers aberrant E2F-dependent gene expression (McLaughlin-Drubin & Munger 2009). By contrast, a similar type of analysis performed with retinoblastoma tumors, whereby both copies of the RB1 gene are inactivated, did not identify any E2F targets among the 27 differentially expressed proteins (Mallikarjuna et al. 2010). In this work, more aggressive tumors showed significantly higher expression of CRABP2, APOA1, PRDX6 and RCVRA, and lower expression of CRABP1. Differentially expressed proteins were shown to be involved in metabolic process, transport activity, response to oxidative stress, development, and cell signaling and transduction, reflecting the important role of these processes during retinoblastoma progression.

In general, 2-DE/MS-based proteomic analyses of cancer cells have barely yielded a handful of E2F-target genes among the differentially expressed proteins. For example, the comprehensive proteome profiles of mouse lung adenocarcinoma cell lines, have revealed 82 and 40 unique proteins significantly up- or down-regulated respectively in highly metastatic cells compared to low metastatic controls (Zhang et al. 2008). Several of the proteins are involved in proteasome, cell-cycle and cell-cell communication pathways. Among them, several E2F targets have previously been associated with cancer development and metastasis: KRT8, the main cytokeratin in lung cancer, MCM7, a highly informative biomarker for cervical cancer, or ANX4, overexpressed in pancreatic adenocarcinoma. Similarly, a comparative proteome analysis of human lung squamous carcinoma and paired normal bronchial epithelial tissues revealed some deregulated E2F target genes in a list of 68 proteins that were identified by MS (LTBP4, GNB1L, MDM2, IRS1)(Li et al. 2006a).

As 2-DE/MS methodology is being replaced by more powerful techniques, the number of proteins that can be identified in a given proteome is increasing rapidly, allowing for a more accurate definition of the pathways involved in cancer. A recent report has described the use of 1-D gel electrophoresis followed by tryptic in-gel digestion and chromatography coupled to MS. This shotgun proteomic approach revealed changes in the expression levels of 281 proteins in meningiomas compared to normal human arachnoidal cells (Saydam et al. 2010). Interestingly, a highly significant functional network involved in DNA replication, recombination and repair, and in cell cycle was exclusively expressed in cancer cells, arguing for a prevalent RB/E2F signature in the meningioma proteome. Similar results have been gathered recently with high-risk neuroblastoma proteomes analyzed by another type of shotgun proteomics approach. Quantitative global protein expression profiling performed using isotope-coded affinity tags (ICAT) followed by LC-MS/MS analysis identified a total of 1,461 proteins that were differentially expressed in neuroblastoma. Again, pathway analysis of these proteins showed enrichment in the RB/E2F regulated network (Chen et al. 2010). These results underscore the power of shotgun proteomics, and suggest that many novel insights regarding RB/E2F function will be unraveled by this approach.

5. Future perspectives

Much has been learned on RB/E2F-mediated regulation of gene transcription by proteomic approaches to date. The identification of E2F interacting proteins as well as transcriptional complexes encompassing RB and E2F has helped elucidating the regulation of this pathway. However, the current knowledge is still too limited to fully understand the complex RB/E2F-regulated network. Further work involving high throughput proteomic approaches should help elucidate the nature of the diverse macromolecular complexes that are thought to harbor RB/E2F, and the role of these complexes in different biological settings.

Development of modified peptide enrichment methods together with recent advances in MS has allowed large-scale analyses of PTMs, providing a large pool of new PTM identifications. With regard to E2Fs, MS-based phosphorylation analyses have greatly increased the number of phosphorylated residues identified within this transcription factor family, and many more will probably be identified in the future. However, they will need to be validated and functionally characterized *in vivo* in order to decipher the influence of each individual PTM on E2F activity. As works focused on MS-based identification are gaining relevance, other types of PTMs such as acetylations and ubiquitinations, will probably be identified on E2Fs in a short period of time. Furthermore, multiple PTMs should be possible to analyze in the same system, producing direct data on their crosstalk at the global level in regulating E2F function. In addition, implementation of quantitative methods will allow studying the dynamics of site-specific PTMs on E2Fs, which was almost unachievable a decade ago. Defining their kinetics will be crucial to understand how PTMs influence on protein regulation and function. This explosion of information, still very descriptive, opens a huge range of possible new studies in the field of RB/E2F network.

Several differential proteomic analyses have been performed to examine how the presence/absence of each individual E2F is reflected in the proteome. The strategy to accomplish this objective will surely move from the low scale approach that represents 2-DE/MS used so far, to gel-free high throughput strategies. This approach has been widely adopted in proteomics lately, owing to its superior performance compared to 2-DE technology. Advances in sample preparation, including novel fractionation methods, together with more powerful mass spectrometers have been proved to qualitatively and quantitatively assess changes in large scale protein analyses. Indeed, large-scale protein expression analysis of cancer cell proteomes by shotgun proteomics promises to be valuable for investigating mechanisms of cancer transformation (Chen & Yates, III 2007). Nonetheless, the limitations of global proteomic analyses in identifying and quantifying low abundant proteins such as transcription factors will push the emergence of hypothesis-driven strategies based on targeted proteomic approaches.

6. Acknowledgments

This work was supported by grants from the Spanish Ministry of Science and Innovation (SAF2009-12037 and Consolider-Ingenio Programme CSD2007-00017 to AMZ) and the Basque Government Department of Industry (ETORTEK-IE09-256 and SAIOTEK-S-PE10UN82 to AMZ and JMA). JM is supported by a Basque Government fellowship for graduate studies, and NO is supported by a UPV/EHU fellowship for graduate studies.

7. References

Attwooll, C., Lazzerini, D. E., & Helin, K. (2004). The E2F family: specific functions and overlapping interests. *EMBO J.*, 23 (24): 4709-4716.

Attwooll, C., Oddi, S., Cartwright, P., Prosperini, E., Agger, K., Steensgaard, P., Wagener, C., Sardet, C., Moroni, M. C., & Helin, K. (2005). A novel repressive E2F6 complex containing the polycomb group protein, EPC1, that interacts with EZH2 in a proliferation-specific manner. *J.Biol.Chem.*, 280 (2): 1199-1208.

Azkargorta, M., Arizmendi, J. M., Elortza, F., Alkorta, N., Zubiaga, A. M., & Fullaondo, A. (2006). Differential proteome profiles in E2F2-deficient T lymphocytes. *Proteomics*, 6 Suppl (1): S42-S50.

Azkargorta, M., Fullaondo, A., Laresgoiti, U., Aloria, K., Infante, A., Arizmendi, J. M., & Zubiaga, A. M. (2010). Differential proteomics analysis reveals a role for E2F2 in the regulation of the Ahr pathway in T lymphocytes. *Mol.Cell Proteomics,* 9 (10): 2184-2194.

Balciunaite, E., Spektor, A., Lents, N. H., Cam, H., Te, R. H., Scime, A., Rudnicki, M. A., Young, R., & Dynlacht, B. D. (2005). Pocket protein complexes are recruited to distinct targets in quiescent and proliferating cells. *Mol.Cell Biol.,* 25 (18): 8166-8178.

Bandara, L. R. & La Thangue, N. B. (1991). Adenovirus E1a prevents the retinoblastoma gene product from complexing with a cellular transcription factor. *Nature,* 351 (6326): 494-497.

Baumann, P. & West, S. C. (1998). Role of the human RAD51 protein in homologous recombination and double-stranded-break repair. *Trends Biochem.Sci.,* 23 (7): 247-251.

Beausoleil, S. A., Jedrychowski, M., Schwartz, D., Elias, J. E., Villen, J., Li, J., Cohn, M. A., Cantley, L. C., & Gygi, S. P. (2004). Large-scale characterization of HeLa cell nuclear phosphoproteins. *Proc.Natl.Acad.Sci.U.S.A,* 101 (33): 12130-12135.

Boersema, P. J., Divecha, N., Heck, A. J., & Mohammed, S. (2007). Evaluation and optimization of ZIC-HILIC-RP as an alternative MudPIT strategy. *J.Proteome Res.,* 6 (3): 937-946.

Brehm, A., Miska, E. A., McCance, D. J., Reid, J. L., Bannister, A. J., & Kouzarides, T. (1998). Retinoblastoma protein recruits histone deacetylase to repress transcription. *Nature,* 391 (6667): 597-601.

Bunker, C. A. & Kingston, R. E. (1994). Transcriptional repression by Drosophila and mammalian Polycomb group proteins in transfected mammalian cells. *Mol.Cell Biol.,* 14 (3): 1721-1732.

Burkhart, D. L. & Sage, J. (2008). Cellular mechanisms of tumour suppression by the retinoblastoma gene. *Nat.Rev.Cancer,* 8 (9): 671-682.

Cartwright, P., Muller, H., Wagener, C., Holm, K., & Helin, K. (1998). E2F-6: a novel member of the E2F family is an inhibitor of E2F-dependent transcription. *Oncogene,* 17 (5): 611-623.

Chellappan, S. P., Hiebert, S., Mudryj, M., Horowitz, J. M., & Nevins, J. R. (1991). The E2F transcription factor is a cellular target for the RB protein. *Cell,* 65 (6): 1053-1061.

Chen, E. I. & Yates, J. R., III (2007). Cancer proteomics by quantitative shotgun proteomics. *Mol.Oncol.,* 1 (2): 144-159.

Chen, H. Z., Tsai, S. Y., & Leone, G. (2009a). Emerging roles of E2Fs in cancer: an exit from cell cycle control. *Nat.Rev.Cancer,* 9 (11): 785-797.

Chen, Q. R., Song, Y. K., Yu, L. R., Wei, J. S., Chung, J. Y., Hewitt, S. M., Veenstra, T. D., & Khan, J. (2010). Global genomic and proteomic analysis identifies biological pathways related to high-risk neuroblastoma. *J.Proteome Res.,* 9 (1): 373-382.

Chen, R. Q., Yang, Q. K., Lu, B. W., Yi, W., Cantin, G., Chen, Y. L., Fearns, C., Yates, J. R., III, & Lee, J. D. (2009b). CDC25B mediates rapamycin-induced oncogenic responses in cancer cells. *Cancer Res.,* 69 (6): 2663-2668.

Chittenden, T., Livingston, D. M., & Kaelin, W. G., Jr. (1991). The T/E1A-binding domain of the retinoblastoma product can interact selectively with a sequence-specific DNA-binding protein. *Cell,* 65 (6): 1073-1082.

Choi, Y. P., Kang, S., Hong, S., Xie, X., & Cho, N. H. (2005). Proteomic analysis of progressive factors in uterine cervical cancer. *Proteomics,* 5 (6): 1481-1493.

Choudhary, C., Olsen, J. V., Brandts, C., Cox, J., Reddy, P. N., Bohmer, F. D., Gerke, V., Schmidt-Arras, D. E., Berdel, W. E., Muller-Tidow, C., Mann, M., & Serve, H. (2009). Mislocalized activation of oncogenic RTKs switches downstream signaling outcomes. *Mol.Cell,* 36 (2): 326-339.

DeGregori, J., Leone, G., Miron, A., Jakoi, L., & Nevins, J. R. (1997). Distinct roles for E2F proteins in cell growth control and apoptosis. *Proc.Natl.Acad.Sci.U.S.A,* 94 (14): 7245-7250.

DeGregori, J. & Johnson, D. G. (2006). Distinct and Overlapping Roles for E2F Family Members in Transcription, Proliferation and Apoptosis. *Curr.Mol.Med.,* 6 (7): 739-748.

Dephoure, N., Zhou, C., Villen, J., Beausoleil, S. A., Bakalarski, C. E., Elledge, S. J., & Gygi, S. P. (2008). A quantitative atlas of mitotic phosphorylation. *Proc.Natl.Acad.Sci.U.S.A,* 105 (31): 10762-10767.

Dimova, D. K. & Dyson, N. J. (2005). The E2F transcriptional network: old acquaintances with new faces. *Oncogene,* 24 (17): 2810-2826.

Escher, N., Kob, R., Tenbaum, S. P., Eisold, M., Baniahmad, A., von, E. F., & Melle, C. (2007). Various members of the E2F transcription factor family interact in vivo with the corepressor alien. *J.Proteome Res.,* 6 (3): 1158-1164.

Fagan, R., Flint, K. J., & Jones, N. (1994). Phosphorylation of E2F-1 modulates its interaction with the retinoblastoma gene product and the adenoviral E4 19 kDa protein. *Cell,* 78 (5): 799-811.

Fay, D. S. & Han, M. (2000). The synthetic multivulval genes of C. elegans: functional redundancy, Ras-antagonism, and cell fate determination. *Genesis.,* 26 (4): 279-284.

Field, S. J., Tsai, F. Y., Kuo, F., Zubiaga, A. M., Kaelin, W. G., Jr., Livingston, D. M., Orkin, S. H., & Greenberg, M. E. (1996). E2F-1 functions in mice to promote apoptosis and suppress proliferation. *Cell,* 85 (4): 549-561.

Fields, S. & Song, O. (1989). A novel genetic system to detect protein-protein interactions. *Nature,* 340 (6230): 245-246.

Florens, L. & Washburn, M. P. (2006). Proteomic analysis by multidimensional protein identification technology. *Methods Mol.Biol.,* 328: 159-175.

Freedman, J. A., Chang, J. T., Jakoi, L., & Nevins, J. R. (2009). A combinatorial mechanism for determining the specificity of E2F activation and repression. *Oncogene,* 28 (32): 2873-2881.

Frolov, M. V. & Dyson, N. J. (2004). Molecular mechanisms of E2F-dependent activation and pRB-mediated repression. *J.Cell Sci.,* 117 (Pt 11): 2173-2181.

Garcia, I., Murga, M., Vicario, A., Field, S. J., & Zubiaga, A. M. (2000). A role for E2F1 in the induction of apoptosis during thymic negative selection. *Cell Growth Differ.,* 11 (2): 91-98.

Gaubatz, S., Wood, J. G., & Livingston, D. M. (1998). Unusual proliferation arrest and transcriptional control properties of a newly discovered E2F family member, E2F-6. *Proc.Natl.Acad.Sci.U.S.A,* 95 (16): 9190-9195.

Gavin, A. C., Bosche, M., Krause, R., Grandi, P., Marzioch, M., Bauer, A., Schultz, J., Rick, J. M., Michon, A. M., Cruciat, C. M., Remor, M., Hofert, C., Schelder, M., Brajenovic, M., Ruffner, H., Merino, A., Klein, K., Hudak, M., Dickson, D., Rudi, T., Gnau, V.,

Bauch, A., Bastuck, S., Huhse, B., Leutwein, C., Heurtier, M. A., Copley, R. R., Edelmann, A., Querfurth, E., Rybin, V., Drewes, G., Raida, M., Bouwmeester, T., Bork, P., Seraphin, B., Kuster, B., Neubauer, G., & Superti-Furga, G. (2002). Functional organization of the yeast proteome by systematic analysis of protein complexes. *Nature,* 415 (6868): 141-147.

Giangrande, P. H., Hallstrom, T. C., Tunyaplin, C., Calame, K., & Nevins, J. R. (2003). Identification of E-box factor TFE3 as a functional partner for the E2F3 transcription factor. *Mol.Cell Biol.,* 23 (11): 3707-3720.

Görg, A., Weiss, W., & Dunn, M. J. (2004). Current two-dimensional electrophoresis technology for proteomics. *Proteomics,* 4 (12): 3665-3685.

Gygi, S. P., Rist, B., & Aebersold, R. (2000). Measuring gene expression by quantitative proteome analysis. *Curr.Opin.Biotechnol.,* 11 (4): 396-401.

Hallstrom, T. C. & Nevins, J. R. (2003). Specificity in the activation and control of transcription factor E2F-dependent apoptosis. *Proc.Natl.Acad.Sci.U.S.A,* 100 (19): 10848-10853.

Hallstrom, T. C. & Nevins, J. R. (2006). Jab1 is a specificity factor for E2F1-induced apoptosis. *Genes Dev.,* 20 (5): 613-623.

Harrison, M. M., Ceol, C. J., Lu, X., & Horvitz, H. R. (2006). Some C. elegans class B synthetic multivulva proteins encode a conserved LIN-35 Rb-containing complex distinct from a NuRD-like complex. *Proc.Natl.Acad.Sci.U.S.A,* 103 (45): 16782-16787.

Ho, Y., Gruhler, A., Heilbut, A., Bader, G.D., Moore, L., Adams, S.L., Millar, A., Paul Taylor, Bennett, K., Boutilier, K., Yang, L., Wolting, C., Donaldson, I., Schandorff, S., Shewnarane, J., Vo, M., Taggart, J., Goudreault, M., Muskat, B., Alfarano, C., Dewar, D., Lin, Z., Michalickova, K., Willems, A.R., Sassi, H., Nielsen, P.A., Rasmussen, K.J., Andersen, J.R., Johansen, L.E., Hansen, L.H., Jespersen, H., Podtelejnikov, A., Nielsen, E., Crawford, J., Poulsen, V., Sørensen, B.D., Matthiesen, J., Hendrickson, R.C., Gleeson, F., Pawson, T., Moran, M.F., Durocher, D., Mann, M., Hogue, C.W.V., Figeys, D., & Tyers, M. (2002). Systematic identification of protein complexes in *Saccharomyces cerevisiae* by mass spectrometry. *Nature,* 415 (6868): 180-183.

Hofmann, F., Martelli, F., Livingston, D. M., & Wang, Z. (1996). The retinoblastoma gene product protects E2F-1 from degradation by the ubiquitin-proteasome pathway. *Genes Dev.,* 10 (23): 2949-2959.

Hong, S., Paulson, Q. X., & Johnson, D. G. (2008). E2F1 and E2F3 activate ATM through distinct mechanisms to promote E1A-induced apoptosis. *Cell Cycle,* 7 (3): 391-400.

Hornbeck, P. V., Chabra, I., Kornhauser, J. M., Skrzypek, E., & Zhang, B. (2004). PhosphoSite: A bioinformatics resource dedicated to physiological protein phosphorylation. *Proteomics,* 4 (6): 1551-1561.

Horsley, D., Hutchings, A., Butcher, G. W., & Singh, P. B. (1996). M32, a murine homologue of Drosophila heterochromatin protein 1 (HP1), localises to euchromatin within interphase nuclei and is largely excluded from constitutive heterochromatin. *Cytogenet.Cell Genet.,* 73 (4): 308-311.

Hurlin, P. J., Steingrimsson, E., Copeland, N. G., Jenkins, N. A., & Eisenman, R. N. (1999). Mga, a dual-specificity transcription factor that interacts with Max and contains a T-domain DNA-binding motif. *EMBO J.,* 18 (24): 7019-7028.

Huttlin, E. L., Jedrychowski, M. P., Elias, J. E., Goswami, T., Rad, R., Beausoleil, S. A., Villen, J., Haas, W., Sowa, M. E., & Gygi, S. P. (2010). A tissue-specific atlas of mouse protein phosphorylation and expression. *Cell,* 143 (7): 1174-1189.

Iaquinta, P. J. & Lees, J. A. (2007). Life and death decisions by the E2F transcription factors. *Curr.Opin.Cell Biol.,* 19 (6): 649-657.

Iglesias, A., Murga, M., Laresgoiti, U., Skoudy, A., Bernales, I., Fullaondo, A., Moreno, B., Lloreta, J., Field, S. J., Real, F. X., & Zubiaga, A. M. (2004). Diabetes and exocrine pancreatic insufficiency in E2F1/E2F2 double-mutant mice. *J.Clin.Invest.,* 113 (10): 1398-1407.

Infante, A., Laresgoiti, U., Fernandez-Rueda, J., Fullaondo, A., Galan, J., Diaz-Uriarte, R., Malumbres, M., Field, S. J., & Zubiaga, A. M. (2008). E2F2 represses cell cycle regulators to maintain quiescence. *Cell Cycle,* 7 (24): 3915-3927.

Jirawatnotai, S., Hu, Y., Michowski, W., Elias, J. E., Becks, L., Bienvenu, F., Zagozdzon, A., Goswami, T., Wang, Y. E., Clark, A. B., Kunkel, T. A., van, H. T., Xia, B., Correll, M., Quackenbush, J., Livingston, D. M., Gygi, S. P., & Sicinski, P. (2011). A function for cyclin D1 in DNA repair uncovered by protein interactome analyses in human cancers. *Nature,* 474 (7350): 230-234.

Johnson, D. G. & DeGregori, J. (2006). Putting the Oncogenic and Tumor Suppressive Activities of E2F into Context. *Curr.Mol.Med.,* 6 (7): 731-738.

Kaelin, W. G., Jr. (2003). E2F1 as a target: promoter-driven suicide and small molecule modulators. *Cancer Biol.Ther.,* 2 (4 Suppl 1): S48-S54.

Ko, M., Huang, Y., Jankowska, A. M., Pape, U. J., Tahiliani, M., Bandukwala, H. S., An, J., Lamperti, E. D., Koh, K. P., Ganetzky, R., Liu, X. S., Aravind, L., Agarwal, S., Maciejewski, J. P., & Rao, A. (2010). Impaired hydroxylation of 5-methylcytosine in myeloid cancers with mutant TET2. *Nature,* 468 (7325): 839-843.

Kontaki, H. & Talianidis, I. (2010). Lysine methylation regulates E2F1-induced cell death. *Mol.Cell,* 39 (1): 152-160.

Korenjak, M., Taylor-Harding, B., Binne, U. K., Satterlee, J. S., Stevaux, O., Aasland, R., White-Cooper, H., Dyson, N., & Brehm, A. (2004). Native E2F/RBF complexes contain Myb-interacting proteins and repress transcription of developmentally controlled E2F target genes. *Cell,* 119 (2): 181-193.

Kowalik, T. F., DeGregori, J., Leone, G., Jakoi, L., & Nevins, J. R. (1998). E2F1-specific induction of apoptosis and p53 accumulation, which is blocked by Mdm2. *Cell Growth Differ.,* 9 (2): 113-118.

Krogan, N. J., Cagney, G., Yu, H., Zhong, G., Guo, X., Ignatchenko, A., Li, J., Pu, S., Datta, N., Tikuisis, A. P., Punna, T., Peregrin-Alvarez, J. M., Shales, M., Zhang, X., Davey, M., Robinson, M. D., Paccanaro, A., Bray, J. E., Sheung, A., Beattie, B., Richards, D. P., Canadien, V., Lalev, A., Mena, F., Wong, P., Starostine, A., Canete, M. M., Vlasblom, J., Wu, S., Orsi, C., Collins, S. R., Chandran, S., Haw, R., Rilstone, J. J., Gandi, K., Thompson, N. J., Musso, G., St, O. P., Ghanny, S., Lam, M. H., Butland, G., Altaf-Ul, A. M., Kanaya, S., Shilatifard, A., O'Shea, E., Weissman, J. S., Ingles, C. J., Hughes, T. R., Parkinson, J., Gerstein, M., Wodak, S. J., Emili, A., & Greenblatt, J. F. (2006). Global landscape of protein complexes in the yeast Saccharomyces cerevisiae. *Nature,* 440 (7084): 637-643.

Lang, S. E., McMahon, S. B., Cole, M. D., & Hearing, P. (2001). E2F transcriptional activation requires TRRAP and GCN5 cofactors. *J.Biol.Chem.,* 276 (35): 32627-32634.

Larsen, M. R., Thingholm, T. E., Jensen, O. N., Roepstorff, P., & Jorgensen, T. J. (2005). Highly selective enrichment of phosphorylated peptides from peptide mixtures using titanium dioxide microcolumns. *Mol.Cell Proteomics,* 4 (7): 873-886.

Lazzerini, D. E., Attwooll, C., Pasini, D., & Helin, K. (2005). Deregulated E2F activity induces hyperplasia and senescence-like features in the mouse pituitary gland. *Mol.Cell Biol.,* 25 (7): 2660-2672.

Lee, B. K., Bhinge, A. A., & Iyer, V. R. (2011). Wide-ranging functions of E2F4 in transcriptional activation and repression revealed by genome-wide analysis. *Nucleic Acids Res.,* 39 (9): 3558-3573.

Lehmann, R., Melle, C., Escher, N., & von, E. F. (2005). Detection and identification of protein interactions of S100 proteins by ProteinChip technology. *J.Proteome Res.,* 4 (5): 1717-1721.

Lewis, P. W., Beall, E. L., Fleischer, T. C., Georlette, D., Link, A. J., & Botchan, M. R. (2004). Identification of a Drosophila Myb-E2F2/RBF transcriptional repressor complex. *Genes Dev.,* 18 (23): 2929-2940.

Li, C., Xiao, Z., Chen, Z., Zhang, X., Li, J., Wu, X., Li, X., Yi, H., Li, M., Zhu, G., & Liang, S. (2006a). Proteome analysis of human lung squamous carcinoma. *Proteomics,* 6 (2): 547-558.

Li, S. & Dass, C. (1999). Iron(III)-immobilized metal ion affinity chromatography and mass spectrometry for the purification and characterization of synthetic phosphopeptides. *Anal.Biochem.,* 270 (1): 9-14.

Li, Z., Kreutzer, M., Mikkat, S., Mise, N., Glocker, M. O., & Putzer, B. M. (2006b). Proteomic analysis of the E2F1 response in p53-negative cancer cells: new aspects in the regulation of cell survival and death. *Proteomics,* 6 (21): 5735-5745.

Liao, C. C., Tsai, C. Y., Chang, W. C., Lee, W. H., & Wang, J. M. (2010). RB.E2F1 complex mediates DNA damage responses through transcriptional regulation of ZBRK1. *J.Biol.Chem.,* 285 (43): 33134-33143.

Lin, W. C., Lin, F. T., & Nevins, J. R. (2001). Selective induction of E2F1 in response to DNA damage, mediated by ATM-dependent phosphorylation. *Genes Dev.,* 15 (14): 1833-1844.

Liontos, M., Niforou, K., Velimezi, G., Vougas, K., Evangelou, K., Apostolopoulou, K., Vrtel, R., Damalas, A., Kontovazenitis, P., Kotsinas, A., Zoumpourlis, V., Tsangaris, G. T., Kittas, C., Ginsberg, D., Halazonetis, T. D., Bartek, J., & Gorgoulis, V. G. (2009). Modulation of the E2F1-driven cancer cell fate by the DNA damage response machinery and potential novel E2F1 targets in osteosarcomas. *Am.J.Pathol.,* 175 (1): 376-391.

Litovchick, L., Sadasivam, S., Florens, L., Zhu, X., Swanson, S. K., Velmurugan, S., Chen, R., Washburn, M. P., Liu, X. S., & Decaprio, J. A. (2007). Evolutionarily conserved multisubunit RBL2/p130 and E2F4 protein complex represses human cell cycle-dependent genes in quiescence. *Mol.Cell,* 26 (4): 539-551.

Liu, F. & Lee, W. H. (2006). CtIP activates its own and cyclin D1 promoters via the E2F/RB pathway during G1/S progression. *Mol.Cell Biol.,* 26 (8): 3124-3134.

Luo, R. X., Postigo, A. A., & Dean, D. C. (1998). Rb interacts with histone deacetylase to repress transcription. *Cell,* 92 (4): 463-473.

Ma, Y., Croxton, R., Moorer, R. L., Jr., & Cress, W. D. (2002). Identification of novel E2F1-regulated genes by microarray. *Arch.Biochem.Biophys.,* 399 (2): 212-224.

Magnaghi-Jaulin, L., Groisman, R., Naguibneva, I., Robin, P., Lorain, S., Le Villain, J. P., Troalen, F., Trouche, D., & Harel-Bellan, A. (1998). Retinoblastoma protein represses transcription by recruiting a histone deacetylase. *Nature,* 391 (6667): 601-605.

Mallikarjuna, K., Sundaram, C. S., Sharma, Y., Deepa, P. R., Khetan, V., Gopal, L., Biswas, J., Sharma, T., & Krishnakumar, S. (2010). Comparative proteomic analysis of differentially expressed proteins in primary retinoblastoma tumors. *Proteomics.Clin.Appl.,* 4 (4): 449-463.

Martinez, L. A., Goluszko, E., Chen, H. Z., Leone, G., Post, S., Lozano, G., Chen, Z., & Chauchereau, A. (2010). E2F3 is a mediator of DNA damage-induced apoptosis. *Mol.Cell Biol.,* 30 (2): 524-536.

Martinez-Balbas, M. A., Bauer, U. M., Nielsen, S. J., Brehm, A., & Kouzarides, T. (2000). Regulation of E2F1 activity by acetylation. *EMBO J.,* 19 (4): 662-671.

Marzio, G., Wagener, C., Gutierrez, M. I., Cartwright, P., Helin, K., & Giacca, M. (2000). E2F family members are differentially regulated by reversible acetylation. *J.Biol.Chem.,* 275 (15): 10887-10892.

Mayya, V., Lundgren, D. H., Hwang, S. I., Rezaul, K., Wu, L., Eng, J. K., Rodionov, V., & Han, D. K. (2009). Quantitative phosphoproteomic analysis of T cell receptor signaling reveals system-wide modulation of protein-protein interactions. *Sci.Signal.,* 2 (84): ra46.

McLaughlin-Drubin, M. E. & Munger, K. (2009). The human papillomavirus E7 oncoprotein. *Virology,* 384 (2): 335-344.

Meloni, A. R., Smith, E. J., & Nevins, J. R. (1999a). A mechanism for Rb/p130-mediated transcription repression involving recruitment of the CtBP corepressor. *Proc.Natl.Acad.Sci.U.S.A,* 96 (17): 9574-9579.

Meloni, A. R., Smith, E. J., & Nevins, J. R. (1999b). A mechanism for Rb/p130-mediated transcription repression involving recruitment of the CtBP corepressor. *Proc.Natl.Acad.Sci.U.S.A,* 96 (17): 9574-9579.

Meng, Z., Camalier, C. E., Lucas, D. A., Veenstra, T. D., Beck, G. R., Jr., & Conrads, T. P. (2006). Probing early growth response 1 interacting proteins at the active promoter in osteoblast cells using oligoprecipitation and mass spectrometry. *J.Proteome Res.,* 5 (8): 1931-1939.

Min, S. W., Cho, S. H., Zhou, Y., Schroeder, S., Haroutunian, V., Seeley, W. W., Huang, E. J., Shen, Y., Masliah, E., Mukherjee, C., Meyers, D., Cole, P. A., Ott, M., & Gan, L. (2010). Acetylation of tau inhibits its degradation and contributes to tauopathy. *Neuron,* 67 (6): 953-966.

Monetti, M., Nagaraj, N., Sharma, K., & Mann, M. (2011). Large-scale phosphosite quantification in tissues by a spike-in SILAC method. *Nat.Methods,* 8 (8): 655-658.

Morris, L., Allen, K. E., & La Thangue, N. B. (2000). Regulation of E2F transcription by cyclin E-Cdk2 kinase mediated through p300/CBP co-activators. *Nat.Cell Biol.,* 2 (4): 232-239.

Mueller, T., Breuer, P., Schmitt, I., Walter, J., Evert, B. O., & Wullner, U. (2009). CK2-dependent phosphorylation determines cellular localization and stability of ataxin-3. *Hum.Mol.Genet.,* 18 (17): 3334-3343.

Muller, H., Bracken, A. P., Vernell, R., Moroni, M. C., Christians, F., Grassilli, E., Prosperini, E., Vigo, E., Oliner, J. D., & Helin, K. (2001). E2Fs regulate the expression of genes involved in differentiation, development, proliferation, and apoptosis. *Genes Dev.,* 15 (3): 267-285.

Murga, M., Fernandez-Capetillo, O., Field, S. J., Moreno, B., Borlado, L. R., Fujiwara, Y., Balomenos, D., Vicario, A., Carrera, A. C., Orkin, S. H., Greenberg, M. E., & Zubiaga, A. M. (2001). Mutation of E2F2 in mice causes enhanced T lymphocyte proliferation, leading to the development of autoimmunity. *Immunity,* 15 (6): 959-970.

Nevins, J. R. (2001). The Rb/E2F pathway and cancer. *Hum.Mol.Genet.,* 10 (7): 699-703.

Novy, M., Pohn, R., Andorfer, P., Novy-Weiland, T., Galos, B., Schwarzmayr, L., & Rotheneder, H. (2005). EAPP, a novel E2F binding protein that modulates E2F-dependent transcription. *Mol.Biol.Cell,* 16 (5): 2181-2190.

Ogawa, H., Ishiguro, K., Gaubatz, S., Livingston, D. M., & Nakatani, Y. (2002). A complex with chromatin modifiers that occupies E2F- and Myc-responsive genes in G0 cells. *Science,* 296 (5570): 1132-1136.

Olsen, J. V., Blagoev, B., Gnad, F., Macek, B., Kumar, C., Mortensen, P., & Mann, M. (2006). Global, in vivo, and site-specific phosphorylation dynamics in signaling networks. *Cell,* 127 (3): 635-648.

Ong, S. E., Blagoev, B., Kratchmarova, I., Kristensen, D. B., Steen, H., Pandey, A., & Mann, M. (2002). Stable isotope labeling by amino acids in cell culture, SILAC, as a simple and accurate approach to expression proteomics. *Mol.Cell Proteomics,* 1 (5): 376-386.

Peeper, D. S., Keblusek, P., Helin, K., Toebes, M., van der Eb, A. J., & Zantema, A. (1995). Phosphorylation of a specific cdk site in E2F-1 affects its electrophoretic mobility and promotes pRB-binding in vitro. *Oncogene,* 10 (1): 39-48.

Pinkse, M. W., Uitto, P. M., Hilhorst, M. J., Ooms, B., & Heck, A. J. (2004). Selective isolation at the femtomole level of phosphopeptides from proteolytic digests using 2D-NanoLC-ESI-MS/MS and titanium oxide precolumns. *Anal.Chem.,* 76 (14): 3935-3943.

Polager, S., Ofir, M., & Ginsberg, D. (2008). E2F1 regulates autophagy and the transcription of autophagy genes. *Oncogene,* 27 (35): 4860-4864.

Rabinovich, A., Jin, V. X., Rabinovich, R., Xu, X., & Farnham, P. J. (2008). E2F in vivo binding specificity: comparison of consensus versus nonconsensus binding sites. *Genome Res.,* 18 (11): 1763-1777.

Ren, B., Cam, H., Takahashi, Y., Volkert, T., Terragni, J., Young, R. A., & Dynlacht, B. D. (2002). E2F integrates cell cycle progression with DNA repair, replication, and G(2)/M checkpoints. *Genes Dev.,* 16 (2): 245-256.

Rigbolt, K. T., Prokhorova, T. A., Akimov, V., Henningsen, J., Johansen, P. T., Kratchmarova, I., Kassem, M., Mann, M., Olsen, J. V., & Blagoev, B. (2011). System-wide temporal characterization of the proteome and phosphoproteome of human embryonic stem cell differentiation. *Sci.Signal.,* 4 (164): rs3.

Ross, P. L., Huang, Y. N., Marchese, J. N., Williamson, B., Parker, K., Hattan, S., Khainovski, N., Pillai, S., Dey, S., Daniels, S., Purkayastha, S., Juhasz, P., Martin, S., Bartlet-Jones, M., He, F., Jacobson, A., & Pappin, D. J. (2004). Multiplexed protein quantitation in Saccharomyces cerevisiae using amine-reactive isobaric tagging reagents. *Mol.Cell Proteomics,* 3 (12): 1154-1169.

Saydam, O., Senol, O., Schaaij-Visser, T. B., Pham, T. V., Piersma, S. R., Stemmer-Rachamimov, A. O., Wurdinger, T., Peerdeman, S. M., & Jimenez, C. R. (2010).

Comparative protein profiling reveals minichromosome maintenance (MCM) proteins as novel potential tumor markers for meningiomas. *J.Proteome Res.,* 9 (1): 485-494.

Schlisio, S., Halperin, T., Vidal, M., & Nevins, J. R. (2002). Interaction of YY1 with E2Fs, mediated by RYBP, provides a mechanism for specificity of E2F function. *EMBO J.,* 21 (21): 5775-5786.

Schmit, F., Korenjak, M., Mannefeld, M., Schmitt, K., Franke, C., von, E. B., Gagrica, S., Hanel, F., Brehm, A., & Gaubatz, S. (2007). LINC, a human complex that is related to pRB-containing complexes in invertebrates regulates the expression of G2/M genes. *Cell Cycle,* 6 (15): 1903-1913.

Sellers, W. R., Novitch, B. G., Miyake, S., Heith, A., Otterson, G. A., Kaye, F. J., Lassar, A. B., & Kaelin, W. G., Jr. (1998). Stable binding to E2F is not required for the retinoblastoma protein to activate transcription, promote differentiation, and suppress tumor cell growth. *Genes Dev.,* 12 (1): 95-106.

Song, Y., Willer, J. R., Scherer, P. C., Panzer, J. A., Kugath, A., Skordalakes, E., Gregg, R. G., Willer, G. B., & Balice-Gordon, R. J. (2010). Neural and synaptic defects in slytherin, a zebrafish model for human congenital disorders of glycosylation. *PLoS.One.,* 5 (10): e13743.

Stanelle, J., Stiewe, T., Theseling, C. C., Peter, M., & Putzer, B. M. (2002). Gene expression changes in response to E2F1 activation. *Nucleic Acids Res.,* 30 (8): 1859-1867.

Stevens, C., Smith, L., & La Thangue, N. B. (2003). Chk2 activates E2F-1 in response to DNA damage. *Nat.Cell Biol.,* 5 (5): 401-409.

Stirewalt, D. L. & Radich, J. P. (2003). The role of FLT3 in haematopoietic malignancies. *Nat.Rev.Cancer,* 3 (9): 650-665.

Takasaki, A., Hayashi, N., Matsubara, M., Yamauchi, E., & Taniguchi, H. (1999). Identification of the calmodulin-binding domain of neuron-specific protein kinase C substrate protein CAP-22/NAP-22. Direct involvement of protein myristoylation in calmodulin-target protein interaction. *J.Biol.Chem.,* 274 (17): 11848-11853.

Tenbaum, S. P., Papaioannou, M., Reeb, C. A., Goeman, F., Escher, N., Kob, R., von, E. F., Melle, C., & Baniahmad, A. (2007). Alien inhibits E2F1 gene expression and cell proliferation. *Biochim.Biophys.Acta,* 1773 (9): 1447-1454.

Tevosian, S. G., Shih, H. H., Mendelson, K. G., Sheppard, K. A., Paulson, K. E., & Yee, A. S. (1997). HBP1: a HMG box transcriptional repressor that is targeted by the retinoblastoma family. *Genes Dev.,* 11 (3): 383-396.

Thingholm, T. E., Jensen, O. N., Robinson, P. J., & Larsen, M. R. (2008). SIMAC (sequential elution from IMAC), a phosphoproteomics strategy for the rapid separation of monophosphorylated from multiply phosphorylated peptides. *Mol.Cell Proteomics,* 7 (4): 661-671.

Trimarchi, J. M., Fairchild, B., Verona, R., Moberg, K., Andon, N., & Lees, J. A. (1998). E2F-6, a member of the E2F family that can behave as a transcriptional repressor. *Proc.Natl.Acad.Sci.U.S.A,* 95 (6): 2850-2855.

Trimarchi, J. M., Fairchild, B., Wen, J., & Lees, J. A. (2001). The E2F6 transcription factor is a component of the mammalian Bmi1-containing polycomb complex. *Proc.Natl.Acad.Sci.U.S.A,* 98 (4): 1519-1524.

Trimarchi, J. M. & Lees, J. A. (2002). Sibling rivalry in the E2F family. *Nat.Rev.Mol.Cell Biol.,* 3 (1): 11-20.

Trouche, D., Cook, A., & Kouzarides, T. (1996). The CBP co-activator stimulates E2F1/DP1 activity. *Nucleic Acids Res.*, 24 (21): 4139-4145.

Van, H. D., Munoz, J., Braam, S. R., Pinkse, M. W., Linding, R., Heck, A. J., Mummery, C. L., & Krijgsveld, J. (2009). Phosphorylation dynamics during early differentiation of human embryonic stem cells. *Cell Stem Cell*, 5 (2): 214-226.

Vandel, L. & Kouzarides, T. (1999). Residues phosphorylated by TFIIH are required for E2F-1 degradation during S-phase. *EMBO J.*, 18 (15): 4280-4291.

Weinberg, R. A. (1995). The retinoblastoma protein and cell cycle control. *Cell*, 81 (3): 323-330.

Weinmann, A. S., Yan, P. S., Oberley, M. J., Huang, T. H., & Farnham, P. J. (2002). Isolating human transcription factor targets by coupling chromatin immunoprecipitation and CpG island microarray analysis. *Genes Dev.*, 16 (2): 235-244.

Whitfield, M. L., George, L. K., Grant, G. D., & Perou, C. M. (2006). Common markers of proliferation. *Nat.Rev.Cancer*, 6 (2): 99-106.

Xie, Q., Bai, Y., Wu, J., Sun, Y., Wang, Y., Zhang, Y., Mei, P., & Yuan, Z. (2011). Methylation-mediated regulation of E2F1 in DNA damage-induced cell death. *J.Recept.Signal.Transduct.Res.*, 31 (2): 139-146.

Yamasaki, L., Jacks, T., Bronson, R., Goillot, E., Harlow, E., & Dyson, N. J. (1996). Tumor induction and tissue atrophy in mice lacking E2F-1. *Cell*, 85 (4): 537-548.

Yao, Q., Li, H., Liu, B. Q., Huang, X. Y., & Guo, L. (2011). SUMOylation-regulated Protein Phosphorylation, Evidence from Quantitative Phosphoproteomics Analyses. *J.Biol.Chem.*, 286 (31): 27342-27349.

Young, A. P., Nagarajan, R., & Longmore, G. D. (2003). Mechanisms of transcriptional regulation by Rb-E2F segregate by biological pathway. *Oncogene*, 22 (46): 7209-7217.

Zhang, K., Wrzesinski, K., Stephen, J. F., Larsen, P. M., Zhang, X., & Roepstorff, P. (2008). Comparative proteome analysis of three mouse lung adenocarcinoma CMT cell lines with different metastatic potential by two-dimensional gel electrophoresis and mass spectrometry. *Proteomics*, 8 (23-24): 4932-4945.

Zhao, Y. & Jensen, O. N. (2009). Modification-specific proteomics: strategies for characterization of post-translational modifications using enrichment techniques. *Proteomics*, 9 (20): 4632-4641.

Zhu, J. W., Field, S. J., Gore, L., Thompson, M., Yang, H., Fujiwara, Y., Cardiff, R. D., Greenberg, M., Orkin, S. H., & DeGregori, J. (2001). E2F1 and E2F2 determine thresholds for antigen-induced T-cell proliferation and suppress tumorigenesis. *Mol.Cell Biol.*, 21 (24): 8547-8564.

F_0F_1 ATP Synthase: A Fascinating Challenge for Proteomics

Federica Dabbeni-Sala[1], Amit Kumar Rai[1] and Giovanna Lippe[2]
[1]*Department of Pharmacology, University of Padova, Padova*
[2]*Department of Food Science, University of Udine, Udine*
Italy

1. Introduction

The aim of this review is to provide insight and encouragement into the development of new proteomic approaches aimed at analyzing the relationship between structure and function of ATP synthase in different organisms and under different metabolic conditions. Particular attention will be paid to the preparation of the sample for the mass spectrometry (MS) analyses, which is also a critical step and requires a specific competence.

2. The nano-motor enzyme F_0F_1ATP synthase

F_0F_1ATP synthase is the terminal enzyme of the oxidative phosphorylation pathway (named complex V of the OXPHOS system) that is responsible for the majority of ATP synthesis in all living cells (Boyer, 1997). It is an exceptionally complicated protein complex, whose molecular mass varies from 540 to 585 kDa depending on the source, which is organized into a globular catalytic part (F_1) and a membranous moiety (F_0) linked by central and peripheral stalks.

The enzyme is present in bacterial plasma membranes and chloroplast thylakoids, where it contains 8 and 9 subunits, respectively (Borghese et al,. 1998; Richter et al,. 2000), and in mitochondria, where it is located in the inner membrane and consists of at least 15 and 17 different subunits in mammals and yeasts, respectively (Wittig and Schägger, 2008). The F_1 sector always consists of five subunits $\alpha_3\beta_3\gamma_1\delta_1\varepsilon_1$ and the α- and β-subunits are arranged alternatively, forming a hexagonal cylinder around the coiled-coil structure of the γ subunit. The F_0 part, which is responsible for ion translocation across the membrane, has instead a variable composition. The simplest form is present in bacteria and consists of the subunits $ac_{10\text{-}14}$. The c subunits form a ring structure with variable stoichiometry among species connected to F_1 by the central stalk, constituted by the subunits γ and ε, latter being homologous to subunit δ of the mitochondrial enzyme (Vignais and Satre, 1984) and able to modulate the catalysis (Suzuki et al,. 2011). The a subunit associates with the c-ring peripherally and with the lateral stalk, which is formed by the homo-dimer of subunits b and by subunit δ, present in single copy and located at the top of F_1(Walker and Dickson, 2006)(Fig.1A).

In mitochondria the additional subunits d, e, f, g, A6L, F6 and OSCP are associated to the complex, of which the subunits b, d, F6 and OSCP form the lateral stalk in single copies, OSCP homologous to prokaryotic subunit δ (Walker and Dickson, 2006). The so-called

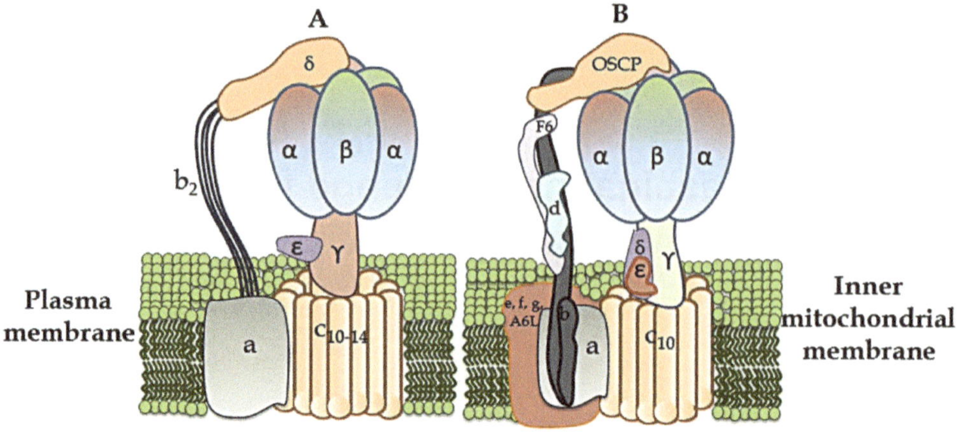

(A) Bacterial (*E.coli*) enzyme is assembled with a stiochiometry of α (3), β (3), γ, δ, ε, b (2), a, c (10-14). The central stalk is composed of γ and ε subunits, the peripheral one is composed of subunits b and δ, the proton channel is formed by the subunits $ac_{10\text{-}14}$.
(B) In the eukaryotic enzyme (*Bos taurus*) the central stalk is formed by subunits γ, δ and ε, the peripheral stalk is composed of subunits OSCP, b, d and F6 and the additional subunits A6L, e, f, g are associated to the proton channel ac_{10}.

Fig. 1. Schematic representation of bacterial and mitochondrial F_0F_1 ATP synthase.

minor subunits e, f, g and A6L all span the membrane and, apart for subunit e (Bisetto et al, 2008), their exact stoichiometries are poorly defined (Fig. 1B). Other subunits are species-specific, such as subunit i and k in *Saccharomyces cerevisiae* (Wittig and Schägger, 2008) and coupling factor B in *Bos taurus* (Lee et al,. 2008).
Besides these subunits, in some mammals such as beef, rat and man two hydrophobic proteins namely MLQ/6.8-kDa proteolipid (Chen et al,. 2007; Meyer et al,. 2007), and AGP/DAPIT (Ohsakaya et al,. 2011) are associated to the F_0 part when phospholipids are not extracted. All together, the mitochondrial membrane domain is constituted by approximately 30 trans-membrane α-helices (Carroll et al,. 2009). In addition, the mitochondrial complex can bind the inhibitor protein IF_1, which reversibly binds to F_1 with a 1:1 stoichiometry and fully inhibits the enzyme activity (Bason et al,. 2011; Harris and Das, 1991). In yeast, along with IF_1, the enzyme can be regulated by two additional proteins, namely Stf1 and Stf2 (stabilizing factor 1 and 2) (Andrianaivomananjaona et al,. 2010). The subunit composition of the ATP synthase from prokaryotic and eukaryotic sources along with the subunit homology and the corresponding nomenclature is reported in Table 1. The molecular masses of the different subunits are reported in Table 2, based on ATP synthase from *Bos taurus* and *Bacillus pseudofirmus*.
Despite the differences in the complexity, functionally important subunits are conserved and in all sources the enzyme catalyses the synthesis of ATP by using the energy of the electrochemical gradient of protons (or less commonly of sodium) generated by the respiratory chain. F_0F_1 is an unusually efficient rotary motor that synthesizes ATP at rates exceeding 100 molecules per second (Senior, 2007). Protons traveling down the H^+ gradient generate the rotation of the F_0 c-ring, making the central stalk also rotates, which in turn drives ATP synthesis from ADP and Pi by forcing different conformations sequentially on each of the catalytic sites in the three F_1 subunits β. The enzyme is able to work in the

Homologous subunits	Stoichiometry	Prokaryotes	Eukaryotes		
		E.coli	*S. cerevisiae*	*B. taurus*	*H. sapiens*
F_1	3	α	α	α	α
	3	β	β	β	β
	1	γ	γ	γ	γ
	1	ε	δ	δ	δ
	1	-	ε	ε	ε
F_0	1	δ	5	OSCP	OSCP
	1	a	6	a	a
	1	-	8	A6L	A6L
	10-14	c	9	c	c
	1-2	b	4	b	b
	1	-	d	d	d
	1	-	h	F6	F6
	1	-	f	f	f
	1-2	-	e	e	e
	n.d*	-	g	g	g
Species specific subunits	1		i	-	-
	n.d*	-	k	-	-
	1	-	-	Coupl. fact.B	-
Inhibitor Protein	0-1	-	Inh1	IF_1	IF_1
Stabilizing factor for IF_1	n.d*		Stf1	-	-
	n.d*	-	Stf2	-	
Associated proteins		-	-	AGP or DAPIT	AGP or DAPIT
		-	-	MLQ or 6.8 PL	MLQ or 6.8 PL

*n.d.- not determined

Table 1. Subunit composition and nomenclature of the ATP synthases from prokaryotes (*Escherichia coli*) and Eukaryotes (*Saccharomyces cerevisiae, Bos taurus* and *Homo sapiens*).

direction of ATP hydrolysis, sustaining the formation of the proton gradient, when there is loss of membrane potential (Fig. 2).

First direct visualization of ATP-driven rotation of *Bacillus* F_1 immobilized on the glass surface via the N-termini of its β-subunits was obtained more than 10 years ago (Noji et al,. 1997). These experiments showed that a fluorescent actin filament attached on the γ-subunit rotates uni-directionally, counterclockwise when viewed from membrane side, upon addition of ATP. A further technical sophistication used a sub-millisecond resolution camera to detect the rotation of gold beads attached to the γ subunit of the $\alpha_3\beta_3\gamma$ sub-complex along with fluorescence changes of an ATP hydrolysable analog. This technique allowed to display in real time the binding and release of nucleotides at the three catalytic sites simultaneously with the γ rotation (Adachi et al,. 2007). The rotation probe reports a pause, which corresponds to the period during which ATP binds to the empty catalytic site,

Subunits	*Bos taurus*		*Bacillus pseudofirmus*	
	Accession Numbers*	Molecular mass+	Accession Numbers*	Molecular mass+
α	P19483	55263.39	AAG48361.1	54674.48
β	P00829	51562.97	AAG48363.1	51752.14
γ	P05631	30255.71	AAG48362.1	31835.49
δ	P05630	15064.93	AAG48360.1	20534.63
ε	P05632	5651.67	AAG48364.1	14327.68
a	P00847	24787.91	AAG48358.1	26863.77
b	P13619	24668.72	AAG48359.1	18510.16
c	P32876	14223	AAC08039.1	6956.06
c	P07926	15029	-	-
c	Q3ZC75	14693	-	-
d	P13620	18561.28	-	-
e	Q00361	8189.47	-	-
f	Q28851	10165.99	-	-
g	Q28852	11286.26	-	-
8 or A6L	P03929	7936.56	-	-
F6	P02721	8958.09	-	-
OSCP	P13621	20929.75	-	-
Total F_0F_1	583442[a]		540290.53[b]	

*Accession numbers were obtained from UniProt

+Molecular masses are shown in Dalton

[a]Assuming the assigned stoichiometry for *Bos taurus* including the subunits e_1 and g_1 (excluding the amino-terminal modifications). If proteins MLQ and AGP are considered, the total protein mass increases to 596579 Da (Wittig and Schägger, 2008).

[b]According to the stoichiometry ($\alpha_3\beta_3\gamma\delta\varepsilon ab_2c_{13}$) for *Bacillus pseudofirmus*

Table 2. Molecular masses of subunits of *Bos taurus* and *Bacillus pseudofirmus* F_0F_1 ATP synthase

and a 120° step rotation, constituted by two sub-steppings, whose duration is still debated, during which ATP hydrolysis and release occur. Single molecule technology studies have been applied also to the whole F_0F_1 complexes from *Propionigenium modestum* and *Escherichia coli.* Rotation was probed with probes attached to the c-ring in the immobilized F_0F_1 and, as expected, occurred in the opposite direction when c-ring rotation was driven by ATP or by proton-flow (Ueno et al,. 2005).

2.1 ATP synthase biogenesis

The mitochondrial F_0F_1 complex is composed of both nuclear and mitochondrial gene products. In yeast the three F_0 core proteins a (Su6), A6L (Su8) and c (Su9) are encoded by mDNA, while in mammals only subunits a and A6L are encoded by mitochondrial genome. This arrangement highlights the complexity of enzyme assembly, which requires accessory factors, whose definition is still under investigation (Wittig and Schägger, 2008). Altogether 9 factors have been identified in yeast, but, until now, the role of only five of them has been defined. Three factors mediate the F_1 formation (Atp11p, Atp12p and possibly Fmc1p) (Ackerman, 2002; Lefebvre-Legendre et al,. 2001) and two the F_0 assembly (Atp10p and

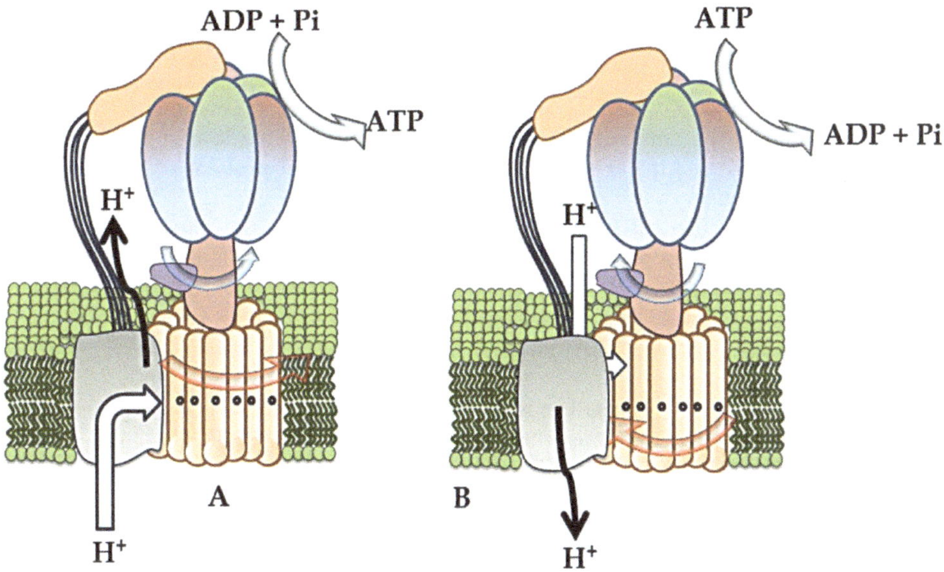

Fig. 2. Schematic representation of ATP synthesis and hydrolysis by F_0F_1 ATP synthase (A) Proton powered rotation of c ring makes the central stalk turn with it, generating torque and conformational changes in the catalytic αβ domain to synthesize ATP from ADP and Pi. (B) The hydrolysis of ATP sustains proton flow in opposite direction.

Eukaryotes	Factors	Mass (Da)	Swiss-Prot Accession
Yeast	Fmc1p	≤18364	P40491
Yeast	Atp10p	32093.91	P18496
Yeast	ATP11p	≤36581	P32453
Yeast	ATP12p	≤36554	P22135
Yeast	ATP22p	≤79756	A6ZYV0
Yeast	ATP23p	26890.37	P53722
Yeast	Mdm38p	58610.83	Q08179
Yeast	Aep3p	70310.03	Q12089
Yeast	Oxa 1p	40000.09	P39952
Human	ATPF2	32772	**Q8N5M1***
Human	ATPF1	36437	Q5TC12*

* UNIPROT accession number

Table 3. Assembly factors of yeast and human F_0F_1 ATP Synthase. The assembly factors for F_1 are in blue and F_0 are in red (Wittig and Schägger, 2008).

Atp22p) (Helfenbein et al,. 2003; Rak et al,. 2011). In mammalian cells only two factors are known, which are orthologus to yeast F_1 assembly factors (Table 3).

The assembly process is best characterized in yeast, where recent *in organello* pulse-labeling and pulse-chase experiments have enabled to identify three different assembly intermediates and to demonstrate that the whole enzyme is formed by two separate pathways that converge to form the ATP synthase from their respective end-products. One pathway leads to the formation of F_1, which was already known to assemble as an independent unit (Tzagoloff, 1969), and of the Su9-ring. These two sub-complexes subsequently combine to constitute the F_1/Su9-ring end-product. The other pathway leads to the formation of the Su6/Su8/stator sub-complex, which, in addition to Su6 and Su8, contains the chaperone Atp10p and additional still undefined proteins of the lateral stalk (Rak et al., 2011) (Fig. 3).

Because in yeast the interaction between Su6 and Su8 is kinetically much more rapid, the entire process is regulated by the control of the Su6 and Su8 translation by F_1 in order to obtain a balanced production of the different intermediates (Rak et al., 2011). Conversely, in mammals the amount of ATP synthase seems to be controlled by the availability of subunit c, as demonstrated in brown fat (Houstek et al,. 1995) and other tissues (Andersson et al,. 1997).

Independent of the mechanism, it has been proposed that the ATP synthase assembly may recapitulate some of the evolutionary events that gave rise to this enzyme. In fact, there is evidence that F_1 evolved from an ATP-dependent helicase (Gomis-Rüth et al,. 2001), while the Su9 derived from an ion channel (Rak et al., 2011), so that their combination converted a passive channel into an active pump.

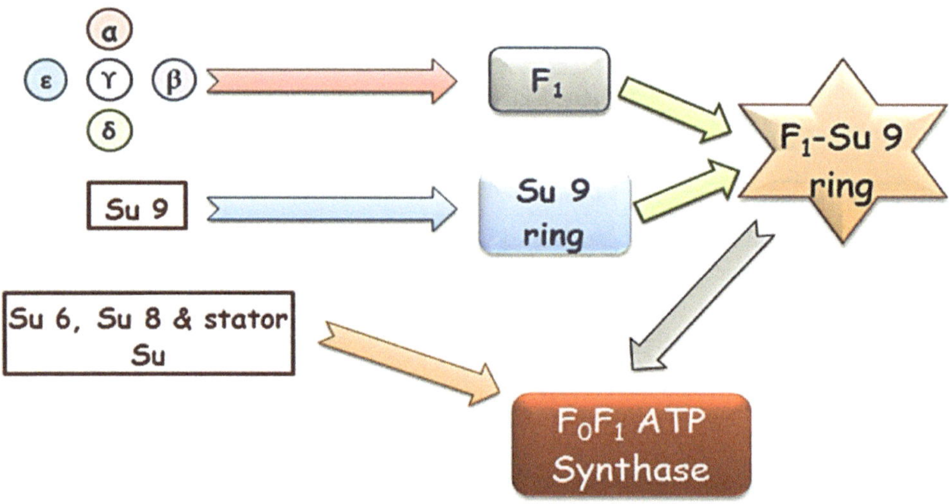

Fig. 3. Assembly of F_0F_1 ATP synthase in yeast. The scheme shows the two separate pathways, leading to two separate end-products, i.e. the F_1/Su9-ring and Su6/Su8/stator sub-complexes that converge at the end to form the whole F_0F_1 complex (Rak et al., 2011).

So far there is little evidence for tissue-specific or developmentally regulated isoforms of ATP synthase subunits. In tobacco plants three isoforms of the F_1 subunit β have been identified, of which only one is exclusively expressed in pollen (Lalanne et al,. 1998). In mammals, two tissue-specific isoforms of the F_1 γ subunit, heart and liver type, were identified in bovine F_0F_1-ATP synthase (Matsuda et al,. 1993). These two isoforms are generated by alternative splicing and their V_{max} and K_m are identical (Matsuda et al,. 1994). In addition, three isoforms (P1, P2, and P3) of the F_0 subunit c have been identified (Vives-

Bauza et al,. 2011). These isoforms differ in their cleavable mitochondrial targeting peptides, whereas the mature peptides are identical. Considering that in mammals c genes determine the ATP synthase content, the existence of iso-genes would be advantageous for regulation of subunit c synthesis, and thus ATP synthase biogenesis, by multiple factors. It appears that much remains to be learned about this argument.

2.2 ATP synthase self-association

Biochemical evidence and electron microscopy studies recently demonstrated that within the inner mitochondrial membrane the enzyme is organized in dimers and oligomers, which possibly associate with other inner mitochondrial membrane proteins, e.g. with phosphate and adenine nucleotide carriers in the "phosphorylating assemblies"- the so called ATP synthasome (Chen et al,. 2004; Wittig and Schägger, 2008). Elucidation of dimer/oligomers structural properties and of their formation process is quite important. In fact, proposed roles of the ATP synthase oligomers are higher efficiency and higher stability. In this regard, we demonstrated that dimers have a greater specific activity than monomers (Bisetto et al,. 2007). In accordance, a recent numerical simulation indicated a significant increase in charge density in regions of high membrane curvature induced by ATP synthase dimerization, thus favoring effective ATP synthesis under proton-limiting conditions (Fig. 4) (Strauss et al,. 2008). Moreover, these oligomers appear to play a special role for mitochondrial morphology, being involved in cristae formation (Couoh-Cardel et al,. 2010; Paumard et al,. 2002).

The structural properties of dimers/oligomers were initially characterized in yeast where genetic approaches, cross-linking analyses and electron microscopy images established preferential interactions within the inner membrane (Thomas et al,. 2008) mainly through the subunits Su6 (Wittig et al,. 2008), Su4 (Spannagel et al,. 1998), e (Everard-Gigot et al,. 2005) and g (Bustos and Velours, 2005), which are conserved in mammals, and also through the F_0 subunits h and i in yeast (Fronzes et al,. 2006). High-resolution images showed that both in yeast and mammals the dimers display angles between two F_1-F_1 ranging from 35° to 180°. Recent images of yeast dimers at 27 Å resolution showed that the dominant angle is 42°, suggesting that this is the most stable conformation (Couoh-Cardel et al., 2010).

We recently demonstrated by a structural proteomic approach that also in mammals the e subunit is essential for ATP synthase self-association in dimers and oligomers. Selective degradation by *in situ* limited proteolysis caused an alteration of the oligomeric distribution of ATP synthase by eliminating oligomers and reducing dimers in favor of monomers (Bisetto et al., 2008).

A critical aspect of F_0F_1 dimerization is related to the role of IF_1, which is still controversial (Wittig and Schägger, 2008). IF_1 is well known to bind ATP synthase under energy deficiency, i.e. at low pH and membrane potential, when the enzyme hydrolyzes rather than synthesizes ATP. Therefore, IF_1 is considered responsible for the beneficial down-regulation of F_0F_1 during ischemia in *in vitro* experimental models, but also *in vivo*, as demonstrated by our group in anaesthetized open-chest goat heart (Di Pancrazio et al,. 2004). Nevertheless, because isolated IF_1 from bovine heart is present in dimeric form in solution where it has been shown to link two F_1-subcomplexes (Cabezón et al,. 2003), it seemed conceivable that dimeric IF_1 might also be able to link two F_0F_1 complexes in the inner mitochondrial membrane. However, in yeast deletion of IF_1 and of the associated proteins Stf1 and Stf2 did not eliminate dimers and oligomers (Dienhart et al,. 2002), thus excluding an essential role of IF_1 in ATP synthase self-association. On the other hand, a very recent study revealed that

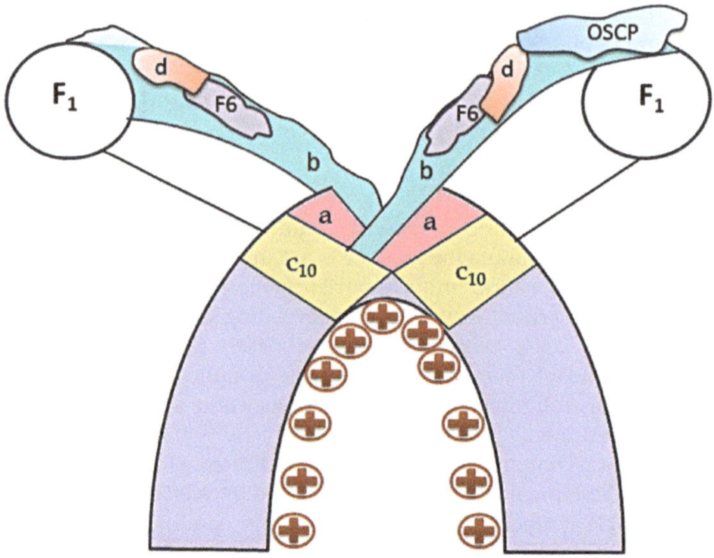

Fig. 4. Model of ATP synthase dimers. Dimers mainly interact through F_0 sector and enforce a strong local curvature on the inner mitochondrial membrane, where an increased charge density favors effective ATP synthesis (Strauss et al., 2008).

also in yeast oligomers contain considerable amounts of IF_1, raising the question of whether bound IF_1 inhibits the oligomer activity (Couoh-Cardel et al., 2010).

In bovine heart mitochondria, we demonstrated that physical release of IF_1 from the inner membrane did not markedly alter the amount of dimers separated by Blue Native electrophoresis (Tomasetig et al,. 2002), suggesting that F_0F_1 dimers could form independently from IF_1. Nevertheless, in human HeLa cells IF_1 overexpression increased ATP synthase dimers, as revealed by native electrophoresis, and this was paralleled by a higher ATP synthesis efficiency (Campanella et al,. 2009). However, it should be noted that in this paper the identification and quantification of ATP synthase dimers, as well as of their IF_1 content, seems questionable due to the use of dodecylmaltoside as detergent, which is well known to alter the dimer/monomer ratio (Tomasetig et al., 2002).

2.3 Disorders related to ATP synthase

In spite of the fact that the assembly process of the mitochondrial ATP synthase is still poorly characterized in humans, its defects have been recognized as a cause of human diseases (Houstek et al,. 2006; Kucharczyk et al,. 2009). Alteration of ATP synthase biogenesis leading to mitochondrial ATP synthase deficiency may cause two types of defects: qualitative when the enzyme is structurally modified and does not function properly, and quantitative when it is present in insufficient amounts. Examples of qualitative defects are those caused by missense mutations in the mitochondrially-encoded subunit a gene. Eight point mutations and a two-nucleotide micro-deletion in the ATP6 gene have been identified, of which the most common and best studied is the T8993G mutation that leads to replacement of a highly conserved leucine by arginine (Kucharczyk et al,. 2009). These mutations prevent ATP synthesis but not ATP hydrolysis because mutated F_0 can translocate protons from the cytosol to the mitochondrial matrix, thus sustaining membrane potential (Sgarbi et al,. 2006). The impaired ATP synthesis mainly affects brain tissue and at high mutation load, up to approximately 95%, the heteroplasmic ATP6 gene mutations manifest as neuropathy, ataxia, retinitis pigmentosa (NARP) or as fatal encephalopathy known as Leigh syndrome (Houstek et al., 2006). Examples of quantitative defects are those in which the cellular content of the enzyme is reduced to less than 30%. Apparently, these disorders are caused by different nuclear genetic defects that remain to be identified, but most of them display a uniform fatal phenotype with onset in newborns characterized by lactic acidosis and hypertrophic cardiomyopathy (Houstek et al., 2006). In both types of ATP synthase disorders, hyperpolarization due to decreased ATP synthesis promotes ROS production by the respiratory chain, an event that can contribute to the clinical phenotypes as suggested by the beneficial effect of antioxidants observed in NARP cells (Mattiazzi et al,. 2004). This finding is quite important, considering that, in spite of the considerable progress in understanding of the molecular mechanisms of ATP synthase disorders, the available therapeutic approaches are still extremely limited (Kucharczyk et al., 2009). It has been proposed that other secondary effects possibly involved in the pathogenic pathways of ATP synthase deficiency could be changes in mitochondrial cristae morphology, which is mediated by ATP synthase oligomerization (Couoh-Cardel et al., 2010; Paumard et al., 2002), and/or a concomitant impairment of an ectopic function of ATP synthase localized on cell surface (see paragraph 4) (Kucharczyk et al., 2009).

Microarray analyses have been performed in an attempt to gain a more global view of the cellular consequences of ATP synthase deficiency. In fibroblast cell lines from 13 genetically heterogeneous patients, 1632 human genes involved in mitochondrial biology, cell cycle regulation, signal transduction and apoptosis have been analysed. Surprisingly, only minor changes in expression of ATP synthase related genes were shown. Moreover, the cellular gene expression phenotypes were different depending on the site (mtDNA vs nuclear DNA) and the severity (ATP synthase content) of the underlying defect, indicating the need for further investigation of these pathways in other ATP synthase disorders (Cížková et al,. 2008). As far as our knowledge is concerned, the proteomic profiles of ATP synthase-related diseases have not yet been reported.

Other intriguing examples of ATP synthase-related diseases are Batten disease in man or ceroid lipofuscinosis in sheep. Both are storage diseases with abnormal accumulation of subunit c in lysosomes occurring in the brain and liver, respectively. MS and protein sequencing have shown that the stored protein is structurally identical to the normal mitochondrial subunit c (Chen et al,. 2004).

Up- and down-regulation of ATP synthase biogenesis has been observed under different pathophysiological conditions (Houstek et al., 2006). We developed polyspecific antibodies directed against the whole human mitochondrial subproteome by hyperimmunization of rabbits with purified skeletal muscle mitochondria, which allowed detection of up-regulation of ATP synthase, in muscle biopsies from patients affected by MELAS (mitochondrial encephalomyopathy with lactic acidosis and stroke-like episodes) which are characterized by a drastic reduction of OXPHOS complex 1 (Loro et al,. 2009). MS approaches have also been applied to compare the ATP synthase expression levels *in vivo* and *in vitro*. Recent examples of ATP synthase down-regulation have been obtained by the mitochondrial proteome analyses in heart from type 2 diabetic patients (Heather and Clarke, 2010) and in pancreatic β-cells exposed to high glucose (Ahmed et al,. 2010).

3. Mass spectrometry data of F_0F_1 ATP synthase

The whole F_0F_1 complex, as well as individual subunits or sub-complexes, have been purified by classical approaches and their amino acid sequences determined almost entirely by direct protein sequence analysis (Walker et al,. 1991). The detailed molecular structures of F_0F_1 from several species have been studied intensively by different groups (Chen et al,. 2006; Cingolani and Duncan, 2011; Dautant et al,. 2010), and the importance of these studies is highlighted by the award of the Nobel Prize to John Walker in 1997. The structural analyses by X-ray diffraction required the identification of the subunit composition by measurement of accurate molecular masses by mass spectrometry, allowing the detection of posttranslational modifications. The exploration of the exposed regions by limited proteolysis had similar analytical requirements.

Mass spectrometry of F_0F_1 has been a methodological challenge due to the presence of both hydrophilic parts and hydrophobic subunits, which are difficult to detect by standard ionization techniques, and the fact that all subunits are bound non-covalently. More than 15 years ago, reverse phase liquid chromatography methods were applied to purify the hydrophilic subunits and also some membrane-bound subunits (b, d, F6, e, f, g and A6L) of the bovine heart enzyme, so as to allow their molecular masses to be measured by a mass spectrometer with electrospray ionization (Collinson et al,. 1994). Over the years, direct identification of all the hydrophilic and most of the hydrophobic subunits of ATP synthase from many sources has been obtained by MALDI- and ESI-MS/MS analyses of the tryptic peptides of individual bands or spots on native polyacrylamide or SDS gels. However, the most hydrophobic membrane proteins, such as subunit c and A6L, could not be detected by these approaches (Wittig et al,. 2010). All of the hydrophobic subunits have been identified by tandem mass spectrometry after optimization of their purification in organic solvents and by fragmenting the intact protein ions by collision induced dissociation (CID) with argon (Carroll et al,. 2007). Moreover, a procedure that allows to measure the molecular masses of all of the 17 subunits of F_0F_1 from bovine heart in a single experiment has been published, this approach is based on the use of a mobile phase during liquid chromatography separation, in which the hydrophilic and hydrophobic components remained soluble, linked directly via an electrospray interface to a triple quadrupole mass spectrometer operated in positive ion mass spectrometry. The method has been used to characterize the ATP synthase subunits from a variety of species and to follow the progress of mild trypsinolysis of the enzyme (Carroll et al., 2009).

3.1 Phosphoproteome of ATP synthase

The measurement of the mass of a protein allows the presence but not the location of any posttranslational modifications (PTMs) to be detected. Phosphorylation of serine, threonine and tyrosine residues is one of the most prominent PTMs and a key regulator of nearly all biological processes including mitochondrial oxidative phosphorylation (Hüttemann et al,. 2007). However, phosphorylation is often a sub-stoichiometric process and usually only a low percentage of a given protein is present in phosphorylated state at a given time, making its observation challenging. In the past, phosphorylation analysis was mostly done by radiolabeling with $^{32/33}P$ (Bendt et al,. 2003; MacDonald et al,. 2002) combined with amino acid analysis. In the last decade, considerable effort has been devoted to improving the analysis of phospho-proteome by MS (Eyrich et al,. 2011; Gerber et al,. 2003). The main criticisms are ion suppression of phosphorylated species in a high background of non-phosphorylated ones, specificity lack of the proteolytic cleavage and lability of phosphoester bonds during MS analysis. Different enrichment strategies for phosphorylated peptides or proteins, such as immunoaffinity chromatography (IMAC) or metal oxide affinity chromatography (MOAC), have been established to reduce sample complexity. Concurrently, attention has been paid to the LC-MS instrumentation to avoid loss of phosphorylated peptides within the analytical system. In addition, specific MS techniques have been developed for the identification and relative quantification of phosphorylation sites down to the femtomole range. Nevertheless, phospho-proteomics still remains far from being routine.

Regarding ATP synthase, in a recent phospho-proteomic study an improved protocol called BEMAD enabled to identify in a cytosolic lysate from mouse brain Ser76 of the F_1 subunit α as being phosphorylated (Vosseller et al,. 2005). This method involved differential isotopic labeling of O-phosphate-modified serine/ threonine residues through Michael addition with normal or deuterated dithiothreitol and enrichment of these peptides by thiol chromatography. Specificity of O-phosphate mapping was achieved by blocking of cysteine labeling by prior oxidation and by subsequent enzymatic dephosphorylation of O-phosphate-modified peptides. In a single mass spectrometry analysis along with αSer76 other 20 phosphorylation sites (5 previously reported) were identified and quantified.

MS allowed to identify phosphorylated tyrosine and serine residues in the F_1 subunits α and β from yeast, which was long considered a "zero background" organism for tyrosine phosphorylation (Krause-Buchholz et al,. 2006). A novel screening technique was applied in combination with Blue Native electrophoresis to separate the ATP synthase complex in native state and second dimension SDS-PAGE to resolve its subunit composition (see below). LA–ICP–MS (Laser ablation inductively coupled plasma mass spectrometry) was used to rapidly screen for the presence of phosphorus in the subunits using sulfur as the internal standard element for quantification. The subunits containing phosphorus were then identified by MALDI–FTICR–MS (matrix-assisted laser desorption/ionization Fourier transform ion cyclotron resonance mass spectrometry) as Tyr434, Ser 413 and Ser426 of the α subunit and Tyr7 of the β subunit (Krause-Buchholz et al., 2006).

At variance from yeast, by combining Blue Native electrophoresis and second/third dimension SDS-PAGEs with LC-ESI/MS analysis we found that in bovine heart mitochondria only the F_1 γ subunit contained one phosphorylated tyrosine (Di Pancrazio et al,. 2006). Moreover, the tyrosine residue was phosphorylated only in the monomeric form of ATP synthase and was present in low amount (about 6% of the total protein monomer), while the ATP synthase dimers were lacking. Interestingly, this finding suggested that the oligomerization process might be regulated through cell signaling (Di Pancrazio et al., 2006), but the pathway is still to be clarified. To obtain these results a novel procedure was developed because, due to the low percentage of the phosphorylated species, standard MS/MS analysis failed to detect phosphorylated peptides. The screening of the phosphorylated subunits was done by immunoblotting using anti-phosphotyrosine antibody after the third SDS-PAGE and after trypsin digestion the phosphorylated fragment of γ subunit was identified and quantified by a novel LC-ESI/MS method. This latter was based on the use of two different de-clustering potential values that allowed to obtain, with a single LC-ESI/MS run, the pattern of the phosphorylated and unphosphorylated species. These species were further analyzed by tracing back the origin of the HPO_3-deprived forms using tandem MS (Alverdi et al,. 2005).

Several other studies have shown that phoshorylation can occur on different sites of ATP synthase in mammals (HÃ¸jlund et al,. 2003; Ko et al,. 2002), yeast and plants (Struglics et al,. 1998). Nevertheless, a comprehensive mapping is still lacking. The constant technological progress might soon enable to generate the quantitative and temporal phosphorylation pattern of the enzyme in all organisms and under different pathophysiological conditions, thus allowing understanding of the regulation of ATP synthase in light of cell signaling.

3.2 Native mass spectrometry

ESI-MS and the novel LILBID-MS (laser induced liquid bead ion desorption mass spectrometry) are two techniques that can be used under native conditions to determine the molecular mass of non-covalently assembled complexes up to the MDa-range with high accuracy. The techniques are complementary, LILBID being more tolerant than nESI to addition of detergents, which are necessary to solubilise membrane proteins such as ATP synthase. Very recently, LILBID-MS combined with Blue Native electrophoresis was successfully applied to compare the subunit composition of the whole F_0F_1 from *Bacillus pseudofirmus* and from bovine and human heart (Hoffmann et al,. 2010), but also to determine the subunit composition of other even larger membrane complexes such as the NADH-dehydrogenase (complex I of the OXPHOS system) from *Yarrowia lipolytica* (Sokolova et al,. 2010). LILBID-MS can be applied in several modes, from soft laser desorption (yielding the intact macromolecular complexes) to medium to high laser intensity (which disassembles the protein complexes partially into sub-complexes and these latter into the single subunits). The analysis of the bacterial enzyme revealed at low laser intensity the masses of the F_1 sub-complex, the F_1 sub-complex lacking the δ-subunit and the F_0 sub-complex, while at high laser energy the signal of the 8 subunits appeared. In the case of the mammalian enzymes, the spectra evidenced all of the 15 subunits, of which the masses agreed within ± 150 Da with theoretical masses (see Table 2). While functionally important subunits are conserved, others, such as the so-called minor F_0 subunits, show differences in their masses among the species. Determination of their masses from many sources might help to clarify their structural and functional roles, which are still only partially known, and LILBID-MS certainly offers a novel and rapid way to obtain such results using very low material and in detergent solution.

LILBID-MS has also provided an accurate determination of stoichiometry (c_n) of the sub-complex formed by the c-ring from the thermoalkaliphilic bacterium *Bacillus sp.* (Meier et al,. 2007). This result is particularly interesting, considering the difficulty to detect c subunit by classical MALDI-MS and LC-MS/MS (Bisetto et al., 2008; Wittig et al., 2010). Moreover, it represents an important MS application in cell bioenergetics, the number of c-subunits being in principle equals to the number of H^+ transported across the membrane for every 360° rotation of the rotor in which three ATP molecules are synthesized in the three β subunits. Hence the H^+/ATP ratio can be expressed by $c_n/3$.

At variance from LILBID, nESI is ideal for soluble complexes and we recently applied this technique to determine the exact molecular mass of the non-covalent complex formed in solution by the ATP synthase inhibitor IF_1 and Calmodulin, the archetypal EF-hand calcium sensor. Interestingly, nESI established a 1:1 stoichiometry between IF_1 and Calmodulin, suggesting that binding to Calmodulin promotes the dissociation of the pre-existing dimeric form of IF_1 (Cabezon et al,. 2001). Furthermore, native mass analysis was paralleled to the definition of the IF_1-CaM complex topology by combining limited proteolysis and cross-linking data with MALDI-MS and LC-MS/MS analyses (Pagnozzi et al,. 2010).

3.3 AQUA workflow

Native mass spectrometry is a powerful technique to define the stoichiometry of protein complexes, but this can be defined also by quantifying the absolute amounts of the different subunits and therefore by calculating their molar ratio. An interesting approach is the AQUA workflow, which is a variation of isotope dilution MS techniques used for decades for quantification of small molecules and more recently successfully applied in the proteomics context to the absolute quantification of proteins and their modification states in whole cell lysates (Gerber et al., 2003). This approach is based on the addition of synthetic isotopically labeled reference peptides in known amounts to a protein sample in solution prior to tryptic digestion and LC-MS analysis. Being gel-free, this approach avoids errors due to incomplete peptide extraction from the gel or impaired protein digestion within the gel matrix.

Regarding ATP synthase, we recently applied the AQUA workflow to determine the stoichiometry of the F_0 subunit e in bovine heart mitochondria (Bisetto et al., 2008). This subunit is involved in dimer/oligomer formation both in yeast (Fronzes et al., 2006) and mammals (Bisetto et al., 2008), but its stoichiometry was still unknown (Arakaki et al,. 2001; Hong and Pedersen, 2003). A critical point of the AQUA approach is the design of the heavy-labeled peptides, which must be unique to the proteins of interest and show high ionization efficiency (proteotypic peptides). In addition, such peptides should have a good fragmentation pattern with reliable matching of b- and y- ion series, a preferable length between 7 and 15 amino acid residues and contain no chemically unstable residues (M,W, C or N-terminal Q or N) or unstable peptide bonds (e.g. D-P). Moreover, it is necessary to choose reference subunits, whose stoichiometry is already known, to validate the method. We have chosen the F_0 subunit b and the F_1 subunit γ as reference subunits which are present in single copies in the whole F_0F_1 complex, as defined by crystal structures. After having chosen among the proteotypic peptides characterized by LC-MS/MS three peptides - one from subunits e, b and γ-, the corresponding isotopically labeled analogues were added in known amounts to the detergent extracts of bovine heart mitochondria prior to tryptic digestion. The absolute quantification of the three subunits was then achieved by comparison of the areas under the curve (AUC) of the extracted ion chromatograms of the endogenous and labeled peptides in LC-MS mode. Accuracy of the method was demonstrated by confirming the 1:1 stoichiometry of subunit γ and b and by the low coefficients of variation which were <12% for technical and biological replicates. In the samples analyzed, which contained extracts of mitochondria in resting state, subunit e was present in 1:1 molar ratio with respect to subunit b or γ, demonstrating that in F_0F_1 it is contained as unique copy.

4. Native electrophoresis of F_0F_1 ATP synthase

Classical 2D IEF-SDS-PAGE do not resolve all the subunits of ATP synthase, because they are quite often small, hydrophobic and basic (pI>9). For this reason, in some studies MS analysis has been run on peptide mixtures obtained after in-solution trypsinization of sample extracts (Bisetto et al., 2008). Alternatively, a powerful approach for efficient separation from tissue homogenates, tissue biopsies and cell cultures of the whole complex of ATP synthase, as well as of assembly intermediates and supra-molecular structures is the native polyacrylamide gel electrophoresis after mild detergent extraction (Wittig et al,. 2006). Following native PAGE, proteins of interest can be extracted in native state and analyzed by MS or electroblotted for immunodetection or analyzed by in-gel catalytic activity assays. In addition, subunit composition of the complexes can be identified by various denaturating techniques: SDS-PAGE, doubled SDS-PAGEs, as we used to detect phosphotyrosine in monomer/dimers of ATP synthase (Di Pancrazio et al., 2006) and IEF/SDS PAGEs (Wittig et al., 2006), as shown in Fig. 5. These advantages make this approach superior for functional proteomic analyses. For this reason, a brief introduction to native electrophoresis will be presented.

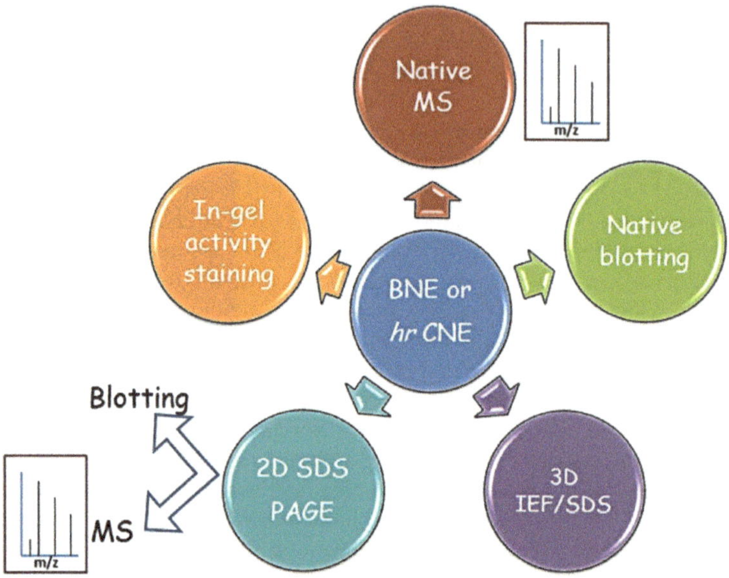

Fig. 5. Applications of native electrophoresis for functional proteomic analyses.

Blue native electrophoresis, abbreviated as BNE, was developed to isolate native membrane proteins and complexes on micro-scale. It separates proteins in the mass range of 10 kDa to 10 MDa. It is a one step technique to isolate proteins from mitochondria, whole cell lysates and tissue homogenates (Wittig et al., 2006). BNE has also been used for the identification of protein-protein interactions, as we recently did to define the new interaction between ATP synthase and Cyclophilin D in mammalian mitochondria (Giorgio et al,. 2009). Besides BNE a similar native electrophoresis method was developed that is called Clear native electrophoresis (CNE) with its variant high resolution CNE (*hr* CNE). Fig. 6 depicts the resolution of the five OXPHOS complexes including ATP synthase with its dimeric form obtained by BNE and *hr* CNE. All these methods are quite similar and have been used for MS analyses, but differ in few aspects, which are discussed below, with their drawbacks and applications.

From a practical stand point BNE, CNE and hr CNE differ in the composition of cathode buffers as well as in the mechanisms by which proteins migrate in the gel. What makes BNE different from CNE and *hr* CNE is the incorporation of Coomassie Brilliant Blue G-250 both in the cathode buffer as well as in loading dye. Coomassie is an anionic dye, it binds to the proteins and imparts negative charge over their surface. In this way proteins migrate with

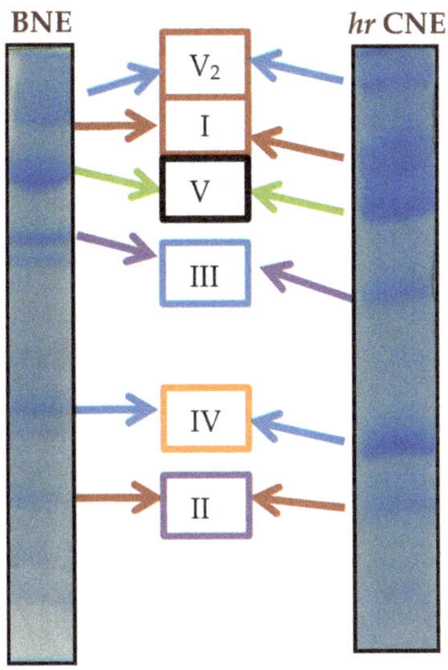

Fig. 6. BNE and *hr* CNE of DDM extracts of bovine heart mitochondria showing OXPHOS complexes.

respect to their native masses independently of their p*I*. Negative charge also helps in preventing protein aggregation as negative charges repel each other and this is the reason for its very good resolution. Furthermore, upon binding the previously detergent-solubilised membrane, proteins lose their hydrophobic character and become water soluble hence no further detergent is required in these gels minimising the risk of detergent-dependent protein denaturation (Wittig et al., 2006). Besides Coomassie, the presence of Imidazole in anode and cathode buffer (BNE, CNE, *hr* CNE) helps in maintaining pH in the range 7.0-7.5, and incorporation of high concentration of 6-aminohexanoic acid (a zwitterionic substance) improves the solubilisation of membranes (Wittig and Schägger, 2008). Separation of proteins as blue bands helps in gel excision and recovery of blue stained native proteins by electroelution (Wittig et al., 2006) for further MS analysis, as recently applied for LILBID MS (Hoffmann et al., 2010).

A rapid way to identify ATP synthase in BNE is to monitor ATP hydrolysis by in-gel activity staining, which was developed in our lab and is based on the formation of a white lead phosphate precipitate from phosphate (Pi) released during the reaction (Fig. 7) (Zerbetto et al,. 1997). The catalytic activity can be obtained by incubating the gels in glycine buffer supplemented with Mg-ATP in the presence of 0.2% $Pb(NO_3)_2$. The native staining of ATP synthase is reproducible and the white bands on gel can be easily quantified by densitometry (Bisetto et al., 2007). Moreover, the bands can be excised and easily destained in acetic acid solution giving a colourless protein complex ready for MS analysis. This method had been successfully applied by our group to analyse skeletal muscle and heart biopsies from patients with oxidative phosphorylation enzyme deficiencies (Zerbetto et al., 1997)

Detection limits of in-gel activity staining are in the microgram range of protein or micromolar phosphate and the resulting white bands are challenging for detection and documentation of low activity due to interference of Coomassie dye. Different strategies of optimization for activity staining of BNE have been applied by us (Bisetto et al., 2007) and others (Suhai et al,. 2009; Wittig and Schägger, 2005). Alternatively, CNE can be used that was introduced to circumvent this disadvantage of BNE. In fact, it uses the same buffers and conditions for electrophoresis but the difference lies on the absence of Coomassie dye both in cathode buffer as well as in sample buffer. In this way, much higher activity staining has been obtained (Wittig et al,. 2007). However, due to the absence of Coomassie there is no negative charge shift and the movement of proteins totally depends on their intrinsic mass and p*I*. Therefore CNE suffers from a poor resolution and is limited to proteins having a p*I*<7 unlike BNE where even proteins having pI>10.5 migrate towards anode (Wittig and Schägger, 2008). Anyway, CNE offers advantage over BNE for isolation of supra-molecular structures, including ATP synthase dimers and oligomers, being the mildest technique to separate mitochondrial membrane proteins.

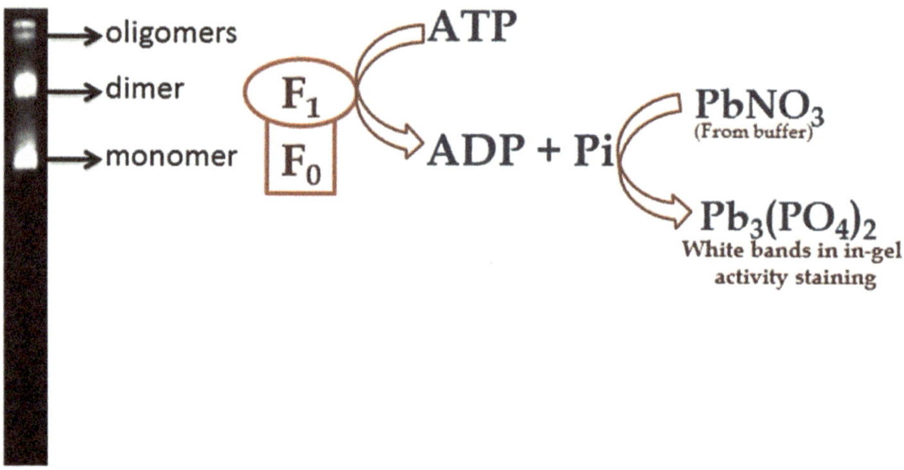

Fig. 7. In-gel ATPase activity staining of the different oligomeric forms of ATP synthase extracted by Digitonin (0.5 g/g protein) from mouse heart mitochondria and analyzed by BNE.

To preserve the advantages of both the techniques Wittig et al introduced *hr* CNE. In this technique cathode buffer is supplemented with a combination of colourless anionic and neutral detergents such as Triton X-100, Deoxycholate, or Dodecyl-β-D-maltoside (DDM). This leads to a charge shift over the surface of the proteins and helps them in migration with a resolution comparable with BNE. Also there is no interference in in-gel assays due to absence of Coomassie.

An interesting recent application of *hr* CNE is related to the molecular characterization of assembly intermediates of ATP synthase in mammals. In fact, using particularly mild detergent conditions and *hr* CNE, Wittig et al. were able to separate the assembly intermediate in human ρ_0 cells, which lack the mitochondrial DNA encoding subunits a and A6L (Wittig et al., 2010). By analyzing its subunit composition by ESI-MS/MS after excising the native band from 1D *hr* CN-PAGE or by MALDI-MS (MS/MS) after 2D *hr* CN-/SDS-PAGE they established that this intermediate contains all the nuclear-encoded subunits. These results allowed to propose that in mammals, differently from yeast (Hoffmann et al., 2010), the assembly of the whole enzyme is a linear process and the subunits of the lateral

stalk combine with the F_1 sector and the c-ring independently from the mitochondrial encoded subunits a and A6L which bind at the late stage. Conversely it has been proposed that in yeast the subunits Su6/Su8, homologous to subunits a and A6L, first combine to the subunits of the lateral stalk, forming the sub-complex Su6/Su8/stator, which finally binds to the sub-complex F_1/c-ring, as already shown in Fig. 3. Moreover, the finding that ρ_0 mitochondria still contain dimers/oligomers of ATP synthase although in lower amounts than control mitochondria, supported the idea that subunits a/A6L contribute, together with subunits e/g (Bisetto et al., 2008), to stabilize the supra-molecular structures, but they are not the most important interface as previously proposed in yeast (Wittig et al., 2008).
Recently Yan et al., using rat brain mitochondria, demonstrated that a non-gradient highly porous BNE of 8% polyacrilamide is an efficient technique to resolve all OXPHOS complex along with other mitochondrial proteins, such as DLDH and Hsp60 polymer. Further, the gel strips can be even used to perform 2D BN-/SDS PAGE or the bands can be excised for MS peptide sequencing (Yan and Forster, 2009).

4.1 Types of detergents and their use in native electrophoresis

The choice of detergent for protein extraction is an integral part of a successful native electrophoresis. The principal effect of detergents during solubilisation is the breaking of lipid-lipid and lipid-protein interactions present on biomembranes. Competing with lipids for the occupation of the surface of integral hydrophobic proteins, they form mixed micelles containing detergent, lipids and proteins. The solubilisation effect is maximum when the detergent is used at a concentration equal or higher to the Critical Micelle Concentration (CMC), the concentration at which the detergent molecules form micelles. These are detergent self associating structures with hydrophobic ends facing inside and hydrophilic groups facing outside the aqueous phase. CMC is a characteristic of each detergent and depends on pH, temperature and ionic strength (Reisinger and Eichacker, 2008).
The anionic SDS is, in principle, not suitable for native electrophoresis as besides solubilising membranes, it dissociates and denatures the enzyme complex leading to loss of activity. Non-ionic detergents are uncharged and milder and hence can be used in membrane solubilisation to isolate mitochondrial complexes with varying degrees of association dependent on the kind of detergent used and its concentration. The most commonly used non-ionic detergents are Triton X-100, Digitonin and Dodecyl-β-D-maltoside (DDM) which form micelles at very low concentration, thus avoiding protein denaturation (Wittig and Schägger, 2008). Regarding isolation of OXPHOS complexes, these non-ionic detergents behave very differently from each other. For example, Digitonin can be used in a very broad concentration range (from 0.5 to 8 g/g proteins), as compared to Triton and DDM which work in the range of 1-2 g/g proteins (Schägger and Pfeiffer, 2000). Besides this, Digitonin is the best candidate for the isolation of supercomplexes due to its milder nature (Reisinger and Eichacker, 2008). They can be used to extract OXPHOS complexes from bacteria, yeast and mammals, as well as from subcellular fractions or total membranes (Wittig et al., 2006). The quantity of detergent required to solubilise membrane proteins vary in the different cells/tissues and optimal solubilisation conditions for each membrane and each membrane complex should be experimentally investigated.
Recently, an interesting modification of classical native PAGE has been proposed. Klodmann et al. reported the treatment of the samples with low amounts of SDS before BNE. This allowed to destabilize the OXPHOS complexes in sub-complexes in a very defined and reproducible manner and to study their internal architectures. SDS was added

to the mitochondrial Digitonin extracts from *Arabidopsis* in the range of 0.05-1.0% just before BNE loading. By combining with 2D BN-/ SDS or 2D BN/BN PAGE, the authors clearly demonstrated the variable effect of SDS on the OXPHOS complexes. As an example, at 0.2% SDS concentration, the ATP synthase complex dissociated in to F_0 and F_1. At 0.3% F_0 even dissociated in to a sub-complex composed of c-ring (Klodmann et al,. 2011).

5. Ectopic F_0F_1ATP synthase of mammalian cells

The application of proteomic analyses to sub-cellular mammalian fractions other than mitochondria revealed the presence of mitochondrial membrane components in unexpected cellular locations, such as plasma membranes or nuclei. Some of these studies ascribed it to cross-contamination, due to the contiguity of the different membranes within the cell and to the high sensitivity of MS which identifies the proteins up to subfentomolar levels, but in others cases the parallel demonstration of such unusual locations obtained in cells and tissues by immunofluorescence and functional studies led the scientists to consider the proteomics results a mainstay to discover new scenarios in the intracellular traffic connections.

Regarding ATP synthase, many proteomics studies have recently reported that subunits of this complex, along with other OXPHOS complexes, are expressed in extra-mitochondrial membranes of different mammalian cell types - especially on the cell surface, but also in the endoplasmic reticulum and nuclear envelope (Panfoli et al,. 2011). In human apoptotic T-leukemia cells the presence of eight ATP synthase subunits was revealed in the nucleus fraction obtained by differential extraction and stable isotope labeling of cell culture followed by LC-MS/MS analysis and it has been ascribed to a dynamic recruitment of mitochondria into nuclear invaginations during apoptosis (Hwang et al,. 2006). In mouse brain a proteomics analysis of microsomal fraction obtained both by 2D-LC-MS/MS and shotgun LC-MS/MS found many subunits of the OXPHOS complexes, including ATP synthase, which were proposed to represent mitochondrial proteins with high turnover rates in the cell (Stevens Jr et al,. 2008). Conversely, ATP synthase is now considered a true resident on the plasma membranes. In fact, the identification by MS of ATP synthase subunits in plasma membrane preparations from different sources has been paralleled by the demonstration of the enzyme expression with the F_1 sector facing outside (and for this reason the enzyme is named ecto-F_0F_1) obtained by cytometry, confocal microscopy and functional studies (Vantourout et al,. 2010). ATP synthase subunits were identified in plasma membranes isolated from cell culture, i.e. in hypoxia-adapted tumor cells where differential $^{16}O/^{18}O$ stable isotopic labeling and multidimensional LC-MS/MS revealed an increased expression of ATP synthase α subunit with respect to normoxia (Stockwin et al,. 2006), and in tissues that were characterized by high purity, i.e. obtained by combining subcellular fractionation with immunoisolation strategies so that no proteins from endoplasmic reticulum and nuclear envelope were detected (Zhang et al,. 2007). In other studies, the presence of ATP synthase subunits was found in the detergent-resistant fragments of plasma membranes, i.e. in the lipid rafts which are cholesterol and sphingolipid-rich microdomains involved in signal trasduction. In particular, in lipid rafts isolated from rat liver and subjected to an efficient *in solution* digestion followed by cRPLC/MS/MS four subunits both of F_1 and F_0 sector were identified (Bae et al,. 2004).

The major limit of the proteomic studies related to plasma membranes is that in no one the complete subunit composition of ecto-F_0F_1 has been recognized, leaving open the possibility of a different assembly of the ectopic enzyme with respect to the mitochondrial ATP synthase. We recently separated by detergent extraction and BNE the whole ecto- F_0F_1 from plasma membranes of rat liver (Giorgio et al,. 2010) and we found that the low, but constant amounts of F_0F_1 complexes display a similar molecular weight to the monomeric form of the mitochondrial F_0F_1 ATP synthase, as evidenced by in-gel ATPase activity staining and immunoblotting. This suggests that the plasma membranes of normal liver do contain complete, functional F_0F_1 ATP synthase complexes, which display very similar subunit composition and assembly of the mitochondrial enzymes for which MS analysis is in progress in our laboratory.

All together these studies support the view that ATP synthase is mainly located in lipid rafts of plasma membranes, is enzymatically active and functions as a cell-surface receptor involved in different biological effects depending on the cell types (Fig. 8). In hepatocytes ecto-F_0F_1 functions as high affinity ApoA1 receptor and regulates HDL metabolism, in endothelial cells it functions as angiostatin receptor thus mediating angiogenesis, in tumour cells it functions as a pH regulator and participates in tumor recognition by cytotoxic Vγ9/Vδ2 T lymphocytes (Vantourout et al., 2010). Various independent studies have reported that ecto-F_0F_1 can synthesize ATP from ADP and Pi extruding protons from cytoplasm in different cell types, such as endothelial cells or hepatocytes. The resulting ATP can triggers cation influx into the cells through ATP-gated ion channels (P2X purinoreceptors) or can bind to G-protein coupled receptors (P2Y purinoreceptors) activating a downstream signaling pathways (Mowery and Pizzo, 2010). However, whether or not ecto-F_0F_1 can synthesize ATP is still debated, as there are several conflicting reports. Conversely, it is widely accepted that ecto-F_0F_1 catalyses the hydrolysis of ATP, potentially affecting purinergic signaling (Fig. 8). As an example, in hepatocytes, ADP generated by

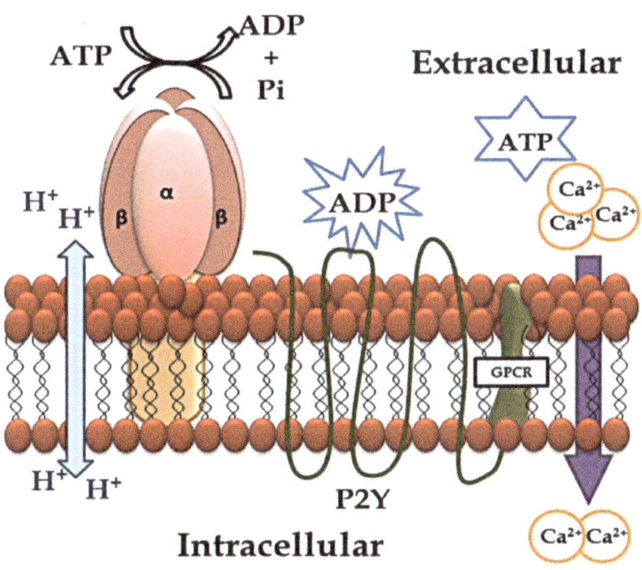

Fig. 8. The model depicts the orientation of ectopic F_0F_1 ATP synthase in eukaryotes with the F_1 sector facing outside. In some cells the ATP synthesized by the enzyme leads to influx of cations such as Ca^{2+} through P2X receptors and in others the ADP generated by ATP hydrolysis triggers signaling pathways through activation of G-protein coupled P2Y receptors.

ecto-F_0F_1 upon binding of ApoA1 activates the P2Y receptors resulting in HDL endocytosis and downstream the small GTPase RhoA and its effector ROCK I (Malaval et al,. 2009).
The mechanism used by ATP synthase to reach the plasma membrane is still unknown (Vantourout et al., 2010). The hypothesis that the single ATP synthase subunits are routed to plasma membrane instead of the mitochondria seems unlikely, because different mRNA isoforms of ATP synthase subunits have not been found in mammals apart for the bovine subunit c (Vives-Bauza et al., 2011). The simpler explanation seems that once assembled into mitochondria, the whole complex reaches the cell surface *via* vescicular transport or fusion of mitochondrial membranes with plasma membranes (Vantourout et al., 2010). It is tempting to hypothesize that the new technology of imaging MS (MALDI MS profiling/imaging), which can acquire individual spectra from the surface of frozen tissue sections (Chaurand et al,. 2006), could give important answers regarding the trafficking of the enzyme to cell surface.

6. Conclusions

F_0F_1 ATP synthase is an intensely studied enzyme complex, for which single molecule studies have allowed to define the fascinating catalysis in great detail. In addition, high-resolution molecular structures have been obtained mainly by X-ray crystal analyses. In spite of this tremendous progress, many aspects of ATP synthase physiology, such as biogenesis or super-complex formation, and its role in pathology are still unknown. The omni-comprehensive nature of proteomics, unlike the more reductionistic approaches of classical biochemistry and genetics, makes it the best candidate for revealing changes in the expression level of the whole complex and/or of its single subunits, but also to define the quantitative and temporal phosphorylation pattern of the enzyme in all organisms and under different physiopathological conditions, thus allowing the understanding of the ATP synthase regulation in a better way. In addition, the constant technological progress will enable to define the intriguing enzyme intracellular trafficking and its translocation to cell surface. In this context, native electrophoresis combined with MS techniques offers a powerful top-down approach for functional and structural analyses of such complicated enzyme using minimal amount of cell lysates or tissue homogenates and making this approach useful also for clinical investigation.

7. Acknowledgements

Authors acknowledge Prof. Paolo Bernardi, Dept. of Biomedical Sciences, University of Padova and Dr. Paola Picotti, Institute of Biochemistry, ETH, Zürich for critical reading of the manuscript.

8. References

Ackerman, S. H. (2002). Atp11p and Atp12p are chaperones for F1-ATPase biogenesis in mitochondria. *Biochimica et Biophysica Acta (BBA)-Bioenergetics*, Vol.1555, No.1-3, pp. 101-105

Adachi, K.; Oiwa, K.; Nishizaka, T.; Furuike, S.; Noji, H.; Itoh, H.; Yoshida, M. & Kinosita Jr, K. (2007). Coupling of rotation and catalysis in F1-ATPase revealed by single-molecule imaging and manipulation. *Cell*, Vol.130, No.2, pp. 309-321

Ahmed, M.; Muhammed, S. J.; Kessler, B. & Salehi, A. (2010). Mitochondrial proteome analysis reveals altered expression of voltage dependent anion channels in pancreatic -cells exposed to high glucose. *Islets*, Vol.2, No.5, pp. 283-292

Alverdi, V.; Di Pancrazio, F.; Lippe, G.; Pucillo, C.; Casetta, B. & Esposito, G. (2005). Determination of protein phosphorylation sites by mass spectrometry: a novel electrospray based method. *Rapid communications in mass spectrometry*, Vol.19, No.22, pp. 3343-3348

Andersson, U.; Houstek, J. & Cannon, B. (1997). ATP synthase subunit c expression: physiological regulation of the P1 and P2 genes. *Biochemical Journal*, Vol.323, No.Pt 2, pp. 379-385

Andrianaivomananjaona, T.; Moune-Dimala, M.; Herga, S.; David, V. & Haraux, F. (2010). How the N-terminal extremity of Saccharomyces cerevisiae IF1 interacts with ATP synthase: A kinetic approach. *Biochimica et Biophysica Acta (BBA)-Bioenergetics*, Vol.1807, No.2, pp. 197-204

Arakaki, N.; Ueyama, Y.; Hirose, M.; Himeda, T.; Shibata, H.; Futaki, S.; Kitagawa, K. & Higuti, T. (2001). Stoichiometry of subunit e in rat liver mitochondrial H+-ATP synthase and membrane topology of its putative Ca2+-dependent regulatory region. *Biochimica et Biophysica Acta (BBA)-Bioenergetics*, Vol.1504, No.2-3, pp. 220-228

Bae, T. J.; Kim, M. S.; Kim, J. W.; Kim, B. W.; Choo, H. J.; Lee, J. W.; Kim, K. B.; Lee, C. S.; Kim, J. H. & Chang, S. Y. (2004). Lipid raft proteome reveals ATP synthase complex in the cell surface. *Proteomics*, Vol.4, No.11, pp. 3536-3548

Bason, J. V.; Runswick, M. J.; Fearnley, I. M. & Walker, J. E. (2011). Binding of the Inhibitor Protein IF1 to Bovine F1-ATPase. *Journal of Molecular Biology*, Vol.406, No.3, pp. 443-453

Bendt, A. K.; Burkovski, A.; Schaffer, S.; Bott, M.; Farwick, M. & Hermann, T. (2003). Towards a phosphoproteome map of Corynebacterium glutamicum. *Proteomics*, Vol.3, No.8, pp. 1637-1646

Bisetto, E.; Giorgio, V.; Di Pancrazio, F.; Mavelli, I. & Lippe, G. (2007). Characterization of oligomeric forms from mammalian F0F1ATP synthase by BN-PAGE: the role of detergents. *The Italian journal of biochemistry*, Vol.56, No.4, pp. 254-258

Bisetto, E.; Picotti, P.; Giorgio, V.; Alverdi, V.; Mavelli, I. & Lippe, G. (2008). Functional and stoichiometric analysis of subunit e in bovine heart mitochondrial F 0 F 1 ATP synthase. *Journal of bioenergetics and biomembranes*, Vol.40, No.4, pp. 257-267

Borghese, R.; Turina, P.; Lambertini, L. & Melandri, B. A. (1998). The atpIBEXF operon coding for the F0 sector of the ATP synthase from the purple nonsulfur photosynthetic bacterium Rhodobacter capsulatus. *Archives of microbiology*, Vol.170, No.5, pp. 385-388

Boyer, P. D. (1997). The ATP synthase-a splendid molecular machine. *Annual review of biochemistry*, Vol.66, No.1, pp. 717-749

Bustos, D. M. & Velours, J. (2005). The modification of the conserved GXXXG motif of the membrane-spanning segment of subunit g destabilizes the supramolecular species of yeast ATP synthase. *Journal of Biological Chemistry*, Vol.280, No.32, pp. 29004-29010

Cabezón, E.; Montgomery, M. G.; Leslie, A. G. W. & Walker, J. E. (2003). The structure of bovine F1-ATPase in complex with its regulatory protein IF1. *Nature structural biology*, Vol.10, No.9, pp. 744-750

Cabezon, E.; Runswick, M. J.; Leslie, A. G. W. & Walker, J. E. (2001). The structure of bovine IF1, the regulatory subunit of mitochondrial F-ATPase. *The EMBO journal*, Vol.20, No.24, pp. 6990-6996

Campanella, M.; Parker, N.; Tan, C. H.; Hall, A. M. & Duchen, M. R. (2009). IF1: setting the pace of the F1Fo-ATP synthase. *Trends in biochemical sciences*, Vol.34, No.7, pp. 343-350

Carroll, J.; Altman, M. C.; Fearnley, I. M. & Walker, J. E. (2007). Identification of membrane proteins by tandem mass spectrometry of protein ions. *Proceedings of the National Academy of Sciences*, Vol.104, No.36, pp. 14330-14335

Carroll, J.; Fearnley, I. M.; Wang, Q. & Walker, J. E. (2009). Measurement of the molecular masses of hydrophilic and hydrophobic subunits of ATP synthase and complex I in a single experiment. *Analytical Biochemistry*, Vol.395, No.2, pp. 249-255

Chaurand, P.; Cornett, D. S. & Caprioli, R. M. (2006). Molecular imaging of thin mammalian tissue sections by mass spectrometry. *Current opinion in biotechnology*, Vol.17, No.4, pp. 431-436

Chen, C.; Ko, Y.; Delannoy, M.; Ludtke, S. J.; Chiu, W. & Pedersen, P. L. (2004). Mitochondrial ATP Synthasome. *Journal of Biological Chemistry*, Vol.279, No.30, pp. 31761-31768

Chen, C.; Saxena, A. K.; Simcoke, W. N.; Garboczi, D. N.; Pedersen, P. L. & Ko, Y. H. (2006). Mitochondrial ATP Synthase. *Journal of Biological Chemistry*, Vol.281, No.19, pp. 13777-13783

Chen, R.; Fearnley, I. M.; Palmer, D. N. & Walker, J. E. (2004). Lysine 43 is trimethylated in subunit c from bovine mitochondrial ATP synthase and in storage bodies associated with Batten disease. *Journal of Biological Chemistry*, Vol.279, No.21, pp. 21883-21887

Chen, R.; Runswick, M. J.; Carroll, J.; Fearnley, I. M. & Walker, J. E. (2007). Association of two proteolipids of unknown function with ATP synthase from bovine heart mitochondria. *FEBS letters*, Vol.581, No.17, pp. 3145-3148

Cingolani, G. & Duncan, T. M. (2011). Structure of the ATP synthase catalytic complex (F1) from Escherichia coli in an autoinhibited conformation. *Nature Structural & Molecular Biology*, Vol.18, No.6, pp. 701-707

Cížková, A.; Stránecký, V.; Ivánek, R.; Hartmannová, H.; Nosková, L.; Piherová, L.; Tesa ová, M.; Hansíková, H.; Honzík, T. & Zeman, J. (2008). Development of a human mitochondrial oligonucleotide microarray (h-MitoArray) and gene expression analysis of fibroblast cell lines from 13 patients with isolated F1Fo ATP synthase deficiency. *BMC genomics*, Vol.9, No.1, pp. 38

Collinson, I. R.; Fearnley, I. M.; Skehel, J. M.; Runswick, M. J. & Walker, J. E. (1994). ATP synthase from bovine heart mitochondria: identification by proteolysis of sites in F0 exposed by removal of F1 and the oligomycin-sensitivity conferral protein. *Biochemical Journal*, Vol.303, No.Pt 2, pp. 639-645

Couoh-Cardel, S. J.; Uribe-Carvajal, S.; Wilkens, S. & García-Trejo, J. J. (2010). Structure of dimeric F1F0-ATP synthase. *Journal of Biological Chemistry*, Vol.285, No.47, pp. 36447-36455

Dautant, A.; Velours, J. & Giraud, M. F. (2010). Crystal Structure of the Mg·ADP-inhibited State of the Yeast F1c10-ATP Synthase. *Journal of Biological Chemistry*, Vol.285, No.38, pp. 29502-29510

Di Pancrazio, F.; Bisetto, E.; Alverdi, V.; Mavelli, I.; Esposito, G. & Lippe, G. (2006). Differential steady-state tyrosine phosphorylation of two oligomeric forms of mitochondrial F0F1ATPsynthase: A structural proteomic analysis. *Proteomics*, Vol.6, No.3, pp. 921-926

Di Pancrazio, F.; Mavelli, I.; Isola, M.; Losano, G.; Pagliaro, P.; Harris, D. A. & Lippe, G. (2004). In vitro and in vivo studies of F0F1ATP synthase regulation by inhibitor protein IF1 in goat heart. *Biochimica et Biophysica Acta (BBA)-Bioenergetics*, Vol.1659, No.1, pp. 52-62

Dienhart, M.; Pfeiffer, K.; Schägger, H. & Stuart, R. A. (2002). Formation of the yeast F1F0-ATP synthase dimeric complex does not require the ATPase inhibitor protein, Inh1. *Journal of Biological Chemistry*, Vol.277, No.42, pp. 39289-39295

Everard-Gigot, V.; Dunn, C. D.; Dolan, B. M.; Brunner, S.; Jensen, R. E. & Stuart, R. A. (2005). Functional analysis of subunit e of the F1Fo-ATP synthase of the yeast Saccharomyces cerevisiae: importance of the N-terminal membrane anchor region. *Eukaryotic cell*, Vol.4, No.2, pp. 346-355

Eyrich, B.; Sickmann, A. & Zahedi, R. P. (2011). Catch me if you can: Mass spectrometry based phosphoproteomics and quantification strategies. *Proteomics*, Vol.11, No.4, pp. 554-570

Fronzes, R.; Weimann, T.; Vaillier, J.; Velours, J. & Brèthes, D. (2006). The peripheral stalk participates in the yeast ATP synthase dimerization independently of e and g subunits. *Biochemistry*, Vol.45, No.21, pp. 6715-6723

Gerber, S. A.; Rush, J.; Stemman, O.; Kirschner, M. W. & Gygi, S. P. (2003). Absolute quantification of proteins and phosphoproteins from cell lysates by tandem MS. *Proceedings of the National Academy of Sciences of the United States of America*, Vol.100, No.12, pp. 6940-6945

Giorgio, V.; Bisetto, E.; Franca, R.; Harris, D. A.; Passamonti, S. & Lippe, G. (2010). The ectopic F O F 1 ATP synthase of rat liver is modulated in acute cholestasis by the inhibitor protein IF 1. *Journal of bioenergetics and biomembranes*, pp. 1-7

Giorgio, V.; Bisetto, E.; Soriano, M. E.; Dabbeni-Sala, F.; Basso, E.; Petronilli, V.; Forte, M. A.; Bernardi, P. & Lippe, G. (2009). Cyclophilin D modulates mitochondrial F0F1-ATP synthase by interacting with the lateral stalk of the complex. *Journal of Biological Chemistry*, Vol.284, No.49, pp. 33982-33988

Gomis-Rüth, F. X.; Moncalián, G.; Pérez-Luque, R.; González, A.; Cabezón, E.; de la Cruz, F. & Coll, M. (2001). The bacterial conjugation protein TrwB resembles ring helicases and F1-ATPase. *Nature*, Vol.409, No.6820, pp. 637-641

HÃ¸jlund, K.; Wrzesinski, K.; Larsen, P. M.; Fey, S. J.; Roepstorff, P.; Handberg, A.; Dela, F.; Vinten, J. r.; McCormack, J. G.; Reynet, C. & Beck-Nielsen, H. (2003). Proteome Analysis Reveals Phosphorylation of ATP Synthase Î²-Subunit in Human Skeletal Muscle and Proteins with Potential Roles in Type 2 Diabetes. *Journal of Biological Chemistry*, Vol.278, No.12, pp. 10436-10442

Harris, D. A. & Das, A. M. (1991). Control of mitochondrial ATP synthesis in the heart. *Biochemical Journal*, Vol.280, No.Pt 3, pp. 561-573

Heather, L. C. & Clarke, K. (2010). Metabolism, hypoxia and the diabetic heart. *Journal of Molecular and Cellular Cardiology*, Vol.50, No.4, pp. 529-540

Helfenbein, K. G.; Ellis, T. P.; Dieckmann, C. L. & Tzagoloff, A. (2003). ATP22, a nuclear gene required for expression of the F0 sector of mitochondrial ATPase in Saccharomyces cerevisiae. *Journal of Biological Chemistry*, Vol.278, No.22, pp. 19751-19756

Hoffmann, J.; Sokolova, L.; Preiss, L.; Hicks, D. B.; Krulwich, T. A.; Morgner, N.; Wittig, I.; Schägger, H.; Meier, T. & Brutschy, B. (2010). ATP synthases: cellular nanomotors characterized by LILBID mass spectrometry. *Phys. Chem. Chem. Phys.*, Vol.12, No.41, pp. 13375-13382

Hong, S. & Pedersen, P. L. (2003). Subunit e of mitochondrial ATP synthase: a bioinformatic analysis reveals a phosphopeptide binding motif supporting a multifunctional regulatory role and identifies a related human brain protein with the same motif. *Proteins: Structure, Function, and Bioinformatics*, Vol.51, No.2, pp. 155-161

Houstek, J.; Andersson, U.; Tvrdík, P.; Nedergaard, J. & Cannon, B. (1995). The expression of subunit c correlates with and thus may limit the biosynthesis of the mitochondrial F0F1-ATPase in brown adipose tissue. *Journal of Biological Chemistry*, Vol.270, No.13, pp. 7689-7694

Houstek, J.; Pícková, A.; Vojtísková, A.; Mrácek, T.; Pecina, P. & Jesina, P. (2006). Mitochondrial diseases and genetic defects of ATP synthase. *Biochimica et Biophysica Acta (BBA)-Bioenergetics*, Vol.1757, No.9-10, pp. 1400-1405

Hüttemann, M.; Lee, I.; Samavati, L.; Yu, H. & Doan, J. W. (2007). Regulation of mitochondrial oxidative phosphorylation through cell signaling. *Biochimica et Biophysica Acta (BBA)-Molecular Cell Research*, Vol.1773, No.12, pp. 1701-1720

Hwang, S. I.; Lundgren, D. H.; Mayya, V.; Rezaul, K.; Cowan, A. E.; Eng, J. K. & Han, D. K. (2006). Systematic characterization of nuclear proteome during apoptosis. *Molecular & Cellular Proteomics*, Vol.5, No.6, pp. 1131-1145

Klodmann, J.; Lewejohann, D. & Braun, H. P. (2011). Low SDS Blue native PAGE. *Proteomics*, pp. 1-6

Ko, Y. H.; Pan, W.; Inoue, C. & Pedersen, P. L. (2002). Signal transduction to mitochondrial ATP synthase: Evidence that PDGF-dependent phosphorylation of the [delta]-subunit occurs in several cell lines, involves tyrosine, and is modulated by lysophosphatidic acid. *Mitochondrion*, Vol.1, No.4, pp. 339-348

Krause-Buchholz, U.; Becker, J. S.; Zoriy, M.; Pickhardt, C.; Przybylski, M. & Rodel, G. (2006). Detection of phosphorylated subunits by combined LA-ICP-MS and MALDI-FTICR-MS analysis in yeast mitochondrial membrane complexes separated by blue native/SDS-PAGE. *International Journal of Mass Spectrometry*, Vol.248, No.1-2, pp. 56-60

Kucharczyk, R.; Salin, B. & Di Rago, J. P. (2009). Introducing the human Leigh syndrome mutation T9176G into Saccharomyces cerevisiae mitochondrial DNA leads to severe defects in the incorporation of Atp6p into the ATP synthase and in the mitochondrial morphology. *Human molecular genetics*, Vol.18, No.15, pp. 2889

Kucharczyk, R.; Zick, M.; Bietenhader, M.; Rak, M.; Couplan, E.; Blondel, M.; Caubet, S. D. & di Rago, J. P. (2009). Mitochondrial ATP synthase disorders: molecular mechanisms and the quest for curative therapeutic approaches. *Biochimica et Biophysica Acta (BBA)-Molecular Cell Research*, Vol.1793, No.1, pp. 186-199

Lalanne, E.; Mathieu, C.; Vedel, F. & De Paepe, R. (1998). Tissue-specific expression of genes encoding isoforms of the mitochondrial ATPase subunit in Nicotiana sylvestris. *Plant molecular biology*, Vol.38, No.5, pp. 885-888

Lee, J. K.; Belogrudov, G. I. & Stroud, R. M. (2008). Crystal structure of bovine mitochondrial factor B at 0.96-Å resolution. *Proceedings of the National Academy of Sciences*, Vol.105, No.36, pp. 13379-13384

Lefebvre-Legendre, L.; Vaillier, J.; Benabdelhak, H.; Velours, J.; Slonimski, P. P. & di Rago, J. P. (2001). Identification of a nuclear gene (FMC1) required for the assembly/stability of yeast mitochondrial F1-ATPase in heat stress conditions. *Journal of Biological Chemistry*, Vol.276, No.9, pp. 6789-6796

Loro, E.; Gianazza, E.; Cazzola, S.; Malena, A.; Wait, R.; Begum, S.; Brizio, C.; Dabbeni Sala, F. & Vergani, L. (2009). Development and characterization of polyspecific anti mitochondrion antibodies for proteomics studies on in toto tissue homogenates. *Electrophoresis*, Vol.30, No.8, pp. 1329-1341

MacDonald, J. A.; Mackey, A. J.; Pearson, W. R. & Haystead, T. A. J. (2002). A strategy for the rapid identification of phosphorylation sites in the phosphoproteome. *Molecular & Cellular Proteomics*, Vol.1, No.4, pp. 314-322

Malaval, C.; Laffargue, M.; Barbaras, R.; Rolland, C.; Peres, C.; Champagne, E.; Perret, B.; Tercé, F.; Collet, X. & Martinez, L. O. (2009). RhoA/ROCK I signalling downstream of the P2Y13 ADP-receptor controls HDL endocytosis in human hepatocytes. *Cellular signalling*, Vol.21, No.1, pp. 120-127

Matsuda, C.; Endo, H.; Hirata, H.; Morosawa, H.; Nakanishi, M. & Kagawa, Y. (1993). Tissue-specific isoforms of the bovine mitochondrial ATP synthase [gamma]-subunit. *FEBS letters*, Vol.325, No.3, pp. 281-284

Matsuda, C.; Muneyuki, E.; Endo, H.; Yoshida, M. & Kagawa, Y. (1994). Comparison of the ATPase Activities of Bovine Heart and Liver Mitochondrial ATP Synthases with Different Tissue-Specific [gamma] Subunit Isoforms. *Biochemical and biophysical research communications*, Vol.200, No.2, pp. 671-678

Mattiazzi, M.; Vijayvergiya, C.; Gajewski, C. D.; DeVivo, D. C.; Lenaz, G.; Wiedmann, M. & Manfredi, G. (2004). The mtDNA T8993G (NARP) mutation results in an impairment of oxidative phosphorylation that can be improved by antioxidants. *Human molecular genetics*, Vol.13, No.8, pp. 869-879

Meier, T.; Morgner, N.; Matthies, D.; Pogoryelov, D.; Keis, S.; Cook, G. M.; Dimroth, P. & Brutschy, B. (2007). A tridecameric c ring of the adenosine triphosphate (ATP) synthase from the thermoalkaliphilic Bacillus sp. strain TA2. A1 facilitates ATP synthesis at low electrochemical proton potential. *Molecular microbiology*, Vol.65, No.5, pp. 1181-1192

Meyer, B.; Wittig, I.; Trifilieff, E.; Karas, M. & Schägger, H. (2007). Identification of two proteins associated with mammalian ATP synthase. *Molecular & Cellular Proteomics*, Vol.6, No.10, pp. 1690-1699

Mowery, Y. M. & Pizzo, S. V. (2010). Cell Surface ATP Synthase: A Potential Target for Anti-Angiogenic Therapy. *Extracellular ATP and Adenosine as Regulators of Endothelial Cell Function*, pp. 139-159

Noji, H.; Yasuda, R.; Yoshida, M. & Kinosita, K. (1997). Direct observation of the rotation of F1-ATPase. *Nature*, Vol.386, No.6622, pp. 299-302

Ohsakaya, S.; Fujikawa, M.; Hisabori, T. & Yoshida, M. (2011). Knockdown of DAPIT (diabetes-associated protein in insulin-sensitive tissue) results in loss of ATP synthase in mitochondria. *Journal of Biological Chemistry*, Vol.286, No.23, pp. 20292-20296

Pagnozzi, D.; Birolo, L.; Leo, G.; Contessi, S.; Lippe, G.; Pucci, P. & Mavelli, I. (2010). Stoichiometry and Topology of the complex of the endogenous ATP Synthase Inhibitor Protein IF1 with Calmodulin. *Biochemistry*, Vol.49, No.35, pp. 7542-7552

Panfoli, I.; Ravera, S.; Bruschi, M.; Candiano, G. & Morelli, A. (2011). Proteomics unravels the exportability of mitochondrial respiratory chains. *Expert Review of Proteomics*, Vol.8, No.2, pp. 231-239

Paumard, P.; Vaillier, J.; Coulary, B.; Schaeffer, J.; Soubannier, V.; Mueller, D. M.; Brèthes, D.; Di Rago, J. P. & Velours, J. (2002). The ATP synthase is involved in generating mitochondrial cristae morphology. *The EMBO journal*, Vol.21, No.3, pp. 221-230

Rak, M.; Gokova, S. & Tzagoloff, A. (2011). Modular assembly of yeast mitochondrial ATP synthase. *The EMBO journal*, Vol.30, pp. 920-930

Reisinger, V. & Eichacker, L. A. (2008). Solubilization of membrane protein complexes for blue native PAGE. *Journal of Proteomics*, Vol.71, No.3, pp. 277-283

Richter, M. L.; Hein, R. & Huchzermeyer, B. (2000). Important subunit interactions in the chloroplast ATP synthase. *Biochimica et Biophysica Acta (BBA)-Bioenergetics*, Vol.1458, No.2-3, pp. 326-342

Schägger, H. & Pfeiffer, K. (2000). Supercomplexes in the respiratory chains of yeast and mammalian mitochondria. *The EMBO journal*, Vol.19, No.8, pp. 1777-1783

Senior, A. E. (2007). ATP synthase: Motoring to the finish line. *Cell*, Vol.130, No.2, pp. 220-221

Sgarbi, G.; Baracca, A.; Lenaz, G.; Valentino, L. M.; Carelli, V. & Solaini, G. (2006). Inefficient coupling between proton transport and ATP synthesis may be the pathogenic mechanism for NARP and Leigh syndrome resulting from the T8993G mutation in mtDNA. *Biochemical Journal*, Vol.395, No.Pt 3, pp. 493-500

Sokolova, L.; Wittig, I.; Barth, H. D.; Schägger, H.; Brutschy, B. & Brandt, U. (2010). Laser induced liquid bead ion desorption MS of protein complexes from blue native gels, a sensitive top down proteomic approach. *Proteomics*, Vol.10, No.7, pp. 1401-1407

Spannagel, C.; Vaillier, J.; Arselin, G.; Graves, P. V.; Grandier-Vazeille, X. & Velours, J. (1998). Evidence of a subunit 4 (subunit b) dimer in favor of the proximity of ATP synthase complexes in yeast inner mitochondrial membrane. *Biochimica et Biophysica Acta (BBA)-Biomembranes*, Vol.1414, No.1-2, pp. 260-264

Stevens Jr, S. M.; Duncan, R. S.; Koulen, P. & Prokai, L. (2008). Proteomic analysis of mouse brain microsomes: identification and bioinformatic characterization of endoplasmic reticulum proteins in the mammalian central nervous system. *Journal of proteome research*, Vol.7, No.3, pp. 1046-1054

Stockwin, L. H.; Blonder, J.; Bumke, M. A.; Lucas, D. A.; Chan, K. C.; Conrads, T. P.; Issaq, H. J.; Veenstra, T. D.; Newton, D. L. & Rybak, S. M. (2006). Proteomic analysis of plasma membrane from hypoxia-adapted malignant melanoma. *Journal of proteome research*, Vol.5, No.11, pp. 2996-3007

Strauss, M.; Hofhaus, G.; Schröder, R. R. & Kühlbrandt, W. (2008). Dimer ribbons of ATP synthase shape the inner mitochondrial membrane. *The EMBO journal*, Vol.27, No.7, pp. 1154-1160

Struglics, A.; Fredlund, K. M.; Møller, I. M. & Allen, J. F. (1998). Two Subunits of the FoF1-ATPase Are Phosphorylated in the Inner Mitochondrial Membrane. *Biochemical and biophysical research communications*, Vol.243, No.3, pp. 664-668

Suhai, T.; Heidrich, N. G.; Dencher, N. A. & Seelert, H. (2009). Highly sensitive detection of ATPase activity in native gels. *Electrophoresis*, Vol.30, No.20, pp. 3622-3625

Suzuki, T.; Wakabayashi, C.; Tanaka, K.; Feniouk, B. A. & Yoshida, M. (2011). Modulation of nucleotide specificity of thermophilic FoF1-ATP synthase by -subunit. *Journal of Biological Chemistry*, Vol.286, No.19, pp. 16807-16813

Thomas, D.; Bron, P.; Weimann, T.; Dautant, A.; Giraud, M.; Paumard, P.; Salin, B.; Cavalier, A.; Velours, J. & Brethes, D. (2008). Supramolecular organization of the yeast F1Fo-ATP synthase. *Biology of the Cell*, Vol.100, pp. 591-601

Tomasetig, L.; Di Pancrazio, F.; Harris, D. A.; Mavelli, I. & Lippe, G. (2002). Dimerization of F0F1ATP synthase from bovine heart is independent from the binding of the inhibitor protein IF1. *Biochimica et Biophysica Acta (BBA)-Bioenergetics*, Vol.1556, No.2-3, pp. 133-141

Tzagoloff, A. (1969). Assembly of the mitochondrial membrane system. II. Synthesis of the mitochondrial adenosine triphosphatase. F1. *The Journal of biological chemistry*, Vol.244, No.18, pp. 5027-5033

Ueno, H.; Suzuki, T.; Kinosita, K. & Yoshida, M. (2005). ATP-driven stepwise rotation of FoF1-ATP synthase. *Proceedings of the National Academy of Sciences of the United States of America*, Vol.102, No.5, pp. 1333-1338

Vantourout, P.; Radojkovic, C.; Lichtenstein, L.; Pons, V.; Champagne, E. & Martinez, L. O. (2010). Ecto-F1-ATPase: A moonlighting protein complex and an unexpected apoA-I receptor. *World Journal of Gastroenterology: WJG*, Vol.16, No.47, pp. 5925-5935

Vignais, P. V. & Satre, M. (1984). Recent developments on structural and functional aspects of the F 1 sector of H+-linked ATPases. *Molecular and cellular biochemistry*, Vol.60, No.1, pp. 33-70

Vives-Bauza, C.; Magrane, J.; Andreu, A. L. & Manfredi, G. (2011). Novel Role of ATPase Subunit C Targeting Peptides Beyond Mitochondrial Protein Import. *Molecular Biology of the Cell*, Vol.21, No.1, pp. 131-139

Vosseller, K.; Hansen, K. C.; Chalkley, R. J.; Trinidad, J. C.; Wells, L.; Hart, G. W. & Burlingame, A. L. (2005). Quantitative analysis of both protein expression and serine/threonine post translational modifications through stable isotope labeling with dithiothreitol. *Proteomics*, Vol.5, No.2, pp. 388-398

Walker, J. E. & Dickson, V. K. (2006). The peripheral stalk of the mitochondrial ATP synthase. *BBA-Bioenergetics*, Vol.1757, No.5-6, pp. 286-296

Walker, J. E.; Lutter, R.; Dupuis, A. & Runswick, M. J. (1991). Identification of the subunits of F1F0-ATPase from bovine heart mitochondria. *Biochemistry*, Vol.30, No.22, pp. 5369-5378

Wittig, I. & Schägger, H. (2005). Advantages and limitations of clear native PAGE. *Proteomics*, Vol.5, No.17, pp. 4338-4346

Wittig, I. & Schägger, H. (2008). Features and applications of blue-native and clear-native electrophoresis. *Proteomics*, Vol.8, No.19, pp. 3974-3990

Wittig, I. & Schägger, H. (2008). Structural organization of mitochondrial ATP synthase. *Biochimica et Biophysica Acta (BBA)-Bioenergetics*, Vol.1777, No.7-8, pp. 592-598

Wittig, I.; Braun, H. P. & Schägger, H. (2006). Blue native PAGE. *Nature protocols*, Vol.1, No.1, pp. 418-428

Wittig, I.; Carrozzo, R.; Santorelli, F. M. & Schagger, H. (2007). Functional assays in high-resolution clear native gels to quantify mitochondrial complexes in human biopsies and cell lines. *Electrophoresis*, Vol.28, No.21, pp. 3811-3820

Wittig, I.; Meyer, B.; Heide, H.; Steger, M.; Bleier, L.; Wumaier, Z.; Karas, M. & Schägger, H. (2010). Assembly and oligomerization of human ATP synthase lacking mitochondrial subunits a and A6L. *Biochimica et Biophysica Acta (BBA)-Bioenergetics*, Vol.1797, No.6-7, pp. 1004-1011

Wittig, I.; Velours, J.; Stuart, R. & Schägger, H. (2008). Characterization of domain interfaces in monomeric and dimeric ATP synthase. *Molecular & Cellular Proteomics*, Vol.7, No.5, pp. 995-1004

Yan, L. J. & Forster, M. J. (2009). Resolving mitochondrial protein complexes using nongradient blue native polyacrylamide gel electrophoresis. *Analytical Biochemistry*, Vol.389, No.2, pp. 143-149

Zerbetto, E.; Vergani, L. & Dabbeni Sala, F. (1997). Quantification of muscle mitochondrial oxidative phosphorylation enzymes via histochemical staining of blue native polyacrylamide gels. *Electrophoresis*, Vol.18, No.11, pp. 2059-2064

Zhang, L.; Xi'e, W.; Peng, X.; Wei, Y.; Cao, R.; Liu, Z.; Xiong, J.; Ying, X.; Chen, P. & Liang, S. (2007). Immunoaffinity purification of plasma membrane with secondary antibody superparamagnetic beads for proteomic analysis. *Journal of proteome research*, Vol.6, No.1, pp. 34-43

8

Comparative Proteomics: An Approach to Elucidating the Function of a Novel Gene Called BRE

Kenneth Ka Ho Lee[1,2] et al.*

[1]Stem Cell and Regeneration Thematic Research Programme, School of Biomedical Sciences, Chinese University of Hong Kong, Shatin, N.T.

[2]Joint JUN-CUHK Key Laboratories for Regenerative Medicine, Ministry of Education, JiNan University, Guangzhou

[1]Hong Kong

[2]China

1. Introduction

Proteomics was developed in the early 1990s to allow proteins expressed by cells and tissues to be systematically studied (Celis et al., 1999; Arrell et al., 2001). The word proteome was coined by Marc Wilkins et al (Wilkins et al, 1996) from the words "protein and genome". It is therefore defined as protein equivalent of the genome. Generally, unique spectrum of proteins is only synthesized by specific cell types, for example amylase is secreted by the parotid gland, insulin by the pancreas and thyroxin by thyroid follicles. Protein synthesis is a complicated process formed by the different combination and length of the 20 unique amino acids found in our body (Arnstein, 1965). For example, following the transcription of genes encoded in the DNA, the mRNAs translocate into the cytoplasm where they are translated into a specific type of protein by the ribosomes (Lengyel, 1966). This is then followed by post-translational modification of the peptide chain to configure the protein so that it becomes biologically active. Post-translational modifications of proteins involve glycosylation, alkylation, methylation and sulfation (Blundell et al., 1993, Fleischer, 1983). The co- and post-translational modifications allow the protein to be transported and secreted during cellular homeostasis (Finnerty et al., 1979; Mao et al., 2011). In this chapter, we have described the comparative 2-dimensional electrophoresis (2-DE) proteomics workflow for protein identification by mass spectometry. Comparative proteomics was used

* Mei KuenTang[1], John Yeuk-Hon Chan[2], Yiu Loon Chui[3], Elve Chen[1], Yao Yao[1], Olivia Miu Yung Ngan[4] and Henry Siu Sum Lee[1]

[1]Stem Cell and Regeneration Thematic Research Programme, School of Biomedical Sciences, Chinese University of Hong Kong, Shatin, N.T., Hong Kong

[2]Joint JUN-CUHK Key Laboratories for Regenerative Medicine, Ministry of Education, JiNan University, Guangzhou, China

[3]Department of Chemical Pathology, Sir Y.K. Pao Centre for Cancer, Prince of Wales Hospital, Chinese University of Hong Kong, Shatin, N.T., Hong Kong

[4]Department of Biology, University of Michigan, Ann Arbor, USA

to identify proteins that were differentially expressed in the tissues after treatment with various small molecules and siRNAs.

2. Proteomics research and applications

Protein properties are diverse and complex. They are dynamically influenced by physiological change in their environment, such as hormones, factors present in inflammatory response and enzymes activated by the presence of drugs. Proteomics is founded on three basic procedures: (1) the isolation and separation of proteins from cells and tissues, (2) the identification of the proteins by mass spectrometry and (3) the resolution of analyzed protein peptides by bioinformatics. Advancement in proteomic technologies has allowed researchers to investigate the proteome of many diverse biological systems - allowing breakthroughs to be made in biomedical and biological sciences. Proteomics has also enabled the identification of important biomarkers of many human diseases and allows the discovery of novel targets for drugs. In this section, we will to discuss how proteomic technologies have been applied in biomedical sciences research and the limitations encountered.

2.1 History of protein research

Swedish biochemist Pehr Victor Edman first developed the technique called Edman Degradation which allowed the amino acid sequence in peptides to be elucidated (Edman, 1950). Determination of the protein structure could be performed under micro scale. Pehr Victor Edman also developed an instrument, the protein sequenator, which allowed the amino acids sequence to be determined following Edman degradation reaction (Edman and Begg, 1967). This sequenator was commercialized by the company Beckman. The discovery popularized the studying of protein chemistry. However, there are several disadvantages associated with this method. Firstly, the technique can only accurately determine amino acid sequences up to 50-60 residuals after using Edman reagent, phenyl isothiocyanate for degradation. Secondly, the peptide N-terminal, with NH_2-group, has to react with the Edman reagent. Thirdly, sequencing can only work on a single pure peptide and not a protein mixture. Finally, only the primary peptide structure can be determined but not information on the secondary structure, such as the position of disulfide bridge. Nevertheless, it has the advantage that only small quantity (10-100 pico-moles) of peptide is needed for the Edman reaction and can be performed directly from PVDF membranes. For its time, it was a pioneering and sophisticated method for studying protein chemistry, allowing the important amino acid sequence of hormones to be discovered (Niall et al., 1969 and Birr and Frank, 1975).

In the early 1970s, mass spectrometry was used to try and resolve all the peptide sequences derived from a protein mixture (Lucas et al., 1969; Morris et al, 1971). This early work has now developed leaps and bounds and protein mixtures can routinely be analyzed by computer aided high resolution mass spectrometry (MS). Consequently, John Fenn was awarded the 2002 Nobel Prize for his work in developing the electrospray ionization for mass spectrometry which provided a new platform for protein research (Fenn et al., 1989, 2002). The electrospray ionization mass spectrometer can rapidly, accurately and sensitively analyze peptide sequences from recombinant proteins, large biomolecules, protein mixture and body fluids (Chowdhury et al., 1990; Andersen et al., 1996; Bergquist et al., 2002). The parallel development of protein databases, search engines and new softwares has made it now even easier to conduct proteomic studies. Protein databases are essential tools that allow the matching and identification of peptides from peak spectrums obtained from MS studies. In particular, the Protein Prospector (Chalkley et al., 2005) and Mascot (Perkins et al., 1999) databases are user-friendly and contain many years of interpreted MS data for protein identification.

2.2 New era in studying the protein profile

Protein chemistry has now shifted to studying the proteome which permits a better understanding of interaction between cells, hormones with cells and bioactive molecules with cells. Profiling of protein mixtures is still difficult, despite recent development in using a partial enzyme digestion strategy and advancement in instrumentation - such as electrospray ionization tandem (triple quadrupole) and mass spectrometry (ESI-MS/MS) (Ceglarek et al. 2009), quadrupole ion trap MS (Schwartz and Jardine, 1996) and Matrix-assisted laser desorption/ionization-time of flight mass spectrophotometer (Maldi-TOF MS) (Hillenkamp et al., 1991; Andersen et al., 1996). Studying the proteome also depends on the use of two dimensional electrophoresis (2-DE) (O'Farrell, 1975). This technique allows complex mixture of proteins found in cells to be separated into individual protein spots by isoelectrical focusing (IEF) and sodium dodecyl sulfate polyacrylamide gel electrophoresis (SDS-PAGE). Proteinase inhibitors are always added to protein lysates freshly prepared from cells or tissues to prevent protein degradation. Contaminants such as phospholipids, nucleic acid and ionic molecules are also present and can be removed by gel filtration, dialysis and protein precipitation. Although O'Farell improved the IEF procedure, he used non-equilibrium pH gradient electrophoresis which cannot be reproducible from batch to batch - as the pH gradient is difficult to maintain during IEF. However, Bjellqvist et al. (1982) developed the immobilized pH gradients (IPG) method which replaced the use of the carrier-ampholyte. Development of the IPG strip was a milestone in proteomics and is now widely used in resolving individual proteins from complex protein mixtures (Weiss and Görg, 2009). In the IPG strip, proteins migrate under a high electrical field (up to 5000V) but always stop at same pI point. If several protein spots co- exist within the same pI, then a wider range of IPG strip could be flexibly used. SDS-PAGE is used to separate the protein spots according to their molecular weight. The limitation with this method is that it can only resolve proteins ranging from 120 kDa to 10 kDa. The protein spots resolved in the 2-DE gel need to be stained before it can be analyzed. Gels are most commonly stained with coomassie blue because it is inexpensive, and compatible for MS analysis. However, the sensitivity of this staining method is limited and cannot stain-up protein spots lower than 30 ηg. Silver staining is also another method widely used for revealing the resolved protein spots in the gel and only need 1 ηg of protein. Fluorescent dyes (CyDyes) have now been developed to label protein samples for Difference Gel Electrophoresis (DIGE). The DIGE technique is very sensitive, with protein detection range down to 125 pg per spot, giving it high precision in terms of protein quantification and use in comparative proteomics (Conrotto and Souchelnytskyi, 2008; Larbi and Jefferies, 2009). 2-DE/MS is now a well-established technique for large-scale protein expression studies. However, there are drawbacks with the method which hold it back from being developed for clinical diagnosis. Drawbacks such as the high abundance of plasma and albumin present in biofluids which interfere with detection of lower abundant proteins. Resolving hydrophobic, very acidic and basic proteins is also a major deficiency with the 2-DE/MS technique (Altland et al., 1988; Görg et al., 2009).

3. Breakthroughs in proteomics

Proteins are separated according to their isoelectrical points and molecular weights by 2-DE. In addition, their m/s ratio and peptide sequences in MS can resolve up to 2,000-4,000 single protein spots at a time (Görg et al., 2004). Moreover, proteins that cause abbreviated changes in normal tissues may be identified and use as potential biomarkers in medical diagnosis. This is especially important in oncology where early detection of the cancer could be properly treated and not metastasize. In the last decade, advancement in 2-DE, mass spectrometry and bioinformatics has allowed potential cancer biomarkers to be identified in serum and biofluids in the blood (Voss, et al., 2001; Gioia et al., 2011), colon (McKerrow et al., 2000), breast (Sauter et al., 2002; Lau et al., 2007; Galvão et al., 2011), ovaries (Zhang et al., 2004; Tung et al., 2008) and prostate (Ornstein et al., 2004; Ornstein and Tyson, 2006). However, the 2-DE technique still has its limitation - where proteins with extreme isoelectric point and molecular mass are not resolvable and identified. Also, it is very difficult to resolve membrane proteins and non-water soluble proteins by 2-DE. Another approach is to use non-gel based proteomic techniques (for example, ionic exchange affinity, reverse-phase and liquid chromatography) followed by MS/MS provide a novel platform for identifying proteins and therefore it can resolve the disadvantage of 2-DE technique. Now, the development of laser capture micro-dissection and MALDI-MS has allowed proteomics to be performed on a specific cell population isolated from heterogeneous tissues (Marko-Varga, 2003). It is possible to surgically isolate cancer tissue from normal tissues in histological sections of biopsies for proteomic analysis. This will accelerate the discovery of cancer biomarkers as the laser capture micro-dissection will remove "background noise" generated by normal tissues.

4. Comparative proteomics

Comparative Proteomics is the identification of the differentially expressed proteins from comparison of two or more 2-DE protein profiles, for example, isolated from cells that were treated and untreated with a drug. This method allows proteins that are differentially expressed to be identified and quantified. It is a very powerful technique for identifying the molecular targets of drugs and understanding the function of novel genes. The comparative proteomic technique is schematically summarized in Figure 1. Basically, it involves image analysis of 2-DE by matching different sets of gels together; identifying and isolating of proteins which are differentially expressed; mass spectrometry and bioinformatics. The proteome of a wide variety of biological systems can be investigated that includes cells, tissues, organs, fractionated cell lysates, and immuno-precipitated cell lysates. Since the technique only requires micrograms of materials to create a complex protein profile, the proteomes of bacteria, yeast and insect have also been investigated (Chen and Snyder, 2010; Han et al., 2011; Novak et al., 2011; Sirot et al., 2011).

5. As an example of the usefulness of comparative proteomics in identifying gene function, a gene called BRE which has anti-apoptotic properties, was analyzed

We have been interested in genes that are responsive to DNA damage (Li et al., 1995; Dong et al., 2003), and identified a novel human gene which we named BRE in this context. The

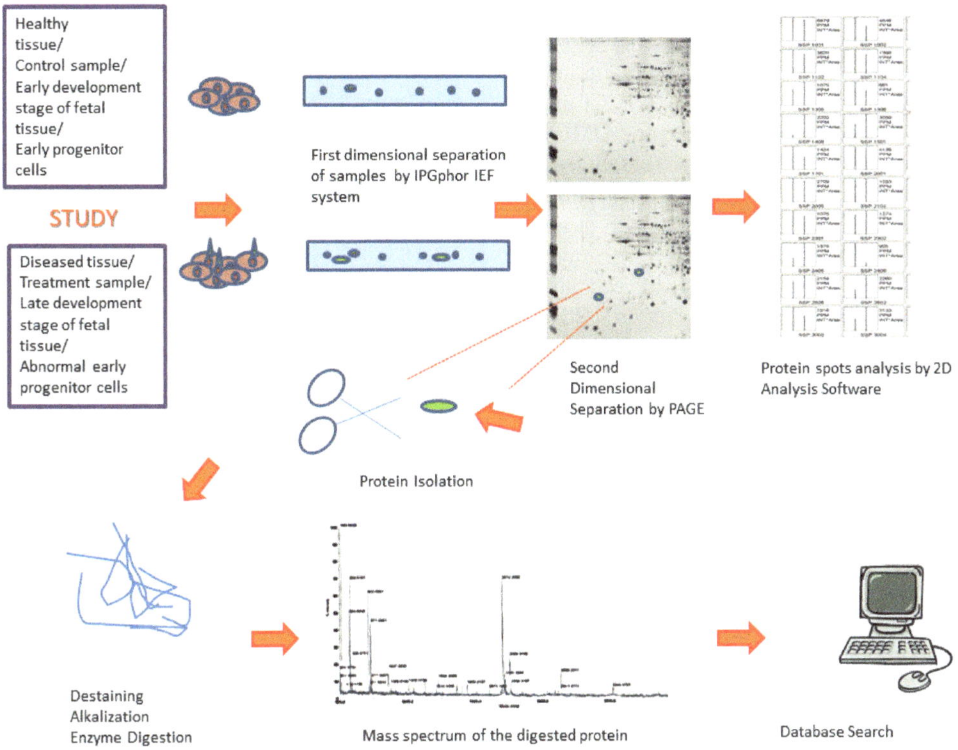

Fig. 1. The principle and workflow involved in comparative proteomics.

gene is highly Expressed in Brain and Reproductive organs and that is why we named it, BRE. The gene is down-regulated after treatment of cells with DNA damaging agents such as ultraviolet light (UV), 4-nitroquinoline-1-oxide and all-trans retinoic acid (Li et al., 1995). The BRE gene encodes a 1.7-1.9 kb mRNA which give rise to a protein with 383 amino acid residues and a molecular weight of 44 kDa. Using the yeast two-hybrid assay, it was reported that BRE interacts with the juxtamembrane (JM) region of p55-TNFR, but has no affinity for the p75-TNFR, Fas or p75-NGFR of the TNFR family (Gu et al., 1998). Meanwhile, over-expression of BRE in the human 293 embryonic kidney cells that was treated with TNF-α could inhibit the activation of the transcriptional factor NF-κB (Gu et al., 1998). Since NF-κB is known to induce the survival pathway associated with TNF receptor, it is likely that BRE can modulate the cell death process. The expression of the BRE gene has been investigated in various biological models including adrenal glands (Miao et al., 2001), testis (Miao et al., 2005) and hepatocellular carcinoma cells (Chan et al., 2008), but the function of BRE has still not been clarified - the protein structure of BRE do not have identifiable functional domain. It has been suggested the BRE contained 2 ubiquitin-conjugating enzyme family-like regions (Hu et al., 2011). However, these regions lacked the critical Cys residues required for ubiquitination but retain the ability to bind ubiquitin. The multifunctional nature of BRE and the lack of positive identifiable functional domains on BRE, make it an ideal candidate for study using proteomics. We therefore used comparative proteomics to examine the function of this novel gene in different cell types and also in vivo.

5.1 Materials and methods

5.1.1 Tissue cultures

All of the cell cultures were maintained at 37°C and 5% CO_2 in a humidified cultured chamber. C2C12 myoblasts (ATCC) and D122 Lewis lung carcinoma cells (gift from Lea Eisenbach) were cultured in DMEM medium supplemented with 10% FBS and penicillin/streptomycin. Two stably transfected cell lines were produced from D122 using a pcDNA3.1 expression vector. D122v3B harbor the empty vector, while D122αa4 cells over-express the full length *BRE* (Chan et al., 2005). D122v3B and D122αa4 were maintained in DMEM plus 10% FBS and 400 mg/mL of G418 (Invitrogen), Immortalized human esophageal epithelial (SHEE) cell line and the malignantly transformed esophageal carcinoma cell line (SHEEC) were cultured in DMEM medium plus F-12 Nutrient Mixture (1:1) supplemented with 10% FBS (GibcoBRL) and penicillin/streptomycin (Shen et al., 2000). Chang cells (ATCC, CCL-13) were cultured in Minimum Essential Medium Eagle plus 10% FBS.

5.1.2 Transgenic mice

The transgenic mice were generated carrying the full-length BRE gene and the transthyretin (TTR) promoter. The TTR promoter is specifically expressed in hepatocytes in the liver (Ching et al, 2001). All mice were maintained in the Laboratory Animal Services Centre, Chinese University of Hong Kong. Ethical approval has been obtained from the animal ethics committee, Chinese University of Hong Kong before performing the animal experiments.

5.1.3 Subcellular fractioning of soluble proteins

SHEE and SHEEC cells were extracted in lysis buffer (8M Urea, 2M Thiourea, 2% CHAPS, 0.01% TBP, 0.01% NP-40) containing protease inhibitors (GE Healthcare). After extraction, the lysates were incubated on ice for 30 min and then centrifuged at 8000 rpm for 15 min to remove all cell debris. The fractions (cytosol, membrane, and nucleoplasm) were obtained using a ProteoExtract Subcellular Proteome Extraction Kit (Calbiochem) following instructions provided by the manufacturer. The total protein concentration for each fraction was determined using a Bio-Rad Protein Assay kit (Bio-Rad, Richmond).

5.1.4 BRE gene silencing analysis

Two BRE-specific siRNAs were designed corresponding to 5′-TCTGGCTGCACATCATTGA-3′ (nucleotides 124–142, nucleotide position number 1 being the start of the initiation codon), and 5′-CTGGACTGGTGAATTTTCA-3′ (nucleotides 491–509). siRNA sequence 5′-AAGCCUCGAAAUAUCUCCU-dTT-3′ with no known mRNA targets was used as a control.

5.1.5 Semi-quantitative RT-PCR analysis

The total RNA was isolated and purified by using TRIzol solution (Invitrogen Corporation, United States). 1 μg of the total RNA was used for reverse-transcription to synthesize the complementary DNA (cDNA) according to the procedures of ImProm-II™ Reverse Transcription System. cDNA was used as the template for PCR amplification. 20 μl of PCR mixture containing 1 μl of cDNA, 2.5 μl of PCR 10X buffer (Bio-firm, Hong Kong), 0.75 μl of magnesium chloride solution (25 mM, Bio-firm, Hong Kong), 1 μl of dNTP mix (10 mM,

Promega Corporation, United States), 1 µl of forward primer, 1 µl of reverse primer, 0.25 µl of Taq polymerase (Bio-firm, Hong Kong) and DEPC-treated water in a PCR microcentrifuge tube was placed into the thermal cycler for PCR amplification. All of the primers used in this study were manufactured and desalted by Invitrogen Corporation. The primers' sequences and the annealing temperature and duration shown in Table 1 were designed with Primer3

Primers	Sequences	Annealing temp & duration
mouse β-actin	Forward: 5′-TGAGACCTTCAACACCCCAG-3′ and	59 °C , 45s
	Reverse: 5′-TTCATGAGGTAGTCTGTCAGGTCC-3′	55 °C , 60s
	or	
	forward: 5′-TGAGACCTTCAACACCCCAG-3′	
	reverse: 5′-TTCATGAGGTAGTCT GTCAGGTCC-3′	
mouse BRE	Forward: 5′-CTAGTCGCCGGTTACTGA-3′	56 °C, 45s
	Reverse: 5′-TTCATGAGGTAGTCTGTCA-3′	
	or	55 °C, 60s
	Forward: 5′-CCACATTCCCACATACCTTCTC-3′	
	Reverse: 5′ – GCCATTTCATTTCCATCCCATC-3′	
mouse Mdm4	Forward: 5′-CTCCAAGCAAGAGGTACTG-3′	54 °C, 60s
	Reverse: 5′-AATGACCTGGTCCTCCTAG-3′	
Mouse Akt-3	Forward: 5′- CTGGCACCAGAGGTATTAGA-3′	56 °C, 60s
	Reverse: 5′-AGGAGAACTGAGGGAAGTGT-3′	
Mouse 26S Proteasome	Forward: 5′-TGATCTGTAACCTGGCCTAC-3′	57 °C, 60s
	Reverse: 5′-GTTACCCTCAGTGTCTTGGA-	
mouse Prohibitin	Forward: 5′-TGAGTGATGACCTCACAGA-3	54 °C, 45s
	Reverse: 5′-CAGTCTGCATAGGCACTTG-3′	
mouse p53	Forward:5′-ACTCTCCTCCCCTCAATAAG-3′	54 °C, 60s
	Reverse: 5′-CTGGAGTCTTCCAGTGTGAT-3′	
human β-actin	Forward: 5′-ATGGATGATGATATCGCCGCG-3′	55 °C, 45s
	Reverse: 5′-CTCCATGTCGTCCCAGTTG GT-3′	
human BRE	Forward: 5′-ATCTTGCCTCCTGGAATCCT-3′	57 °C, 60s
	Reverse: 5′-CACGTACTGCACCTTGTTGG-3′	
human Prohibitin	Forward: 5′- CGGAG AGGACTATGATGAGC-3′	57 °C, 60s
	Reverse: 5′- GGTAGGTGATGTTCCGAGAG-3′	
human cyclin A	Forward: 5′-TCCTGTCTTCCATGTCAGTG-3′	57 °C,60s
	Reverse: 5′- TAGGTCTGGTGAAGGTCCAT-3′	
Human TNF-R1	Forward: 5′- ACCAAGTGCCACAAAGGAACC -3′	56 °C, 60s
	Reverse: 5′-TACACACGGTGTTCTGTTTCTCC -3′	
human p53	Forward: 5′-GCCTGACTCAGACTGACATT-3′	54 °C, 60s
	Reverse 5′-GACAGCTTCCCTGGTTAGTA-3′	
mouse TUSC4	Forward: 5′-CTGGTATCC ATCCTCCAGTA-3′	53 °C, 60s
	Reverse: 5′-GTCTTGCAGCAGATCTCATC-3′	
mouse ENO1	Forward: 5′-CTACGAGGCCCTCTAAGAACTCC-3′	58 °C, 60s
	Reverse: 5′-TCCTTCCCGTACTTCTCCTT-3′	
mouse DPF2	Forward: 5′-TCCTTGGCGAGC AATACTAC-3′	53 °C, 60s
	Reverse: 5′-GCTGCCATCCTGAGAGATAA -3′	
mouse HSPA7	Forward: 5′-GCAGTCGGATATGAAGCACT-3′	58 °C, 60s
	Reverse: 5′-CTCCTCCCAAGTGGGTATCT-3′	
mouse HSPA2	Forward: 5′-GACGAATGTCAGGAGGTGAT-3′	58 °C, 60s
	Reverse: 5′-CTAAGTTGTTGCACCTCTCC-3′	

Table 1. Primers used in the study.

software (version 0.4.0, Rozen and Skaletsky; http://frodo.wi.mit.edu). The PCR mixtures were reacted in a PTC-100 thermal cycler (MJ Research, Watertown, MA, USA) set under the following amplification conditions: initial denaturation at 95°C for 2 min, followed by a total of 35 cycles of denaturation at 95°C for 1 min, annealing at different temperature according to the primer' conditions as shown in Table 1 and extension at 72°C for 1 min. An additional 7 min extension step at 72°C was performed at the end of the last cycle. After the electrophoresis, the PCR products were analyzed on a 1.5% agarose gel with ethidium bromide staining, the intensities of the PCR products were visualized and determined using the GelDoc-It imaging system (UVP, BioImaging System, USA). β-actin was used as a house keeping gene for internal control and normalization. The experiments were repeated three times.

5.1.6 Western blot analysis

Control and treated cells were lysed in 200 µl of lysis buffer (50 mM NaCl, 20 mM Tris, pH 7.6, 1% NP-40, 1 X protease inhibitor mixture) for 60 min. The lysates were cleared by centrifugation at 16 000×g at 4 °C for 10 min. Crude protein concentration was measured by using a protein assay kit (Bio-Rad). 30 to 50 µg of total protein lysate were resolved on 10 to 12% SDS-PAGE, with Rainbow molecular weight markers and electroblotted onto Hybond NC membranes (GE Healthcare). The blots were incubated with Akt-3 (1:100, sc-11521 Santa Cruz Biotechnology), Bre (1:500 to 1000, Chan et al,. 2008), mdmX (1:100, sc-14738, Santa Cruz Biotechnology), prohibitin (1:000, sc-18196, Santa Cruz Biotechnology),p53 (1:000, sc-6243, Santa Cruz Biotechnology) or β-tubulin (1:1000 to 1500, Zymed Laboratories), α-tubulin (1:1500, Zymed Laboratories), cyclin A (1:1000, sc-11521, Santa Cruz Biotechnology), prohibitin (1:600, sc-18196, Santa Cruz Biotechnology), TNF-R1 (1:800, sc-8436, Santa Cruz Biotechnology), CDK2 (M2) (1:800, sc-163 Santa Cruz Biotechnology). Bound antibodies were detected using the appropriate horseradish peroxidase-conjugated secondary antibodies (Southern biotechnology), followed by development with an ECL Western blotting Detection kit (GE Healthcare). The blots were analyzed using Quantity One software (Bio-Rad) and the intensity of the bands produced for each antibody was normalized against the tubulin band (internal control) produced from each sample. Three replicates of each sample were studied.

5.1.7 In situ hybridization

All of the procedures performed were according to Lee et al. (2001). The liver samples were fixed in 4% paraformaldehyde (w/v, Sigma, United States) for 24 hrs. The fixed samples were washed in Dulbecco's Phosphate Buffered Saline (DPBS, Invitrogen Corporation, United States) for 15 min with three changes. The samples were then dehydrated, cleared and embedded in paraffin wax. Finally, the specimens were sectioned at 7 µm and mounted onto TESPA treated slides. The riboprobe was prepared from pGEM-T plasmid containing 1,205 bp encoding BRE sequence. The plasmid cDNA was linearized by EcoRI and in-vitro transcribed to generate digoxigenin (DIG)-labeled sense and antisense BRE riboprobe using a DIG RNA labeling kit (Roche Applied Science, United States). After dewaxing the paraffin sections, the specimens were rehydrated and equilibrated in DPBS for 10 min. The sections were digested with 10 µg/ml of proteinase K (Fermentas Life Science, Canada) for 7 min and post-fixed in 2% paraformaldehyde for 5 min. After washing in DPBS for 10 minutes twice, the samples were incubated in pre-hybridization buffer (2X SSC, 1X Denhardt's reagent, 5mM EDTA , 0.1% sodium dodecyl sulfate, 10X Dextran sulfate (Chemicon, United

States), 50 μg/ml salmon sperm DNA and 50% formamide) for 2 hrs. The samples were then added and hybridized in 0.5 μg/ml of DIG-labeled antisense riboprobe. The sense probe was used as a negative control. The hybridization temperature was 55°C and the incubation time was 16 hrs. Following hybridization, the samples were washed in 2X SSC at 42°C for 20 mins with two changes, 0.1% SDS (w/v) in 0.2X SSC buffer for 15 min and then 0.2X SSC buffer for 10 mins. The alkaline phosphatase-conjugated digoxigenin antibody (1:50, Roche Applied Science, United States) was added to the specimens for 2 hrs and then washed in DPBS for 10 min with four changes. Nitroblue tetrazolium salt and 5-bromo-4-chloro-3-indolylphosphate (NBT/BCIP, Roche Applied Science, United States) were used as the color substrates. After color development, the sections were mounted in 50% glycerol (v/v, USB, United States). The experiment was performed in triplicates.

5.1.8 BrdU (Bromodeoxyuridine) labeling assay

Chang liver cells were cultured in 8-well glass slide (Nalge Nunc international, Naperville) with Minimum Essential Medium Eagle plus 10% FBS. After 80% confluent, the cultures were transfected with Ctl-siRNA or BRE-siRNA respectively according to maufacturers' instructions. Forty-eight hours after transfection, BrdU was added into the cultures to a final concentration of 20 μM and incubated at 37°C for 4 hrs. The treated cultures were then fixed with 2% paraformaldehyde for 24 hr. The fixed cultures were processed for immunohistochemistry by using mouse BrdU antibodies (1:1000, Sigma-Aldrich, United States). The BrdU positive and negative cells were counted and analysed by Spot Digital Camera & Carl Zeiss Microscope Axiophot 2 Integrated Biological Imaging System.

5.1.9 First dimensional separation of samples – Isoelectric focusing

The cell lysate for the first DE was performed on an IPGphor IEF system using 11-cm long IPG electrode strip with 4-7 pH gradient (Amersham Biosciences, United Kingdom) and an Ettan IPGphor Strip Holder (Amersham Biosciences, United Kingdom). 150 μg of protein was applied for each IPG strip. The total volume of protein sample and rehydration buffer (8M Urea, 2% CHAPS (w/v), 1% IPG buffer (v/v, Amersham Biosciences, United Kingdom), 40 mM DTT loaded onto the strip holder was 210 μl. 1ml of IPG Cover Fluid (Amersham Biosciences, United Kingdom) was applied to each strip so as to minimize evaporation and urea crystallization. The rehydration step was done under voltage and followed by a separation process. The electrophoresis condition for step 1 was 30 V for 13 hrs; step 2 was 500 V for 1 hr; step 3 was 2000 V for 1 hr and step 4 was 5000 V for 20 hrs. The program was stopped when the total volt-hours reached 40000.

5.1.10 Second dimensional separation – Sodium dodecyl sulphate polyacrylamide-gel

After first DE was completed, the IPG strips were removed from the strip holders. Each strip was then treated with 1% DTT in 6.5 ml of equilibration buffer (50 mM Tris, 6M of urea, 30% glycerol, 2% SDS, 0.1% bromophenol blue) for 30 min. The strips were further treated with 1% iodoacetamide (IAA, w/v, Sigma-Aldrich, United States) dissolved in the 6.5 ml of the same equilibration buffer. The strips were treated in the solution for 30 min. The equilibrated strips were then loaded on the 12% SDS-acrylamide separating gels. The 2-DE was performed in an ISO-DALT apparatus (Hoefer Scientific Instruments). Prestained protein molecular weight marker (Fermentas Life Science, Canada) with the range of 20 to 120 kDa was used to determine the sizes of the proteins on the gel.

5.1.11 Gel to gel matching

The gels were stained and scanned by using a GS 800 Densitometer (Bio-Rad Laboratories, United States) and images were captured for further analysis. The protein spots on the gel were analyzed by the discovery series, PDQuest 2D Analysis Software (Bio-Rad Laboratories, United States) version 7.13 PC. The experiment was performed in triplicate.

5.1.12 Protein identification by mass fingerprinting

All protein spots of interest were isolated from the gel and processed for destaining. The gel pieces were first washed in MilliQ water, immersed in 200 µl of destaining solution (15 mM potassium ferricyanide and 50 mM sodium thiosulphate) and then incubated at room temperature until they turned into colorless. Each gel piece was then washed with 400 µl of MilliQ water for 15 min, three times. The destained gel pieces were equilibrated in 200 µl of 10 mM ammonium bicarbonate/50% acetonitrile each for about 15 min. The solution was discarded and the equilibrated gel pieces were dehydrated by incubating in 200 µl of acetonitrile for 15 min. The solution was then poured off and the spots were dried in an incubator at 30°C for 5 min. Fifteen µg/ml trypsin working solution in 40 mM ammonium bicarbonate/50% acetonitrile (v/v) was used for in-gel digestion. Twelve µl of the working solution was added to each gel sample. The samples were then incubated at 35°C for 16 hrs. After trypsinization, 3 µl of extraction solution (50% acetonitrile (v/v) and 5% trifluoroacetic acid (Fluka Chemika, Switzerland) were added to each gel piece to stop the reaction. They are then centrifuged at 3,000 rpm for 2 min at room temperature. Three µl of reaction mixture from each sample was mixed with α-cyano-4-hydroxycinnamic acid matrix and then spotted onto a sample plate (Applied Biosystems, United States) for the MALDI-TOF mass spectroscopy. The mass spectrums generated were analyzed using the software Data Explorer Version 4.0.0.0 (Applied Biosystems, United States) and by mass fingerprinting search using the search engine provided by Protein prospector (http://prospector.ucsf.edu/ucsfhtml4.0/msfit.htm). To determine the significance of variance in the experiments, data were analyzed using the two-tailed, paired student's t-test. $P<0.05$ was considered to be statistically significant. All statistical analysis was performed using the SPSS software.

5.2 Results and discussions of the comparative proteomic analysis of BRE

5.2.1 Comparative proteomic analysis reveals BRE regulates prohibitin and p53 expression

BRE gene encodes a highly conserved stress-modulating protein. To gain further insight into the function of this gene, we used comparative proteomics to investigate the protein profiles of C2C12 and D122 cells resulting from small interfering RNA (siRNA)-mediated silencing as well as overexpression of BRE. It was found that silencing BRE expression in C2C12 cells would up-regulate Akt-3 and carbonic anhydrase III expression. In contrast, 26S proteasome regulatory subunit S14 and prohibitin expressions were down-regulated as shown in Figures 2 (2-DE gel) and 3 (semiquantitative RT-PCR and Western blot analyses). It has been reported that prohibitin is normally expressed in different cellular compartments involved in regulating cell proliferation, mitochondrial activities and protein processing (Mishra, 2010). Prohibitin can apparently directly interact with p53 in response to stress (Fusaro et al., 2003; Joshi et al., 2007). We established that cell proliferation was significantly increased after silencing BRE expression and this was accompanied by a reduction in p53 and

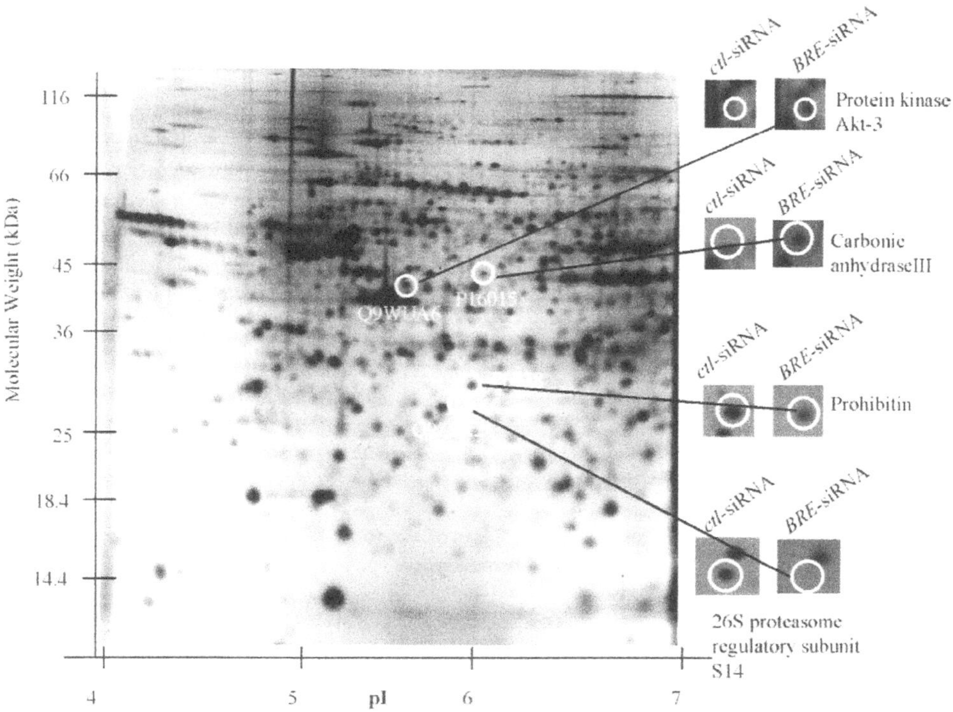

Fig. 2. Representative 2-DE gel of protein extracts from C2C12 cells that had been transfected with CTL- or BRE-siRNAs. Four differentially expressed proteins were identified (Swiss-Prot accession number provided). Silencing BRE expression up-regulated protein spots Q9WUA6 and P16015, but P6778 and Q9Z2X2 were down-regulated. pI 4–7 (x-axis) and MW in kDa (y-axis) (Tang et al., 2006).

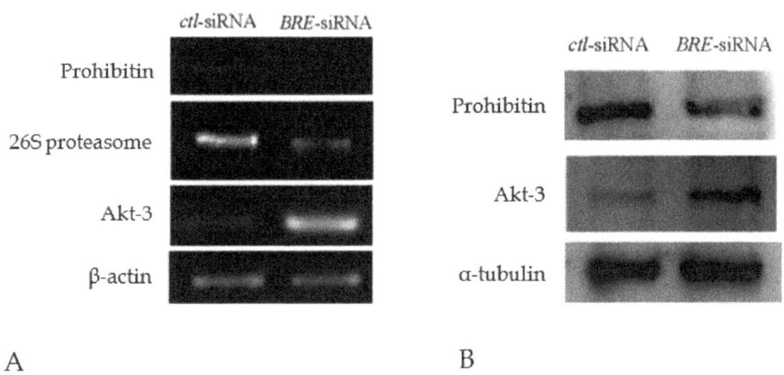

Fig. 3. Semiquantitative RT-PCR (A) and Western blots (B) analyses confirming the comparative proteomic results that silencing *BRE*, down-regulated p*rohibitin* and *26S proteasome regulatory subunit S14* expression, while *Akt-3* expression was up-regulated. *β-actin* and α-tubulin serve as internal controls (Tang et al., 2006).

prohibitin expression. We also identified Akt-3 that was affected by BRE silencing which suggests BRE might be involved in the P13/AKT signaling pathway (Madhunapantula et al., 2009). We observed that cell proliferation was suppressed when BRE was overexpressed in the D122αa4 cell line as shown in Figure 4. This was accompanied by an increase in p53 and prohibitin expression as shown in Figure 5. It has been reported that in the nucleus BRE is

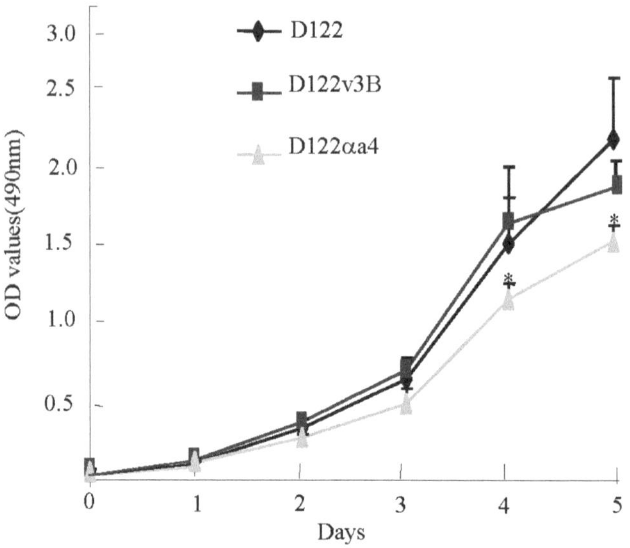

Fig. 4. MTT assay of D122, D122v3B and D122αa4 cell lines. The chart shows *BRE* overexpression in D122αa4 inhibited cell proliferation. Values = means ±SEM, *P*, ≤0.01, * D122αa4 significantly different from D122 and D122v3B (Tang et al., 2006).

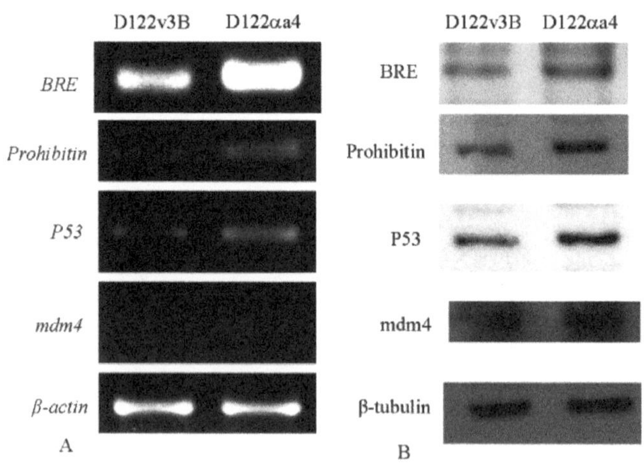

Fig. 5. Semiquantitative RT-PCR (A) and Western blot (B) showing that D122αa4 cells overexpressed *prohibitin, p53* and *mdm4*. β-*actin* and α-tubulin serve as internal controls (Tang et al., 2006) .

one of the components of BRCA1 A complex that is essential for tumor suppression (Harris and Khanna, 2011). BRE peptide has an ubiquitin E2 variant domain which has been determined to bind ubiquitin in co-immunoprecipitation experiments (Hu et al., 2011; Li et al., 2004). Coincidently, a 26S proteasome regulatory subunit S14 was one of the proteins found to be down-regulated by BRE over-expression. It is now known that the ubiquitin-proteasome pathway plays an important role in regulating the proteolytic processes that occur during signal transduction, transcriptional regulation and cell-cycle progression (Clague and Urbé, 2010). In this context, we speculate that BRE participates in the ubiquitin-proteasome pathway to regulate protein turnover within cells. In the 2-DE profiling of D122α4 cells, where BRE was stably overexpressed, we identified five proteins that were up-regulated. They were granulin precursor, TNF receptor associated factor 6 (TRAF6), mitogen protein kinase 8, Mdm4 and baculoviral IAP repeat-containing protein 4 as shown in Figures 6 (2 DE gel) and 7 (semiquantitative RT-PCR and Western blot analyses).

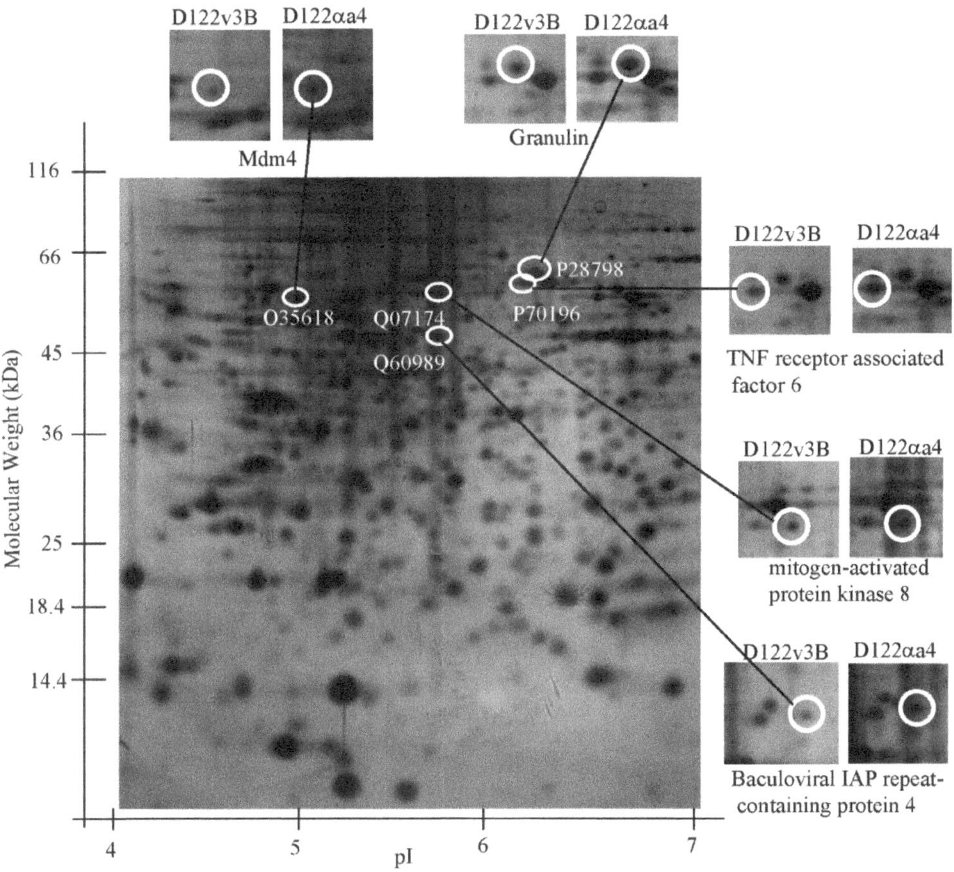

Fig. 6. Representative 2-DE gel of protein extracts from D122v3B and D122αa4 cell lines. Five protein spots (O35618, P28798, Q07174, P70196 and Q60989) were up-regulated in D122αa4 cells (Swiss-Prot accession number provided) (Tang et al., 2006).

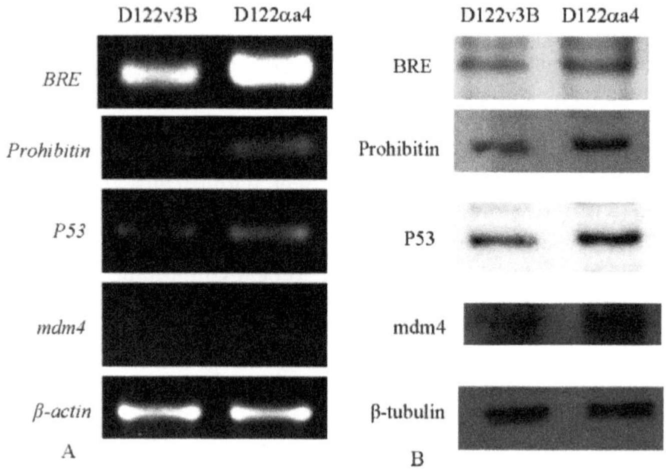

Fig. 7. Semiquantitative RT-PCR (A) and Western blot (B) showing that D122αa4 cells overexpressed *prohibitin, p53* and *mdm4*. β-*actin* and α-tubulin serve as internal controls (Tang et al., 2006).

Interestingly, TRAF6 is a unique member of the TRAF family of adaptor protein. It is associated with a diverse range of cellular responses to pathogens, growth factors or intracellular stress (Chung et al., 2007). Recent finding also showed that TRAF6 was involved in the RANK-TRAF6-NF-κB pathways during osteoclastogenesis (Inoue et al., 2007). Overexpression of BRE in human 293 embryonic kidney cells has been reported to inhibit NF-κB activation in response to TNFα (Gu et al., 1998). This finding suggests that BRE indirectly cross-talk with TRAF6 and NF-κβ, where it may play a central role in regulating cell proliferation, differentiation and survival. BRE may also mediate in post-translational sumoylation, similar to the action of PML and MO25α proteins (Kretz-Remy and Tanguay, 1999). Our results established a crucial function for BRE in regulating key proteins of cellular stress-response and provided an explanation for the multifunctional nature of BRE.

5.2.2 Comparative proteomic analysis reveals differentially expressed proteins regulated by a potential tumor promoter, BRE, in human esophageal carcinoma cells

Esophageal cancer is one of the most common malignancies that cause high mortality. Esophageal carcinogenesis is a complex and cascading process that involve the interaction of many genes and proteins (Kuwano et al., 2005). In this study, we have used comparative proteomic approaches to identify proteins that maybe involved in esophageal carcinogenesis. Two dimensional electrophoresis (2-DE) and MALDI-TOF-MS analyses of esophageal carcinoma, SHEEC and control cells SHEE revealed 10 proteins that were up-regulated as shown in Figure 8 of the 2-DE. Additional 10 proteins were down-regulated as shown in Figure 9. Interestingly, BRE, prohibitin, cyclin A and p53

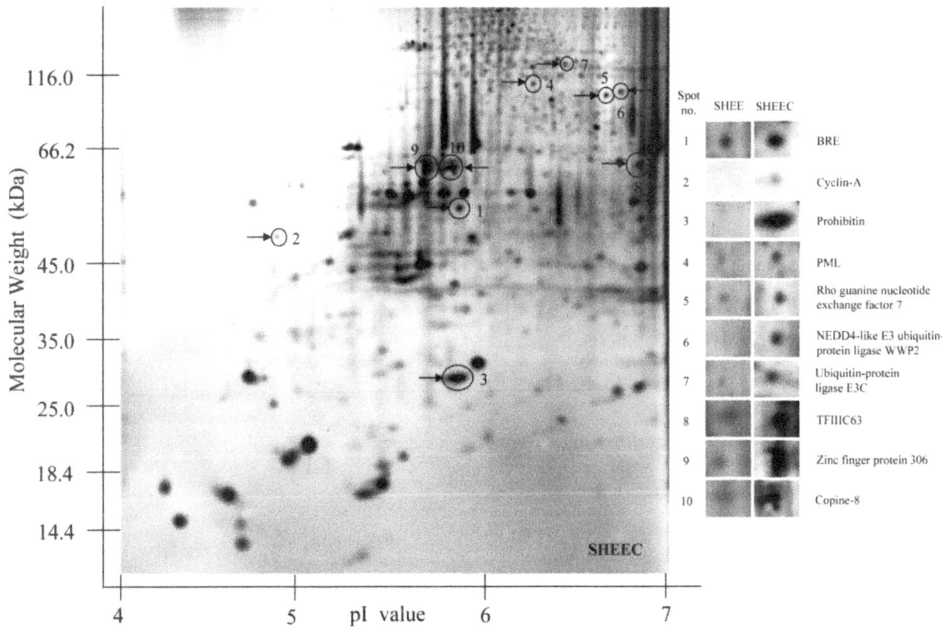

Fig. 8. Representative 2-DE gel of nucleic proteins extracted from SHEE and SHEEC cells. Ten silver-stained protein spots were found to be up-regulated in SHEEC cells (Chen et al., 2008).

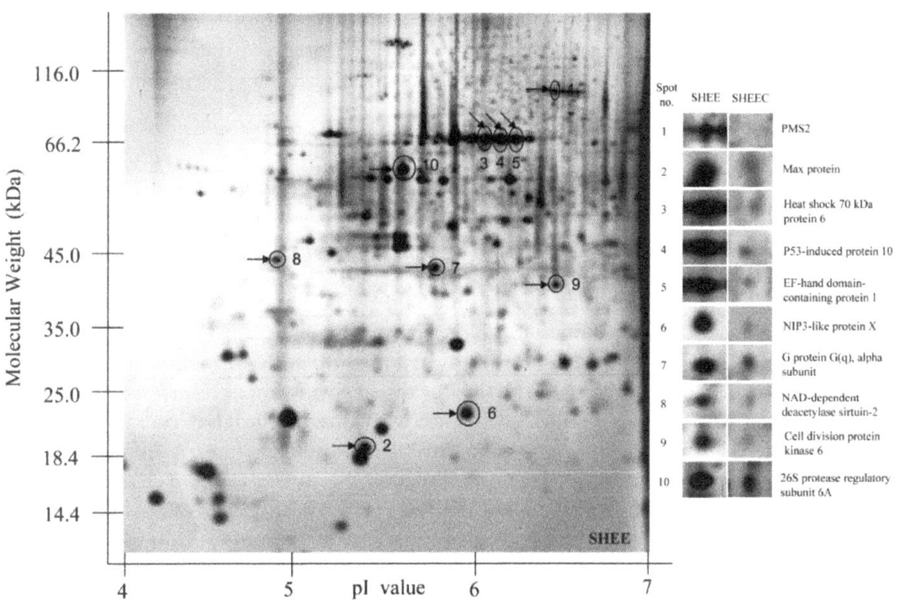

Fig. 9. Representative 2-DE gel of nucleic proteins extracted from SHEE and SHEEC cells. Ten silver-stained protein spots were found to be down-regulated in SHEEC cells (Chen et al., 2008).

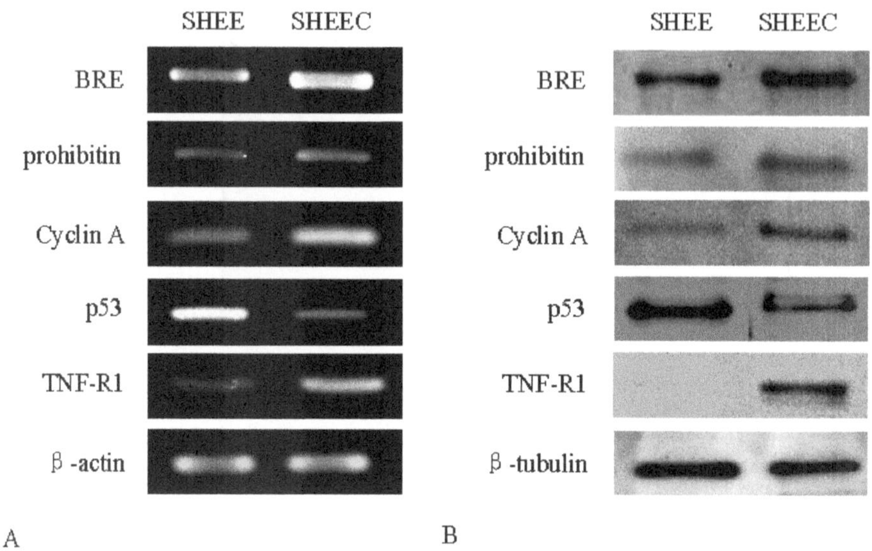

Fig. 10. Semiquantitative RT-PCR (A) and Western Blot (B) analyses of SHEE and SHEEC cells. The results confirmed the proteomic data that BRE, prohibitin and cyclin A were highly expressed in SHEEC cells. The SHEEC cells also expressed relatively higher levels of TNF-R1 but lower levels of p53, when compared with SHEE cells. *β-actin* and α-tubulin serve as internal controls (Chen et al., 2008).

expression were up-regulated in the cancer cells and this was confirmed by both semiquantitative RT-PCR and western blot analyses (Figure 10). Among these 20 differentially expressed proteins, BRE protein was identified as a potential tumor promoter. Furthermore, we have also determined p53 expression was down-regulated; whereas TNF-R1 expression was up-regulated in SHEEC cells (Figure 10). It has been reported that BRE can interact with the intracellular juxtamembrane domain TNF-R1 and inhibit the TNF-α induced activation of NF-κB (Gu et al., 1998). Therefore, we propose that BRE plays an anti-apoptotic role in SHEEC cells. To gain more insight into BRE's function, we silenced BRE expression in esophageal carcinoma cells using BRE-specific small interference RNA. It was found that silencing BRE expression corresponds to down-regulated prohibitin expression but up-regulated tumor-suppressor gene, p53 as shown in Figure 11. These findings contradicted the results with previous data (Tang, et al., 2006) that may due to multifunctional nature of BRE. Besides BRE, cyclin A and CDK2 expressions were suppressed in the SHEEC cells. Cyclin A is an important regulator of the cell cycle that rises in early S phase and falls in mid M phase (Parwaresch and Rudolph, 1996). Recent finding showed the cyclin A might be a prognostic marker in early breast cancer (Ahlin, et al. 2007). In summary, these results imply that BRE may be a survival factor and plays a proliferative role in esophageal carcinoma.

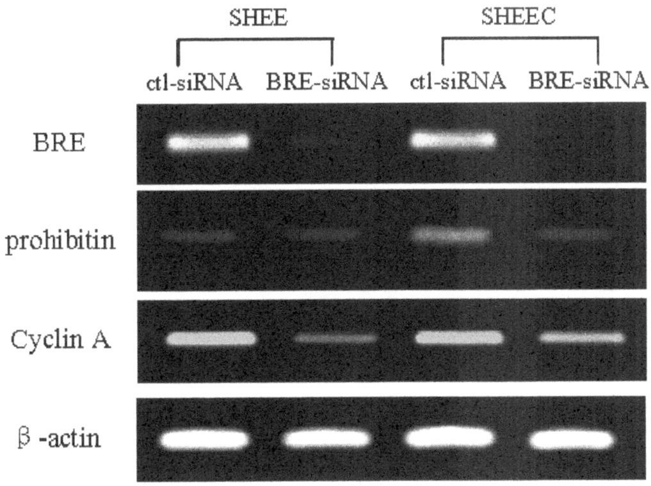

Fig. 11. Semiquantitative RT-PCR analysis of SHEE and SHEEC cells transfected with CTL- and BRE-siRNAs. The results showed that our BRE construct can silence BRE expression, as well as suppressed prohibitin and cyclin A expressions. *β-actin* served as an internal control (Chen et al., 2008).

5.2.3 Livers over-expressing BRE transgene are under heightened state of stress-response, as revealed by comparative proteomics

BRE is normally expressed at very low levels in the liver (Chan, et al., 2008). It binds to TNF-R1 and Fas, and modulates the actions of these cytokines (Li, et al., 2004; Chan et al., 2010). In this study, we demonstrated that BRE expression was rapidly induced when the liver was insulted with carbon tetrachloride (CCl_4) or in human hepatocellular carcinoma (HCC) as shown in Figure 12. We produced transgenic mice that specifically over-expressed BRE in the liver to determine the effect of high levels of BRE in the liver. The livers of these transgenic mice were determined to be histologically normal. Because of the lack of a phenotype, we conducted comparative proteomics to determine whether there were any differences at the protein level (Figure 13). The 2-DE revealed four up-regulated protein spots and nine down-regulated protein spots as summarized in Table 2. It was established that several stress responsive proteins were up-regulated in the BRE-transgenic liver including: Alpha enolase (ENO 1), Heat shock-related 70 kDa protein 2 (HSPA2), Putative heat shock 70 kDa protein 7 (HSPA7), Zinc-finger protein Ubid 4 (DPF2) and Tumor suppressor candidate 4 G21 protein (TUSC4) as shown in Figure 14. Recently, it has been reported that HSPA7 is a biomarker for early detection of HCC (Park, 2011). In addition, we have silenced BRE expression in Chang liver cells and inversely demonstrated that it did not affect cell proliferation rate as confirmed by BrdU Labelling assay (Table 3). We have previously reported that BRE is not only expressed in the cytoplasm but also in the nuclei of HCC cells. BRE also accumulates in the nuclei of esophagus cancer SHEEC cells (Chen, et al., 2008). Since BRE is one of the components of BRCA1 A complex, it could be involved in DNA repair, as well as responding to environmental stress. We propose that the livers in our BRE transgenic mice were under a heighten state of stress response and this may explain why the transgenic mice was more resistant to liver toxic drugs.

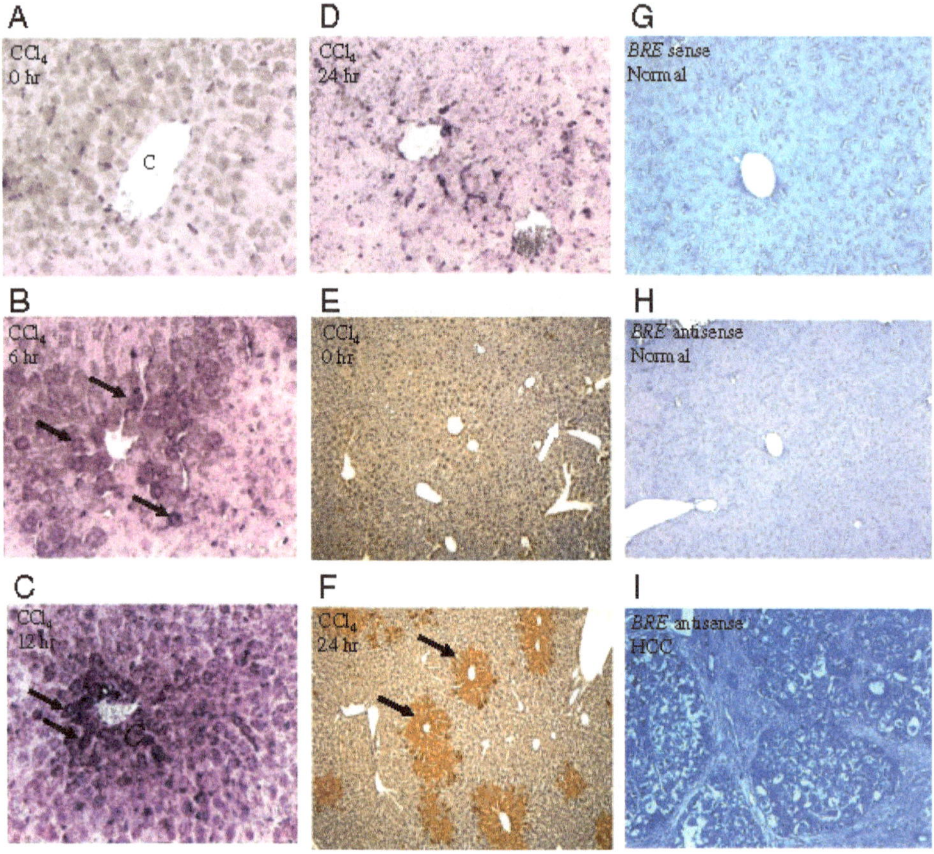

Fig. 12. In situ hybridization (A–D and G–I). BRE is normally expressed at very low levels in normal mouse liver (A). CCl4 insult induced increased BRE expression in the affected hepatocytes at 6 h (B) and 12h (C). Twenty-four hours after CCl4 insult, BRE expression declined. This was probably the result of the affected hepatocytes starting to die off (D). Immunohistological staining revealed that BRE expression was strongly induced in the affected hepatocytes by CCl4 (E, F). BRE expression remained low in the unaffected cells. We also examined BRE expression in HCC cells. BRE was expressed at low levels in non-tumor human liver tissues (H). In HCC tissues, all the cells strongly expressed BRE (I). Sense control (G). Arrows, hepatocytes overexpressing BRE. C, liver central veins (Tang et al., 2009).

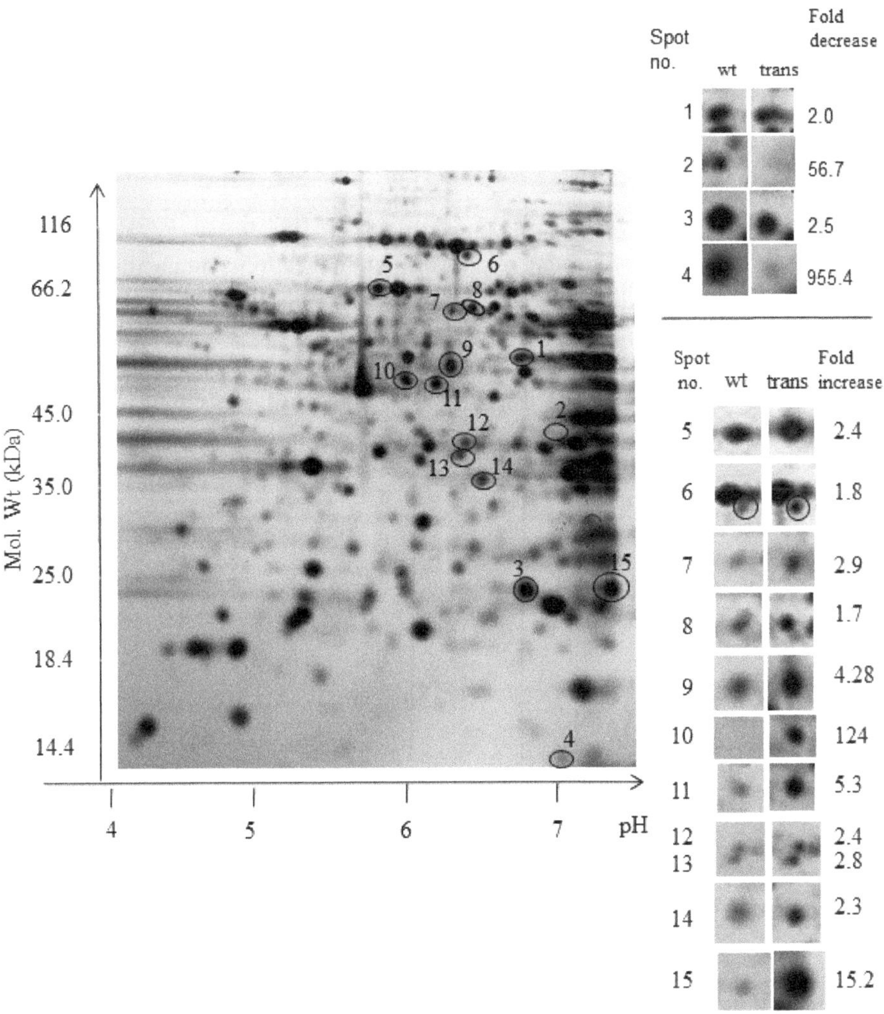

Fig. 13. A representative 2-DE gel of BRE transgenic liver. Protein spots 1–15 were identified to be differentially expressed when compared with control gels. Protein spots 1–4 were downregulated in the transgenic (trans) liver, while protein spots 5–15 were upregulated in the wild type (wt) liver. These results were acquired from three independent liver samples and 2-DE was correspondingly performed three times (Tang et al., 2009).

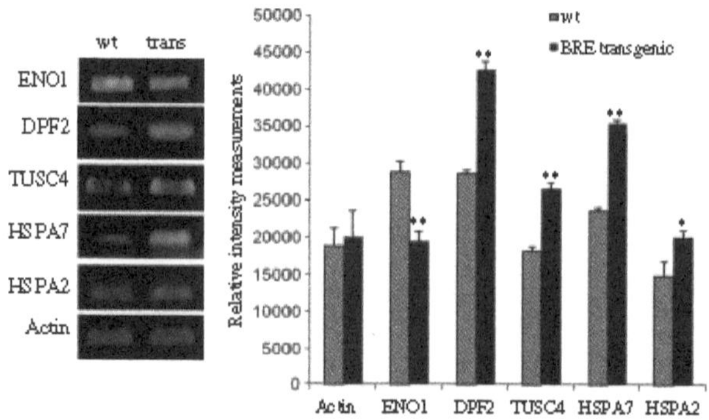

Fig. 14. Semi-quantitative RT-PCR revealed that the proteins identified were differentially expressed in BRE transgenic livers were also correspondingly affected at the transcriptional level. *p<0.05, **p<0.01, denote significant difference in the staining intensity of wt and BRE transgenic PCR bands (Tang et al., 2009).

Spot no.	Proteins identified	Swissprot accession no.	Mowse Score	Actual MW (kDa)/pI	No. of peptide mass match (%)	Functions
1	Alpha enolase	P17182	2.65e+008	47.1/6.37	18/165 (10%)	Multifunctional enzyme involved in various processes such as growth control, hypoxia tolerance and allergic responses
2	Zinc-finger protein	Q9QX66	6.74e+003	44.2/6.73	8/121 (6%)	May play a role as a neurospecific transcription for developing neurons by participating in regulation of cell survival
3	ARF-related protein	Q8BXL7	1.07e+006	22.7/6.17	16/272 (5%)	Possibly involved in plasma membrane-related signaling events
4	Hepatocellular carcinoma associated antigen 127	Q9NQZ6	4.22e+003	26.2/6.68	9/77 (11%)	Unknown
5	Heat shock-related 70kDa Protein 2	P54652	4.77e+008	70.0/5.56	28/274 (10%)	Cooperate with other chaperones, it stabilizes preexistent proteins against aggregation and mediates the folding of newly translated polypeptides in the cytosol or within organelles
6	Tumor suppressor candidate 4 (G21 protein)	Q9WUE4	1.01e+005	43.6/6.23	9/119 (6%)	May act as a tumor suppressor
7	Nuclear receptor ROR-alpha	P35398	1.23e+006	63.0/5.97	9/119 (6%)	Might be an orphan nuclear receptor that binds DNA as a monomer to hormone response elements
8	Leucine-rich repeat LG1 family member 2	Q8K4Z0	1.61e+008	63.0/6.10	10/165 (6%)	Might be a potential secreted protein
9	Mitogen-activated protein kinase 12	P53778	7.17e+008	41.9/5.98	28/197 (14%)	Responds to activation of environmental stress or pro-inflammatory cytokines by phosphorylating downstream targets
10	Ankyrin repeat domain protein	Q99LW0	7.81e+005	44.0/5.85	15/205 (5%)	Plays a wide variety of roles in protein–protein interaction and in the signal pathways
11	Caspase-2 precursor	P29594	1.12e+003	48.9/5.80	5/68 (7%)	Might be involved in regulation of proteins in cell death
12	Protein FAM54A	Q8VED8	6.66e+004	40.8/6.05	11/149 (7%)	Unknown
13	CD209 antigen-like protein B	Q8CJ91	4.77e+004	37.1/6.10	8/121 (6)	Might be a pathogen-recognition receptor and mediate the endocytosis of pathogens
14	Zinc-finger protein Ubid4	Q61103	4.75e+006	44.2/6.06	16/280 (5%)	Might be a transcription factor in apoptosis response; it also plays a role in the development and maturation of lymphoid cells
15	Heat shock 70 kDa protein	P48741	1.52e+006	25.9/6.97	4/37 (10%)	May act as chaperones in presenting tumor antigens

Table 2. Proteins that are differentially expressed in BRE transgenic liver (Tang et al., 2009).

Treatments	BrdU⁻ cells	BrdU⁺ cells	Total	Percentage Brdu⁺ cells
Ctl-siRNA	293±30	293±32	585±36	50.04±0.02
BRE-siRNA	276±32	265±16	541±24	49.09±0.03

Table 3. Effects of silencing BRE expression on Chang liver cell proliferation (Tang et al., 2009).

6. Future perspective of proteomics

Conventional "gel-based" electrophoresis and improved mass spectrometry have provided useful tools for revealing molecular changes in cells and tissues that otherwise maybe missed by morphological observation alone (Vercauteren et al., 2007). Nevertheless, the 2-DE protocol is still to be refined and improved so that 2-DE is more reproducible and sensitive. Therefore, it has still some distance to go before it can be adopted as a standard "diagnostic tool" in the 21st century (Colucci-D'Amato et al., 2011). The "shotgun" methodology has been used as a high-throughput screen to identify proteins that are differentially expressed in cells or tissues, as a result of some experimental procedure or changes in environmental condition (Lill, 2003; Zhu et al., 2010). Liu et al. (2011) recently described the SELDI-TOF-MS technology that could be used to screen and detect differentially expressed proteins in the serum of patients with cancer. Liquid chromatography interfaced plasma mass spectrometry has now been developed for absolute quantitation of proteins (Esteban-Fernández et al., 2011). Furthermore, latest development of computational tools for analyzing high-throughput 'shotgun' proteomic data also play a vital role in moving proteomic research forward (Dowsey et al., 2010). All of these improvements will allow proteomics to be rapidly developed as a practical, robust, accurate and inexpensive analytical tool for routine use in the clinical setting. The proteomics will also allow many novel disease biomarkers to be discovered and also lead to the discovery of new drugs.

7. References

[1] Ahlin C, Aaltonen K, Amini RM, Nevanlinna H, Fjällskog ML, Blomqvist C. (2007) Ki67 and cyclin A as prognostic factors in early breast cancer. What are the optimal cut-off values? Histopathology. 51(4):491-8.

[2] Altland K, Becher P, Rossmann U, Bjellqvist B. (1988) Isoelectric focusing of basic proteins: the problem of oxidation of cysteines. Electrophoresis. (9):474-85.

[3] Andersen JS, Svensson B, Roepstorff P. (1996) Electrospray ionization and matrix assisted laser desorption/ionization mass spectrometry: powerful analytical tools in recombinant protein chemistry. Nat Biotechnol. 14(4):449-57.

[4] Arnstein, HR (1965). Mechanism of protein biosynthesis. Br Med Bull. 21(3):217-22.

[5] Arrell DK, Neverova I, Van Eyk JE. (2001) Cardiovascular proteomics: evolution and potential. Circ Res. 88(8):763-73.

[6] Bergquist J, Palmblad M, Wetterhall M, Håkansson P, Markides KE. (2002) Peptide mapping of proteins in human body fluids using electrospray ionization Fourier transform ion cyclotron resonance mass spectrometry. Mass Spectrom Rev. 21(1):2-15.

[7] Birr C, Frank R. (1975) Control for uniformity of synthetic peptides: quantitative evaluation of the Edman degradation of support-bound human insulin B 22-30 synthetized by the Merrifield method. FEBS Lett. 55(1):68-71.

[8] Bjellqvist B, Ek K, Righetti PG, Gianazza E, Görg A, Westermeier R, Postel W. (1982) Isoelectric focusing in immobilized pH gradients: principle, methodology and some applications. J Biochem Biophys Methods. 6(4):317-39.

[9] Blundell TL, Johnson MS. (1993) Catching a common fold. Protein Sci. 2(6):877-83.

[10] Ceglarek U, Kortz L, Leichtle A, Fiedler GM, Kratzsch J, Thiery J. (2009) Rapid quantification of steroid patterns in human serum by on-line solid phase extraction combined with liquid chromatography-triple quadrupole linear ion trap mass spectrometry. Clin Chim Acta.401(1-2):114-8.

[11] Celis JE, Celis P, Ostergaard M, Basse B, Lauridsen JB, Ratz G, Rasmussen HH, Orntoft TF, Hein B, Wolf H, Celis A.(1999) Proteomics and immunohistochemistry define some of the steps involved in the squamous differentiation of the bladder transitional epithelium: a novel strategy for identifying metaplastic lesions. Cancer Res. 59(12):3003-9.

[12] Chalkley RJ, Baker PR, Huang L, Hansen KC, Allen NP, Rexach M, Burlingame AL.(2005) Comprehensive analysis of a multidimensional liquid chromatography mass spectrometry dataset acquired on a quadrupole selecting, quadrupole collision cell, time-of-flight mass spectrometer: II. New developments in Protein Prospector allow for reliable and comprehensive automatic analysis of large datasets. Mol Cell Proteomics 4(8):1194-204.

[13] Chan BC, Ching AK, To KF, Leung JC, Chen S, Li Q, Lai PB, Tang NL, Shaw PC, Chan JY, James AE, Lai KN, Lim PL, Lee KK, Chui YL. (2008) BRE is an antiapoptotic protein in vivo and overexpressed in human hepatocellular carcinoma. Oncogene. 27(9):1208-17.

[14] Chan BC, Li Q, Chow SK, Ching AK, Liew CT, Lim PL, Lee KK, Chan JY, Chui YL.(2005). BRE enhances in vivo growth of tumor cells. Biochem Biophys Res Commun 326(2):268-73.

[15] Chan JY, Li L, Miao J, Cai DQ, Lee KK, Chui YL.(2010) Differential expression of a novel gene BRE (TNFRSF1A modulator/BRCC45) in response to stress and biological signals. Mol Biol Rep. 37(1):363-8.

[16] Chen HB, Pan K, Tang MK, Chui YL, Chen L, Su ZJ, Shen ZY, Li EM, Xie W, Lee KK. (2008) Comparative proteomic analysis reveals differentially expressed proteins regulated by a potential tumor promoter, BRE, in human esophageal carcinoma cells. Biochem Cell Biol. 86(4):302-11.

[17] Chen R, Snyder M. (2010) Yeast proteomics and protein microarrays. J Proteomics. 73(11):2147-57.

[18] Ching, A.K., Li, P.S., Li, Q., Chan, B.S., Chan, J.Y., Lim, P.L., Pang, J.C., Chui, Y.L. (2001). Expression of human BRE in multiple isoforms. Biochem. Biophys. Res. Commun. 288, 535-545.

[19] Chowdhury SK, Katta V, Chait BT. (1990) An electrospray-ionization mass spectrometer with new features. Rapid Commun Mass Spectrom. 4(3):81-7.
[20] Chung JY, Lu M, Yin Q, Lin SC, Wu H. (2007) Molecular basis for the unique specificity of TRAF6. Adv Exp Med Biol. 597:122-30.
[21] Clague MJ, Urbé S. (2010) Ubiquitin: same molecule, different degradation pathways. Cell. 143(5):682-5.
[22] Colucci-D'Amato L, Farina A, Vissers JP, Chambery A. (2011) Quantitative neuroproteomics: classical and novel tools for studying neural differentiation and function. Stem Cell Rev. 7(1):77-93.
[23] Conrotto P, Souchelnytskyi S. (2008) Proteomic approaches in biological and medical sciences: principles and applications. Exp Oncol. 30(3):171-80.
[24] Dong Y, Hakimi MA, Chen X, Kumaraswamy E, Cooch NS, Godwin AK, Shiekhattar R. (2003) Regulation of BRCC, a holoenzyme complex containing BRCA1 and BRCA2, by a signalosome-like subunit and its role in DNA repair. Mol Cell. 12(5):1087-99.
[25] Dowsey AW, English JA, Lisacek F, Morris JS, Yang GZ, Dunn MJ. (2010) Image analysis tools and emerging algorithms for expression proteomics. Proteomics. 10(23):4226-57.
[26] Edman, P. (1950) Method for Determination of the Amino Acid Sequence in Peptides. Acta Chem Scand 10: 283-293.
[27] Edman, P. and Begg, G. (1967) A protein Sequenator. European J. Biochem. 1: 80-91.
[28] Esteban-Fernández D, Scheler C, Linscheid MW. (2011) Absolute protein quantification by LC-ICP-MS using MeCAT peptide labeling. Anal Bioanal Chem. 401(2):657-66.
[29] Fenn JB, Mann M, Meng CK, Wong SF, Whitehouse CM. (1989) Electrospray ionization for mass spectrometry of large biomolecules. Science. 246(4926):64-71.
[30] Fenn JB. (2002) Electrospray ionization mass spectrometry: How it all began. J Biomol Tech. 13(3):101-18.
[31] Finnerty V, Johnson G. (1979) Post-Translational Modification as a Potential Explanation of High Levels of Enzyme Polymorphism: Xanthine Dehydrogenase and Aldehyde Oxidase in DROSOPHILA MELANOGASTER. Genetics. 91(4):695-722.
[32] Fleischer, B. (1983) Mechanism of glycosylation in the Golgi apparatus. J Histochem Cytochem. 31(8):1033-40.
[33] Fusaro G, Dasgupta P, Rastogi S, Joshi B, Chellappan S. (2003) Prohibitin induces the transcriptional activity of p53 and is exported from the nucleus upon apoptotic signaling. J Biol Chem. 278(48):47853-61.
[34] Galvão ER, Martins LM, Ibiapina JO, Andrade HM, Monte SJ. (2011) Breast cancer proteomics: a review for clinicians. J Cancer Res Clin Oncol. 137(6):915-25.
[35] Gioia R, Leroy C, Drullion C, Lagarde V, Etienne G, Dulucq S, Lippert E, Roche S, Mahon FX, Pasquet JM. (2011) Quantitative phosphoproteomics revealed interplay between Syk and Lyn in the resistance to nilotinib in chronic myeloid leukemia cells. Blood. 118(8):2211-21.
[36] Görg A, Drews O, Lück C, Weiland F, Weiss W.(2009) 2-DE with IPGs. Electrophoresis. 30 Suppl 1:S122-32.
[37] Görg A, Weiss W, Dunn MJ. (2004) Current two-dimensional electrophoresis technology for proteomics. Proteomics. 4(12):3665-85.

[38] Gu C, Castellino A, Chan JY, Chao MV. (1998) BRE: a modulator of TNF-alpha action. FASEB J. 12(12):1101-8.
[39] Han MJ, Lee JW, Lee SY. (2011) Understanding and engineering of microbial cells based on proteomics and its conjunction with other omics studies. Proteomics. 11(4):721-43.
[40] Harris JL, Khanna KK. (2011) BRCA1 A-complex fine tunes repair functions of BRCA1. Aging (Albany NY). 3(5):461-3.
[41] Hillenkamp F, Karas M, Beavis RC, Chait BT. (1991) Matrix-assisted laser desorption/ionization mass spectrometry of biopolymers. Anal Chem. 63(24):1193A-1203A.
[42] Hu X, Kim JA, Castillo A, Huang M, Liu J, Wang B. (2011) NBA1/MERIT40 and BRE interaction is required for the integrity of two distinct deubiquitinating enzyme BRCC36-containing complexes. J Biol Chem. 286(13):11734-45.
[43] Inoue J, Gohda J, Akiyama T, Semba K. (2007) NF-kappaB activation in development and progression of cancer. Cancer Sci. 98(3):268-74.
[44] Joshi B, Rastogi S, Morris M, Carastro LM, DeCook C, Seto E, Chellappan SP. (2007) Differential regulation of human YY1 and caspase 7 promoters by prohibitin through E2F1 and p53 binding sites. Biochem J. 401(1):155-66.
[45] Kretz-Remy C, Tanguay RM. (1999) SUMO/sentrin: protein modifiers regulating important cellular functions. Biochem Cell Biol. 77(4):299-309.
[46] Kuwano H, Kato H, Miyazaki T, Fukuchi M, Masuda N, Nakajima M, Fukai Y, Sohda M, Kimura H, Faried A. (2005) Genetic alterations in esophageal cancer. Surg Today. 35(1):7-18.
[47] Larbi, NB and Jefferies, C. (2009) 2D-DIGE: Comparative Proteomics of Cellular Signalling Pathways. Methods Mol Biol. 517:105-32.
[48] Lau TY, O'Connor DP, Brennan DJ, Duffy MJ, Pennington SR, Gallagher WM.(2007) Breast cancer proteomics: clinical perspectives. Expert Opin Biol Ther. 7(2):209-19.
[49] Lee KK, Leung AK, Tang MK, Cai DQ, Schneider C, Brancolini C, Chow PH (2001). Functions of the growth arrest specific 1 gene in the development of the mouse embryo. Dev Biol 234(1):188-203.
[50] Lengyel P. (1966) Problems in protein biosynthesis. J Gen Physiol. 49(6):305-30.
[51] Li Q, Ching AK, Chan BC, Chow SK, Lim PL, Ho TC, Ip WK, Wong CK, Lam CW, Lee KK, Chan JY, Chui YL. (2004) A death receptor-associated anti-apoptotic protein, BRE, inhibits mitochondrial apoptotic pathway. J Biol Chem. 279(50):52106-16.
[52] Li, L., Yoo, H., Becker, F.F., Ali-Osman, F. and Chan, J.Y. (1995). Identification of a brain- and reproductive-organs-specific gene responsive to DNA damage and retinoic acid. Biochem. Biophys. Res. Commun. 206, 764-774.
[53] Lill, J (2003) Proteomic Tools for Quantitation by Mass Spectrometry. Mass Spect Rev. 22: 182-194.
[54] Liu C, Pan C, Wang H, Yong L. (2011) Effect of surface-enhanced laser desorption/ionization time-of-flight mass spectrometry on identifying biomarkers of laryngeal carcinoma. Tumour Biol. 2011 Aug 9.
[55] Lucas F, Barber M, Wolstenholme WA, Geddes AJ, Graham GN, Morris HR. (1969) Mass-spectrometric determination of the amino acid sequences in peptides isolated from the protein silk fibroin of Bombyx mori. Biochem J. 114(4):695-702.

[56] Madhunapantula SV, Robertson GP. (2009) The PTEN-AKT3 signaling cascade as a therapeutic target in melanoma. Pigment Cell Melanoma Res. 22(4):400-19.

[57] Mao LM, Guo ML, Jin DZ, Fibuch EE, Choe ES, Wang JQ. (2011) Post-translational modification biology of glutamate receptors and drug addiction. Front Neuroanat. 5:19.

[58] Marko-Varga G, Berglund M, Malmström J, Lindberg H, Fehniger TE. (2003) Targeting hepatocytes from liver tissue by laser capture microdissection and proteomics expression profiling. Electrophoresis. 24(21):3800-5.

[59] McKerrow JH, Bhargava V, Hansell E, Huling S, Kuwahara T, Matley M, Coussens L, Warren R. (2000) A functional proteomics screen of proteases in colorectal carcinoma. Mol Med. 6(5):450-60.

[60] Miao J, Chan KW, Chen GG, Chun SY, Xia NS, Chan JY, Panesar NS. (2005) Blocking BRE expression in Leydig cells inhibits steroidogenesis by down-regulating 3beta-hydroxysteroid dehydrogenase. J Endocrinol. 185(3):507-17.

[61] Miao, J., Panesar, N.S., Chan, K.T., Lai, F.M., Xia, N., Wang, Y., Johnson, P.J. and Chan, J.Y. (2001). Differential expression of a stress-modulating gene, BRE, in the adrenal gland, in adrenal neoplasia, and in abnormal adrenal tissues. J. Histochem. Cytochem. 49, 491-500.

[62] Mishra S, Ande SR, Nyomba BL. (2010) The role of prohibitin in cell signaling. FEBS J. 277(19):3937-46.

[63] Morris, HR, Williams, DH, Ambler RP. (1971) Determination of the Sequences of Protein-Derived Peptides and Peptide Mixtures by Mass Spectrometry. Biochem. J. 125: 189-201.

[64] Niall HD, Keutmann HT, Copp DH, Potts JT Jr. (1969) Amino acid sequence of salmon ultimobranchial calcitonin. Proc Natl Acad Sci U S A. 64(2):771-8.

[65] Novak A, Amit M, Ziv T, Segev H, Fishman B, Admon A, Itskovitz-Eldor J. (2011). Proteomics Profiling of Human Embryonic Stem Cells in the Early Differentiation Stage. Stem Cell Rev. 2011 Jul 6.

[66] O'Farrell PH.(1975) High resolution two-dimensional electrophoresis of proteins. J Biol Chem. 250(10):4007-21.

[67] Ornstein DK, Rayford W, Fusaro VA, Conrads TP, Ross SJ, Hitt BA, Wiggins WW, Veenstra TD, Liotta LA, Petricoin EF 3rd. (2004) Serum proteomic profiling can discriminate prostate cancer from benign prostates in men with total prostate specific antigen levels between 2.5 and 15.0 ng/ml. J Urol. 172(4 Pt 1):1302-5.

[68] Ornstein DK, Tyson DR. (2006) Proteomics for the identification of new prostate cancer biomarkers. Urol Oncol. 24(3):231-6.

[69] Park YN. (2011) Update on precursor and early lesions of hepatocellular carcinomas. Arch Pathol Lab Med. 135(6):704-15.

[70] Parwaresch R, Rudolph P. (1996) The Cell Cycle - Theory and Application to Cancer. Onkologie 19:464-472.

[71] Perkins DN, Pappin DJ, Creasy DM, Cottrell JS. (1999) Probability-based protein identification by searching sequence databases using mass spectrometry data. Electrophoresis. 20(18):3551-67.

[72] Sauter ER, Zhu W, Fan XJ, Wassell RP, Chervoneva I, Du Bois GC. (2002) Proteomic analysis of nipple aspirate fluid to detect biologic markers of breast cancer. Br J Cancer. 86(9):1440-3.

[73] Schwartz JC, Jardine I. (1996) Quadrupole ion trap mass spectrometry. Methods Enzymol. 270:552-86.

[74] Shen Z, Cen S, Shen J, et al. 2000. Study of immortalization and malignant transformation of human embryonic esophageal epithelial cells induced by HPV18 E6E7. J Cancer Res Clin Oncol, 126(10):589-94.

[75] Sirot LK, Hardstone MC, Helinski ME, Ribeiro JM, Kimura M, Deewatthanawong P, Wolfner MF, Harrington LC. (2011) Towards a semen proteome of the dengue vector mosquito: protein identification and potential functions. PLoS Negl Trop Dis. 5(3):e989.

[76] Tang, M.K., Wang, C.M., Shan, S.W., Chui, Y.L., Ching, A.K., Chow, P.H., Grotewold, L., Chan, J.Y. and Lee, K.K. (2006). Comparative proteomic analysis reveals a function of the novel death receptor-associated protein BRE in the regulation of prohibitin and p53 expression and proliferation. Proteomics 6, 2376-2385.

[77] Tang, MK, Liu, G, Hou, Z., Chui, YL, Chan, JYH, Lee, KKH (2009) Livers overexpressing BRE transgene are under heightened state of stress-response, as revealed by comparative proteomics. Proteomics Clin. Appl. 3(12):1362-70.

[78] Tung CS, Wong KK, Mok SC. (2008) Biomarker discovery in ovarian cancer. Womens Health (Lond Engl). 4:27-40.

[79] Vercauteren FG, Arckens L, Quirion R. (2007) Applications and current challenges of proteomic approaches, focusing on two-dimensional electrophoresis. Amino Acids. 33(3):405-14.

[80] Voss T, Ahorn H, Haberl P, Döhner H, Wilgenbus K. (2001) Correlation of clinical data with proteomics profiles in 24 patients with B-cell chronic lymphocytic leukemia. Int J Cancer. 91(2):180-6.

[81] Weiss W, Görg A. (2009) High-resolution two-dimensional electrophoresis. Methods Mol Biol. 564:13-32.

[82] Wilkins MR, Sanchez JC, Gooley AA, Appel RD, Humphery-Smith I, Hochstrasser DF, Williams KL.(1996) Progress with proteome projects: why all proteins expressed by a genome should be identified and how to do it. Biotechnol Genet Eng Rev. 13:19-50.

[83] Zhang Z, Bast RC Jr, Yu Y, Li J, Sokoll LJ, Rai AJ, Rosenzweig JM, Cameron B, Wang YY, Meng XY, Berchuck A, Van Haaften-Day C, Hacker NF, de Bruijn HW, van der Zee AG, Jacobs IJ, Fung ET, Chan DW. (2004) Three biomarkers identified from serum proteomic analysis for the detection of early stage ovarian cancer. Cancer Res. 64(16):5882-90.

[84] Zhu, W, Smith, JW and Hung, CM (2010). Mass Spectrometry-Based Label-Free Quantitative Proteomics. J. Biomed and Biotech 2010: 840518.

9

Identification of the Novel Plasminogen Receptor, Plg-R_{KT}

Lindsey A. Miles[1], Nicholas M. Andronicos[2], Emily I. Chen[3], Nagyung Baik[1], Hongdong Bai[4], Caitlin M. Parmer[5], Shahrzad Lighvani[1], Samir Nangia[4,6], William B. Kiosses[1], Mark P. Kamps[6], John R. Yates III[1] and Robert J. Parmer[4,6]

1. Introduction

1.1 The plasminogen activation system

Initiation of the plasminogen activation system results in generation of the broad spectrum serine protease, plasmin, from the circulating zymogen, plasminogen. Plasminogen is activated to plasmin by plasminogen activators (PA's), either urokinase type-plasminogen activator (u-PA) or tissue-type plasminogen activator (t-PA), via specific proteolytic cleavage (Castellino & Ploplis, 2005). Plasmin is the major enzyme responsible for degradation of fibrin clots (fibrinolysis) to maintain normal blood homeostasis (Bugge et al., 1995; Ploplis et al., 1995). Dysregulation of the plasminogen activation system can result in hemorrhage (excess fibrinolysis) or thrombosis (insufficient fibrinolysis). The plasminogen activation system is regulated by direct inhibition of plasmin (by the circulating serpin, α_2-antiplasmin) and by synthesis and secretion of plasminogen activators and the serpin, plasminogen activator inhibitor 1 (PAI-1)] (Collen, 1999). In a key regulatory step, plasminogen activation is promoted when plasminogen and its activator, t-PA, bind concomitantly to lysine residues on the surface of fibrin clots, resulting in a marked reduction in the Km for activation of plasminogen compared with the reaction in solution (Hoylaerts et al., 1982).

1.2 Functions of plasminogen receptors

In the past 25 years an additional mechanism for positive regulation of plasminogen activation has been recognized: co-localization of plasminogen and PA's on cell surfaces markedly decreases the Km for plasminogen activation in a mechanism analogous to assembly of components of the plasminogen activation system on fibrin (Miles et al., 2005). The plasmin produced is retained on the cell surface where it is protected from its inhibitor, α_2-antiplasmin (Figure 1) (Hall et al., 1991; Plow et al., 1986). Thus, the cell surface becomes

[1]*The Scripps Research Institute, USA*
[2]*CSIRO Livestock Industries, Armidale, NSW, Australia*
[3]*Stony Brook University, USA*
[4]*Veterans Administration San Diego Healthcare System, USA*
[5]*Yale University, USA*
[6]*University of California, San Diego, USA*

armed with the broad spectrum proteolytic activity of plasmin. Cell surface plasmin plays a key role in processes in which cells must degrade an extracellular matrix in order to migrate, including inflammation (Busuttil et al., 2004; Ploplis et al., 1998; Plow et al., 1999), wound healing (Creemers et al., 2000; Romer et al., 1996), metastasis (Palumbo et al., 2003; Ranson et al., 1998) and neurite outgrowth (Gutierrez-Fernandez et al., 2009; Jacovina et al., 2001). Cell surface plasmin also plays a key role in myogenesis (Lopez-Alemany et al., 2003) and prohormone processing (Jiang et al., 2001, 2002).

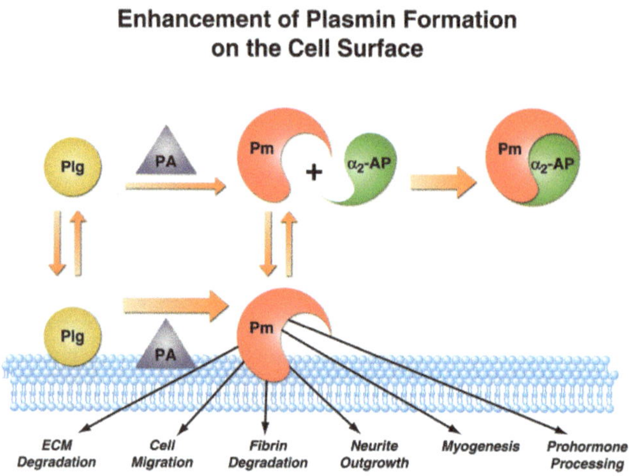

Activation of cell-associated plasminogen (Plg) to plasmin (Pm) by cell-associated plasminogen activators (PA) is markedly enhanced compared to the reaction in solution. The Pm formed remains on the cell surface where it is relatively protected from its inhibitor, α_2-antiplasmin (α_2-AP).

Fig. 1. Enhancement of plasminogen activation on the cell surface.

1.3 Characteristics of plasminogen receptors

Cellular plasminogen binding sites are very broadly distributed on both prokaryotic and eukaryotic cells. Of the many cell types examined to date, only red cells do not exhibit detectable plasminogen binding ability (Miles et al., 2005). The interactions of plasminogen with cells are of very high capacity, reaching 3 X 10^7 molecules/cell on lung fibrolasts (Plow et al., 1986), for example. Thus, the plasminogen binding capacity of a cell is made up of contributions from a set of distinct cell surface proteins.

An important aspect of the mechanism of promotion of plasminogen activation on cell surfaces is that a subset of carboxypeptidase-B-sensitive plasminogen binding proteins is responsible for enhancement of plasminogen activation on eukaryotic cells. When cells are treated with carboxypeptidase B, the ability to stimulate plasminogen activation is lost (Félez et al., 1996). Since carboxypeptidase B removes C-terminal basic residues, these results imply that proteins exposing C-terminal basic residues on cell surfaces are responsible for stimulation of plasminogen activation (Figure 2,A). Known carboxypeptidase-B-sensitive cell surface plasminogen receptors could previously be divided into two classes: 1) proteins synthesized with C-terminal lysines and having additional known intracellular functions, including α-enolase (Miles et al., 1991; Redlitz et al., 1995), cytokeratin 8 (Hembrough et al., 1995, 1996), S100A10 (Choi et al., 2003; Kassam et al., 1998), TIP49a (Hawley et al., 2001) and histone H2B (Herren et al., 2006) and; 2) proteins requiring proteolytic processing in order to reveal a C-terminal basic residue (lysine), including actin (Dudani & Ganz, 1996; Miles et al., 2006) and annexin 2 (Hajjar et al., 1994). However, until recently, no integral membrane plasminogen binding proteins synthesized with a C-terminal basic residue had been identified. The existence of a plasminogen receptor with the latter characteristics would reveal a novel mechanism for stimulation of plasminogen activation because release and rebinding of intracellular proteins or proteolytic cleavage of membrane proteins to expose C-terminal basic residues would not be required.

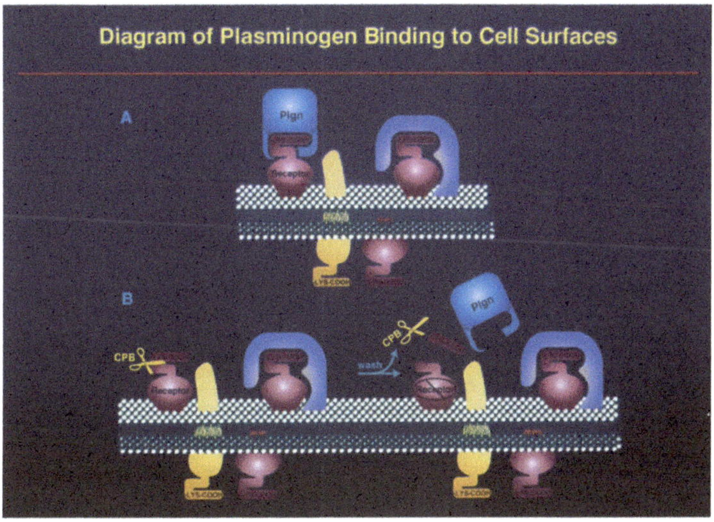

Plasminogen binding to carboxyl terminal lysines on the cell surface. Panel A) The binding of plasminogen to cell surface proteins occurs via receptors exposing carboxyl terminal lysines to the extracellular environment. Cell surface proteins with carboxyl terminal lysines that are masked or in other inaccessible orientations on the cell surface, or membrane-associated proteins with carboxyl terminal lysines that are located on the inner face of the membrane, cannot serve as plasminogen receptors. Panel B) CpB treatment of intact cells removes carboxyl terminal lysines from plasminogen receptors, and plasminogen binding to the cell surface is reduced. Reprinted with permission from (Hawley, Green, and Miles 2000, 84:882-890).

Fig. 2. Plasminogen binding to carboxyl terminal lysines on the cell surface.

1.4 Need for a proteomics approach to identify integral membrane plasminogen receptor(s) with C-terminal basic residues

Previous methodologies and characteristics of plasminogen binding proteins may have precluded identification of an integral membrane plasminogen binding protein with a C-terminal basic residue. The identification of plasminogen receptors has relied previously on cell surface labeling followed by affinity chromatography on plasminogen-Sepharose columns and N-terminal sequencing of fractions eluted from SDS gels. Thus, many intracellular proteins that are also present on the cell surface were readily identified because protein fractions that bound to plasminogen-Sepharose included the labeled, surface-associated protein, as well as nonlabeled intracellular protein. Using these methods, a lower abundance integral membrane plasminogen binding protein might not have been detectable.

Previously, we used a proteomics approach to examine monocytoid cell membranes for the presence of proteins exposing carboxyl terminal lysines on the extracellular face of the cell membrane (Hawley et al., 2000). We compared plasminogen ligand blots of 2-D gels of membrane fractions of intact cells treated with carboxypeptidase B with untreated membranes (e.g. Figure 2,B). We eluted a prominent carboxypeptidase B-sensitive protein from the 2-D gels and obtained two peptide sequences using tandem mass spectrometry. These peptide sequences corresponded to TATA-binding protein-interacting protein (TIP49a) (Hawley et al., 2001). However, TIP49a is a member of the class of cell surface plasminogen receptors synthesized with a C-terminal lysine and also having intracellular functions and is not an integral membrane protein.

The methodology used to identify TIP49a and other plasminogen receptors has required elution of candidate proteins from 2-D SDS polyacrylamide gels. However, many membrane proteins are not well resolved on SDS polyacrylamide gels. Therefore, we used an isolation method that used column chromatography instead of SDS polyacrylamide gel analysis: We took advantage of the exquisite sensitivity of multidimensional protein identification technology (MudPIT) to search for integral membrane plasminogen receptor(s) exposing a C-terminal basic residue on the cell surface and present on viable cells.

2. Methods

2.1 Plasminogen receptor isolation

Plasminogen receptor isolation was performed as described (Andronicos et al., 2010). Briefly, progenitor and M-CSF-differentiated Hoxa9-ER4 cells were separately biotinylated, using EZ-Link Amine-PEO$_3$-Biotin. The cells were then subjected to dead cell removal on annexin V-coated magnetic microspheres that resulted in a 99% enrichment of viable cells. Membrane fractions were prepared from the viable cells by dounce homogenization in the presence of Complete Protease Inhibitor Cocktail in Invitrosol, followed by centrifugation steps as used in our laboratory (Hawley et al., 2000, 2001) and were applied to a plasminogen-Sepharose affinity column as described (Miles et al., 1991). The column was washed in phosphate buffered saline containing 1 X Invitrosol until no protein was detected at 280 nm followed by elution with the washing buffer containing 0.2 M ε-aminocaproic acid (EACA). The eluant from the plasminogen-Sepharose column was incubated with 50μl of immobilized avidin for 30 minutes at 4°C. The proteins bound to the immobilized avidin were resuspended in Invitrosol and heated at 60°C. Then, 80% acetonitrile was added and the samples were digested with trypsin. After 24 h, the solvent was evaporated in a speedvac, and peptides were dissolved in buffer A (95% H_2O, 5% acetonitrile, and 0.1% formic acid).

2.2 Multidimensional chromatography and tandem mass spectrometry

Multidimensional chromatography and tandem mass spectrometry were performed as described (Andronicos et al., 2010). Briefly, the protein digest was subjected to MudPIT [reviewed in (Eng et al., 1994)]. Peptide mixtures were resolved by strong cation exchange liquid chromatography upstream of reversed phase liquid chromatography (Larmann, Jr. et al., 1993; Link et al., 1999; Opiteck & Jorgenson, 1997; Wolters et al., 2001). Eluting peptides were electrosprayed onto an LTQ ion trap mass spectrometer equipped with a nano-LC electrospray ionization source. Full MS spectra were recorded over a 400–1600 m/z range, followed by three tandem mass (MS/MS) events sequentially generated in a data-dependent manner on the first, second, and third most intense ions selected from the full MS spectrum (at 35% collision energy). Mass spectrometer scan functions and HPLC solvent gradients were controlled by the Xcalibur data system.

2.3 Database search and interpretation of MS/MS datasets

Database searching and interpretation of MS/MS Datasets were performed as described (Andronicos et al., 2010). Briefly, tandem mass spectra were extracted from raw files, and a binary classifier (Bern et al., 2004), previously trained on a manually validated data set, was used to remove low quality MS/MS spectra. Remaining spectra were searched against a mouse protein database containing 50,370 protein sequences downloaded as FASTA-formatted sequences from EBI-IPI and 124 common contaminant proteins, for a total of 66,743 target database sequences (Peng et al., 2003). To calculate confidence levels and false positive rates, a decoy database containing the reverse sequences of the 66,743 proteins appended to the target database and the SEQUEST algorithm (Yates, III, 1998) were used to find the best matching sequences from the combined database.

SEQUEST searches were done on an Intel Xeon 80-processor cluster running under the Linux operating system. The peptide mass search tolerance was set to 3 Da. No differential modifications were considered. No enzymatic cleavage conditions were imposed on the database search, so the search space included all candidate peptides whose theoretical mass fell within the 3 Da mass tolerance window, despite their tryptic status.

The validity of peptide/spectrum matches was assessed in DTASelect2 (Tabb et al., 2002) using SEQUEST-defined parameters, the cross-correlation score (XCorr) and normalized difference in cross-correlation scores (DeltaCN). The search results were grouped by charge state (+1, +2, and +3) and tryptic status (fully tryptic, half-tryptic, and non-tryptic), resulting in 9 distinct sub-groups. In each one of the sub-groups, the distribution of XCorr and DeltaCN values for direct and decoy database hits was obtained, and the two subsets were separated by quadratic discriminant analysis. Outlier points in the two distributions (for example, matches with very low Xcorr but very high DeltaCN) were discarded. Full separation of the direct and decoy subsets is not generally possible; therefore, the discriminant score was set such that a false positive rate of 5% was determined based on the number of accepted decoy database peptides. This procedure was independently performed on each data subset, resulting in a false positive rate independent of tryptic status or charge state.

3. Results

3.1 Isolation of an integral membrane plasminogen receptor exposing a C-terminal lysine on the cell surface

We used specific proteolysis followed by MudPIT to probe the membrane proteome of differentiated mouse monocyte progenitor cells (Hoxa9-ER4) for the presence of integral membrane plasminogen receptor(s) exposing a C-terminal basic residue on the cell surface, as outlined in Figure 3. [The Hoxa9-ER4 cell line was derived from primary murine bone marrow myeloid precursors immortalized with an estrogen regulated conditional oncoprotein, HoxA9-ER4 (Wang et al., 2006). The Hoxa9-ER4 line is factor-dependent and differentiates to monocytes when estrogen is removed from the medium, thereby inactivating the Hoxa9-ER protein. The mature monocytes respond to M-CSF (Odegaard et al., 2007)]. First, the Hoxa9-ER4 monocyte progenitor cells were differentiated with macrophage colony stimulating factor (M-CSF), which induces plasminogen receptors on these cells (Andronicos et al., 2010). Then intact cells were biotinylated. Because early apoptotic and non-viable/necrotic cells exhibit markedly enhanced plasminogen binding ability (Mitchell et al., 2006; O'Mullane & Baker, 1998, 1999) we passed the biotinylated cells over a dead cell removal column to enrich for live cells. Cells were then lysed and membrane fractions prepared and passed over a plasminogen-Sepharose affinity column and specifically eluted with ε-aminocaproic acid (EACA), a lysine analog that blocks the binding of plasminogen to cells (Miles & Plow, 1985). Biotinylated proteins bound to the avidin column and were digested with trypsin while still on the column. The peptide digest was then subjected to MudPIT.

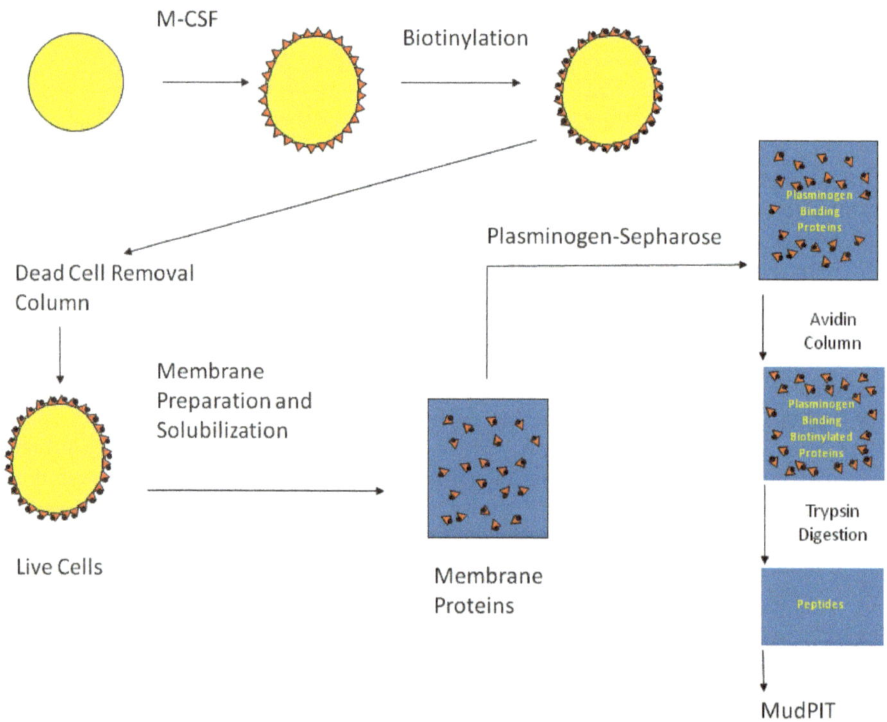

Monocyte (Hoxa9-ER4) progenitor cells were differentiated with macrophage colony stimulating factor (M-CSF), which induces plasminogen receptors (▲) on these cells. Then intact cells were biotinylated (•) and passed over a dead cell removal column. Live cells were then lysed and membrane fractions prepared and passed over a plasminogen-Sepharose affinity column and specifically eluted. Biotinylated plasminogen receptors (▲•) were then bound to an avidin column and digested with trypsin.

Fig. 3. Isolation of plasminogen receptors.

In MudPIT, the peptide mixtures were first resolved by strong cation exchange liquid chromatography followed by reversed phase liquid chromatography. Eluting peptides were electrosprayed onto an LTQ ion trap mass spectrometer and full MS spectra were recorded over a 400-1600 m/z range, followed by three tandem mass events. The spectra obtained were searched against a mouse protein database. Using this method, only one protein with a predicted transmembrane sequence and a C-terminal basic residue was identified: the hypothetical protein, C9orf46 homolog (IPI00136293), homologous to the protein predicted to be encoded by human chromosome 9, open reading frame 46. The peptides corresponding to C9orf46 homolog that were obtained in the MudPIT analysis are shown in Table 1. We have designated the protein, Plg-R_{KT}, to indicate a plasminogen receptor with a C-terminal lysine and having a transmembrane domain (see below). [A limitation of shotgun proteomics, such as MudPIT, is that they typically under sample a proteome because they use data dependent data acquisition (a computer-driven data acquisition approach). This can lead to variations in the proteins identified, particularly amongst the lower abundant proteins. Thus, we cannot exclude the possibility that other membrane proteins exposing C-terminal lysines were present in the membrane proteome.]

Xcorr	DeltCN	Conf%	ObsM+H+	CalcM+H+	Peptide Sequences
3.8378	0.2884	99.8%	2195.8743	2196.4788	K.SMNENMKNQQEFMVTHAR.L (3+)
2.6749	0.1167	95.2%	1359.5521	1361.5181	K.NQQEFMVTHAR.L (2+)
2.6771	0.2534	99.8%	1160.4321	1160.3514	R.HLTMQNEMR.E (2+)
4.7468	0.3052	100%	1523.5322	1523.6954	R.MKSEAEDILETEK.T (2+)
5.1774	0.3788	100%	2335.5544	2333.6997	R.MKSEAEDILETEKTKLELPK.G (3+)
3.775	0.3164	100%	1264.0922	1264.3287	K.SEAEDILETEK.T (2+)
2.995	0.0655	96.8%	1137.2722	1137.3184	K.GLITFESLEK.A (2+)
2.893	0.2591	99.7%	1364.4922	1364.5848	K.GLITFESLEKAR.R (2+)

SEQUEST-defined parameters (Xcorr, DeltCN, and Conf%) are shown for each peptide. (core: cross-correlation score; DeltCN: normalized difference in cross-correlation scores; Conf%: confidence level of the peptide; ObsM+H+: observed peptide mass; CalcM+H+: theoretical peptide mass). Observed peptide mass, theoretical peptide mass, and charges of the peptide identified (3+ or 2+) are also shown to demonstrate accurate peptide identification. This research was originally published in Blood, Andronicos, N.M., Chen, E.I., Baik, N., Bai, H., Parmer, C.M., Kiosses, W.B., Kamps, M.P., Yates, J.R., III, Parmer, R.J., Miles, L.A., Proteomics-based discovery of a novel, structurally unique, and developmentally regulated plasminogen receptor, Plg-R_{KT}, a major regulator of cell surface plasminogen activation, Blood. 2010, 115: 1319-30.

Table 1. Peptides obtained corresponding to C9orf46 homolog

A key advantage of MudPIT is that proteins in a given proteome can be identified simultaneously. As proof of principle of our isolation method, peptides corresponding to other proteins previously identified as plasminogen binding proteins on monocytes were also detected in the membrane preparations: α-enolase, gamma actin, S100A10, histone H2B, annexin 2, and β_2 integrin.

	10	20	30	40	50	60
Mouse	MGFIFSKSMN	ENMKNQQEFM	VTHARLQLER	HLTMQNEMRE	RQMAMQIAWS	REFLKYFGTF
Human	MGFIFSKSMN	ESMKNQKEFM	LMNARLQLER	QLIMQSEMRE	RQMAMQIAWS	REFLKYFGTF
Rat	MGFIFSKSMN	ENMKNQQEFM	VMHARLQLER	QLIMQNEMRE	RQMAMQIAWS	REFLKYFGTF
Dog	MGFIFSKSMN	ENMKNQQEFM	LMNARLQMER	QLMMQNEMRE	RQMAMQIAWS	REFLKYFGTF
Cow	MGFIFSKSMN	ENLKSQQEFM	LMNSRLQLER	QLIMQNEMRE	RQMAMQIAWS	REFLKYFGTF
Alpaca	MGFIFSKSMN	ENMKSQQEFM	LMNARLQLER	QLMMQNEMRE	RQMAMQIAWS	REFLKYFGTF
Chimpanzee	MGFIFSKSMN	ESMKNQKEFM	LMNARLQLER	QLIMQSEMRE	RQMAMQIAWS	REFLKYFGTF
Dolphin	MGFIFSKSMN	ENMKSQQEFM	LMNARLQLER	QLMMQNETRE	RQMAMQIAWS	REFLKYFGTF
Gibbon	MGFIFSKSMN	ESMKNQKEFM	LMNARLQLER	QLIMQSEMRE	RQMAMQIAWS	REFLKYFGTF
Guinea Pig	MGFMLSKSMN	ENMKNQQEFM	LMNARLQLER	QLLLQNEMRE	RQMAMQIAWS	REFLKYFGTF
Horse	MGFIFSKSMN	ENMKNQQEFM	LMNARLQLER	QLTMQNEMRE	RQMAMQIAWS	REFLKYFGTF
Lemur	MGFIFSKSMK	ENAQNQQEFM	LMNARLQLER	QLTMQNEMRE	RQMAMQIAWS	REFMKYFGTF
Opossum	MGFLFSKHMN	ENMKQQQEFM	LMNARLQMER	QLTIQNEMRE	RQMAMQIAWT	REFLKYFGTF
Orangutan	MGFIFSKSMN	ESMKNQKEFM	LMNARLQLER	QLIMQSEMRE	RQMAMQIAWS	REFLKYFGTF
Panda (Giant)	MGFIFSKSMS	ENMKNQQEFM	LMNARLQLER	QLMMQNEMRE	RQMALQIAWS	REFLKYFGTF
Pig	MGFIFSKSMN	ENMKRQQEFM	LMNTRLQLER	QLIMQNEMRE	RQMAMQIAWS	REFLKYFGTF
Rabbit	MGFIFSKSMN	ENLKNQQEFM	LMNARLQLER	QLMLQNEMRE	RQMAMQIAWS	REFLKYFGTF
Rhesus Monkey	MGFIFSKSMN	ESMKNQKEFM	LMSARLQLER	QLIMQSEMRE	RQMAMQIAWS	REFLKYFGTF
Tarsier	MGFIF-KSMN	ENMKHQQEFM	LMNAQLQLER	QLTMQNEMRE	RQMAMQIAWS	REFLKYFGTF
Tree Shrew	MGFIFSKSMN	ENMKNQQEFM	LMNARLQLER	QLMMQNEMRE	RQMAMQIAWS	REFLKYFGTF
Lizard (arborial)	MGFIFSKSMN	ENLKNQQEFM	IMNSRLQLER	QLLMQNQMRE	RQMAMQIAWT	REFLKYFGAF
Frog (xenopus)	MGSLISKATE	TQMKKQQELM	QMNAQIQLER	QIIMQNMMRE	RQMAMQIAWS	REFLKYYGSF

	70	80	90	100	110	120
Mouse	FGIATISLAT	GALKRKKPAF	LVPIVPLSFI	FTYQYDLGYG	TLLQRMKSEA	EDILETEKTK
Human	FGLAAISLTA	GAIKKKKPAF	LVPIVPLSFI	LTYQYDLGYG	TLLERMKGEA	EDILETEKSK
Rat	FGIATISLAA	GAIKRKKPAF	LIPIVPLSFI	FTYQYDLGYG	TLLQRMKSEA	EDILETEKTK
Dog	FGIAAISLTA	GAIRKKKPAF	LFPIIPLSFI	FTYQYDLGYG	TLLQRMKGEA	ENILETEKSK
Cow	FGITAVSLTA	GAIKGKKPVL	IFPIVPLGFV	LAYQYDMGYG	TLIHRMKGEA	ENILETEKSK
Alpaca	FGIAAISLTA	GAIKRKKPAF	IFPIVPLGFV	LTYQFDLGYG	TLLQRMKGEA	ENILETEKSK
Chimpanzee	FGLAAISLTA	GAIKKKKPAF	LVPIVPLSFI	LTYQYDLGYG	TLLERMKGEA	EDILETEKSK
Dolphin	FGIAAISLTA	GAIKKKKPAF	VFPIVPLGFV	LAYQYDMGYG	TLIQRMKGEA	DNILETEKSK
Gibbon	FGLAAISLTA	GAIKKKKPAF	LVPIVPLSFI	LTYQYDLGYG	TLLERMKGEA	EDILETEKSK
Guinea Pig	FGISAISLTA	RAIKQKKPAF	FIPIVPLSFV	LAYQYDLGYG	TLLQRMKGEA	EDILETEKNK
Horse	FGIAAISLTA	GALKRKKPAF	LFPIVPLGFV	LTYQYDLGYG	TLLQRMKGEA	ENILETEKSK
Lemur	FGITAISLTA	GAIKSKKPGF	LFPIVPLSFV	LAYQYDLGYG	TLLQRMKGEA	EDILETEKSK
Opossum	FGIAAISLTA	GAIKKKQPGL	FFPIVPLSFI	LAYQYDMGYG	TLLQRMKGEA	ENILETENSK
Orangutan	FGLAAISLTA	GAIKKKKPAF	LVPIVPLSFI	LTYQYDLGYG	TLLERMKGEA	EDILETEKSK
Panda (Giant)	FGITAISLTA	GAIRRKKPAF	LFPIIPLSFI	FTYQYDLGYG	TLLQRMKGEA	ENILETEKSK
Pig	FGIASVALTA	GAIKRKKPAF	FLPIIPLGFV	FTYQYDLGYG	TLLQRMKGEA	ENILETETSK
Rabbit	FGVATISLTA	GAMRRKKPAF	LLPIVPLSFI	FIYQCDLGYG	TLLQRMKGEA	EDILETEKSK
Rhesus Monkey	FGFAAISLTA	GAIKKKKPAF	LVPIVPLSFI	LTYQYDLGYG	TLLERMKGEA	EDILETEKSK
Tarsier	FGITAISLTA	GAIKRKKPAL	LLPIVPLSFI	FTYQYDLGYG	TLLERMKGEA	EEILEAEKNM
Tree Shrew	FGIAAISLTA	GAIKKKNPAF	FFPIVPLSFI	LTYQYDLGYG	TLLPRMKSEA	EDILETEKSK
Lizard (arborial)	SGLAAVGLTV	GAIKRKKPAF	FLPMVPLSFI	LAYQYDMGYG	SLLKRMKSEA	ESILDTESTT
Frog (xenopus)	FSLAVIGLTV	GAVKNKKPAL	FTPVIPLTFV	FAYQFDMGYG	TLVTRMKGEA	ENILEKEHIL

	130	140	147
Mouse	LELPKGLITF	ESLEKARREQ	SKLFSDK
Human	LQLPRGMITF	ESIEKARKEQ	SRFFIDK
Rat	LELPKGLITF	ESLEKARREQ	SKFFSDK
Dog	LQLPRGMITF	ESLEKARREQ	SKFFIDK
Cow	LQLPKGMITF	ESLEKARKEQ	SKFFIDK
Alpaca	LQLPKGIITF	ESLEKARKEQ	SKFFIDK
Chimpanzee	LQLPRGMITF	ESIEKARKEQ	SRFFIDK
Dolphin	LQLPKGMITF	ENLEKARREQ	SKFFIDK
Gibbon	LQLPRGMITF	ESIEKARKEQ	SKFFIDK
Guinea Pig	LELPKGVITF	ESLEKARREQ	SKFFLGK
Horse	LQLPKGMITF	ESLEKARREQ	SKFFIDK
Lemur	LQLPKGMITF	ESLEKARREQ	SKFFIEK
Opossum	LQLPRGSITF	ETLEKARKAQ	SKFFIEK
Orangutan	LQLPRGMITF	ESIEKARKEQ	SRFFIDK
Panda (Giant)	LQLPRGMITF	ENLEKARREQ	SKFFIDK
Pig	LQLPKGMITF	EGLEKARREQ	SKFFIDK
Rabbit	LQLPGGMITF	ESLEKARREQ	SKFFIDK
Rhesus Monkey	LQLPRGMITF	ESIEKARKEQ	SKFFIDK
Tarsier	LQLPKGMITF	ESLEKTRREQ	SKFFTDK
Tree Shrew	LELPRGMITF	ESLEKARREQ	SKFFVDK
Lizard (arborial)	LEMPKGPLTF	ESIEKARRAQ	SKFFIEK
Frog (xenopus)	LEMPQGLPTF	EGIEKTRKAH	RSLLL-K

Table 2. Alignment of Orthologs of Plg-R_{KT}

3.2 Conservation of Plg-R_{KT} across species

The C9orf46 homolog/Plg-R_{KT} murine DNA sequence encodes a protein of 147 amino acids with a molecular mass of 17,261 Da and a C-terminal lysine (Table 2, first line). We blasted the C9orf46 homolog/Plg-R_{KT} sequence against all species using NCBI Blast and obtained unique human, rat, dog, cow, dog, giant panda, gibbon, horse, pig, rabbit, and rhesus monkey predicted orthologs, with high identity and homology (e.g. human versus rhesus monkey = 99% similarity), high identity (e.g. human vs rhesus monkey = 98% identity) and no gaps in the sequence (Table 2). Of key importance, a C-terminal lysine was predicted for all of the mammalian orthologs obtained in the blast search. In a query of the Ensembl Gene Report, DNA sequences of all 10 other sequenced mammalian orthologs encoded C-terminal lysines (Table 2).

In addition, the DNA sequences of xenopus and the green lizard also encoded C-terminal lysines (Table 2). Furthermore, Plg-R_{KT} orthologs with 149 amino acids with a C-terminal lysine were encoded in bony fish (salmon and zebrafish) and the high similarity with a mammalian ortholog is illustrated in the alignment of the mouse and zebrafish proteins in Table 3.

The Plg-R_{KT} sequence also encodes a putative conserved DUF2368 domain (encompassing amino acids 1-135), an uncharacterized protein with unknown function conserved from nematodes to humans. Notably, Plg-R_{KT} orthologs of lower organisms were of different predicted lengths and did not consistently predict C-terminal lysines. It is interesting to note that the evolutionary origin of plasminogen is currently believed to originate with protochordates (Liu & Zhang, 2009), so that lower organisms without plasminogen would not utilize the C-terminal lysine of Plg-R_{KT} to bind plasminogen.

Mouse	1	MGFIFSKSMNENMKNQQEFMVTHARLQLERHLTMQNEMRERQMAMQIAWSREFLKYFGTF	60
Zebrafish	1	MGFVLSKGMEQNFQKQQEFMLLNARLQLERQLAMQNQMRERQMAMQLAWSREFLKYFGSF	60
Mouse	61	FGIATISLATGALKRKKPAFLVPIVPLSFIFTYQYDLGYGTLLQRMKSEAEDILETEKTK	120
Zebrafish	61	FGLATLGLTVGAVKKRKPALLAPVIPLSFILVYQMDAAYGTMLQRMRAEAESIMVSECER	120
Mouse	121	LELPKGLITFESLEKARREQSKL--FSDK	147
Zebrafish	121	LDVPHGMPTFESIEKSRRAKAHLTTLTEK	149

Table 3. Alignment of Mouse and Zebrafish Plg-R_{KT} Sequences

It is also noteworthy that the primary sequence of C9orf46 homolog/Plg-R_{KT} is apparently tightly conserved in humans, with no validated polymorphisms (cSNPs) within the 6 exons encoded by the gene (on chromosome 9p24.1) in the NCBI human genome sequence variation database (dbSNP, http://www.ncbi.nlm.nih.gov/SNP).

3.3 Topology of Plg-R_{KT}

The C9orf46 homolog/Plg-R_{KT} sequence was analyzed in the TMpred site (www.ch.embnet.org/cgi-bin/TMPRED). The model predicted two transmembrane helices extending from F_{53}-L_{73} (secondary helix, oriented from outside the cell to inside the cell) and P_{78}-Y_{99} (primary helix, oriented from inside the cell to outside the cell) (Figure 4). Hence a 52 amino acid N-terminal region and a 48 amino acid C-terminal tail with a C-terminal lysine were predicted to be exposed on the cell surface.

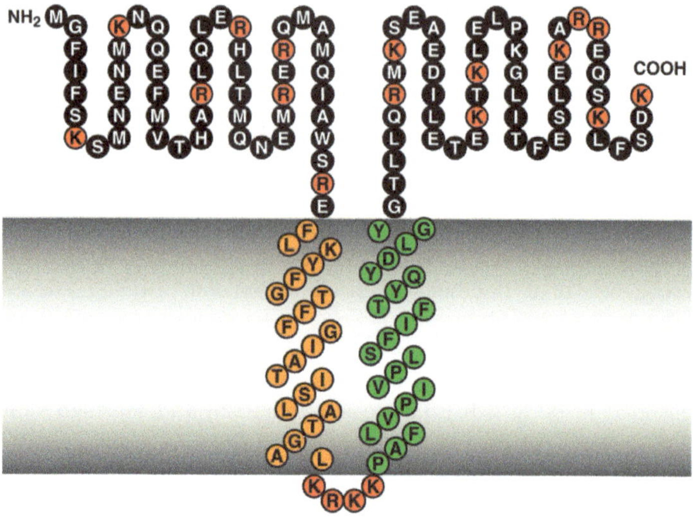

Green indicates amino acids within the predicted primary transmembrane helix. Orange indicates amino acids within the predicted secondary transmembrane helix. Red indicates basic amino acids. This research was originally published in *Blood,* Andronicos, N.M., Chen, E.I., Baik, N., Bai, H., Parmer, C.M., Kiosses, W.B., Kamps, M.P., Yates, J.R., III, Parmer, R.J., Miles, L.A., Proteomics-based discovery of a novel, structurally unique, and developmentally regulated plasminogen receptor, Plg-R_{KT}, a major regulator of cell surface plasminogen activation, *Blood.* 2010, 115: 1319-30.

Fig. 4. Structural model of Plg-R_{KT}.

We experimentally tested predictions of the model. First, we raised a monoclonal antibody against the synthetic peptide, CEQSKLFSDK (corresponding to the nine C-terminal amino acids of murine Plg-R_{KT} with an amino terminal cysteine added for coupling). To examine subcellular localization, membrane and cytoplasmic fractions from progenitor and differentiated Hoxa9-ER4 monocyte progenitor cells were electrophoresed and western blotted with anti-Plg-R_{KT} mAb or isotype control mAb. A specific immunoreactive band migrating with an Mr_{app} of ~17,000, was detected in membrane fractions of differentiated monocyte progenitor cells, clearly demonstrating the existence of this new protein (Figure 5,A). The protein was not detected in undifferentiated cells or in the cytoplasmic fraction of the differentiated cells.

To test the prediction that Plg-R_{KT} is an integral membrane protein, membranes from differentiated monocyte progenitor cells were subjected to phase separation in Triton X-114 as described (Bordier, 1981; Estreicher et al., 1989). In this method, integral membrane proteins form mixed micelles with the nonionic detergent and are recovered in the Triton X-114 detergent phase, whereas hydrophilic proteins remain in the aqueous phase. An immunoreactive band migrating with an Mr_{app} of ~17,000 was detected in the detergent phase in western blotting with anti-Plg-R_{KT} mAb, but was not detected in the aqueous phase (Figure. 5,B). These data support the prediction that Plg-R_{KT} is an integral membrane protein.

To experimentally test whether the C-terminal lysine of Plg-R_{KT} was exposed on the cell surface, we treated intact biotinylated cells with carboxypeptidase B prior to performing our isolation procedure. Under this condition, C-terminal lysines exposed on the cell surface are

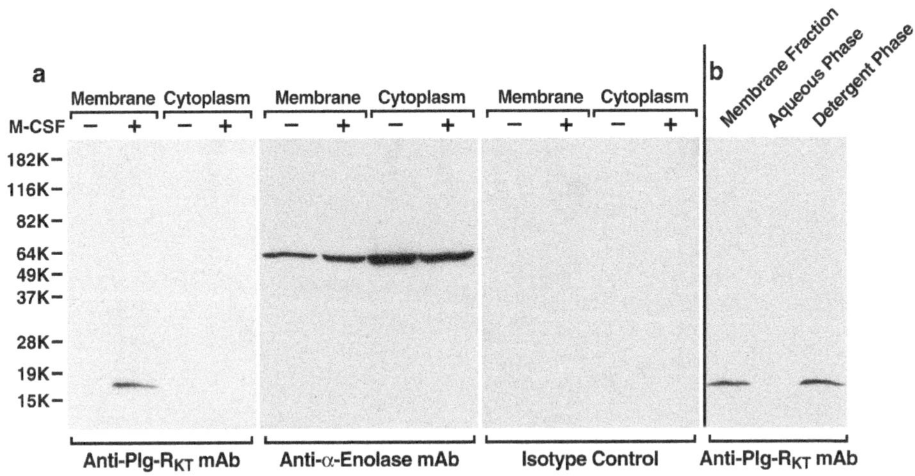

A. Membrane fractions or cytoplasmic fractions from either undifferentiated or M-CSF-treated Hoxa9-ER4 cells were electrophoresed on 12% sodium dodecyl sulfate polyacrylamide gels under reducing conditions and western blotted with either anti-Plg-R_{KT} mAb, anti-α-enolase mAb as a loading control, or isotype control mAb. B. M-CSF-treated Hoxa9-ER4 cell membranes were solubilized in 3% Triton X-114. After heating at 37°C and separation of the phases by centrifugation, an aliquot of both phases was electrophoresed and western blotted with anti-Plg-R_{KT} mAb. This research was originally published in *Blood,* Andronicos, N.M., Chen, E.I., Baik, N., Bai, H., Parmer, C.M., Kiosses, W.B., Kamps, M.P., Yates, J.R., III, Parmer, R.J., Miles, L.A., Proteomics-based discovery of a novel, structurally unique, and developmentally regulated plasminogen receptor, Plg-R_{KT}, a major regulator of cell surface plasminogen activation, *Blood.* 2010, 115: 1319-30.

Fig. 5. Plg-R_{KT} behaves as a regulated integral membrane protein.

removed but intracellular C-terminal lysines are protected (see Figure 2,B). Under this condition, no peptides corresponding to Plg-R_{KT} were obtained in the MudPIT analysis, consistent with cell surface exposure of the C-terminal lysine of Plg-R_{KT}.

In order to experimentally evaluate whether the N-terminus of Plg-R_{KT} was exposed on the cell surface, PC12 (rat pheochromocytoma) cells were stably transfected with V5-pCIneo-Plg-R_{KT} that expressed a V5 tag at the N-terminus of Plg-R_{KT}. (The V5 sequence was added in front of the mammalian expression vector, pCIneo using PCR and then the full-length 443 bp Plg-R_{KT} cDNA was subcloned into the V5-pCIneo vector using the Xho1 and Sma1 cloning sites. Constructs were transfected into cells using Lipofectamine 2000 and stable transfectants were selected with G418.)

A specific band migrating with a M_{rapp} of 17,000 was detected in cell membranes of the stably transfected cells with both anti-V5 mAb and anti-Plg-R_{KT} mAb (Figure 6, lane 1). The band was not detected by either mAb after trypsin digestion of the isolated membrane fraction (lane 2). When intact cells were incubated with trypsin and the trypsin neutralized with SBTI prior to preparation of the membrane fraction, the majority of the band detectable with either anti-V5 or anti-Plg-R_{KT} was lost (lane 4). In controls, treatment with soybean trypsin inhibitor (SBTI) fully neutralized the ability of trypsin to degrade the V5-tagged Plg-R_{KT} in purified membrane fractions (lane 3), demonstrating that the trypsin had been neutralized prior to membrane fractionation of the treated cells. These results suggest that the N- terminus of Plg-R_{KT} is accessible to trypsin proteolysis of intact cells and is, therefore,

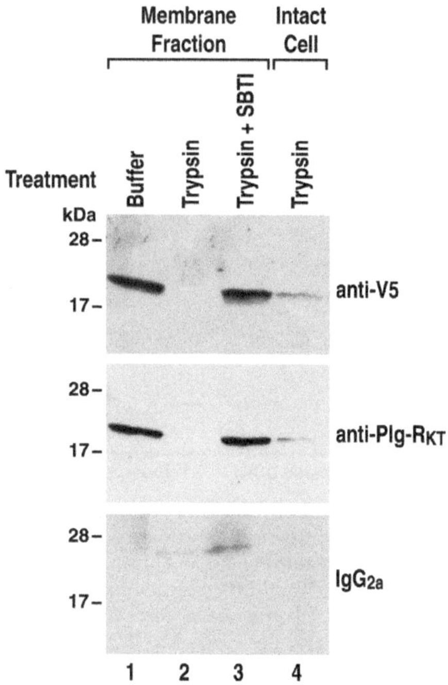

Membrane fractions of PC12 cells stably transfected with V5-pCIneo-Plg-R_{KT} were incubated with either buffer (lane 1), trypsin (1mg/ml) (lane 2) or trypsin 1 mg/ml + soybean trypsin inhibitor (SBTI) (2 mg/ml) (lane 3) for 30 minutes at 37°C or intact PC12 cells were incubated with 1 mg/ml trypsin for 2 hr at 37°C, followed by 2 mg/ml SBTI for 15 min . Following neutralization of trypsin with SBTI, the membrane fraction was prepared from the treated, intact cells (lane 4). 30 µg/lane of membrane fractions were electrophoresed on 18% SDS PAGE under reducing conditions and western blotted with either anti-V5, anti-Plg-R_{KT} mAb or isotype control.

Fig. 6. The N-termini and C-termini of Plg-R_{KT} are exposed on the cell surface.

exposed on the extracellular face. Furthermore, because the anti-Plg-R_{KT} mAb reacts with the C-terminus of Plg-R_{KT}, these data also confirm the exposure of the C-terminus on the extracellular face of the cell membrane.

3.4 Role of the C-terminal lysine of Plg-R_{KT} in plasminogen binding

We further addressed the exposure of the C-terminus of Plg-R_{KT} on the cell surface using confocal microscopy with a mAb raised against the Plg-R_{KT} C-terminal peptide. (The mAb reacted with the C-terminal peptide of murine Plg-R_{KT} and blocked plasminogen binding to CEQSKLFSDK). When cells were incubated with anti-Plg-R_{KT} mAb and a polyclonal anti-plasminogen antibody, Plg-R_{KT} and plasminogen were both immunodetected in small aggregates dispersed over the cell surface (Figure 7,A), in a similar distribution to that published for confocal analyses of monocyte-associated plasminogen (Das et al., 2007). Most importantly, after preincubation of monocytes with plasminogen, immunodetection of Plg-R_{KT} was reduced by half (Figure 7,A,B). These results demonstrate that the C-terminus of Plg-R_{KT} is exposed on the cell surface. Furthermore, these results show that plasminogen binds to the C-terminal domain of Plg-R_{KT} on the cell surface.

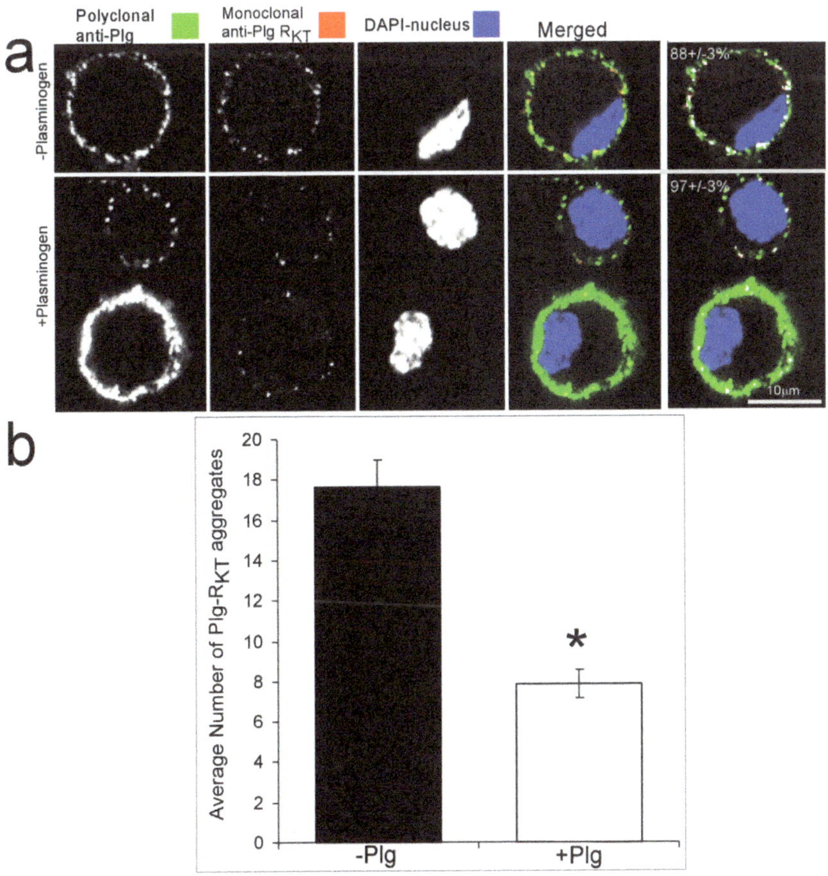

A. M-CSF-differentiated (Hoxa9-ER4) cells were grown on coverslips and preincubated with either phosphate buffered saline (- plasminogen) or 2 µM plasminogen (+ plasminogen), then fixed in 1% formaldehyde, washed and stained with polyclonal anti-plasminogen IgG or anti-Plg-R_{KT} mAb and stained with a combination of Alexa 488- F(ab')$_2$ of goat anti-rabbit IgG and Alexa 568- F(ab')$_2$ fragment of goat anti-mouse IgG.
B. The number and size of each labeled aggregate was determined. The results reflect counts from over 40 cells in 2 independent experiments. Data represent mean ± SEM. *$p < 0.001$. This research was originally published in *Blood,* Andronicos, N.M., Chen, E.I., Baik, N., Bai, H., Parmer, C.M., Kiosses, W.B., Kamps, M.P., Yates, J.R., III, Parmer, R.J., Miles, L.A., Proteomics-based discovery of a novel, structurally unique, and developmentally regulated plasminogen receptor, Plg-R_{KT}, a major regulator of cell surface plasminogen activation, *Blood*. 2010, 115: 1319-30.

Fig. 7. Plg-R_{KT} binds plasminogen on the cell surface.

To further address the plasminogen binding function of the C-terminus of Plg-R_{KT} , we tested whether the synthetic peptide, corresponding to the C-terminus of Plg-R_{KT} could bind plasminogen. The peptide, CEQSKLFSDK, was coupled to BSA and then coated onto wells of microtiter plates. Biotinylated Glu-plasminogen was incubated with the wells and specific binding was detected with HRP-streptavidin (Figure 8). We tested the ability of the soluble C-terminal peptide to inhibit Glu-plasminogen binding under solution phase equilibrium conditions. The soluble peptide competed for Glu-plasminogen binding in a dose-dependent manner with an IC_{50} of 2 μM (Figure 8), similar to the Kd values we have previously determined for Glu-plasminogen binding to cells (Miles et al., 2005). In addition, a mutated peptide with the C-terminal lysine substituted with alanine did not compete for plasminogen binding at concentrations up to 1 mM (Figure 8), further supporting the role of the C-terminal lysine in the interaction of Plg-R_{KT} with plasminogen.

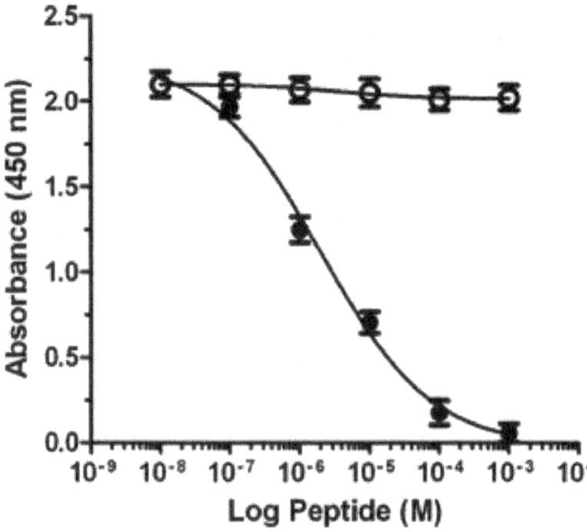

The peptide, CEQSKLFSDK, was coupled to BSA and immobilized on microtiter wells. Biotinylated-Glu-plasminogen (25 nM) was incubated with immobilized CEQSKLFSDK in the presence of increasing concentrations of CEQSKLFSDK (•) or a K147A mutant peptide, CEQSKLFSDA (○). Biotinylated Glu-plasminogen binding was detected with HRP-streptavidin. Data are as mean ± SEM, n=3, for each determination. This research was originally published in Blood, Andronicos, N.M., Chen, E.I., Baik, N., Bai, H., Parmer, C.M., Kiosses, W.B., Kamps, M.P., Yates, J.R., III, Parmer, R.J., Miles, L.A., Proteomics-based discovery of a novel, structurally unique, and developmentally regulated plasminogen receptor, Plg-R_{KT}, a major regulator of cell surface plasminogen activation, Blood. 2010, 115: 1319-30.

Fig. 8. Plasminogen binds to the C-terminal peptide of Plg-R_{KT}.

3.5 Plg-R_{KT} regulates cell surface plasminogen activation

We verified that plasminogen activation was promoted in the presence of differentiated Hoxa9-ER4 cells. Plasminogen activation was stimulated 12.7-fold in the presence of differentiated monocyte progenitor cells, compared to the reaction in the absence of cells (Figure 9). In order to test the role of Plg-R_{KT} in plasminogen activation, we tested the effect of anti-Plg-R_{KT} mAb raised against the synthetic peptide, CEQSKLFSDK . Anti-Plg-R_{KT} mAb substantially suppressed cell-dependent plasminogen activation (Figure 9). In controls, plasminogen activation in the absence of cells was not affected by anti-Plg-R_{KT} mAb.

3.6 Tissue and cellular distribution and regulation of the Plg-R_{KT} transcript

We searched results of gene expression array analyses for expression of the C9orf46 homolog/Plg-R_{KT} transcript. The transcript is broadly expressed in normal human and mouse tissues [as determined in high-throughput gene expression profiling in which RNA samples from human and murine tissues were hybridized to high-density gene expression arrays (Su et al., 2002; Su et al., 2004)]. The C9orf46 homolog/Plg-R_{KT} transcript has been

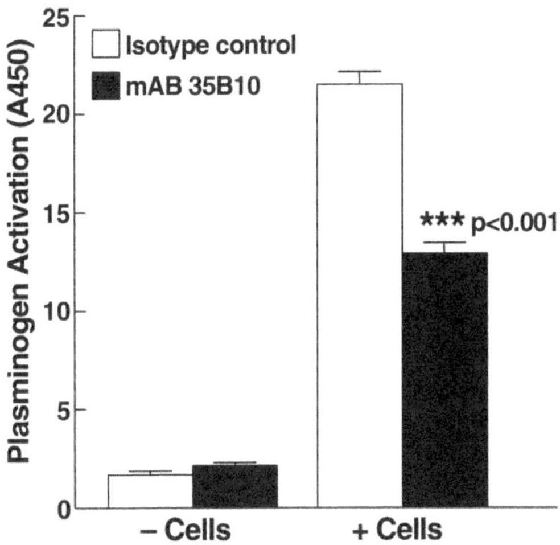

Plasminogen activation was determined in either the presence or absence of differentiated Hoxa9-ER4 cells and in the presence of either anti-Plg-R_{KT} mAb (filled bars) or isotype control rat IgG2a (open bars). ***$p < 0.001$, compared to the corresponding isotype control. This research was originally published in Blood, Andronicos, N.M., Chen, E.I., Baik, N., Bai, H., Parmer, C.M., Kiosses, W.B., Kamps, M.P., Yates, J.R., III, Parmer, R.J., Miles, L.A., Proteomics-based discovery of a novel, structurally unique, and developmentally regulated plasminogen receptor, Plg-R_{KT}, a major regulator of cell surface plasminogen activation, Blood. 2010, 115: 1319-30.

Fig. 9. Plg-R_{KT} regulates cell surface plasminogen activation.

detected in spleen, lymph node, thymus, bone marrow, lung, intestine, adrenal, pituitary, and other endocrine tissues, vascular tissue, kidney, liver, stomach, bladder, and neuronal tissue (hippocampus, hypothalamus, cerebellum, cerebral cortex, olfactory bulb and dorsal root ganglion) (Table 4).

We also searched for C9orf46 homolog/Plg-R_{KT} mRNA microarray expression data at http://www.ebi.ac.uk/microarray-as/aew/. C9orf46 homolog/Plg-R_{KT} mRNA is present in monocytes, leukocytes, natural killer (NK) cells, T cells, myeloid, dendritic, and plasmacytoid cells, breast cancer, acute lymphoblastic leukemia and Molt-4 acute lymphoblastic leukemia cells (Table 5).

• Spleen	• Liver
• Thymus	• Stomach
• Lymph Node	• Bladder
• Lung	• Hippocampus
• Intestine	• Hypothalamus
• Bone Marrow	• Cerebellum
• Adrenal	• Cerebral Cortex
• Pituitary	• Olfactory Bulb
• Vascular Tissue	• Dorsal Root Ganglion
• Kidney	

Results of high-throughput gene expression profiling (54).

Table 4. Tissue Distribution of Plg-R_{KT} mRNA

• Monocytes	• B-cell precursor cells
• NK cells	• Acute lymphoblastic leukemia cells
• T cells	• Molt-4 acute lymphoblastic leukemia cells
• Myeloid cells	• Breast cancer cells, SKBR3, MDA468, BT474, T47D
• Dendritic cells	
• Plasmacytoid cells	

www.ebi.ae.uk/microarray-as/aew/

Table 5. Microarray Expression Data for Plg-R_{KT} mRNA

These data are consistent with previous reports documenting expression of plasminogen binding sites on peripheral blood leukocytes (Miles & Plow, 1987), breast cancer cells (Correc et al., 1990; Ranson et al., 1998) and other tissues [reviewed in (Miles et al., 2005)]. In addition, results obtained by searching the ArrayExpress Warehouse (http://www.ebi.ac.uk/microarray) indicated that the C9orf46 homolog gene is also regulated in other tissues by lipopolysaccharide, aldosterone, canrenoate, H_2O_2, and dexamethasone (Table 6).

In a previously published genome-scale quantitative image analysis, overexpression of a cDNA that we now recognize to be the Plg-R_{KT} cDNA, resulted in dramatic increases in cell proliferation whereas knockdown of the corresponding mRNA resulted in apoptosis (Harada et al., 2005). Consistent with an anti-apoptotic role of Plg-R_{KT}, we have shown that cell-bound plasminogen inhibits TNFα-induced apoptosis (Mitchell et al., 2006). In microarray studies, C9orf46 homolog mRNA expression has a high power to predict cervical lymph node metastasis in oral squamous cell carcinoma (Nguyen et al., 2007).

Experiment	Tissue	Agonist	Effect*
E-MEXP-420	Hippocampal microglial cells	lipopolysaccharide	↓
E-TABM-229	Kidney	aldosterone	↓
E-TABM-229	Kidney	canrenoate	↓
E-MEXP-710	Cholinergic cells	H_2O_2	↓
E-MEXP-774	Preadipocytes	Dexamethasone	↓

Data were obtained from ArrayExpress Warehouse (http://www.ebi.ac.uk/microarray).
* ↓ = downregulation. This research was originally published in Blood, Andronicos, N.M., Chen, E.I., Baik, N., Bai, H., Parmer, C.M., Kiosses, W.B., Kamps, M.P., Yates, J.R., III, Parmer, R.J., Miles, L.A., Proteomics-based discovery of a novel, structurally unique, and developmentally regulated plasminogen receptor, Plg-R_{KT}, a major regulator of cell surface plasminogen activation, Blood. 2010, 115: 1319-30.

Table 6. Regulation of C9orf46 homolog/Plg-R_{KT} mRNA in Tissues

4. Conclusions

In conclusion, MudPIT has allowed us to identify a new protein, Plg-R_{KT}, a novel plasminogen receptor with unique characteristics: integral to the cell membrane and exposing a C-terminal lysine on the cell surface in an orientation to bind plasminogen and promote plasminogen activation. Thus, Plg-R_{KT} is likely to play a key role in plasminogen-dependent functions of cells including inflammation, wound healing, development, metastasis, neurite outgrowth, fibrinolysis, myogenesis and prohormone processing. The broad distribution of the Plg-R_{KT} transcript and its regulation in tissues that have been demonstrated to express plasminogen binding sites, suggest that Plg-R_{KT} provides plasminogen receptor function that may serve to modulate plasmin proteolytic functions (both physiologic and pathologic) specific to a large number of tissues. Furthermore, the potential function of Plg-R_{KT} in the regulation of apoptosis and proliferation may play a key role in cancer and metastasis. Future studies with knockout mice should build on our initial results using MudPIT to elucidate the role of Plg-R_{KT}.

5. Acknowledgments

Supported by National Institutes of Health Grants (HL38272, Hl45934, and HL081046 to L.A.M., HL50398 to R.J.P., NIH P41 RR011823 to J.R.Y., NIAID sub-contract grant UCSD/MCB0237059 to E.I.C.) and Department of Veterans Affairs to R.J.P. S.L was supported by NIH training grant, T32 HL007195. We thank Dr. Ray Stevens at The Scripps Research Institute and Dr. Nuala Booth and Dr. Ian Booth, University of Aberdeen, for helpful discussions. We thank Ms. Linda Bonafede for manuscript preparation. This is publication #21378 from The Scripps Research Institute.

6. References

Andronicos, N. M., E. I. Chen, N. Baik, H. Bai, C. M. Parmer, W. B. Kiosses, M. P. Kamps, J. R. Yates, III, R. J. Parmer, and L. A. Miles. 2010. Proteomics-based discovery of a novel, structurally unique, and developmentally regulated plasminogen receptor, Plg-RKT, a major regulator of cell surface plasminogen activation. *Blood* 115, no. 7:1319-1330.

Bern, M., D. Goldberg, W. H. McDonald, and J. R. 3rd Yates. 2004. Automatic quality assessment of peptide tandem mass spectra. *Bioinformatics* 20, Suppl 1:I49-I54.

Bordier, C. 1981. Phase separation of integral membrane proteins in Triton X-114 solution. *Journal of Biological Chemistry* 256, no. 4:1604-1607.

Bugge, T. H., M. J. Flick, C. C. Daugherty, and J. L. Degen. 1995. Plasminogen deficiency causes severe thrombosis but is compatible with development and reproducton. *Genes and Development* 9:794-807.

Busuttil, S. J., V. A. Ploplis, F. J. Castellino, L. Tang, J. W. Eaton, and E. F. Plow. 2004. A central role for plasminogen in the inflammatory response to biomaterials. *J.Thromb.Haemost.* 2, no. 10:1798-1805.

Castellino, F. J. and V. A. Ploplis. 2005. Structure and function of the plasminogen/plasmin system. *Thrombosis and Haemostasis* 93, no. 4:647-654.

Choi, K. S., D. K. Fogg, C. S. Yoon, and D. M. Waisman. 2003. p11 regulates extracellular plasmin production and invasiveness of HT1080 fibrosarcoma cells. *FASEB J* 17, no. 2:235-246.

Collen, D. 1999. The plasminogen (fibrinolytic) system. *Thrombosis and Haemostasis* 82:259-270.

Correc, P., M.-C. Fondanèche, M. Bracke, and P. Burtin. 1990. The presence of plasmin receptors on three mammary carcinoma MCF-7 sublines. *International Journal of Cancer* 46:745-750.

Creemers, E., J. Cleutjens, J. Smits, S. Heymans, L. Moons, D. Collen, M. Daemen, and P. Carmeliet. 2000. Disruption of the plasminogen gene in mice abolishes wound healing after myocardial infarction. *American Journal of Pathology* 156, no. 6:1865-1873.

Das, R., T. Burke, and E. F. Plow. 2007. Histone H2B as a functionally important plasminogen receptor on macrophages. *Blood* 110, no. 10:3763-3772.

Dudani, A. K. and P. R. Ganz. 1996. Endothelial cell surface actin serves as a binding site for plasminogen, tissue plasminogen activator and lipoprotein(a). *British Journal of Haematology* 95:168-178.

Eng, J. K., A. L. McCormick, and J. R. III Yates. 1994. An approach to correlate tandem mass spectral data of peptides with amino acid sequences in a protein database. *J.Am.Soc.Mass Spectrom.* 5:976-989.

Estreicher, A., A. Wohlwend, D. Belin, W-D. Scleuning, and J. D. Vassalli. 1989. Characterization of the cellular binding site for the urokinase-type plasminogen activator. *Journal of Biological Chemistry* 264:1180-1189.

Félez, J., L. A. Miles, P. Fábregas, M. Jardi, E. F. Plow, and R. H. Lijnen. 1996. Characterization of cellular binding sites and interactive regions within reactants required for enhancement of plasminogen activation by tPA on the surface of leukocytic cells. *Thrombosis and Haemostasis* 76:577-584.

Gutierrez-Fernandez, A., N. A. Gingles, H. Bai, F. J. Castellino, R. J. Parmer, and L. A. Miles. 2009. Plasminogen enhances neuritogenesis on laminin-1. *Journal of Neuroscience* 29, no. 40:12393-12400.

Hajjar, K. A., A. T. Jacovina, and J. Chacko. 1994. An endothelial cell receptor for plasminogen/tissue plasminogen activator. I. Identity with annexin II. *Journal of Biological Chemistry* 269:21191-21197.

Hall, S. W., J. E. Humphries, and S. L. Gonias. 1991. Inhibition of cell surface receptor-bound plasmin by a_2- antiplasmin and a_2-macroglobulin. *Journal of Biological Chemistry* 266:12329-12336.

Harada, J. N., K. E. Bower, A. P. Orth, S. Callaway, C. G. Nelson, C. Laris, J. B. Hogenesch, P. K. Vogt, and S. K. Chanda. 2005. Identification of novel mammalian growth regulatory factors by genome-scale quantitative image analysis. *Genome Res.* 15, no. 8:1136-1144.

Hawley, S. B., M. A. Green, and L. A. Miles. 2000. Discriminating between cell surface and intracellular plasminogen- binding proteins: heterogeneity in profibrinolytic plasminogen-binding proteins on monocytoid cells. *Thrombosis and Haemostasis* 84, no. 5:882-890.

Hawley, S. B., T. Tamura, and L. A. Miles. 2001. Purification, cloning, and characterization of a profibrinolytic plasminogen-binding protein, TIP49a. *Journal of Biological Chemistry* 276:179-186.

Hembrough, T. A., K. R. Kralovich, L. Li, and S. L. Gonias. 1996. Cytokeratin 8 released by breast carcinoma cells *in vitro* binds plasminogen and tissue-type plasminogen activator and promotes plasminogen activation. *Biochemical Journal* 317:763-769.

Hembrough, T. A., J. Vasudevan, M. M. Allietta, W. F. Glass, and S. L. Gonias. 1995. A cytokeratin 8-like protein with plasminogen-binding activity is present on the external surfaces of hepatocytes, HepG2 cells and breast carcinoma cell lines. *J.Cell Sci.* 108 (Pt 3):1071-1082.

Herren, T., T. A. Burke, R. Das, and E. F. Plow. 2006. Identification of histone H2B as a regulated plasminogen receptor. *Biochemistry* 45, no. 31:9463-9474.

Hoylaerts, M., D. C. Rijken, H. R. Lijnen, and D. Collen. 1982. Kinetics of the activation of plasminogen by human tissue plasminogen activator. *Journal of Biological Chemistry* 257:2912-2919.

Jacovina, A. T., F. Zhong, E. Khazanova, E. Lev, A. B. Deora, and K. A. Hajjar. 2001. Neuritogenesis and the nerve growth factor-induced differentiation of PC-12 cells requires annexin II-mediated plasmin generation. *Journal of Biological Chemistry* 276, no. 52:49350-49358.

Jiang, Q., L. Taupenot, S. K. Mahata, M. Mahata, D. T. O'Connor, L. A. Miles, and R. J. Parmer. 2001. Proteolytic cleavage of chromogranin A (CgA) by plasmin. Selective liberation of a specific bioactive CgA fragment that regulates catecholamine release. *J Biol.Chem.* 276, no. 27:25022-25029.

Jiang, Q., S. Yasothornsrikul, L. Taupenot, L. A. Miles, and R. J. Parmer. 2002. The local chromaffin cell plasminogen/plasmin system and the regulation of catecholamine secretion. *Annals of the New York Academy of Sciences* 971:445-449.

Kassam, G., B. H. Le, K. S. Choi, H. M. Kang, S. L. Fitzpatrick, P. Louie, and D. M. Waisman. 1998. The p11 subunit of the annexin II tetramer plays a key role in the stimulation of t-PA-dependent plasminogen activation. *Biochemistry* 37, no. 48:16958-16966.

Larmann, J. P., Jr., A. V. Lemmo, A. W. Moore, Jr., and J. W. Jorgenson. 1993. Two-dimensional separations of peptides and proteins by comprehensive liquid chromatography-capillary electrophoresis. *Electrophoresis* 14, no. 5-6:439-447.

Link, A. J., J. Eng, D. M. Schieltz, E. Carmack, G. J. Mize, D. R. Morris, B. M. Garvik, and J. R. Yates, III. 1999. Direct analysis of protein complexes using mass spectrometry. *Nat.Biotechnol.* 17, no. 7:676-682.

Liu, M. and S. Zhang. 2009. A kringle-containing protease with plasminogen-like activity in the basal chordate Branchiostoma belcheri. *Biosci.Rep.* 29, no. 6:385-395.

Lopez-Alemany, R., M. Suelves, and P. Munoz-Canoves. 2003. Plasmin generation dependent on alpha-enolase-type plasminogen receptor is required for myogenesis. *Thrombosis and Haemostasis* 90, no. 4:724-733.

Miles, L. A., N. M. Andronicos, N. Baik, and R. J. Parmer. 2006. Cell-surface actin binds plasminogen and modulates neurotransmitter release from catecholaminergic cells. *Journal of Neuroscience* 26, no. 50:13017-13024.

Miles, L. A., C. M. Dahlberg, J. Plescia, J. Felez, K. Kato, and E. F. Plow. 1991. Role of cell-surface lysines in plasminogen binding to cells: Identification of alpha-Enolase as a candidate plasminogen receptor. *Biochemistry* 30:1682-1691.

Miles, L. A., S. B. Hawley, N. Baik, N. M. Andronicos, F. J. Castellino, and R. J. Parmer. 2005. Plasminogen receptors: the sine qua non of cell surface plasminogen activation. *Front Biosci.* 10:1754-1762.

Miles, L. A. and E. F. Plow. 1985. Binding and activation of plasminogen on the platelet surface. *Journal of Biological Chemistry* 260:4303-4311.

Miles, L. A. and E. F. Plow. 1987. Receptor mediated binding of the fibrinolytic components, plasminogen and urokinase, to peripheral blood cells. *Thrombosis and Haemostasis* 58:936-942.

Mitchell, J. W., N. Baik, F. J. Castellino, and L. A. Miles. 2006. Plasminogen inhibits TNF{alpha}-induced apoptosis in monocytes. *Blood* 107, no. 11:4383-4390.

Nguyen, S. T., S. Hasegawa, H. Tsuda, H. Tomioka, M. Ushijima, M. Noda, K. Omura, and Y. Miki. 2007. Identification of a predictive gene expression signature of cervical lymph node metastasis in oral squamous cell carcinoma. *Cancer Sci.* 98, no. 5:740-746.

O'Mullane, M. J. and M. S. Baker. 1998. Loss of cell viability dramatically elevates cell surface plasminogen binding and activation. *Experimental Cell Research* 242:153-164.

O'Mullane, M. J. and M. S. Baker. 1999. Elevated plasminogen receptor expression occurs as a degradative phase event in cellular apoptosis. *Immunol.Cell Biol.* 77, no. 3:249-255.

Odegaard, J. I., D. Vats, L. Zhang, R. Ricardo-Gonzalez, K. L. Smith, D. B. Sykes, M. P. Kamps, and A. Chawla. 2007. Quantitative expansion of ES cell-derived myeloid progenitors capable of differentiating into macrophages. *Journal of Leukocyte Biology* 81, no. 3:711-719.

Opiteck, G. J. and J. W. Jorgenson. 1997. Two-dimensional SEC/RPLC coupled to mass spectrometry for the analysis of peptides. *Anal.Chem.* 69, no. 13:2283-2291.

Palumbo, J. S., K. E. Talmage, H. Liu, C. M. La Jeunesse, D. P. Witte, and J. L. Degen. 2003. Plasminogen supports tumor growth through a fibrinogen-dependent mechanism linked to vascular patency. *Blood* 102, no. 8:2819-2827.

Peng, J., J. E. Elias, C. C. Thoreen, L. J. Licklider, and S. P. Gygi. 2003. Evaluation of multidimensional chromatography coupled with tandem mass spectrometry (LC/LC-MS/MS) for large-scale protein analysis: the yeast proteome. *J.Proteome.Res.* 2, no. 1:43-50.

Ploplis, V. A., P. Carmeliet, S. Vazirzadeh, Vlaenderen Van, I, L. Moons, E. F. Plow, and D. Collen. 1995. Effects of disruption of the plasminogen gene on thrombosis, growth, and health in mice. *Circulation* 92, no. 9:2585-2593.

Ploplis, V. A., E. L. French, P. Carmeliet, D. Collen, and E. F. Plow. 1998. Plasminogen deficiency differentially affects recruitment of inflammatory cell populations in mice. *Blood* 91:2005-2009.

Plow, E. F., D. E. Freaney, J. Plescia, and L. A. Miles. 1986. The plasminogen system and cell surfaces: Evidence for plasminogen and urokinase receptors on the same cell type. *Journal of Cell Biology* 103:2411-2420.

Plow, E. F., V. A. Ploplis, S. Busuttil, P. Carmeliet, and D. Collen. 1999. A role of plasminogen in atherosclerosis and restenosis models in mice. *Thrombosis and Haemostasis* 82 Suppl 1:4-7.

Ranson, M., N. M. Andronicos, M. J. O'Mullane, and M. S. Baker. 1998. Increased plasminogen binding is associated with metastatic breast cancer cells: differential expression of plasminogen binding proteins. *British Journal of Cancer* 77:1586-1597.

Redlitz, A., B. J. Fowler, E. F. Plow, and L. A. Miles. 1995. The role of an enolase-related molecule in plasminogen binding to cells. *European Journal of Biochemistry* 227:407-415.

Romer, J., T. H. Bugge, C. Pyke, L. R. Lund, M. J. Flick, J. L. Degen, and K. Dano. 1996. Impaired wound healing in mice with a disrupted plasminogen gene. *Nat.Med.* 2, no. 3:287-292.

Su, A. I., M. P. Cooke, K. A. Ching, Y. Hakak, J. R. Walker, T. Wiltshire, A. P. Orth, R. G. Vega, L. M. Sapinoso, A. Moqrich, A. Patapoutian, G. M. Hampton, P. G. Schultz, and J. B. Hogenesch. 2002. Large-scale analysis of the human and mouse transcriptomes. *Proc.Natl.Acad.Sci.U.S.A* 99, no. 7:4465-4470.

Su, A. I., T. Wiltshire, S. Batalov, H. Lapp, K. A. Ching, D. Block, J. Zhang, R. Soden, M. Hayakawa, G. Kreiman, M. P. Cooke, J. R. Walker, and J. B. Hogenesch. 2004. A gene atlas of the mouse and human protein-encoding transcriptomes. *Proc.Natl.Acad.Sci.U.S.A* 101, no. 16:6062-6067.

Tabb, D. L., W. H. McDonald, and J. R. Yates, III. 2002. DTASelect and Contrast: tools for assembling and comparing protein identifications from shotgun proteomics. *J.Proteome.Res.* 1, no. 1:21-26.

Wang, G. G., K. R. Calvo, M. P. Pasillas, D. B. Sykes, H. Hacker, and M. P. Kamps. 2006. Quantitative production of macrophages or neutrophils ex vivo using conditional Hoxb8. *Nat.Methods* 3, no. 4:287-293.

Wolters, D. A., M. P. Washburn, and J. R. Yates, III. 2001. An automated multidimensional protein identification technology for shotgun proteomics. *Anal.Chem.* 73, no. 23:5683-5690.

Yates, J. R., III. 1998. Database searching using mass spectrometry data. *Electrophoresis* 19, no. 6:893-900.

10

Proteomic Analysis of Wnt-Dependent Dishevelled-Based Supermolecular Complexes

Noriko Yokoyama
State University of New York at Stony Brook, Stony Brook, New York USA

1. Introduction

Wnt signaling is critical and indispensable for numerous cellular pathways including embryonic development and adult tissue homeostasis such as determination, proliferation, migration and differentiation (Clevers, 2006; Glass and Karsenty, 2006; Nusse, 2005; Wang and Wynshaw-Boris, 2004). There are three independent branches of the Wnt signaling cascade, Wnt canonical beta-catenin/Lef-Tcf-sensitive transcriptional response, the planar cell polarity (PCP) response, and the Wnt5a/Frizzled-2/Ca^{2+}/cGMP response (He et al., 2004; Katanaev et al., 2005; Liu et al., 2001; Malbon, 2005; Wallingford and Habas, 2005; Willert et al., 2003). Dishevelleds (Dvls) are essential components in three major Wnt signaling pathways. Dvls function as scaffold protein bridging the receptors and distinct downstream signaling components. Through formation of dynamic multiprotein complexes, signal is transduced to inside cells.

In Wnt/beta-catenin signaling pathway, Wnts bind to members of the Frizzled (Fz) family of G protein-coupled receptors and to co-receptor low density lipoprotein receptor related protein LRP5 and LRP6 (LRP5/6). Binding of Wnt3a to these receptors facilitates a variety of intracellular events. Phosphorylation of LRP5/6 triggers the interaction of Fz-LRP5/6 complex with dynamic multiprotein complexes, including *adenomatous polyposis coli* (APC), Dishevelled (Dsh/Dvl), Axin, glycogen synthase kinase-3β (GSK3β) and casein kinase 1α (Hart, 1998; Kishida et al., 1998). Scaffold protein Dvl facilitates destruction of multiprotein complexes (Hart, 1998 ; Kishida et al., 1998; Malbon, 2005). As a results, stabilized β-catenin, translocates to nuclear and enhances Lef/Tcf-sensitive transcription (Angers & Moon, 2009; Clevers, 2006; van Amerongen and Nusse, 2009).

Fly Dsh and three isoforms of mammals Dvls (Dvl1-3) all share several prominent, highly-conserved domains: a Dsh homology domain called DIX; a conserved sequence element with homology to the postsynaptic density protein *P*SD-95, *D*iscs-large, and *Z*O-1, termed PDZ; and *D*isheveled, *E*gl-10, *P*leckstrin domain, termed DEP (Wharton, 2003). In addition, there are conserved sequence regions harboring basic amino acids residues and a proline-rich putative Src homology 3 (SH3) binding domain (Penton et al., 2002). Dvl3 knockout mouse is lethal, whereas Dvl1 or Dvl2 knockout mouse is viable (Hamblet et al., 2002; Etheridge et al., 2008; Lijam et al., 1997). The isoforms of mammals Dvl are not truly "redundant" with respect to function (Hamblet et al., 2002; Etheridge et al., 2008; Lee et al., 2008), although functions of each isoform of Dvls are not fully resolved. Previous studies reveal distinct localization of Dvl isoforms in totipotent mouse F9 embryonal teratocarcinoma (F9) cells. Dvl1 and Dvl2 are found in the cytosol-enriched fraction (80 %), the least amount of each of these isoforms is observed in the nuclear-enriched fraction (5 %). Dvl3 content in the cytosol-enriched fraction is reduced to 60 %, whereas content of Dvl3 in the nuclear-enriched fraction is several fold greater than that for either Dvl1 or Dvl2 (20 %). Abundance of Dvl3 and Dvl1 following Wnt3a stimulation is increased and Wnt3a stimulates dramatic Dvl3 trafficking to the plasma membrane. Thus, Dvl3 has a role in Wnt/β-catenin signaling that is distinct from those of the Dvl1 and Dvl2 (Yokoyama et al., 2007). Dvl3 has unique roles in Wnt/β-catenin signaling pathway (Lee et al., 2008; Yokoyama et al., 2007). Dvls are believed to be recruited Fz receptor through their PDZ domain. Many Dvls associating proteins also interact with Dvls via their PDZ domain (Wong et al., 2003). The DIX domain is critical for the ability of Dvl to recruit Axin and for the dynamic self-association of Dvls. Fluorescence microscopy in cells suggests that Dvls undergo dynamic oligomerization associated with activation of Wnt/β-catenin signaling by Wnt3a (Axelrod et al., 1998; Kishida et al., 1999; Rothbacher et al., 2000). Properties of dynamic polymerization correlate with the activation of Wnt/β-catenin signaling (Schwarz-Romond et al., 2007a; Schwarz-Romond et al., 2007b). Wnt induces LRP6 aggregation and phosphorylation in a Dvl-dependent manner. Furthermore, Dvl mutants that lack normal oligomerization also influence the formation of LRP6 complexes (Bilic et al., 2007).

Thus, Dvls scaffold many interacting proteins temporally/spatially to transduce Wnt signaling. To define a regulation of Wnt signaling, it is necessary to establish the regulatory mechanism of assembly of Dvls-based supermolecular complexes. Tight regulation of Wnt signaling by protein-protein interaction involves many post-translational modifications such as phosphorylation, ubiquitination, sumoylation and methylation. Phosphorylation is a crucial and central mechanism of regulating docking of signal molecules to Dvl scaffold. Phosphorylation of protein regulates protein activities, binding affinities, stability and its trafficking to distinct cellular compartments (Yokoyama and Malbon, 2007; Yokoyama et al., 2007; Yokoyama and Malbon, 2009).

To probing Dvls-based complexes, two different approaches were employed. First, our attention is to identify interacting proteins of Dvl2 (most abundant form of Dvl in F9 cells). Dvl2 interacting proteins have been established using glutathione-S-transferase (GST) fusion protein pull down. Interacting proteins were pulled down and eluted from the beads. Eluted proteins were separated by immobilized pH gradient (IPG) strips (pH 3-10, first dimension separation) and subjected to second dimensional SDS-gel electrophoresis. Samples were analyzed by liquid chromatography electrospray ionization mass spectrometry (LC-ESI-MS-MS). Novel Dvls interacting proteins were identified. In addition, immobilized Dvl2 domains pull down is able to find novel roles of Src in Wnt signaling. Identification of tyrosine phosphorylation sites on Dvl2 by Src family tyrosine kinases led to discover that Src family tyrosine kinases are a positive regulator of Wnt/β-catenin signaling (Yokoyama and Malbon, 2009). Second attempt is designed to probe Wnt-dependent assembly of Dvls-based supermolecular complexes. Dishevelled-based "punctae" had been observed earlier by fluorescence microscopy. These "punctae" have been shown to be the assemblies of protein and the size and cellular distribution changed in response to Wnt stimulation. The physical evidence for the existence for these putative "aggregates" or "punctae" of Dvl3-based complexes was established using size-exclusion chromatography (SEC) technique, affinity pull-downs, proteomics, and fluorescent correlation microscopy (*fcs*). Dvl3-based complexes were interrogated physically *in vitro* by SEC analysis of cell extracts and *in vivo* by *fcs* analysis in live cells (Yokoyama et al., 2010). Establishment of physical nature and dynamic character of the Dvls-based complexes is the key to understand Wnt signaling. For the first time, the assembly of supermolecular Dvl3-based complexes is shown in response to Wnt3a. Peak fractions (Dvl3-based supermolecular complexes) separated by SEC were subjected to LC-ESI-MS-MS. To avoid eliminating potential contamination of proteins/complexes, analysis was carried out at distinct time points. These approaches identified both expected and also novel components.

2. Proteomic analysis of Dvls-based multiprotein complexes

Wnt signaling is spatially and temporally transduced through the assembly of dynamic multiprotein complexes. Dvls, scaffold proteins, provide dynamic protein platform including protein kinases, phosphatases, receptors, adaptor molecules, and other signaling molecules. The Wnt home page provides an invaluable frame of Dvls interacting proteins (**http://www.stanford.edu/~rnusse/wntwindow.html**), although real Dvls-based complexes seem much more complicated. Recent measurement of the mass of Dvl3-based complexes showed that the MW of the complexes is >2 MegaDa by SEC and ~35 MegaDa by *fcs* (Yokoyama et al., 2010). Structure and functional analysis of these Dvls-based supermolecular complexes is critical to understanding Wnt signaling. Proteomics provide a portal to identify complex partners assembled into signalsomes. In this study, two distinct approaches are employed.

2.1 Analysis of Dvl2 interacting proteins using glutathione-S-transferase (GST) fusion protein pull down

The pull-down technique is an invaluable tool for studying cellular pathways via protein-protein interactions. GST fusion protein pull down experiments are one approach to identify interaction of between probe protein and unknown targets. GST fusion protein pulls down offers an important biological assay for direct protein-to-protein interactions. In this study, GST fusion proteins of Dvl2 domain are employed to discover novel Dvl2 interacting proteins. Identification of novel Dvls interacting proteins facilitates understanding the regulatory mechanism of Wnt signaling.

2.1.1 Glutathione-S-transferase (GST) fusion protein pulls down

GST fusion proteins of the conserved domains DIX, PDZ, and DEP and the putative SH3 binding domain of Dvl2 were immobilized on glutathione-derivatized agarose matrix. Immobilized GST-PDZ (aa 267-309), GST-DIX (aa 11-93), GST-DEP (aa 433-507), GST-putative SH3 binding containing region (aa 356-378) and GST itself (as a control) were incubated with cell lysates from F9 cells stimulated with or without Wnt 3a. The interacting proteins were pulled down and eluted from the beads. Eluted proteins were separated by immobilized pH gradient (IPG) strips (pH 3-10, first dimension separation) and subjected to second dimensional SDS-gel electrophoresis. Proteins were stained with SYPRO Ruby. Non specific proteins were eliminated by comparing gel patterns obtained with GST-Dvl2 domains with those obtained by GST itself (fig. 1).

To identify Wnt-dependent interacting proteins, spots according in response to Wnt3a stimulation were excised from the gel (fig. 2), digested with trypsin overnight at 37 °C and analyzed by liquid chromatography electrospray ionization mass spectrometry (LC-ESI-MS-MS, Applied Biosystems/MDS SCIEX) using a micro-column reverse phase HPLC interfaced to an LTQ ion trap mass spectrometer. Electrospray tandem mass spectrometry

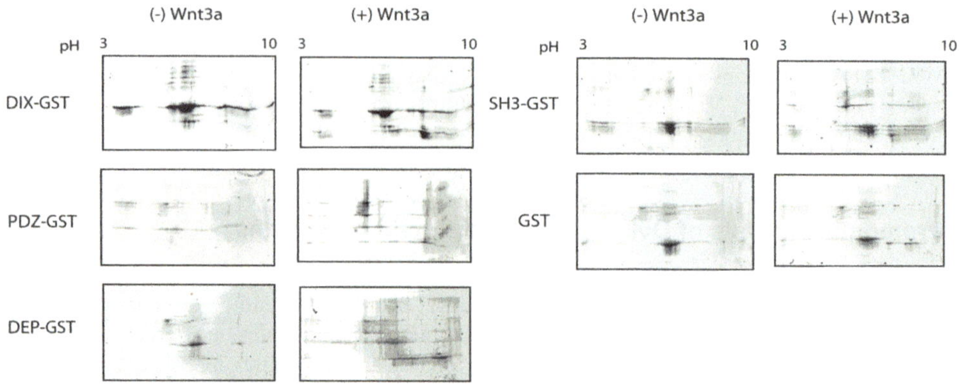

F9 cells were stimulated or unstimulated with Wnt3a for 30 min. Cell lysates were incubated with either GST domain beads or GST beads for 15 min. Bound proteins were eluted by SDS-running buffer and purified using ready prep 2-D cleanup kit. Samples were applied to pH 3-10 IPG strips, and then subjected to second dimensional gel electrophoresis.

Fig. 1. Second dimensional SDS-gel of GST pulls down.

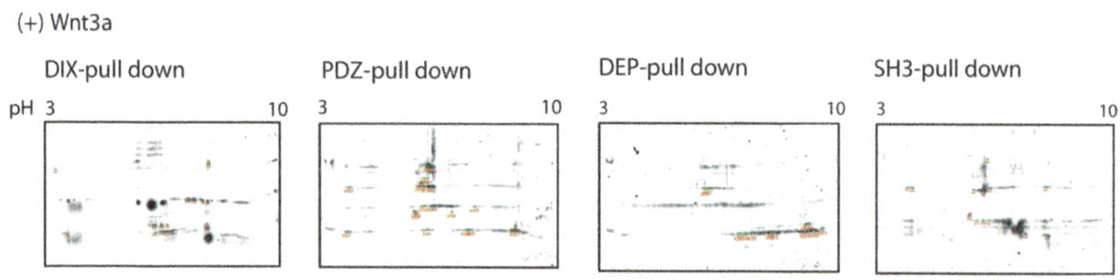

Wnt-dependent spots were selected by comparing gel patterns with or without Wnt stimulation. Spots with red numbers were further analyzed.

Fig. 2. Analysis of Wnt-dependent spots on a second dimensional gel.

based sequencing was performed. Data were analyzed by the Mascot search engine to identify amino acid sequences. LC-ESI-MS-MS analyses were performed at the Stony Brook Proteomics Center.

2.1.2 Identification of Dvl2 interacting proteins

The identified Dvl2 interacting proteins by GST fusion pull down are summarized in Table 1. Dvls are known to oligomerize via their DIX domain. Purified DIX domain polymerizes in vitro to form fibris and to puncta in vivo (Schwarz-Romond et al., 2005). DIX domain mediates dynamic polymerization platform with a high concentration of binding sites for Wnt signaling partners such as Axin and GSK3β. Axin also has a DIX domain at the C-terminus which mediates self-interaction in a head to tail fashion, similar to Dvls (Schwarz-Romond et al., 2007b; Schwarz-Romond et al., 2005). Known interacting proteins pulled down by the DIX domain-GST included all three Dvl isoforms and Axin2. Presence of PDZ and DEP peptides of Dvl2 in GST-DIX pulled down fraction demonstrated that Dvl2 forms homo oligomer. Dvl2 also forms complexes with the other two isoforms, Dvl1 and Dvl3;

Domain	Protein	# of independent peptide identified	# of total peptide	% sequence coverage
DIX	Dvl2	7	38	8
	Dvl1	6	14	6.9
	RGS18	2	5	6.8
	Dvl3	3	4	3.2
	Rho-associated protein kinase	3	3	2.6
	PLK4	2	4	1.45
	Axin 2	2	2	2.42
	PTPRR	1	1	0.8
PDZ	Tropomyosine α	7	9	23.4
	Actin	8	18	21.9
	Cyclin	2	2	5.36
	PKC and casein kinase substrate in neuron protein 1	2	2	4.08
	Axin 2	1	1	1.42
	Axin 1	1	1	1.0
	B-Raf	1	1	0.91
DEP	Actin	6	14	18.1
	Adenylate kinase 1	2	2	8.76
	Ubiquitin-conjugating enzyme E2M	1	1	4.91
	Cyclin	1	1	3.7
SH3 binding	Tropomyosine α	8	12	22.6
	Actin	12	46	31
	HSP 70K	3	4	5.6
	PARD-3	2	14	1.56
	Desmoplakin-3	3	3	1.0
	Junction plakoglobin	2	2	3.4
	Rho-associated protein kinase	2	8	1.0
	Cullin 3	1	1	1.3

Table 1. Identified Dvl2 interacting proteins.

demonstrating Dvls assemble Dvls-based complexes and thus provide a Dvls platform. Polo-like kinase 4 (PLK4), Regulator of G protein signaling (RGS) 18, Rho-associated protein kinase and Receptor-type protein tyrosine phosphatase R (PTPRR) were identified as novel DIX domain interacting proteins.

PDZ domain beads pulled down interacting proteins Axin1 and Axin2. Novel interacting proteins were Tropomyosine α, cyclin, PKC and casein kinase substrate in neuron protein 1 and B-Raf proto-oncogen serine/threonine kinase. Adenylate kinase 1, cyclin and ubiquitin-conjugating enzyme E2M were identified as novel DEP domain interacting proteins. SH3 binding domain pulled down Tropomyosine α, HSP 70K, PARD-3, desmoplakin-3, plakoglobin, Rho-associated protein kinase, and Cullin 3. Actin, known Dvl interacting protein, was pulled down by PDZ, DEP and SH3 binding domains of Dvl2.

2.1.3 Assay for Lef/Tcf-sensitive transcription

Lef/Tcf-sensitive transcription is the read out of Wnt/beta-catenin signaling pathway. F9 cells were grown on 12-well plates and co-transfected with rat Fz1 (Rfz1) and Super8xTOPFlash (M50) (Seto and Bellen, 2006). After 1-2 days of transfection, cells were treated with Wnt3a (20 ng/ml) for up to 8 hours. Cells were lysed in a reporter gene lysis buffer [12.5 mM Tris-H_3PO_4 pH 7.8, 1 mM trans-1, 2-cyclohexanediaminetetraacetic acid (CDTA), 2 mM DTT, 10% glycerol and 1 % Triton X-100] (Promega) and further analyzed. Lef/Tcf-sensitive transcription activity was determined using cell lysates according to the manufacture's instructions (Stratagene) and displayed to relative to unstimulated cells (set to "1").

2.1.4 Evaluation of novel Dvl2 interacting proteins

Dvl proteins are phosphorylated in response to Wnt and display a shift of electrophoretic mobility on SDS-PAGE. Dvl activity itself is reported to be controlled by multiple phosphorylation events (McKay et al., 2001; Sun et al., 2001; Willert et al., 1997). Thus, Dvl phosphorylation is implicated in the Wnt signaling pathway. Many serine/threonine protein kinases and phosphatases are known to interact with Dvls. CK1ε, CK2 and Par1 are proposed to phosphorylate Dvls (Cong et al., 2004; Sun et al., 2001; Willert et al., 1997). Not only serine/threonine kinases, but also Src family tyrosine kinases phosphorylate Dvl2 (Yokoyama and Malbon, 2009). Protein phosphatase 2C (PP2C) and protein phosphatase 2A (PP2A) dock to Dvls (Strovel et al., 2000; Yokoyama and Malbon, 2007).

Treatment with okadaic acid (chemical inhibitor of serine/threonine phosphatases, PP1 and PP2A) mimics Wnt 3a action, increasing the cellular abundance of Axin and GSK3β and β-catenin as well as the trafficking of signaling elements in Wnt/β-catenin signaling pathway. Although mimicking effects of Wnt3a on the cellular abundance and trafficking of key signaling elements in Wnt /β-catenin signaling, suppression of PP2A alone does not provoke activation of Lef/Tcf-sensitive transcription, but potentiates its activation by Wnt3a. PP2A activity declines dramatically after Wnt stimulation and direct binding of Dvl2 to PP2A suppresses a phosphatase activity. PP2A dephosphorylates Dvl2 (Yokoyama and Malbon, 2007). Thus, phosphorylation-dephosphorylation is a central regulatory mechanism of docking proteins–Dvls interaction.

Consistent with the critical roles of phosphorylation-dephosphorylation in Wnt signaling pathway, several kinases and phosphatase were identified as novel Dvl2 interacting proteins. One tyrosine phosphatase PTPRR and two serine/threonine kinases, PLK4 and B-Raf, were further analyzed to confirm their functions in the Wnt/β-catenin signaling pathway.

Receptor-type protein tyrosine phosphatase R (PTPRR), also known as PTP-SL, contains a kinase interacting motif (KIM), located just N-terminal of the phosphatase domain, and associates with the mitogen-activated protein (MAP) kinase. PTPRR associates with MAPKs and inactivates kinases by dephosphorylating tyrosine residue (Hendriks et al., 2009). MAPKs promote Wnt/β-catenin signaling pathway via LRP6 phosphorylation suggesting convergence between Wnt/β-catenin signaling pathway and the mitogenic pathway

(Cervenka et al., 2011). F9 cell extracts from stimulated or unstimulated cells were incubated with GST beads or one of the distinct GST-domain beads. PTPRR displayed prominent docking to DIX and DEP domains, modestly to the PDZ domain and weakly to the putative SH3 binding domain. Wnt stimulation slightly enhanced docking of PTPRR to Dvl2 DIX domain (fig. 3A). Association of Dvl2 and PTPRR was confirmed by Dvl2 immunoprecipitation followed by proved with either anti-Dvl2 antibody or anti-PTPRR antibody. Association of Dvl2 and PTPRR was enhanced by Wnt3a in a time-dependent manner (fig. 3B). Docking of PTPRR to Dvl2 increased over 1hour post Wnt3a stimulation. The functional role of PTPRR in Wnt/β-catenin pathway was investigated by measuring Lef/Tcf-sensitive transcriptional activity, a hallmark of activation of the Wnt/β–catenin pathway, by knocking down of PTPRR. siRNA mediated knockdown of PTPRR resulted in enhancement of Lef/Tcf-sensitive transcription activity, while overexpression of PTPRR attenuated Lef/Tcf-sensitive transcription activity (fig. 3C and 3D) confirming that PTPRR is a novel Dvl2 interacting protein and functions as a negative regulator of the Wnt/β-catenin signaling pathway. Association of tyrosine phosphatase with Dvl2 is a novel finding.

Polo-like kinase 4 (PLK4) is another novel DIX domain interacting protein which was identified in this study. PLK4 is the most structurally divergent Polo family kinase and is essential for mouse embryonic development (Swallow et al., 2005). PLK4 is required for the reproduction of centrosomes during cell cycle (Habedanck et al., 2005). Interaction of PLK4 and Dvl2 was confirmed by co-immunoprecipitation with an anti-Dvl2 antibody. Lef/Tcf-sensitive transcription was enhanced by knockdown of PLK4, while overexpression of PLK4 attenuated Lef/Tcf-sensitive transcription, suggesting negative roles of PLK4 in Wnt/β-catenin signaling pathway (fig. 3E, 3F and 3G). Thus PLK4 is evaluated as functional novel interacting protein of Dvl2.

B-Raf proto-oncogen serine/threonine kinase, which transduces signals from Ras to MEK and ERK/MAPK, was identified as a novel PDZ interacting protein. These pathways regulate many cellular functions, including cell proliferation, differentiation, apoptosis, motility and metabolism (Wellbrock et al., 2004); and implicated in many human diseases such as cancer. (Rapp et al., 2006). Docking of B-Raf to PDZ domain was regulated by Wnt3a (fig. 4A). DIX, DEP and putative SH3 binding domains were also involved in the interaction of the two molecules. Docking of B-Raf to Dvl2 was Wnt-dependent and dramatically increased 15 min after Wnt3a stimulation. The association persisted for 2hours (fig. 4B). Attenuation of Lef/Tcf-sensitive transcription by knocking down of B-Raf demonstrated that B-Raf regulates positively Wnt/β-catenin signaling pathway (fig. 4C). Dose-dependent enhancement of Lef/Tcf-sensitive transcription is occurred by expression of B-Raf (fig. 4D).

Thus, the newly identified Dvl2 interacting proteins, PTPRR, PLK4 and B-Raf are indeed docked to Dvl2 in a Wnt- and time-dependent manner and, regulate Wnt pathway either negatively (PTPRR and PLK4) or positively (B-Raf).

2.2 Tyrosine phosphorylation of Dvl2 regulates Wnt/β-catenin signaling pathway

Dvl proteins are highly phosphorylated in response to Wnt stimulation and Wnt-dependent phosphorylation sites on Dvls have been poorly analyzed. Dvl phosphorylations regulate the Wnt signaling pathway, especially with regard to serine/threonine protein kinases (Kishida et al., 2001; Yanagawa et al., 1995). Involvement of tyrosine kinases in Wnt signaling pathway has not been established, except tyrosine phosphorylation of β-catenin. The phosphorylation sites on Dvls are presumably many and several mechanisms of Dvls

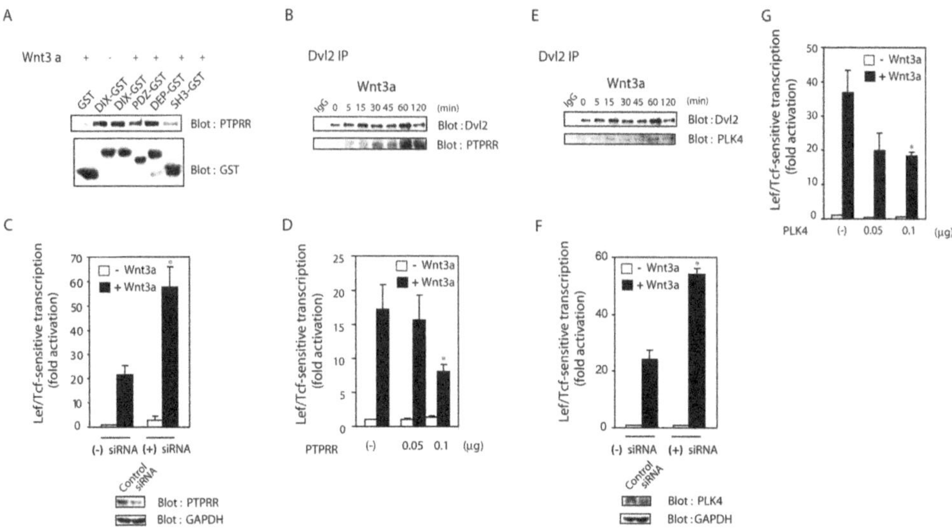

A-D, analysis of PTPRR in Wnt/β-catenin signaling pathway. E-G, analysis of PLK4 in Wnt/β-catenin signaling pathway.
(A) PTPRR docks to Dvl2. Lysates from cell treated or untreated with Wnt3a were incubated with one of the immobilized Dvl2 domains or GST itself. Bound proteins were analyzed by SDS-PAGE and immunoblotting with either anti-PTPRR or anti-GST antibody.
(B) Time course of the association of Dvl2 and PTPRR. Cell lysates were immunoprecipitated with anti-Dvl2 antibody. Bound proteins were analyzed by SDS-PAGE and immunoblotting with either anti-Dvl2 or anti-PTPRR antibody.
(C) Effect of knockdown of PTPRR on Lef/Tcf-sensitive transcription. F9 cells were transfected with siRNA targeting PTPRR one day before co-transfection of the cells with Rfz1 and Super8xTOPFlash reporter (M50). On the following day, the cells were stimulated with Wnt3a for 7 hours and cell lysates were assayed for Lef/Tcf-sensitive transcription. Statistical significance is indicated (*, $p < 0.005$). Cell lysates were analyzed by immunoblotting with either anti-PTPRR or anti-GAPDH antibody (as a control).
(D) Overexpression of PTPRR attenuates Wnt3a-sensitive Lef/Tcf-sensitive transcription. F9 cells were co-transfected with Rfz1, M50, and a PTPRR expression vector one day before cells were stimulated without or with purified Wnt3a for 7 hours. Cell lysates were assayed for Lef/Tcf-sensitive transcription activity. Statistical significance is indicated (*, $p < 0.05$).
(E) Dvl2 docks to PLK4 in a Wnt- and time-dependent manner. Cell lysates were subjected to immunoprecipitation with anti-Dvl2 antibody and analyzed by SDS-PAGE and then immunoblotted with either anti-Dvl2 antibody or anti-PLK4 antibody.
(F) Knockdown of PLK4 enhances Lef/Tcf-sensitive transcription. F9 cells were transfected with siRNA targeting PLK4 one day before co-transfection of the cells with Rfz1 and M50. On the following day, the cells were stimulated with Wnt3a and assay for Lef/Tcf-sensitive transcription was performed as described previously. Statistical significance is indicated (*, $p < 0.005$)
(G) Overexpression of PLK4 attenuates Lef/Tcf-sensitive transcription. Cells were co-transfected with PLK4, Rfz1 and M50 for one day before Wnt stimulation. Assay for Lef/Tcf-sensitive transcription was performed. Statistical significance is indicated (*, $p < 0.005$).

Fig. 3. Analysis of novel Dvl2 interacting proteins.

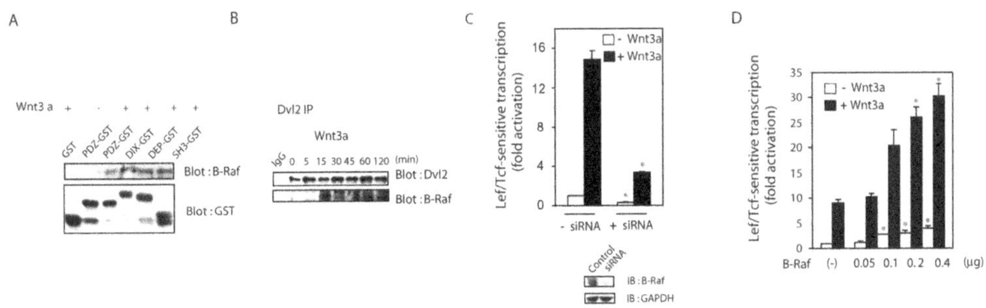

(A) B-Raf docks to Dvl2. Lysates from cells treated or untreated with Wnt3a were incubated with either GST itself or one of the immobilized Dvl2 domains. Bound proteins were proved with either anti-B-Raf antibody or anti-GST antibody.
(B) Time course of the association of Dvl2 and B-Raf. Cell lysates were subjected to Dvl2 immunoprecipitation. Bound proteins were analyzed by SDS-PAGE and immunoblotting with either anti-Dvl2 antibody or anti-B-Raf antibody.
(C) Effect of knockdown of B-Raf on Lef/Tcf-sensitive transcription. F9 cells were transfected with siRNA targeting B-Raf one day before co-transfection of the cells with Rfz1 and M50. On the following day, the cells were stimulated and Lef/Tcf-sensitive transcription was assayed. Statistical significance is indicated (*, $p< 0.005$). Cell lysates were analyzed by immunoblotting with either anti-B-Raf antibody or anti-GAPDH antibody (as a control).
(D) Overexpression of B-Raf enhances Wnt3a-sensitive Lef/Tcf-sensitive transcription. F9 cells were co-transfected with Rfz1, M50, and B-Raf expression vector one day before cells were stimulated with or without purified Wnt3a for 7 hours. Cell lysates were assayed for Lef/Tcf-sensitive luciferase transcription activity. Statistical significance is indicated (*, $p< 0.005$).

Fig. 4. Analysis of B-Raf in Wnt/β-catenin signaling pathway.

phosphorylation may be involved; distributive phosphorylation, sequential priming phosphorylation, processive phosphorylation, and combination of distributive phosphorylation/sequential priming phosphorylation or processive phosphorylation. Similar to LRP5/6, several kinases may phosphorylate same sites on Dvls. Dvl kinases may play multiple opposing roles in Wnt signaling pathway like CK1 and GSK3β do. Thus, regulations by phosphorylation in Wnt signaling pathway are a complicated process, since many important molecules in the pathway are positively or negatively regulated by phosphorylation. To avoid such a complexity, in vitro systems are employed, although functional and physiological analysis *in vivo* is required. The amino acid region 370-376 of Dvl2 displays a consensus sequence for a class I core SH3 protein-binding motif RTEPVRP (Penton et al., 2002). This region is conserved in all three mammalian isoforms of Dvl suggesting that tyrosine phosphorylation may be functional in Dvl biology and Wnt signaling. In developmentally relevant signaling, Src is reported to elevate the expression (Karni et al., 2005) and phosphorylation at Tyr Y654 of β-catenin. The phosphorylation of Tyr654 blocked the E-cadherin-β-catenin interaction (Roura et al., 1999). In addition to Src, other tyrosine kinases such as Fyn, Fer, transmembrane tyrosine kinase EGFR and c-Met, downregulate E-cadherin-mediated adhesion via enhanced tyrosine phosphorylation of β-catenin (Lilien and Balsamo, 2005; Piedra et al., 2001). In chronic myeloid leukemia cells, oncogenic tyrosine kinase Bcr-Abl triggers tyrosine phosphorylation of β-catenin, stabilizes β-catenin levels and enhances nuclear signaling activation (Coluccia et al., 2007). A possible involvement of tyrosine kinases, particularly Src family tyrosine kinases, in Wnt/β-catenin signaling pathway was investigated.

2.2.1 Baculovirus expression and purification of Dvl2

Baculovirus/Sf9 cell system was employed to express Dvl2. Full length Dvl2 was subcloned into plasmid pBACgus-9 (N-terminal T7 tag and C-terminal CBD-tag and poly Histidine-tag, Novagen), and expressed in Sf9 cells using the Bac Vector-3000 DNA transfection kit (Novagen). Sf9 cells were grown in Ex-cell-401 medium supplemented with L-glutamine and 2.5% fetal bovine serum. Sf9 cells were infected with recombinant Dvl2 baculovirus at a MOI (multiplicity of infection) of 5. Cells were harvested after 4 days of infection and lysed in a French pressure cell twice in 20 mM Tris-HCl buffer (pH 8.0) containing 1% deoxycholate, 2 mM Na_3VO_4, 20 mM NaF, 5 mM 2-mercaptoethanol, 10 μg/ml leupeptin, 10μg/ml aprotinin, and 1 mM phenylsulfonyl fluoride (PMSF). After centrifugation, rDvl2 was purified by Ni^{2+}-affinity chromatography.

2.2.2 Phosphorylation of Dvl2 by Src family kinase and identification of tyrosine phosphorylation sites on Dvl2

Phosphorylation of rDvl2 was performed in a kinase buffer (10 mM Tris-HCl, pH7.4, 10mM $MgCl_2$, 10 mM $MnCl_2$, 1 mM Na_3VO_4, 50 mM NaF, 0.5 mM ATP) with purified rSrc (from Sf9 cell) for 1 hour at 30 °C. Phosphorylated rDvl2 was digested with trypsin and subjected to analysis using API QSTAR Pulsar LC/MS/MS (Applied Biosystems/MDS SCIEX) equipped with a Protana nanospray source (Protana Engineering A/S) and an UltiMate capillary high pressure liquid chromatography (LC Packings) with a PepMap C_{18} nano-column (75 μm x 15 cm, LC Packings). Phosphopeptides were detected by a data base search using Pro ID software (Applied Biosystems/MDS SCIEX).

2.2.3 Functional analysis of tyrosine phosphorylation on Dvl2

The functional relevance of the detected tyrosine phosphorylation sites was assessed following site-directed mutagenesis using Qickchange Mutagenesis system (Stratagene). The functional ability of the mutational constructs (YF mutants of Dvl2; Y18F, Y27F, Y275F, Y295F and Y463F) analyzed by Lef/Tcf-sensitive transcription in Dvl2-deficient cells. F9 cell stably expressing Rfz1 and M50 were transfected with siRNA targeting Dvl2 one day before transfection of cells with either wild-type or an YF mutant of Dvl2. On the following day, cells were stimulated with Wnt3a for 7 hours and Lef/Tcf-sensitive transcription was assayed.

2.2.4 Dvl2 docks to and activates Src in a Wnt-dependent manner

F9 cell extracts were incubated with immobilized Dvl2 domains (GST-DIX, GST-DEP, GST-PDZ, GST-putative SH3 binding site, and GST-C-terminus of Dvl2). Src family kinases (Src and Hck) displayed prominent docking on the putative SH3 binding region (aa 356-378) and the proline-rich region of the C-terminus of Dvl2 (aa 511-736) (fig. 5A). The ability of the SH3 domains of Src family tyrosine kinases, but not Nck SH3 domain to enable docking to Dvl2 reflects the specificity of the scaffold-kinase interaction (Yokoyama and Malbon, 2009). Positive roles of Src family tyrosine kinases in the Wnt/β-catenin signaling pathway were confirmed by either treatment with an inhibitor of the Src family tyrosine kinases (PP2) or with a siRNA-induced knockdown of Src. Treatment with PP2 or siRNA targeting Src attenuated the formation of primitive endoderm (another readout of Wnt signaling pathway) as well as Lef/Tcf-sensitive transcription (Yokoyama and Malbon, 2009). Analysis of phosphorylation sites on Dvl2 by Src was performed *in vitro*. Purified rDvl2 from Sf9 cell was phosphorylated by a Src family kinase. The five tyrosine residues (Y18, Y27, Y275, Y295 and Y463) were identified by mass spectrometry. One example was shown in fig. 5B. Src family tyrosine kinases can phosphorylate *in vitro* two tyrosine residues (Y18 and Y27) of the DIX domain, two residues (Y275 and Y295) of the PDZ domain, and a single residue (Y463) in the DEP domain. Dvl2 levels were knocked-down by siRNA targeting Dvl2; the ability of YF mutants (Dvl2 Y18F, Y27F, Y275F, Y295F and Y463F) versus wild-type Dvl2 to rescue Wnt3a-stimulated Lef/Tcf-sensitive transcription was probed. Expression of the wild-type Dvl2 in Dvl2 knockdown cells restored the Wnt3a-stimulated Lef/Tcf-sensitive transcription, whereas the Y18F Dvl2 mutant in particular attenuated the response by more than 50 % (fig. 5C).

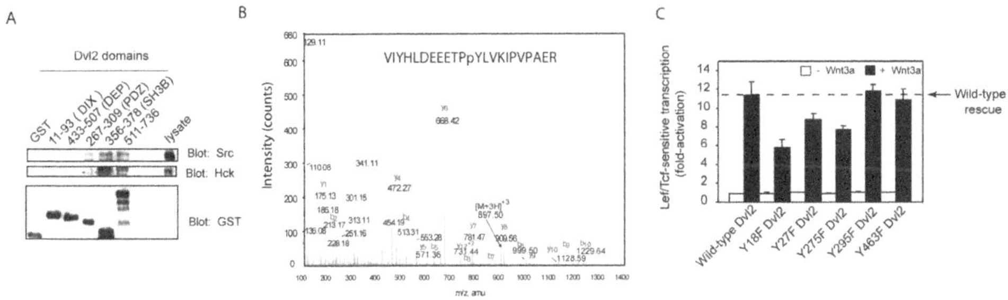

(A) Dvl2 docks to Src and Hck tyrosine kinases. Cell lysates were incubated with one of the immobilized Dvl2 domain, DIX, DEP, PDZ, putative SH3 binding region (SH3B), C-terminus (aa 511-736) and GST itself. Proteins docking to the Dvl2 domains were resolved by SDS-PAGE and analyzed by immunoblotting, staining with: anti-Src, anti-Hck, and anti-GST antibodies (loading control).
(B) Mass spectrum of the Y27 phosphopeptide. Phosphorylated Dvl2 was digested with trypsin and analyzed by LC/MS/MS. Tyrosine 27 was identified as phosphorylation site.
(C) Tyrosine-to-phenylalanine substitution mutants of Dvl2 attenuate Lef/Tcf-sensitive transcription. F9 cells stably expressing Rfz1 and M50 were transfected with siRNA targeting Dvl2 one day before transfection of the cells with either wild-type or one of the YF-mutants of Dvl2 (Y18F, Y27F, Y275F, Y295F and Y463F). On the following day, cells were stimulated with Wnt3a. Assay for Lef/Tcf-sensitive transcription was performed. Data are adapted with permission from the publication (Yokoyama, N. & Malbon, C. C. (2009). J Cell Sci 122, 4439-4451).

Fig. 5. Src family tyrosine kinases are involved in Wnt/β-catenin signaling.

At least two prominent components of the multiprotein complexes, Dvl2 and β-catenin, were phosphorylated on tyrosine residues in response to Wnt stimulation. Tyrosine phosphorylation of Y18, Y27 and Y275 of Dvl2 appears to contribute, in some complex manner, to the ability of Src to enhance Wnt3a/β-catenin signaling. Wnt stimulated Src docking to Dvl2 through the SH3-binding domain and the C-terminus proline-rich domain. Src activity is regulated by intramolecular interactions, an interaction between the SH2 domain and the C-terminal tail as well as an interaction between the SH3 domain and a polyproline-type helix in the SH2-kinase linker region (Sicheri et al., 1997; Williams et al.,

1997; Xu et al., 1997). Docking of Src to Dvl2 SH3 binding domain and C-terminus proline--rich domain disrupts Src autoinhibition, therefore enabling phosphorylation of Src substrates (Brown and Cooper, 1996; Miller, 2003). Activated Src enhances Wnt activation of the canonical pathway via phosphorylation of Dvl2 and β-catenin (Yokoyama and Malbon, 2009). Many Src family kinase substrates themselves possess SH2 and/or SH3 ligands, which couple enzyme activation to substrate phosphorylation (Brown and Cooper, 1996; Miller, 2003; Porter et al., 2000). In deed, total Src activity was increased after Wnt stimulation. Dvl2 bound form of Src showed higher activity than that of free form of Src. Furthermore, knockdown of Dvl2 blocked Wnt3a-induced activation of Src. Previously Y27D mutant of Dvl2 was shown as a polymerization defective mutant (Schwarz-Romond et al., 2007a). Roles of tyrosine residues Y18 and Y27 are the keenest interest. The tyrosine residue in the DIX domain plays an important role in polymerization of Dvl (i.e., form punctae). Application of GST pulled down and proteomics led to discover novel positive roles of Src family tyrosine kinase in Wnt/β-catenin signaling (Yokoyama and Malbon, 2009).

2.3 Assembly of Dvls-based supermolecular complexes in response to Wnt stimulation

Establishment of the physical nature and dynamic character of the Dvls-based complexes is a key to understanding Wnt signaling. The second approach is designed to probe Wnt-dependent assembly of Dvls-based supermolecular complexes. Dishevelled-based "punctae" have been observed earlier by fluorescence microscopy. Wnt treatment resulted in change of size of the "punctae" as well as their cellular localization. The physical evidence for the existence of these putative "aggregates" or "punctae" of Dvl3-based complexes was established using size-exclusion chromatography (SEC), affinity pull-downs, proteomics, and fluorescent correlation microscopy (*fcs*). Dvl3-based complexes were interrogated physically *in vitro* by SEC analysis of cell extracts and *in vivo* by *fcs* analysis in live cells (Yokoyama et al., 2010). *Fcs* enabled to analyze single molecules in live cells and is exploited for the study of the signalsomes mass and dynamic mobility. For the first time, assembly of supermolecular Dvl3-based complexes was shown in response to Wnt3a. Proteomics dissected the compositions of Dvls-based supermolecular complexes in response to Wnt stimulation.

2.3.1 Preparation of Dvl3-based supermolecular complexes and quantification of proteins

F9 cells co-expressing rat fz1(Rfz1) were suspended in ice-cold buffer (20 mM Tris-HCl pH 8.0, 0.2 M NaCl, 1 % NP-40, 1 mM PMSF, 10 μg/ml leupeptin, and 10 μg/ml aprotinin) and disrupted by repeated passage through a 23-gauge needle, and then centrifuged to remove unbroken cells, nucleus and mitochondria. Supernatants were filtered (0.45 μm) and diluted with buffer without detergent. 20 mg proteins were applied to a Superdex 200 gel filtration column (HiLoad Superdex ™ 200 prep grade 26/60, fast-performance liquid chromatography system AKTA, GE Healthcare) which was preequilibrated with 20 mM Tris-HCl (pH 8.0), 0.2 M NaCl, and 10 % glycerol. Each fraction was analyzed by SDS-PAGE and Western immunoblotting. Protein concentration was determined by use of the Bradford assay. The immunoreactive bands were scanned by calibrated Umax 1000 scanner equipped with SilverFast software (LaserSoft Imaging Inc.). The bands were quantified by using Aida software (Raytest, Germany).

2.3.2 High–performance size-exclusion analysis of Dvls-based supermolecular complexes

Size-exclusion chromatography (SEC) is one of the approaches for separating protein mixtures into numerous clusters of reduced complexity. Separation of Dvl3-based signalsomes was established by SEC for the first time. Cell lysates prepared from cells stimulated with or without Wnt3a were subjected to size-exclusion column chromatography. This high-pressure column (very long and well packed, HiLoad Superdex TM 200 prep grade 26/60) permitted high resolution over a M_r range of 43 kDa to ~2.0 MegaDa (i.e., 2,000,000 daltons). The operation was carried out with AKTA system (GE Healthcare). Molecular weight standards showed excellent and reproducible peak separation. The identified peaks are, discrete and highly reproducible M_r (fig. 6A). Thus size-exclusion column chromatography allows separation of Dvls-based supermolecular complexes for a reproducibly and accurate. Individual fractions were subjected to SDS-PAGE and analyzed by immunoblotting with isoform-specific antibodies. Dvl2, the major isoform of Dvls in F9 cell (>95%), displayed two major peaks (one with a peak M_r of ~1.6 MegaDa, and other centered around 0.5 MegaDa-M_r), and a minor peak (~80 kDa of M_r), likely a monomeric Dvl2. Dvl1 revealed the two similar high-M_r supermolecular forms of 1.6 and 0.5 MegaDa-M_r. In contrast, Dvl3 supermolecular complexes appeared a broad peak and the M_r of the resolved complexes spanning from the homodimeric Dvl3 (150-210 kDa) to the well-defined peaks with M_r from 0.8 to 2.0 MegaDa (fig. 6B). All three Dvls isoforms migrated to ~ 2 MegaDa regions without Wnt stimulation. GSK3β and Axin, components of the Dvls-based supermolecular complexes, also migrated to similar positions (Yokoyama et al., 2010).

2.3.3 Wnt stimulation provokes assembly of dynamic Dvl3-based supermolecular complexes

To address the functional significance of Dvls-based supermolecular complexes, we investigated whether their formation was regulated by Wnt3a stimulation. As seen in fig. 7A and 7B, Wnt3a provoked a dramatic shift in the apparent M_r of the Dvl3-based complexes to populations with sharply larger masses (>2.0 MegaDa-M_r). The abundance of Dvl3 based complexes (>2.0 MegaDa-M_r) was increased in a time-dependent manner (30min-60min after Wnt 3a stimulation) (fig. 7A and 7B). The upfield shift of Dvl3-based supermolecular complexes, derived at the expense of lower–M_r peaks, was detected as early as 5 min post-Wnt3a stimulation (unpublished data). In contrast, the shifts of other two isoforms, Dvl1 and Dvl2, to > 2.0 MegaDa-M_r were relatively small in response to Wnt. Dvl1/2-based complexes did not approach the limit size of those formed by Dvl3-based complexes. GSK3β and Axin also migrated with supermolecular complexes of increasing apparent mass (>2 MegaDa-M_r) in response to Wnt3a stimulation for 30 min (Yokoyama et al., 2010).

To ascertain whether mimicking Wnt3a action could result in the assembly of Dvl3-based supermolecular complexes, several distinct approaches were employed. The first approach is overexpression of Dvls. Assembly of Dvl3-based supermolecular complexes varied with the isoform of Dvls. It is known that overexpression of Dvl1 and Dvl3 in mouse F9 cells stimulated Lef/Tcf-sensitive transcription (Lee et al., 2008). Overexpression of Dvls provoked the formation of very large, Dvl3-based supermolecular complexes (fig. 7C), even larger than those observed in response to Wnt3a (fig. 7B). Overexpression of Dvl1 stimulated both activation of the canonical Lef/Tcf-sensitive transcription and an increase in the formation of the very large (>2.0 MegaDa-M_r) Dvl3-based supermolecular complexes

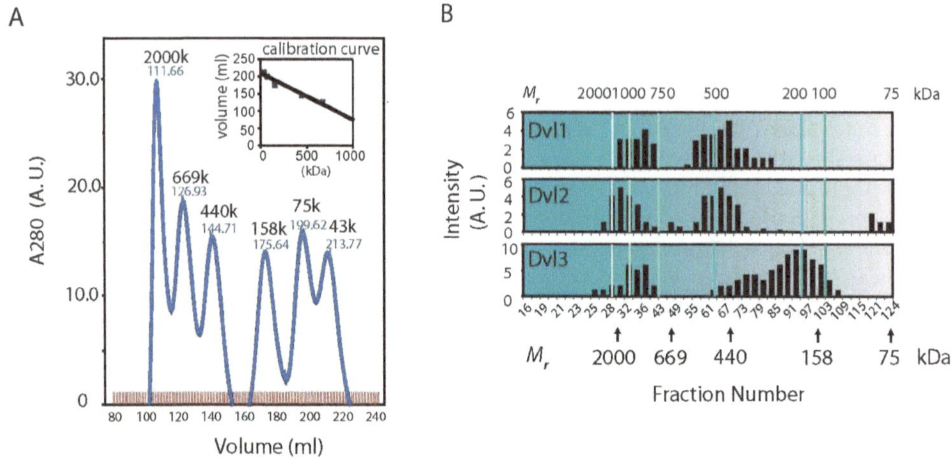

(A) Resolution of Superdex 200 column. Mixtures of molecular weight markers (Blue Dextran 2000, thyroglobulin, ferritin, aldolase, conalbumin and ovaalbumin) were applied to Superdex 200 column. The elution profile was monitored by absorbance at 280 nm.
(B) F9 cells expressing Rfz1 were disrupted and cell lysates were applied to the Superdex 200 column. Proteins were analyzed by SDS-PAGE and immunoblotted with Dvl isoform-specific antibodies. Blots were quantified by the calibrated scanner. The calculated, relative molecular weight (M_r) positions from the calibration curve are labeled at the top, fraction numbers on the bottom. Arrows indicate the precise position at which calibration proteins elute from the Superdex 200 column. Data are adapted with permission from the publication (Yokoyama, N., Golebiewska, U., Wang, H. Y. & Malbon, C. C. (2010) J Cell Sci 123, 3693-3702).

Fig. 6. Separation of Dvls-based supermolecular complexes using size-exclusion column chromatography.

(fig. 7C and Table 2). Overexpression of Dvl3 provoked a prominent activation of Lef/Tcf-sensitive transcription and a sharp increase in the formation of very large (>2.0 MegaDa-M_r) Dvl3-based complexes (fig. 7C and Table 2). In contrast, overexpression of the most abundant Dvl isoform (i.e., Dvl2 which constitutes >95% of Dvls in F9 cell) provoked only a modest Lef/Tcf-sensitive transcriptional response and little formation of the very large, (>2.0 MegaDa-M_r) Dvl3-based complexes (fig. 7C and Table 2). Thus, the formation of the very large Dvl3-based supermolecular complexes can be specifically mimicked by the overexpression of either Dvl1 or Dvl3, which can uniquely activate the Lef/Tcf-sensitive pathway in the absence of Wnt3a. Lef/Tcf-sensitive transcriptional activation (the hallmark of activation of Wnt/beta-catenin pathway) and the assembly of Dvl3-based supermolecular complexes were followed and summarized in Table 2. The second approach to mimicking Wnt stimulation is the expression of constitutively active mutant (CA-delta-N) LRP6. Expression of the constitutively active mutant of LRP6 (CA-delta-N-LRP6) resulted in Wnt stimulation (Tamai et al., 2004). Mimicking Wnt3a action (in the absence of Wnt3a) by CA-delta-N-LRP6 was performed. Overexpression of CA-delta-N-LRP6 likewise provoked formation of the very large, supermolecular Dvl3-based complexes, just like Wnt3a itself (Table 2). Conversely, expression of the dominant-interfering delta-C-LRP6 blocked the canonical pathway and also abolished the formation of Dvl3-based supermolecular complexes. Inhibition of GSK3β activity is a third approach. The chemical inhibition of

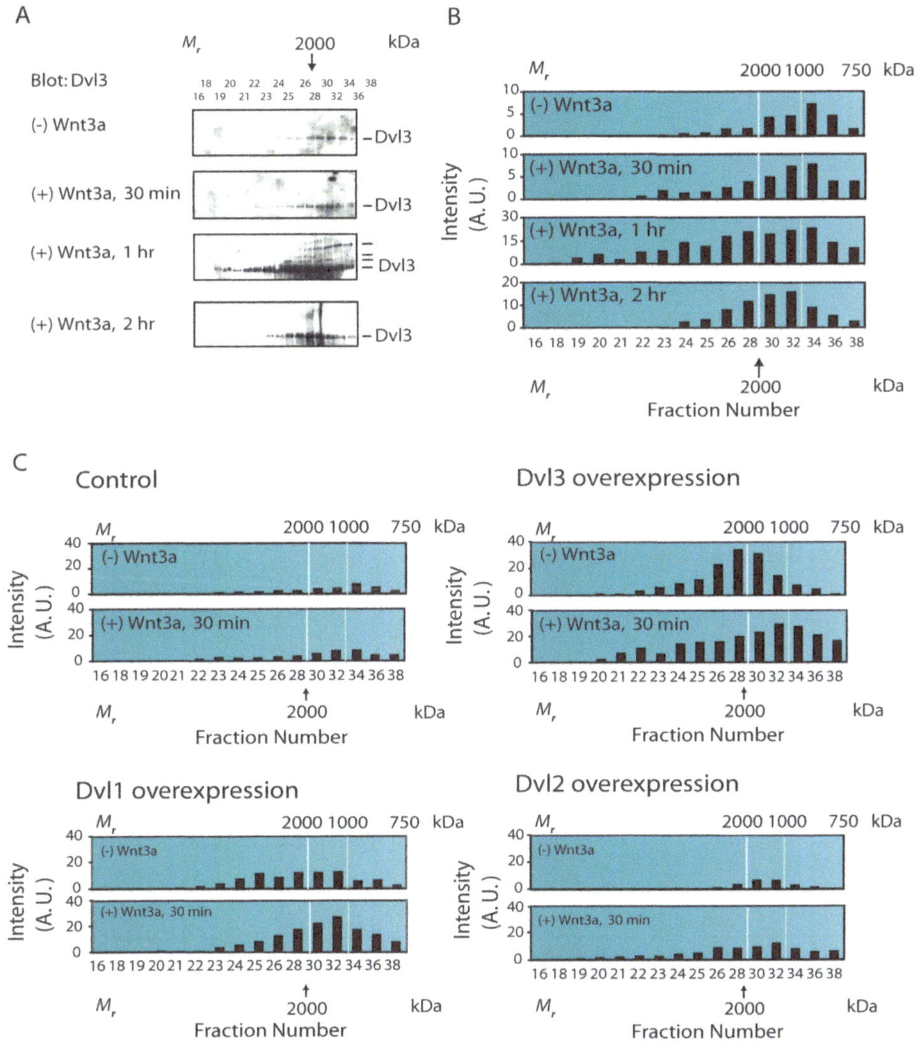

(A, B) Dvl3 assembles supermolecular multi-protein complexes in response to Wnt3a, in a time-dependent manner. F9 cells were stimulated with Wnt3a for the indicated times. Cells were lysed and subject to steric-exclusion chromatography on Superdex 200. Fractions were analyzed by SDS-PAGE and resolved proteins immunoblotted with isoform-specific Dvl antibodies. Dvl3 blot (A) and quantitative analysis of Dvl3 (B) in the region above 750 kDa-M_r.

(C) Overexpression of Dvls provoked formation of supermolecular Dvl3-based complexes without Wnt3a stimulation. F9 cells were co-transfected with Rfz1 and either GFP- and HA-tagged mouse Dvl1, or Dvl2 or Dvl3. F9 cells were either unstimulated or stimulated with Wnt3a for 30 minutes. Cells lysates were applied to Superdex 200 gel filtration column. Fractions were analyzed by SDS-PAGE. Resolved proteins were immunoblotted with anti-Dvl3 antibody and quantified. Data are adapted with permission from the publication (Yokoyama, N., Golebiewska, U., Wang, H. Y. & Malbon, C. C. (2010) J Cell Sci 123, 3693-3702).

Fig. 7. Assembly of Dvl3-based supermolecular complexes by Wnt stimulation and overexpression of Dvls.

GSK3β by LiCl stimulates Lef/Tcf-sensitive transcription (Stambolic et al., 1996). Inhibition of GSK3β provoked increased formation of the very large (>2.0 MegaDa-M_r) Dvl3-based supermolecular complexes (Table 2).

To define precisely roles of Dvl isoforms on the assembly of Dvl3-based supermolecular complexes, the effect of knockdown of each Dvl isoform was investigated (Table 2). Knockdown of each Dvl isoform resulted in attenuation of the assembly of Dvl3-based supermolecular complexes as well as Lef/Tcf-sensitive transcription. Knockdown of Dvl1 and Dvl3, lower abundance of Dvls in F9 cells, was more effective on both parameters. Knockdown of Dvl3 essentially precluded formation of the supermolecular complex in the absence or presence of Wnt3a. Knockdown of Dvl1 had little effect on the abundance of the basal Dvl3-based complex (i.e., without Wnt3a stimulation), but attenuated Wnt3a provoked formation of Dvl3-based supermolecular complexes (>2.0 MegaDa-M_r). Knockdown of the most abundant isoform Dvl2 severely reduced the abundance of the Dvl3-based complexes in the absence of Wnt3a. Wnt3a failed to stimulate the formation of supermolecular Dvl3-based complexes as well as activation of the canonical pathway. Thus, clearly Dvl1 and Dvl2 cooperate in catalyzing the formation of supermolecular, Dvl3-based complexes in either the absence or presence of Wnt3a. Finally, Dickkopf homologue 1 (DKK1), a well known Wnt antagonist (Nusse, 2001), blocked both activation of the Wnt canonical pathway and formation of very large, Dvl3-based supermolecular complexes (Table 2).

	(-) Wnt3a		**(+) Wnt3a**	
	Oligomerization	Lef/Tcf transcription	Oligomerization	Lef/Tcf transcription
Control	-	-	+	+
DKK1	-	-	-	-
delta-N-LRP6	+	+	+	+
delta-C-LRP6	-	-	-	-
LiCl	++	++	++	++
Dvl1 OE	++	++	++	++
Dvl2 OE	+	+	+	+
Dvl3 OE	+++	+++	+++	+++
Dvl1KD	+	-	±	-
Dvl2 KD	±	-	±	-
Dvl3 KD	-	-	-	-

OE: overexpression; KD: knockdown; Data are adapted with permission from the publication (Yokoyama, N., Golebiewska, U., Wang, H. Y. & Malbon, C. C. (2010) J Cell Sci 123, 3693-3702).

Table 2. Summary of Wnt activation and formation of Dvl3-based supermolecular complexes.

Thus, through targeted activation and disruption of Wnt3a signaling, a linkage between the ability to form very large (>2.0 MegaDa-M_r) Dvl3-based supermolecular complexes and the level of activation of Lef/Tcf-sensitive transcription (functional downstream signaling) was established. Unique rolls of Dvl3 in Wnt/β-catenin signaling demonstrate Dvl isoforms are not redundant with respect to function. Several key Dvl-interacting proteins (e.g., Dvl1, Dvl2, Dvl3, GSK3β and Axin) were present in these very large, Dvl3-based supermolecular complexes. Manipulations that provoked the formation of these Dvl3-based complexes also provoked activation of the Wnt/beta-catenin canonical pathway. Mutations of Dvl2 that block punctae formation inhibit the canonical Wnt signaling (Schwarz-Romond et al., 2007a). Dvl2/3 mutants, that do not form punctae, failed to assemble Dvl3-based supermolecular complexes (unpublished data). Phosphorylation-defective mutant of Dvl3 abolished assembly of Dvl3-based supermolecular complexes as well as activation of Wnt/beta-catenin signaling. On the other hand, Phosphorylation-mimetic mutant provoked both assembly of Dvl3-based supermolecular complexes and Lef/Tcf-sensitive transcription (unpublished data). The phosphorylation site was identified by CK1δ *in vitro* followed by proteomics. Data established that phosphorylation of Dvls is a crucial regulatory mechanism for the spatial/temporal assembly of dynamic supermolecular complexes to transduce Wnt signaling. Recent report provided compelling evidence that phosphorylation by CK1δ/ε sequentially regulates activation and de-activation of Dvls. Phosphorylated Dvls stimulate the oligomerization of Dvls, whereas the hyper-phosphorylated Dvls have less ability to oligomerize also form punctae (Bernatik et al., 2011).

2.3.4 Analysis of Dvl3-based supermolecular complexes by fluorescence correlation spectroscopy (*fcs)*

Fluorescence correlation spectroscopy (*fcs)* is used to probe the apparent size of the Dvl3- and Dvl2-based complexes in F9 cell. *Fcs* measurements were performed on a Zeiss LSM 510 Meta/Confocor 2 apparatus (Jena, Germany) fitted with a 40 × NA 1.2 C-Apochromat water immersion objective. *Fcs* of eGFP-tagged Dvl3 or Dvl2 in F9 cells was performed. In live cells the MW of Dvl3- and Dvl2-based supermolecular complexes was calculated. eGFP-tagged Dvl3 was tracked and the molecular weight calculated from the diffusion coefficients (Hess et al., 2002; Lakowicz, 2006; Schwille et al., 1999, Yokoyama et al., 2010). Two populations of eGFP-Dvl3 in unstimulated cells were obtained (Dvl3 dimers, i.e. ~132 kDa, and very large oligomers of ~35 MegaDa). Wnt stimulation slowed down the diffusion of the large complexes and increased the molecular mass of Dvl3-based complexes to ~40 MegaDa. The diffusion of the smaller complexes did not change in response to Wnt treatment. By sharp contrast, Dvl2-based complexes did not change molecular mass before and after stimulation with Wnt3a. This phenomenon is coinciding with those obtained by SEC. Wnt treatment resulted in increase of the mass of Dvl3-based supermolecular complexes, similar to those by SEC. The MW determined by *fcs* is much larger than that reported on the bases of SEC analysis with a Sephacryl S-400 column (HiPrep Sephacryl S400 high-resolution column 16/60, fast-performance AKTA liquid chromatography) (3-7 MegaDa-M_r). The size of Dvl3-based supermolecular complexes by SEC is reassessed and amended to 35 MegaDa, similar to those identified by *fcs* (Patel & Winzor., 2010).

2.3.5 Proteomic analysis of Dvl3-based supermolecular complexes in response to Wnt3a

Thus the assembly of Dvl3-based supermolecular complexes in response to Wnt stimulation is established. Next important questions are "What are the compositions in Dvl3-based supermolecular complexes?" and "How is assembly/disassembly of Dvl3-based complexes regulated?" Proteomic analysis was employed to dissect the compositions of supermolecular

Dvl3-based complexes. Over 3 MegaDa-M_r peak fractions of Dvl3-based supermolecular complexes separated by SEC from Wnt3a treated or untreated cells were subjected to LC-ESI-MS-MS. Dvl3-based supermolecular complexes (>3 MegaDa-M_r) isolated by SEC are distributed in a less populated region of the chromatogram (i.e., near void volume). Limited amount of proteins (~1% of total proteins) migrate to >3 MegaDa-M_r peak without Wnt stimulation. Wnt stimulation enhanced the abundance of these proteins 2-4 times in > 3 MegaDa-M_r region. The low amount of proteins in > 3 MegaDa-M_r region allowed executing proteomic analysis, although a main concerning of this application is potential contamination of proteins/complexes of M_r similar to that of the Dvl3-based supermolecular complexes. However, unrelated proteins/complexes (contamination) would not co-migrate with the Dvl3-based supermolecular complexes and also would not response to Wnt stimulation.

To minimize potential contamination, the analysis was carried out at distinct time points (0, 5, 10 and 30 min). By comparing the proteomic profiles from >3 MegaDa-M_r complexes with Wnt stimulation *versus* without Wnt stimulation, it will be possible to define the relative abundance of partners in >3 MegaDa-M_r peak in a Wnt- and time-dependent manner.

2.3.6 Proteomics of Dvl3-based supermolecular complexes

Pooled peaks (over 3 MegaDa-M_r) were subjected to TCA precipitation. Protein TCA pellets were resuspended in 10 μl of 8M urea, and diluted to 2M urea with 0.1M ammonium bicarbonate. The proteins were reduced with 5mM DTT and alkylated with 10mM iodoacetamide. 2 μg of trypsin was added to the proteins and incubated overnight at 37 °C. The digestion reaction was stopped with formic acid (5% final concentration).

Multidimensional chromatography was applied. Peptide mixtures were pressure-loaded onto a 250 μm inner diameter (i.d.) fused-silica capillary packed first with 3 cm of 5 μm strong cation exchange material (Partisphere SCX, Whatman), followed by 3 cm of 10 μm C18 reverse phase (RP) particles (Magic, Michrom). Loaded and washed microcapillaries were connected to a 100 μm i.d. column, which had been pulled to a 5 μm i.d. tip using a P-2000 CO_2 laser puller (Sutter Instruments), then packed with 13 cm of 3 μm C18 reverse phase (RP) particles (Magic, Michrom) and equilibrated in 2% acetonitrile, 0.1 % formic acid (Buffer A). This split-column was then installed in-line with Thermo Surveyor MS HPLC pump. The flow rate was ~500 nl/min. Fully automated 12-step chromatography runs were carried out. Three different elution buffers were used: 2% acetonitrile, 0.1 % formic acid (Buffer A); 98% acetonitrile, 0.1% formic acid (Buffer B); and 0.5 M ammonium acetate, 2% acetonitrile, 0.1% formic acid (Buffer C). In such sequences of chromatographic events, peptides were sequentially eluted from the SCX resin to the RP resin by increasing salt steps (increase in Buffer C concentration), followed by organic gradients (increase in Buffer B concentration). The last chromatography step consisted in a high salt wash with 100% Buffer C followed by acetonitrile gradient. The application of a 1.8 kV distal voltage electrosprayed the eluting peptides directly into a LTQ mass spectrometer equipped with a nano-LC electrospray ionization source. Full MS spectra were recorded on the peptides over a 400 to 2000 m/z range, followed by five tandem mass (MS/MS) events sequentially generated in a data-dependent manner on the first, second, third, fourth, fifth most intense ions selected from the full MS spectrum (at 35% collision energy). Mass spectrometer scan functions and HPLC solvent gradients were controlled by the Xcalibur data system (ThermoFinnigan).

Tandem mass spectra were extracted by RawXtract version 1.9.7. All MS/MS samples were analyzed using Sequest (Thermo Fisher Scientific). Sequest was set up to search a mouse IPI database (ver. 3.75), including reversed sequences (in total 113990 entries) assuming no specific protease. Sequest was searched with a parent ion tolerance of 1.5Da. Iodoacetamide derivative of cysteine was specified in Sequest as a fixed modification.
Scaffold (version Scaffold_3_00_08, Proteome Software Inc.) was used to validate MS/MS based peptide and protein identifications. Peptide identifications were accepted if they could be established at greater than 95.0% probability as specified by the Peptide Prophet algorithm (Keller et al., 2002). Protein identifications were accepted if they could be established at greater than 99.0% probability and contained at least 2 identified peptides. Protein probabilities were assigned by the Protein Prophet algorithm (Nesvizhskii et al., 2003). Proteins that contained similar peptides and could not be differentiated based on MS/MS analysis alone were grouped to satisfy the principles of parsimony.

2.3.7 Evaluation of compositions of Dvl3-based supermolecular complexes in response to Wnt3a

Data were normalized between distinct time points and positive identification was ascribed to a protein which had at least 30 unique fragments. Proteins, which abundance was changed during Wnt stimulation, were further analyzed. This strategy may identify other supermolecular complexes occurred in advance of Wnt signaling as well. Analysis of proteomics identified both expected and also novel components. Identified compositions of Dvl3-based complexes included protein kinases and phosphatases (serine/threonine and tyrosine), guanine nucleotide binding proteins, inositol phosphate related proteins, Wnt signaling related proteins and other signaling molecules.
Detected known Dvls interacting proteins are listed in Table 3. Presence of Dvls interacting proteins (17 distinct proteins) in the above ~ 3 MegaDa-M_r region strongly indicated these proteins may assemble with Dvl3-based supermolecular complexes.

Identified known Dvls interacting proteins	
PI4kinase	Ephrin B1
CK1γ	aPKC
Src	Par1
PTK7	Calpain
AP-2	Daam 1
Actin	CK1α
LRP6	CK2α
PP2A	CK2β
Ror2	

Table 3. Identified known Dvls interaction proteins.

Identified key molecules involving in Wnt signaling pathway include Rho, Gα family, Gβ1 and mTOR, and abundance of these proteins was changed after Wnt stimulation (Table 4).
Data represent the diversities and complexities of Wnt signaling pathways which Dvls are involved in. Proteomic analysis identified proteins related in the Wnt/β-catenin signaling pathway, but also proteins involved in the planar cell polarity (PCP) pathway, Wnt/Ca^{2+} pathway and other signaling pathway.

Wnt signaling related proteins	
Rho GTPase 2	mTOR
Gαi2	Gαi3
Gαs	Gβ1
Gα13	

Table 4. Identified Wnt signaling related proteins.

Many proteins such as PI4 kinase, CK1γ, Src, LRP6, PP2A, Par1, CK1α, CK2α and CK2β are important key molecules in Wnt/β-catenin signaling pathway and are already known Dvl interacting proteins. Wnt treatment quickly produces plasma-membrane-associated LRP6 aggregates (Bilic et al., 2007). CK1γ phosphorylates LRP5/6 in response to Wnt3a (Davidson et al., 2005). Phosphorylation of LRP5/6 promotes Axin recruitment (Davidson et al., 2005; Tolwinski et al., 2003; Zeng et al., 2005). PI4 kinase together with PI5K kinase enhances PIP2 production and stimulates clustering of Dvls and LRP5/6 receptor (Pan et al., 2008). To see whether key parameters in the Dvl3-based supermolecular complexes will change in response to Wnt stimulation, tentative analysis of these parameters was carried out, although these data are not precisely quantitative (fig. 8A and 8B). First key step after Wnt stimulation is the phosphorylation of LRP6 by CK1γ. The abundance of LRP in the Dvl3-based supermolecular complexes was increased two times 5 min post stimulation by Wnt3a and sustained over 30 min. The abundance of CK1γ in the Dvl3-based supermolecular complexes was increased 5 min post Wnt stimulation and peaked at 10min thereafter decreased (fig. 8A). Thus, similar migration of two components was obtained in response to Wnt3a. These time courses fit quite well to a previous report, which demonstrated that LRP6 starts coalescing into punctate structures at or below the plasma membrane within 15min Wnt stimulation. PI4 kinase, which is involved in the production of PtdIns (4, 5)P_2, dramatically increased 10 min post Wnt stimulation (fig. 8A). Data fits well with a previous report that significant PtdIns (4,5)P_2 formation was detected 15-30 min after Wnt3a stimulation (Pan et al., 2008). In contrast, proteins like actin did not change significantly upon Wnt stimulation. Many Dvls interacting proteins, which are involved in the Wnt/β-catenin signaling, CK1α, CK2α, CK1γ, PI4kinaae and Src migrated at >3 MegaDa-M_r region after 5-10min Wnt stimulation (fig. 8B). Previous data showed that Src docking to Dvl2 is increased after 5-10min Wnt stimulation and sustained for 45min (Yokoyama and Malbon, 2007). Changing of Src abundance in the Dvl3-based supermolecular complexes was matched to the previous finding. Furthermore, not all proteins found in >3 MegaDa-M_r region were increased during Wnt stimulation. Migration of Par1 was decreased upon Wnt stimulation (fig. 8B). Also proteins such as tubulin, HSP60 and 40S ribosomal protein in >3 MegaDa-M_r region were decreased upon Wnt stimulation. Together, migrations of proteins found in the Dvl3-based supermolecular complexes were responsive to Wnt stimulation temporally and some of them were correlated well, suggesting that results obtained by proteomic analysis represent proper variations of compositions.

Interesting observations are several proteins involved in the PCP pathway, Daam 1, PTK7, AP-2, Par1, Ephrin B1 and Rho GTPase, were also found in >3 MegaDa-M_r peak. Therefore, whether or not activation of PCP pathway would provoke assembly of Dvl3-based supermolecular complexes was investigated. Wnt5a has been classified as a non-canonical Wnt family member. Rat Fz2 (Rfz2) expressing F9 cells were stimulated with Wnt5a for 30 min and cell lysates were separated by SEC and further analyzed by immunoblotting with anti-Dvl3

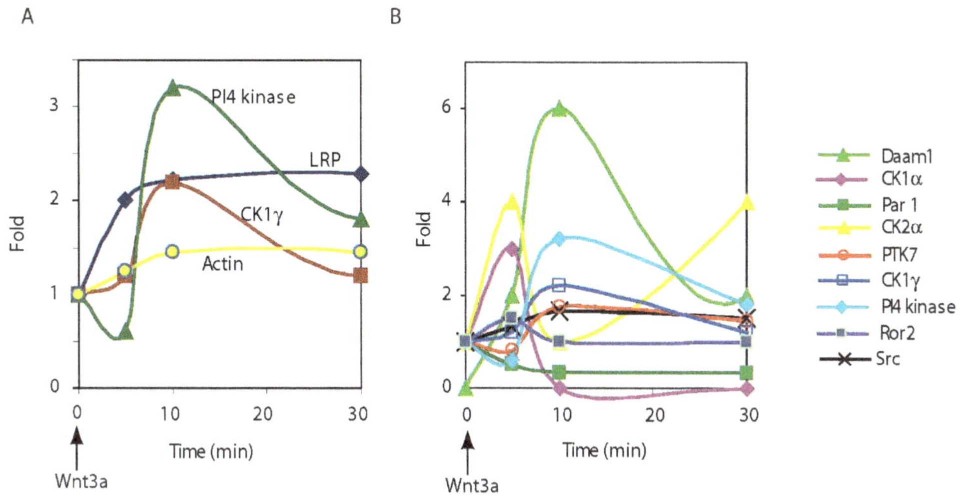

(A) Time courses of LRP, CK1γ and PI4K in >3 MegaDa-M_r peak. Changes of LRP, CK1γ, PI4K and actin in response to Wnt3a stimulation are displayed.
(B) Wnt3a responsive Dvls interacting proteins in >3 MegaDa-M_r peak are displayed.

Fig. 8. Time courses of key components presented in >3 MegaDa-M_r..

antibody. Indeed, assembly of Dvl3-based supermolecular complexes was detected in Rfz2 expressing F9 cell in response to Wnt5a, demonstrating Wnt5a-dependent assembly of the large complexes is provoked in the PCP pathway as well (fig. 9). PCP signaling is pivotal for establishing cell polarity and activation of PCP pathway leads to the activation of Rho-family GTPase and JNK through Dvls and Dishevelled-associated activator of morphogenesis 1 (Daam1) (Wallingford and Habas, 2005). Daam 1 bound to both Rho GTPase and Dvl, mediates Wnt-induced Dvl/Rho complex formation, which in turn activates Rho-associated protein kinase (ROCK) and remodels cytoskeleton (Habas et al., 2001). Daam1 is imprecated in cancer through its regulation of endocytosis of Ephrin B1 (Kida et al., 2007). Furthermore, proteomics also identified Ror2, which is involved in Wnt/Ca^{2+} pathway. Ror2 is a receptor tyrosine kinase. Wnt interaction with Fz and co-receptor Kyn or Ror2 provokes increase of intracellular Ca^{2+} level and subsequently activates calcium/calmodulin-dependent protein kinase II (CaMKII), protein kinase C (PKC) and nuclear factor of activated T cells (NFAT). Ca^{2+} is a central regulator of many cell functions and its downstream targets are numerous. Ror2 also shown as a receptor for Wnt5a, stimulating the non-canonical pathway (Oishi et al., 2003). In addition, Ror2 has a opposing role in the canonical signaling pathway and is able to inhibit Wnt/β-catenin signaling (Mikels and Nusse, 2006). Tyrosine kinase activity of Ror2 is indispensable for Wnt5a-induced inhibition of Wnt/β-catenin signaling (Mikels et al., 2009). Direct interaction of Ror2 with phosphorylated Dvl is required for the inhibition of Wnt/β-catenin signaling (Witte et al., 2010). Thus, Ror2 plays diverse roles in the discrete Wnt signaling pathways.

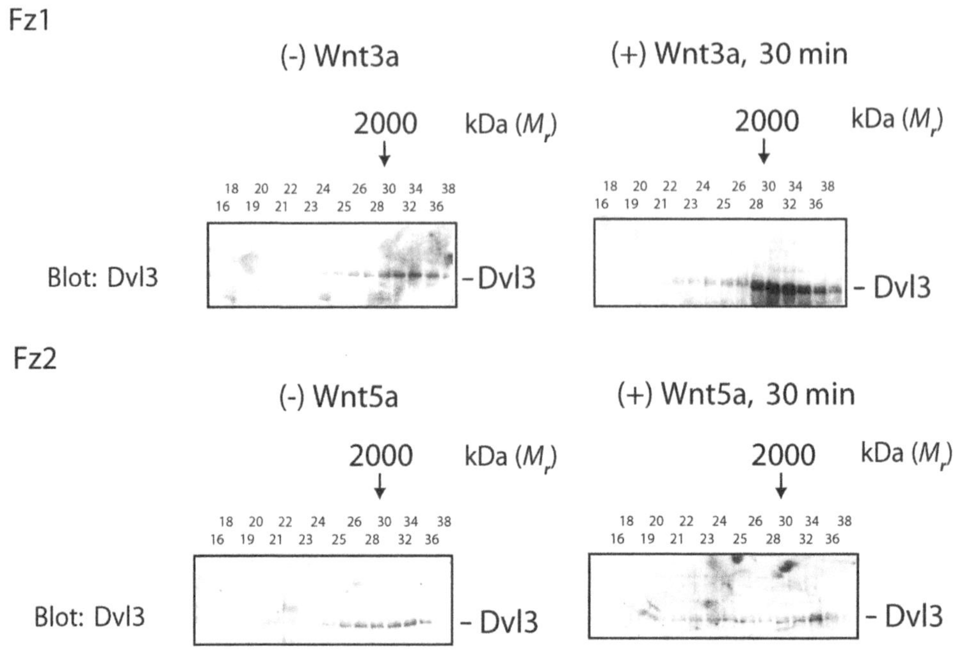

F9 cells expressing either Rfz1 or Rfz2 were stimulated with Wnt3a or Wnt5a for 30min, respectively. Cell lysates were subjected to the gel filtration chromatography and then fractions were analyzed by SDS-PAGE and blotted with anti-Dvl3 antibody. The regions above 750 kDa-M_r were shown.

Fig. 9. Dvl3-based supermolecular complexes are assembled in the PCP pathway.

Similarly, Par1 is discovered as a Dsh-associated kinase in *Drosophila* (Sun et al., 2001) and an essential for canonical signaling pathway, but also functions in non-canonical pathway (Wharton, 2003). Thus, certain molecules are involved in several distinct pathways. Presence of mammalian target of rapamycin (mTOR) in the >3 MegaDa-M_r region also demonstrates diversity of Wnt signaling pathways (Table 4), and supporting a previous finding that Wnt-mediated signaling activates mTOR mediated translational regulation in tumorigenesis (Inoki et al., 2006). Wnt activates mTOR via inhibiting GSK3 (Inoki et al., 2006) and the phosphorylation of tuberous sclerosis complex 2 (TSC2), a tumor-suppressor which negatively regulates mTOR, is suppressed (Mak et al., 2005). These data suggesting that Wnt signaling pathway is integrated to control mTOR activity (Choo et al., 2006).

G proteins found in the Dvl3-based supermolecular complexes are reasonable and expected one. Requirement of Gαo and Gαq in Wnt/β-catenin signaling was established earlier in F9 cell (Liu et al., 1999). Gα13, essential for the formation of the primitive endoderm, induces the activation of Rho protein, mitogen-activated protein kinase kinase (MEKK) and Jun-N-terminal kinase-1 (JNK1) in P19 embryonal carcinoma cells (Jho and Malbon, 1997; Lee et al., 2004). Gα13and Gαi family functions in development and deficiency of these G proteins causes embryonic lethality (Offermanns et al., 1997; Wettschureck et al., 2004). Novel classes of signaling proteins found in this large M_r peak included cAMP-dependent protein kinase, cell division protein kinase, Yes, Fyn, serine/threonine and tyrosine protein phosphatases, inositol 1, 4, 5-triphosphate receptor, phosphoinositide 3-kinase, phosphatidylinositol-4-

phosphate 3-kinase, AKAP 1 and 14-3-3. Many proteolytic targeting proteins including E3 ubiquitin-protein ligase NEDD4, Cullin 4B *etc.* were also found in >3 MegaDa-M_r peak, suggesting an important implication for Wnt-initiated tumorigenesis. Functional analysis demonstrated that Dvls stability is regulated by Cullin 3 ubiquitin ligase complex containing KLH12 (Angers et al., 2006). Some of them were identified by two distinct approaches (GST fusion pulls down and application of proteomics to Dvl3-based supermolecular complexes). Overall, the combined approaches of SEC and proteomics are successful to dissect Dvl3-based supermolecular complexes. Key Dvls interacting proteins, known functions in Wnt/beta-catenin signaling, present in >3 MegaDa-M_r peak, suggesting a compelling evidence that these proteins form complexes with Dvl3. Dvl3-based supermolecular complexes assemble at early stage and their compositions are dynamically changed during Wnt stimulation. Data agrees well with the fact that the size and localization of Dishevelled-based "punctae" have been changed upon Wnt stimulation observed earlier by fluorescence microscopy. Further segregation of unrelated proteins from the enriched Dvl3-based complexes, if possible, will be a benefit to analyze dynamic assembly of molecules central to the function of the Wnt/beta-catenin canonical signaling.

There are at least three major Wnt signaling branches, Wnt/β-catenin (canonical) pathway, PCP pathway (non-canonical) and Wnt/Ca^{2+} pathway. Proteomics in the >3 MegaDa-M_r region have identified proteins, which are involved in Wnt/β-catenin signaling pathway as well as the PCP and Wnt/Ca^{2+} pathways, suggest that these pathways may share a large signaling network. Wnt signaling pathways may not tightly isolate or share intracellular components between pathways. In this way, Wnt signaling pathways can cross talk with each other or other signaling pathways. Accumulated evidences show the cross talk between distinct Wnt pathways as well as other signaling pathways. Diversities of Wnt ligands and its receptors contribute to the complexities of Wnt signaling pathways. Distinct Wnt ligands can initiate discrete signaling pathways through its distinct receptors; however, signaling by different Wnt family members is not only intrinsically regulated by the Wnt proteins themselves, but also by receptor availability (cellular context of the receptor). Some Wnt ligand can bind to non-Frizzled receptor like Ror2 or RYK (an atypical Tyrosine kinase receptor) *etc.* RYK lacks a functional tyrosine kinase domain, but contains a module homologous to the Wnt-binding domain (Lu et al., 2004). Moreover, same Wnt ligand stimulates or inhibits distinct Wnt signaling pathways through its distinct receptors. Certain Wnt ligand activates the PCP and Wnt/Ca^{2+} pathways. Our SEC data demonstrate that Dvl3-based supermolecular complexes (~2 MegaDa-M_r) are assembling at the basal level (i.e., without Wnt stimulation) and Wnt stimulation provokes the upshift of molecular mass of Dvl3-based mutiprotein complexes. Data may suggest that without Wnt stimulation, Wnt signaling pathways may share fundamental platform of Dvls-based complexes, because Dvls are essential scaffold components in all three branches and transduce signals to distinct downstream pathways. In one way, we could say that distinct Wnt ligands provoke assembly of distinct multiprotein complexes. However, more detailed knowledge of the specificity of Wnt ligand and receptor, the receptor availability and protein components mediating signals to downstream are required to answer "How Dvls transduce signals to distinct Wnt signaling pathways?" and "How Wnt signaling integrates with other signaling pathways to form signaling network?" Dvls are a major player in Wnt signaling pathways and scaffold multiproteins to form the platform. Therefore, more precise analysis of protein compositions in the supermolecular complexes, not only Wnt/β-catenin signaling pathway as well as PCP pathway and Wnt/Ca^{2+} pathway, is required. Our data demonstrate that the assembly of Dvl3-based supermolecular complexes is provoked in the PCP pathway. Similar to the Wnt/β-catenin signaling, the molecular mass of Dvl3-based supermolecular complexes is upshifted in the response to Wnt5a. There is no information whether Dvls-based supermolecular complexes form in Wnt/Ca^{2+} signaling pathway. Comparison of proteomic profiles of Dvl3-based supermolecular complexes in the Wnt/β-catenin signaling *versus* the PCP pathway may provide a clearer image of signaling specific compositions of the supermolecular complexes. Precise regulations of Wnt signaling pathway by the Dvls-based supermolecular complexes are needed to analyze more widely in all branches. Advanced proteomic analysis of the Dvls-based supermolecular complexes with high-throughput screening offers an ideal strategy to interrogate the composition of Dvl3-based supermolecular complexes in the Wnt/β-catenin signaling pathway as well as in the non-canonical signaling pathway.

3. Conclusion

Dvls are scaffold proteins and Wnt signaling is transduced through the dynamic assembly/disassembly of protein complexes with Dvls called "signalsomes". Dvls-based supermolecular complexes provide a platform for recruiting many docking proteins and organizing dynamic assembly of proteins. Dvls-based punctae have been visualized by fluorescence microscopy and displayed dynamic protein assemblies. Proteomics of immobilized GST-domain pull down identified several novel and functional Dvl2 interacting proteins. Novel positive roles for Src family tyrosine kinases in Wnt/β-catenin signaling also have been established by GST-domain pull down and proteomics. Identification of tyrosine phosphorylation sites on Dvl2 leads to the discovery of the positive role of Src family kinases in Wnt/β-catenin signaling. Wnt stimulates Src docking to Dvl2 and activates Src tyrosine kinase. Activated Src enhances Wnt activation of the canonical pathway via phosphorylation of Dvl2 and β-catenin.

The physical nature and the dynamic character of the Dvl3-based supermolecular complexes have been established first time. The formation of these very large, supermolecular Dvl3-based complexes in response to Wnt3a is found to be a time-dependent manner and dynamic in character. The assembly of Dvl3-based supermolecular complexes (>3 MegaDa-M_r) occurred at very early stage (detected as early as 5 min post-Wnt3a stimulation) and maximized 30-60 min post-Wnt stimulation, in advances of the Lef/Tcf sensitive-transcription. Formation of very large Dvl3-based supermolecular complexes is essential in Wnt canonical signaling. Data demonstrate "punctae", Lef/Tcf-sensitive transcription (hallmark of activation of Wnt/beta catenin pathway) and dynamically assembled Dvl3-based supermolecular complexes are functionally obligate to Wnt signaling. The mass of very huge Dvl3-based supermolecular complexes reveals MW ranging from 25-35 MegaDa by *fcs*. Reassessed size of Dvl3-based supermolecular complexes is 35 MegaDa by SEC, similar to those obtained by *fcs*. This study demonstrates successful probing of signalsomes by SEC, *fcs*, affinity pull down and advanced proteomics.

Application of the proteomics in Dvl3-based supermolecular complexes provides physical properties of the assemblies. This approach is still experimental and challenging efforts, because cardinal concern is that Dvl3-based supermolecular complexes separated by SEC may contain unrelated proteins. Unsuccessful further separation of pure Dvl3-based supermolecular complexes is the barrier of this approach, because the size of the very huge

Dvl3-based complexes interfered with further purification. Immunoprecipitation might be a useful approach, although there are difficulties to precipitate very large complexes, because epitope sites in the supermolecular complexes are not fully exposed. Under these circumstances, employed proteomics in the Dvl3-based supermolecular complexes provide invaluable information to address "What are the compositions of Dvl3-based supermolecular complexes?" and "How is the assembly/disassembly of Dvl3-based complexes temporally and spatially regulated?" More detailed analysis of the Dvls-based supermolecular complexes in all three Wnt signaling pathways is necessary. Thus, compelling, albeit indirect, studies established the natures of Dvl3-based supermolecular complexes by advanced proteomics. Novel proteins found in Dvl3-based supermolecular complexes need to be validated with functional analysis *in vivo* and *in vitro*.

4. Acknowledgements

The author thanks Dr. Craig. C. Malbon (Department of Pharmacology, School of Medicine, Health Sciences Center, State University of New York at Stony Brook) for helpful discussions and support. The author thanks the staff of the Proteomics Center (State University of New York at Stony Brook) for mass spectrometry analysis. The author acknowledges the contribution of Dr. Weiping Xie (present address: Pioneer Hi-Bred International DuPont Agricultural Biotechnology) in the first half of proteomics work. The author also thanks Drs. Antonius Koller and Emily Chen for technical support in the proteomic analysis. The author acknowledges the contribution of Drs. Urszula Golebiewska and Hsien-yu Wang (Department of Physiology and Biophysics, School of Medicine, Health Sciences Center, State University of New York at Stony Brook) for *fcs* analysis.

5. References

Angers S & Moon RT. (2009). *Proximal events in Wnt signal transduction.* Nat Rev Mol Cell Biol 10:468-477.

Angers S, Thorpe CJ, Biechele TL, Goldenberg SJ, Zheng N, MacCoss MJ & Moon RT. (2006). *The KLHL12-Cullin-3 ubiquitin ligase negatively regulates the Wnt-beta-catenin pathway by targeting Dishevelled for degradation.* Nat Cell Biol 8:348-357.

Axelrod JD, Miller JR, Shulman JM, Moon RT & Perrimon N. (1998). *Differential recruitment of Dishevelled provides signaling specificity in the planar cell polarity and Wingless signaling pathways.* Genes Dev 12:2610-2622.

Bernatik O, Ganji RS, Dijksterhuis JP, Konik P, Cervenka I, Polonio T, Krejci P, Schulte G & Bryja V. (2011). *Sequential activation and inactivation of Dishevelled in the Wnt/beta-catenin pathway by casein kinases.* J Biol Chem 286:10396-10410.

Bilic J, Huang YL, Davidson G, Zimmermann T, Cruciat CM, Bienz M & Niehrs C. (2007). *Wnt induces LRP6 signalosomes and promotes dishevelled-dependent LRP6 phosphorylation.* Science 316:1619-1622.

Brown MT & Cooper JA. (1996). *Regulation, substrates and functions of src.* Biochim Biophys Acta 1287:121-149.

Cervenka I, Wolf J, Masek J, Krejci P, Wilcox WR, Kozubik A, Schulte G, Gutkind JS & Bryja V. (2011). *Mitogen-activated protein kinases promote WNT/beta-catenin signaling via phosphorylation of LRP6.* Mol Cell Biol 31:179-189.

Choo AY, Roux PP & Blenis J. (2006). *Mind the GAP: Wnt steps onto the mTORC1 train.* Cell 126:834-836.

Clevers H. (2006). *Wnt/beta-Catenin Signaling in Development and Disease.* Cell 127:469-480.

Coluccia AM, Vacca A, Dunach M, Mologni L, Redaelli S, Bustos VH, Benati D, Pinna LA & Gambacorti-Passerini C. (2007). *Bcr-Abl stabilizes beta-catenin in chronic myeloid leukemia through its tyrosine phosphorylation.* Embo J 26:1456-1466.

Cong F, Schweizer L & Varmus H. (2004). *Casein kinase Iepsilon modulates the signaling specificities of dishevelled.* Mol Cell Biol 24:2000-2011.

Davidson G, Wu W, Shen J, Bilic J, Fenger U, Stannek P, Glinka A & Niehrs C. (2005). *Casein kinase 1 gamma couples Wnt receptor activation to cytoplasmic signal transduction.* Nature 438:867-872.

Etheridge SL, Ray S, Li S, Hamblet NS, Lijam N, Tsang M, Greer J, Kardos N, Wang J, Sussman DJ, Chen P & Wynshaw-Boris A. (2008). *Murine dishevelled 3 functions in redundant pathways with dishevelled 1 and 2 in normal cardiac outflow tract, cochlea, and neural tube development.* PLoS Genet 4:e1000259.

Glass DA, 2nd & Karsenty G. (2006). *Molecular bases of the regulation of bone remodeling by the canonical Wnt signaling pathway.* Curr Top Dev Biol 73:43-84.

Habas R, Kato Y & He X. (2001). *Wnt/Frizzled activation of Rho regulates vertebrate gastrulation and requires a novel Formin homology protein Daam1.* Cell 107:843-854.

Habedanck R, Stierhof YD, Wilkinson CJ & Nigg EA. (2005). *The Polo kinase Plk4 functions in centriole duplication.* Nat Cell Biol 7:1140-1146.

Hamblet NS, Lijam N, Ruiz-Lozano P, Wang J, Yang Y, Luo Z, Mei L, Chien KR, Sussman DJ & Wynshaw-Boris A. (2002). *Dishevelled 2 is essential for cardiac outflow tract development, somite segmentation and neural tube closure.* Development 129: 5827-5838.

He X, Semenov M, Tamai K & Zeng X. (2004). *LDL receptor-related proteins 5 and 6 in Wnt/beta-catenin signaling: arrows point the way.* Development 131:1663-1677.

Hendriks WJ, Dilaver G, Noordman YE, Kremer B & Fransen JA. (2009). *PTPRR protein tyrosine phosphatase isoforms and locomotion of vesicles and mice.* Cerebellum 8:80-88.

Hess ST, Huang S, Heikal AA & Webb WW. (2002). *Biological and chemical applications of fluorescence correlation spectroscopy*: a review. Biochemistry 41:697-705.

Inoki K, Ouyang H, Zhu T, Lindvall C, Wang Y, Zhang X, Yang Q, Bennett C, Harada Y, Stankunas K, Wang CY, He X, MacDougald OA, You M, Williams BO & Guan KL. (2006). *TSC2 integrates Wnt and energy signals via a coordinated phosphorylation by AMPK and GSK3 to regulate cell growth.* Cell 126:955-968.

Jho EH & Malbon CC. (1997). *Galpha12 and Galpha13 mediate differentiation of P19 mouse embryonal carcinoma cells in response to retinoic acid.* J Biol Chem 272:24461-24467.

Karni R, Gus Y, Dor Y, Meyuhas O & Levitzki A. (2005). *Active Src elevates the expression of beta-catenin by enhancement of cap-dependent translation.* Mol Cell Biol 25:5031-5039.

Katanaev VL, Ponzielli R, Semeriva M & Tomlinson A. (2005). *Trimeric G protein-dependent frizzled signaling in Drosophila.* Cell 120:111-122.

Keller RA, Ambrose WP, Arias AA, Cai H, Emory SR, Goodwin PM & Jett JH. (2002). *Analytical applications of single-molecule detection.* Anal Chem 74:316A-324A.

Kida YS, Sato T, Miyasaka KY, Suto A & Ogura T. (2007). *Daam1 regulates the endocytosis of EphB during the convergent extension of the zebrafish notochord.* Proc Natl Acad Sci U S A 104:6708-6713

Kishida M, Hino S, Michiue T, Yamamoto H, Kishida S, Fukui A, Asashima M & Kikuchi A. (2001). *Synergistic activation of the Wnt signaling pathway by Dvl and casein kinase Iepsilon.* J Biol Chem 276:33147-33155.

Kishida S, Yamamoto H, Hino S, Ikeda S, Kishida M & Kikuchi A. (1999). *DIX domains of Dvl and axin are necessary for protein interactions and their ability to regulate beta-catenin stability.* Mol Cell Biol 19:4414-4422.

Kishida S, Yamamoto H, Ikeda S, Kishida M, Sakamoto I, Koyama S & Kikuchi A. (1998). *Axin, a negative regulator of the wnt signaling pathway, directly interacts with adenomatous polyposis coli and regulates the stabilization of beta-catenin.* J Biol Chem 273:10823-10826.

Lakowicz JR. (2006). *Plasmonics in Biology and Plasmon-Controlled Fluorescence.* Plasmonics 1:5-33

Lee YN, Gao Y, Wang HY. 2008. Differential mediation of the Wnt canonical pathway by mammalian Dishevelleds-1, -2, and -3. Cell Signal 20:443-452.

Lee YN, Malbon CC & Wang HY. (2004). *G alpha 13 signals via p115RhoGEF cascades regulating JNK1 and primitive endoderm formation.* J Biol Chem 279:54896-54904.

Lijam N, Paylor R, McDonald MP, Crawley JN, Deng CX, Herrup K, Stevens KE, Maccaferri G, McBain CJ, Sussman DJ & Wynshaw-Boris A. (1997). *Social interaction and sensorimotor gating abnormalities in mice lacking Dvl1.* Cell 90:895-905.

Lilien J & Balsamo J. (2005). *The regulation of cadherin-mediated adhesion by tyrosine phosphorylation/dephosphorylation of beta-catenin.* Curr Opin Cell Biol 17:459-465.

Liu T, DeCostanzo AJ, Liu X, Wang H, Hallagan S, Moon RT & Malbon CC. (2001). *G protein signaling from activated rat frizzled-1 to the beta-catenin-Lef-Tcf pathway.* Science 292:1718-1722.

Liu T, Liu X, Wang H, Moon RT & Malbon CC. (1999). *Activation of rat frizzled-1 promotes Wnt signaling and differentiation of mouse F9 teratocarcinoma cells via pathways that require Galpha(q) and Galpha(o) function.* J Biol Chem 274:33539-33544.

Lu W, Yamamoto V, Ortega B & Baltimore D. (2004). *Mammalian Ryk is a Wnt coreceptor required for stimulation of neurite outgrowth.* Cell 119:97-108.

Mak BC, Kenerson HL, Aicher LD, Barnes EA & Yeung RS. (2005). *Aberrant beta-catenin signaling in tuberous sclerosis.* Am J Pathol 167:107-116.

Malbon CC. (2005). *G proteins in development.* Nat Rev Mol Cell Biol 6:689-701.

McKay RM, Peters JM & Graff JM. (2001). *The casein kinase I family in Wnt signaling.* Dev Biol 235:388-396.

Mikels A, Minami Y & Nusse R. (2009). *Ror2 receptor requires tyrosine kinase activity to mediate Wnt5A signaling. J Biol Chem 284:30167-30176*

Mikels AJ & Nusse R. (2006). *Purified Wnt5a protein activates or inhibits beta-catenin-TCF signaling depending on receptor context.* PLoS Biol 4:e115.

Miller WT. (2003). *Determinants of substrate recognition in nonreceptor tyrosine kinases.* Acc Chem Res 36:393-400.

Nesvizhskii AI, Keller A, Kolker E & Aebersold R. (2003). *A statistical model for identifying proteins by tandem mass spectrometry.* Anal Chem 75:4646-4658.

Nusse R. (2001). *Developmental biology. Making head or tail of Dickkopf.* Nature 411:255-256.

Nusse R. (2005). *Wnt signaling in disease and in development.* Cell Res 15:28-32.

Offermanns S, Mancino V, Revel JP & Simon MI. (1997). *Vascular system defects and impaired cell chemokinesis as a result of Galpha13 deficiency.* Science 275:533-536.

Oishi I, Suzuki H, Onishi N, Takada R, Kani S, Ohkawara B, Koshida I, Suzuki K, Yamada G, Schwabe GC, Mundlos S, Shibuya H, Takada S & Minami Y. (2003). *The receptor tyrosine kinase Ror2 is involved in non-canonical Wnt5a/JNK signalling pathway.* Genes Cells 8:645-654.

Pan W, Choi SC, Wang H, Qin Y, Volpicelli-Daley L, Swan L, Lucast L, Khoo C, Zhang X, Li L, Abrams CS, Sokol SY & Wu D. (2008). *Wnt3a-mediated formation of phosphatidylinositol 4,5-bisphosphate regulates LRP6 phosphorylation.* Science 321:1350-1353.

Penton A, Wodarz A & Nusse R. (2002). *A mutational analysis of dishevelled in Drosophila defines novel domains in the dishevelled protein as well as novel suppressing alleles of axin.* Genetics 161:747-762.

Piedra J, Martinez D, Castano J, Miravet S, Dunach M & de Herreros AG. (2001). *Regulation of beta-catenin structure and activity by tyrosine phosphorylation.* J Biol Chem 276:20436-20443.

Porter M, Schindler T, Kuriyan J & Miller WT. (2000). *Reciprocal regulation of Hck activity by phosphorylation of Tyr(527) and Tyr(416). Effect of introducing a high affinity intramolecular SH2 ligand.* J Biol Chem 275:2721-2726.

Rapp UR, Gotz R & Albert S. (2006). *BuCy RAFs drive cells into MEK addiction.* Cancer Cell 9:9-12.

Rothbacher U, Laurent MN, Deardorff MA, Klein PS, Cho KW & Fraser SE. (2000). *Dishevelled phosphorylation, subcellular localization and multimerization regulate its role in early embryogenesis.* Embo J 19:1010-1022.

Roura S, Miravet S, Piedra J, Garcia de Herreros A & Dunach M. (1999). *Regulation of E-cadherin/Catenin association by tyrosine phosphorylation.* J Biol Chem 274:36734-36740

Schwarz-Romond T, Fiedler M, Shibata N, Butler PJ, Kikuchi A, Higuchi Y & Bienz M. (2007a). *The DIX domain of Dishevelled confers Wnt signaling by dynamic polymerization.* Nat Struct Mol Biol 14:484-492.

Schwarz-Romond T, Merrifield C, Nichols BJ & Bienz M. (2005). *The Wnt signalling effector Dishevelled forms dynamic protein assemblies rather than stable associations with cytoplasmic vesicles.* J Cell Sci 118:5269-5277.

Schwarz-Romond T, Metcalfe C & Bienz M. (2007b). *Dynamic recruitment of axin by Dishevelled protein assemblies.* J Cell Sci 120:2402-2412.

Schwille P, Haupts U, Maiti S & Webb WW. (1999). *Molecular dynamics in living cells observed by fluorescence correlation spectroscopy with one- and two-photon excitation.* Biophys J 77:2251-2265.

Seto ES & Bellen HJ. (2006). *Internalization is required for proper Wingless signaling in Drosophila melanogaster.* J Cell Biol 173:95-106.

Sicheri F, Moarefi I & Kuriyan J. (1997). *Crystal structure of the Src family tyrosine kinase Hck.* Nature 385:602-609.

Stambolic V, Ruel L & Woodgett JR. (1996). *Lithium inhibits glycogen synthase kinase-3 activity and mimics wingless signalling in intact cells.* Curr Biol 6:1664-1668.

Strovel ET, Wu D& Sussman DJ. (2000). *Protein phosphatase 2Calpha dephosphorylates axin and activates LEF-1-dependent transcription.* J Biol Chem 275:2399-2403.

Sun TQ, Lu B, Feng JJ, Reinhard C, Jan YN, Fantl WJ & Williams LT. (2001). *PAR-1 is a Dishevelled-associated kinase and a positive regulator of Wnt signalling.* Nat Cell Biol 3:628-636.

Swallow CJ, Ko MA, Siddiqui NU, Hudson JW & Dennis JW. (2005). *Sak/Plk4 and mitotic fidelity.* Oncogene 24:306-312.

Tamai K, Zeng X, Liu C, Zhang X, Harada Y, Chang Z & He X. (2004). *A mechanism for Wnt coreceptor activation.* Mol Cell 13:149-156.

Tolwinski NS, Wehrli M, Rives A, Erdeniz N, DiNardo S & Wieschaus E. (2003). *Wg/Wnt signal can be transmitted through arrow/LRP5,6 and Axin independently of Zw3/Gsk3beta activity.* Dev Cell 4:407-418.

van Amerongen R & Nusse R. (2009). *Towards an integrated view of Wnt signaling in development.* Development 136:3205-3214.

Wallingford JB & Habas R. (2005). *The developmental biology of Dishevelled: an enigmatic protein governing cell fate and cell polarity.* Development 132:4421-4436.

Wang J & Wynshaw-Boris A. (2004). *The canonical Wnt pathway in early mammalian embryogenesis and stem cell maintenance/differentiation.* Curr Opin Genet Dev 14:533-539.

Wellbrock C, Karasarides M & Marais R. (2004). *The RAF proteins take centre stage.* Nat Rev Mol Cell Biol 5:875-885.

Wettschureck N, Moers A & Offermanns S. (2004). *Mouse models to study G-protein-mediated signaling.* Pharmacol Ther 101:75-89.

Wharton KA, Jr. (2003). *Runnin' with the Dvl: proteins that associate with Dsh/Dvl and their significance to Wnt signal transduction.* Dev Biol 253:1-17.

Willert K, Brink M, Wodarz A, Varmus H & Nusse R. (1997). *Casein kinase 2 associates with and phosphorylates dishevelled.* Embo J 16:3089-3096.

Willert K, Brown JD, Danenberg E, Duncan AW, Weissman IL, Reya T, Yates JR, 3rd & Nusse R. (2003). *Wnt proteins are lipid-modified and can act as stem cell growth factors.* Nature 423:448-452.

Williams JC, Weijland A, Gonfloni S, Thompson A, Courtneidge SA, Superti-Furga G & Wierenga RK. (1997). *The 2.35 A crystal structure of the inactivated form of chicken Src: a dynamic molecule with multiple regulatory interactions.* J Mol Biol 274:757-775.

Witte F, Bernatik O, Kirchner K, Masek J, Mahl A, Krejci P, Mundlos S, Schambony A, Bryja V & Stricker S. (2010). *Negative regulation of Wnt signaling mediated by CK1-phosphorylated Dishevelled via Ror2.* Faseb J 24:2417-2426.

Wong HC, Bourdelas A, Krauss A, Lee HJ, Shao Y, Wu D, Mlodzik M, Shi DL & Zheng J.(2003). *Direct binding of the PDZ domain of Dishevelled to a conserved internal sequence in the C-terminal region of Frizzled.* Mol Cell 12:1251-1260.

Xu W, Harrison SC& Eck MJ. (1997). *Three-dimensional structure of the tyrosine kinase c-Src.* Nature 385:595-602.

Yanagawa S, van Leeuwen F, Wodarz A, Klingensmith J& Nusse R. (1995). *The dishevelled protein is modified by wingless signaling in Drosophila*. Genes Dev 9:1087-1097.

Yokoyama N, Golebiewska U, Wang HY & Malbon CC. (2010). *Wnt-dependent assembly of supermolecular Dishevelled-3-based complexes*. J Cell Sci 123:3693-3702.

Yokoyama N & Malbon CC. (2007). *Phosphoprotein phosphatase-2A docks to Dishevelled and counterregulates Wnt3a/beta-catenin signaling*. J Mol Signal 2:12.

Yokoyama N & Malbon CC. (2009). *Dishevelled-2 docks and activates Src in a Wnt-dependent manner*. J Cell Sci 122:4439-4451.

Zeng X, Tamai K, Doble B, Li S, Huang H, Habas R, Okamura H, Woodgett J & He X. (2005). *A dual-kinase mechanism for Wnt co-receptor phosphorylation and activation*. Nature 438:873-877.

11

Posttranslational Modifications of Myosin Light Chains Determine the Protein Fate

Virgilio J. J. Cadete and Grzegorz Sawicki
University of Saskatchewan, College of Medicine,
Department of Pharmacology
Canada

1. Introduction

The advances in proteomics over the last decade have made it possible for a more detailed study of protein posttranslational modifications. Posttranslational modification of proteins is an important signaling mechanism regulating vital pathways ranging from transcription to translation, in metabolism, cell survival, and cell death. Posttranslational modification of proteins has commonly been associated with the loss/gain of function and signal transduction with the concept of phosphorylation being the hallmark. However, many other posttranslational modifications of proteins have been detected and their implication to overall cellular homeostasis remains to be elucidated.

The cardiovascular system, in particular the heart due to its high metabolic rates, sensitivity to oxidative stress and necessity to adapt quickly to new environments, is an ideal candidate to the study of posttranslational modifications in physiology and pathology. Cardiac contractile function relies significantly on the integrity of its contractile apparatus, with the myosin light chains being important contractile elements. We have recently described the role of nitration and nitrosylation of ventricular myosin light chains (MLCs) on its degradation by the proteolytic enzyme matrix metalloproteinase-2 (MMP-2) (Doroszko et al. 2010; Doroszko et al. 2009; Polewicz et al. 2010). Using distinct experimental models of oxidative stress, such as hypoxia-reoxygenation or ischemia/reperfusion, we have detected pathological nitration and nitrosylation of MLC induced by oxidative stress. According to our findings, nitration and nitrosylation of MLCs is associated with an increased affinity for MMP-2 and a consequent increase in degradation of these proteins that is associated with a worsening in cardiac contractile function during either reoxygenation or reperfusion.

Since contractile dysfunction is a predictor of patient outcome (Antman et al. 2004), it is crucial to understand the mechanisms behind the development of contractile dysfunction. Moreover, the identification of mechanisms that lead to contractile dysfunction can help and result in the development of new therapeutic approaches aiming at preventing and/or treating contractile dysfunction following oxidative stress.

This review will focus on the current knowledge of posttranslational modification of myosin light chain, a cardiac contractile protein, and how these modifications contribute to protection or pathogenesis in the setting of cardiac injury and contractile dysfunction triggered by oxidative stress. Moreover, this review will deal with the importance of posttranslational modifications of proteins and its determination of protein fate.

2. Proteomics

The term "PROTEOME" (PROTEin complement to the genOME), introduced in 1994, has attracted great attention, as approximately 30,000 human genes correspond to several million different gene products (proteins, peptides). The genome is intrinsically static and basically the same in every cell type, while the proteome is highly dynamic, differs between cell types, and does all the work. Proteins are the most common diagnostic and therapeutic targets in medicine, and the search for the proteome may lead to the discovery of new diagnostic and therapeutic targets. Classical proteomics, or what is now referred as "expression profiling", is a process in which total cellular or tissue proteins are separated on 2D gels and the visible protein spots are identified by peptide mass fingerprinting (Dunn 2000; Pandey and Mann 2000). This approach has been used to generate extensive proteomics online databases containing protein data obtained from the hearts of animals with cardiovascular disease states (Arrell et al. 2001a; Arrell et al. 2001b; Evans et al. 1997; Scheler et al. 1999).

The field of proteomics has its roots in the marriage between 2D electrophoresis and mass spectrometry. In most cases, 2-dimensional electrophoresis is used to separate individual proteins and their modified forms, which are then identified and further characterized/analyzed by mass spectrometry. To date, proteomics has identified changes in more than 40 proteins in heart diseases such as dilated cardiomyopathy, varying degrees of I/R injury, and heart failure (Arrell et al. 2001a; Corbett et al. 1998; Foster and Van Eyk 1999; Jager et al. 2002; Jiang et al. 2001; Schwertz et al. 2002).

Proteomics is an ideal approach to elucidate PTMs associated with kinase activity. Positive and negative modulation of heart contractility by short-term phosphorylation reactions at multiple sites in MLC2, TnI, TnT, α-tropomyosin, and myosin binding protein-C, have been known for almost a decade (Schaub et al. 1998). An example of this modification is the discovery of novel phosphorylation of MLC1 in preconditioned cardiomyocytes (Arrell et al. 2001a). However, the role of this PTM is not known. Phosphorylation of MLC1 was also detected in congestive heart failure (CHF) and this was associated with a decreased sensitivity to 8-Br-cGMP-mediated smooth muscle relaxation (Karim et al. 2004). Similarly, three different PTMs were found in functionally important N-terminal sites of MLC2, two occurred in normal hearts (phosphorylation and deamidation) and one (n-terminal truncation) was associated with I/R injury (White et al. 2003). We have found the same PTMs in MLC1 in our model IR with the exception that phosphorylation and deamidation were associated with truncated forms of MLC1. Thus, the use of the proteomics approach to investigate mechanisms underlying heart disease should result in the generation of new therapeutic strategies and the establishment of precise and sensitive diagnostic markers. A schematic representation of a proteomic workflow is given in figure 1.

2.1 Methodology used in the study of myosin light chains posttranslational modifications

Although new advances have been made recently in the development of new technology for protein separation, the proteomic method relies significantly on 2-dimensional electrophoresis (2-DE) for protein separation for further analysis by mass spectrometry. One of the early limitations of the use of 2-DE for sample generation for mass spectrometry analysis was reproducibility. The problem was generated by the fact that gradient gels are difficult to cast consistently and only 2 gels could be run simultaneously. Recent

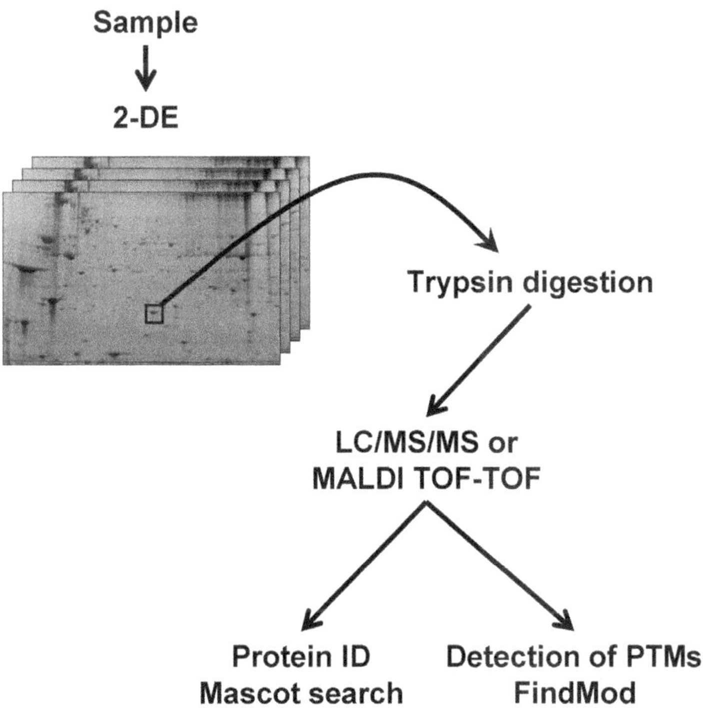

Fig. 1. Schematic representation of a proteomic method workflow. Samples are loaded and separated using 2-dimensional eletrophoresis (2-DE). Following 2-DE, protein spots of interest are identified and subjected to in-gel tryptic digestion followed by a mass spectrometry protocol (typically LC/MS/MS or MALDI TOF-TOF). Data generated from mass spectrometry can be used to identify the protein using the Mascot search database or, after protein identification, for detection of posttranslational modifications (PTMs) using the ExPASy-FindMod tool (http://web.expasy.org/findmod/findmod_masses.html).

technological advances gave rise to commercially available pre-cast gels (Criterion pre-cast gels, BioRad, Hercules, CA, USA) and the development of dodeca electrophoresis systems allowing for the simultaneous run of up to 12 gels (Criterion Dodeca Cell, BioRad, Hercules, CA, USA). These advances were very important in the achievement of reproducibility of sample generation by 2-DE.

The majority of the results here described in terms of the study of posttranslational modifications of myosin light chain 1 and 2 were obtained using the following methodology as described by:

Protein samples for 2-DE were prepared by mixing frozen (-80°C), powdered heart tissue (40 to 60mg wet weight) with 200 μL rehydration buffer (8 mol/L urea, 4% CHAPS, 10 mmol/L DTT, 0.2% Bio-Lytes 3/10 [BioRad, Hercules, CA, USA]) at room temperature. Samples were sonicated for 2X5 seconds and centrifuged (10 minutes at 10,000g) to remove insoluble particles. Protein content of the heart extract in rehydration buffer was measured with the BioRad Bradford protein assay.

Protein samples (400 g) were applied to each of 11 cm immobilized linear pH gradient (5-8) strips (IPG, BioRad, Hercules, CA, USA), with rehydration for 16-18 h at 20°C.

Isoelectrofocusing was performed using the BioRad Protean IEF cell with the following conditions at 20ºC with fast voltage ramping: step 1: 15 min with end voltage at 250 V; step 2: 150 min with end voltage at 8000 V; step 3: 35 000 V-hours (approximately 260 min). Following isoelectrofocusing the strips were equilibrated according to the manufacturer's instructions. The second dimension of 2-DE was performed with Criterion pre-cast gels (8 - 16%) (BioRad). After separation, proteins were detected with Coomassie Briliant Blue R250 (BioRad). To minimize variations in resolving proteins during the 2-DE run, 12 gels were run simultaneously using a Criterion Dodeca Cell (BioRad, Hercules, CA, USA). Because of this limitation for 2-DE analysis we used 4 hearts from each group. All the gels were stained in the same bath and next scanned with a calibrated densitometer GS-800 (BioRad, Hercules, CA, USA). Quantitative analysis of MLC1 and MLC2 spot intensities from 2-DE were measured with PDQuest 7.1 measurement software (BioRad, Hercules, CA, USA).
MLC1 and MLC2 protein spots were manually excised from the 2-DE gel. These spots were then processed using a MassPrep Station (Waters, Milford, MA, USA) using the methods supplied by the manufacturer. The excised gel fragment containing the protein spot was first destained in 200 μl of 50% acetonitrile with 50 mM ammonium bicarbonate at 37°C for 30 minutes. Next, the gel was washed twice with water. The protein extraction was performed overnight at room temperature with 50 μL of a mixture of formic acid, water, and isopropanol (1:3:2, vol:vol). The resulting solution was then analyzed by mass spectrometry (MS). For electrospray, quadruple time-of-flight (Q-TOF) analysis, 1 μl of the solution was used. Liquid chromatography/mass spectrometry (LC/MS) was performed on a CapLC high-performance liquid chromatography unit (Waters, Milford, MA, USA) coupled with Q-TOF-2 mass spectrometer (Waters, Milford, MA, USA). A mass deviation of 0.2 was tolerated and one missed cleavage site was allowed. Resulting values from mass spectrometry (MS/MS) analysis were used to search against the NCBInr and SwissProt databases with Mammalia specified. We used the Mascot (www.matrixscience.com) search engine to search the protein database. Posttranslational modifications were determined using the ExPASy-FindMod tool (http://web.expasy.org/findmod/findmod_masses.html).

3. Cardiac contractile proteins

The heart is the central organ for the circulatory system and is responsible for providing an efficient flow of blood to the whole body in order to meet the metabolic demands of the organism by delivering oxygen and nutrients and, at the same time, removing metabolic waste. Often seen as a pump, the heart relies on the integrity of its contractile machinery in order to efficiently perform its function. The basic unit of contraction is the sarcomere. The sarcomere is constituted of thick and thin filaments that, during contraction, slide over each other leading to the shortening of the sarcomere and contraction. The thick filament is mainly constituted of myosin while the thin filament is mainly constituted of actin, tropomyosin, and troponins (Figure 2). The interaction between thin and thick filaments, the crucial component for the generation of a contractile force, occurs between actin and the myosin head.

3.1 Myosins

Myosin is a large complex molecule. It consists of two heavy chains, an □-helical tail, and four myosin light chains (Craig and Woodhead 2006; Dominguez et al. 1998; Rayment et al. 1993b). The heavy chains (myosin heavy chain, MHC) have the ATPase activity necessary to trigger sliding between filaments and the consequent contraction. The two light chains (myosin light chain 1 and 2, MLC1 and MLC2) confer stability to the myosin head and also have actin binding motifs. MLC1 is also referred to as the essential light chain (ELC) and is present in the hinge of the myosin head for stability purposes. MLC2 is also referred as regulatory light chain (RLC) and together with MLC1 forms the hinge region between the globular head and the α-helical tail of myosin.

The essential light chains (ELC) are expressed by three different genes (MYL1, 3 and 4) which give rise to four isoforms of ELC/MLC (Hernandez et al. 2007). The nomenclature adopted depends on the tissue expressed (ELC_a and ELC_v for atrium and ventricular ELC/MLC, respectively) or whether it is full or short MLC (MLC1 and MLC3 for long and short MLCs, respectively) (Hernandez et al. 2007). The nomenclature for myosin light chains is not always obvious and for this manuscript we will refer to MLC1 as the full length myosin light chain present in the sarcomeres of the ventricle.

It has been described that the amino terminus of MLC1 interacts with the carboxy terminus of actin during contraction (Andreev and Borejdo 1999; Efimova et al. 1998; Henry et al. 1985; Milligan et al. 1990; Miyanishi et al. 2002; Morano et al. 1995; Nieznanska et al. 1998; Nieznanska et al. 2002; Nieznanski et al. 2003; Timson et al. 1999; Trayer et al. 1987; VanBuren et al. 1994). This interaction of MLC1 with actin suggests an important role of MLC1 in the regulation of contraction. Indeed, selective removal of MLC1 from the myosin molecule resulted in a reduction of ~50% of the force generated (VanBuren et al. 1994).

The regulatory light chain (RLC), referred as MLC2 in this review, is involved, as the name suggests, in the regulation of contraction. In the heart, two isoforms are found: a ventricular specific ($MLC2_v$) and an atrium specific ($MLC2_a$) isoform (Collins 2006). MLC2, together with MLC1, contributes to the mechanical stability of the hinge of the head region of the myosin molecule. MLC2 has been better studied and characterized due to the fact that it can be phosphorylated. MLC2 phosphorylation under basal conditions has been demonstrated to regulate Ca^{2+}-dependent contraction (High and Stull 1980; Mizuno et al. 2008; Stull et al. 1980; Sweeney and Stull 1986).

In order for proper sarcomeric contraction, the myosin structure has to be stable and fine tuned. It is the role of the light chains, present in the hinge of the head region, to assure stability of the head region and fine tune contraction by regulating the interaction between MHC and actin.

4. Posttranslational modifications

Virtually all proteins are subjected to posttranslational modifications. In this text, posttranslational modification will refer to the addition of a chemical group to amino acid residue which has a biological functional. Mass spectrometry can be used to determine peptide masses belonging to the native protein. According to the mass of each peptide one can infer about the presence or absence of a posttranslational modification that has a unique mass signature. A useful tool in determining posttranslational modifications by using peptide masses is ExPASy-FindMod tool (available at http://web.expasy.org/findmod/findmod_masses.html). Up to date the available information from ExPASy-FindMod tool, shows seventy one groups of posttranslational modifications that can be detected from analysis of peptide mass fingerprints. Of these, phosphorylation is by far the most studied and well know, mainly due to the identification of enzymes mediating phosphorylation of protein residues: protein kinases.

Phosphorylation is commonly associated with signal transduction, the hallmark of signaling cascades mediated by kinases. Other posttranslational modifications have recently gained more attention, mainly due to the fact that they are associated with oxidative stress. Protein nitration and nitrosylation are common events occurring in cells subjected to oxidative stress. Contrary to phosphorylation, no enzyme has been described to mediate nitration and nitrosylation and these modifications are often seen as a non-enzymatic posttranslational modification dependent on the presence, identity and concentration of reactive nitrogen species. The role of protein nitration on cellular signal transduction pathways has been reviewed by Yakovlev and Mikkelsen (Yakovlev and Mikkelsen 2010). The authors conclude that the gathered evidence supports the notion of protein nitration being a specific reaction. Though not entirely clear, it appears that nitration of protein residues by reactive nitrogen species is dependent on the tertiary structure of the protein and in particular the chemical environment of the tyrosin residues.

Due to the number of possible posttranslational modifications currently identified and the fact that the same posttranslational modification can occur in different amino acids, it is clear that the study of posttranslational modifications of protein under physiological and pathological conditions is a difficult task. Moreover, posttranslational modifications are not isolated reactions. A protein molecule present in physiological or pathological conditions may have more than one posttranslational modification. Also, the same protein can exhibit different types of posttranslational modifications at one time. Hence, the study of posttranslational modifications of proteins is difficult but also of high importance due to the nature of physiological and pathological consequences these modifications often cause. Also of importance is the fact that the study of posttranslational modification of cardiac contractile proteins can result in the identification of disease-specific markers of heart injury, hence contributing to the development of more sensitive and specific biomarkers of heart injury.

4.1 Biomarkers of heart injury

A biomarker is defined as a reproducibly detectable molecular feature, usually present in an accessible bodily fluid or tissue, that is correlated with a disease state. Cardiac enzymes have long been used as front-line diagnostic tools in the detection of myocardial injury caused by myocardial ischemia. However, the most commonly used enzymes (such as creatine kinase (CK) and its myocardial fraction CK myocardial band (MB), aspartic aminotransferase, and lactate dehydrogenase) are limited in their ability to detect myocardial injury by short diagnosis windows, have limited sensitivities, and lack specificity because of their presence in skeletal muscle. Similarly, myoglobin also lacks specificity because its release from skeletal muscle cannot be distinguished from its release from the heart muscle (Christenson and Azzazy 1998). Thus, there is a need to develop novel biomarkers in order to more effectively treat and diagnose myocardial infarction (MI). Using the proteomics approach a time-dependent increase of TnI in the serum from patients with MI was reported (Labugger et al. 2000). This new finding led to the suggestion that MLC1, as a contractile protein, could be considered as a new protein biomarker in I/R injury of the heart (Lee and Vasan 2005; Sato et al. 2004). The list of biomarkers in cardiovascular diseases will grow, particularly when the proteomics approach is used. This method has already identified 177 different proteins (including their different molecular forms) with the potential to be good candidates as biomarkers (Anderson 2005) in cardiovascular disease such as stroke.

4.2 MLCs in heart injury

Muscles contract when filaments containing a molecular motor, myosin, pull against another set of filaments containing mainly actin. The source of energy for this directional movement is provided by the hydrolysis of ATP, which is catalyzed by myosin. Muscle myosin is a hexamer consisting of two heavy chains (MHC), two regulatory (or phoshorylatable) light chains (known as MLC2 or RLC) and two essential chains (known as MLC1, and alkali or ELC). The myosin heavy chain is an elongated molecule where more then 90% of the protein is a coiled coil tail formed by the two heavy chains. However, the N-terminus of MHC is globular and contains ATPase activity, the actin binding site, and MLC1 and MLC2 binding sites (Rayment et al. 1993a; Rayment et al. 1993b). The light chains from cardiac and skeletal muscles are not directly involved in the regulation of contraction. However, both MLC1 and MLC2 can exert a subtle modulatory effect.

The precise molecular basis for myocardial stunning remains unknown, but protein damage within the myofilament is a likely mechanism. It is almost certain that stunning is a multifactoral process. One potential target is ventricular MLC2, which via changes in its phosphorylation status, modulates contractile force generation arising from actin-myosin MHC interaction (the structure, function and malfunction of MLC2 have been reviewed by Szczesna, (Szczesna 2003)). Three years ago an Australian group, using an experimental protocol similar to ours, found changes in phosphorylation of MLC2 and showed how these changes are correlated with the function of stunned myocardium (White et al. 2003). In another model, involving pharmacologically preconditioned isolated cardiomyocytes, altered phosphorylation of MLC1 was also found, but the role of this modification is not yet known (Arrell et al. 2001a).

Not only does heart injury induce chemical modification of MLCs, but during acute congestive heart failure entire MLC molecules, or their degradation products, are released into the circulation (Goto et al. 2003; Hansen et al. 2002). Van Eyk and colleagues have shown that the release of degradation products of MLC1 to coronary effluent is positively correlated with the duration of ischemia (Van Eyk et al. 1998). And White and co-workers found that both to MLC1 and MLC2 are released into the effluent of ischemic hearts (White et al. 2003). There was no evidence as to what proteolytic enzyme could be responsible for MLC degradation or what molecular mechanism could account for the release of their products into the circulation. Our work on the degradation of MLC1 in I/R heart shows that MMP-2 is responsible (at least in part) for the degradation of this protein (Doroszko et al. 2009; Polewicz et al. 2010; Sawicki et al. 2005). Although, the mechanism of release is still unknown, it could result from a loss of cell membrane integrity. Despite the many unanswered questions about the molecular basis of I/R injury in the heart, cardiac MLC1 is becoming a very important candidate as a biomarker of heart injury.

4.3 Phosphorylation

Phosphorylation is a posttranslational modification that consists of the addition of a phosphate group to serine (Ser), threonine (Thr) or tyrosine (Tyr). The addition of the phosphate group to these amino acids is catalyzed by kinases. The currently described mechanism of phosphorylation is that it essentially works as a switch, turning the function the phosphorylated protein on or off. Other consequences of protein phosphorylation may involve subcellular localization of proteins, protein-protein interaction, and proteolytic degradation. In fact, our ongoing studies on role of posttranslational modifications in the development of cardiac contractile dysfunction implies that the phosphorylation of MLC1 during ischemia/reperfusion results in its increase degradation, possibly by MMP-2, contributing to ischemia/reperfusion injury.

Phosphorylation of MLC1 has been demonstrated previously (Arrell et al. 2001a) but it has been associated with stability of the myosin head. The authors reported phosphorylation of rat/human Thr 69/64 and Ser 200/194 or 195. Our unpublished data demonstrates that phosphorylation of MLC1 has direct implications in its degradation by MMP-2. We observed *in vitro* phosphorylation (by myosin light chain kinase) of human recombinant MLC1 at Thr127, Thr129 or Tyr 130, as well as Ser179 and Tyr186. In MLC1 from isolated rat hearts subjected to ischemia/reperfusion we observed six phosphorylated residues: Thr69, Thr77 or Tyr78, Thr132, Thr134 or Tyr135, Thr164, Ser184 and Tyr190. Our data suggests a physiological role for MLC1 phosphorylation of Thr69 and Thr132, Thr134 or Tyr135, since these phosphorylations are present in aerobic control hearts, with the remaining four phosphorylations being induced by ischemia/reperfusion (Table 1). The observed phosphorylations of MLC1 induced by ischemia/reperfusion resulted in an increased degradation of MLC1. In an unpublished *in vitro* study we observed that when MLC1 was phosphorylated by the myosin light chain kinase (MLCK), the affinity of MMP-2 for MLC1 was increased and this increase in affinity resulted in an increase in the degradation of MLC1. Taken together, these observations suggest a role for protein phosphorylation in the induction of proteolytic degradation, namely by MMP-2.

	Identified posttranslational modified residues	
Posttranslational Modification	MLC1	MLC2
Phosphorylation	*in vitro* (human recombinant)	
	Thr127/Thr129/Tyr130, Ser179, Tyr186	
	ex vivo (rat heart)	
	Thr69, Thr77/Tyr78, Thr132/Thr134/Tyr135, Thr164, Ser184, Tyr190	
Tyr nitration	*in vitro* (human recombinant)	
	Tyr73, Tyr130, Tyr185	Tyr152
	in vivo (piglet heart)	
	Tyr141	Tyr118, Tyr152
	ex vivo (rat heart)	
	Tyr78, Tyr190	
Cys S-nitrosylation	*in vitro* (human recombinant)	
	Cys67, Cys76	
	in vivo (piglet heart)	
	Cys138	
	ex vivo (rat heart)	
	Cys81	

Table 1. Identification of MLC1 and MLC2 protein residues subjected to posttranslational modification leading to protein degradation.

To our knowledge these are the first observations concerning phosphorylation of a target protein contributing to the direct proteolytic degradation of that protein. Since it is well known that during several distinct disease processes the activation of phosphorylation cascades occur we speculate that besides up- and down-regulation of protein activity, phosphorylation is responsible for signaling protein degradation contributing directly to the progression of the disease process.

4.4 Nitration and S-nitrosylation

Protein tyrosine nitration has been implicated in many pathological conditions and diseases such as inflammation, chronic hypoxia, myocardial infarction and diabetes among others (Blantz and Munger 2002; Brindicci et al. 2010; Donnini et al. 2008; Giasson et al. 2000; Jones et al. 2009; Kang et al. 2010; Koeck et al. 2009; MacMillan-Crow et al. 1996; Naito et al. 2008; Pacher et al. 2007; Pavlides et al. 2010; Pieper et al. 2009; Reyes et al. 2008; Reynolds et al. 2005; 2007; Smith 2009; Upmacis 2008; Zhang et al. 2010). However, a physiological role for protein tyrosine nitration should not be excluded. Not all the tyrosine residues in a protein are targets for nitration either *in vitro* or *in vivo*. Moreover, the observed nitrations of tyrosine very seldom coincide between *in vitro* and *in vivo* studies. Of importance is the fact that nitration of tyrosine residues is a selective process that appears to be under tight control, even though the exact mechanisms for the regulation of tyrosine nitration remain unknown.

Nitration of protein tyrosine residues (formation of nitrotyrosine) has been suggested to facilitate proteolysis of the nitrated protein (Yakovlev and Mikkelsen 2010). We have recently shown that the contractile proteins MLC1 and MLC2 (part of the thick filament of the sarcomere) are subjected to tyrosine nitration and cysteine s-nitrosylation in cardiac models of oxidative stress (Doroszko et al. 2010; Doroszko et al. 2009; Polewicz et al. 2010). Using an *in vivo* model of neonatal asphyxia in piglets we have shown that both MLC1 and MLC2 are significantly decreased following hypoxia-reoxygenation (Doroszko et al. 2010; Doroszko et al. 2009). Mass spectrometry analysis for nitration and nitrosylation revealed that MLC1 is S-notrosylated at Cys 138 and nitrated at Tyr 141. Interestingly, these residues are located at the positions P3 and P1′ of the cleavage site for MMP-2 and hypoxia-reoxygenation was associated with an increase in MMP-2 activity. Also, MLC2 from hearts subjected to hypoxia-reoxygenation was nitrated at Tyr 118 and Tyr 152, while no nitration was observed for the control group (Table 1). These data suggest a pathological role for MLC2 tyrosine nitration associated with hypoxia-reoxygenation. Using human recombinant mutant MLC2, in which the tyrosine residue is replaced with phenylalanine, (Y152F) the *in vitro* incubation with peroxynitrite as a nitrating agent resulted in the prevention of MLC2 degradation by MMP-2, with no nitration observed at position 152. These observations indicate that although MLC2 has two nitration sites, it is Tyr 152 that mediates the signaling of degradation by MMP-2. MLC1 was also studied in a model of isolated adult rat cardiomyocytes subjected to simulated ischemia. Mass spectrometry analysis revealed nitration of Tyr 190, consistent with what was observed in piglet hearts. However, the Cys in the P3 position of the MMP-2 cleavage site was not S-nitrosylated as observed in MLC1 from piglet hearts. Moreover, MLC1 from rat cardiomyocytes was also nitrated at Tyr 78 and S-nitrosylated at Cys 81. *In vitro* human recombinant MLC1 was nitrated by peroxynitrite (used as a nitrating agent) at Tyr 73 (corresponding to rat MLC1 Tyr 78) Tyr 185 (corresponding to rat MLC1 Tyr 190), Tyr 140 and S-nytrosilated at Cys 76 (corresponding to rat Cys 81) and Cys 67. *In vitro* nitrated and S-nitrosylated MLC1 was more susceptible to degradation by MMP-2.

These data support the concept of highly regulated nitration and S-nitrosylation of proteins previously suggested, even though the exact mechanism remains unknown. Moreover, not only these processes are highly specific, they are also tightly associated with pathophysiological consequences. In this case, nitration and S-nitrosylation of protein residues is associated with an increase in its degradation by the proteolytic enzyme MMP-2 both *in vitro* and *in vivo*.

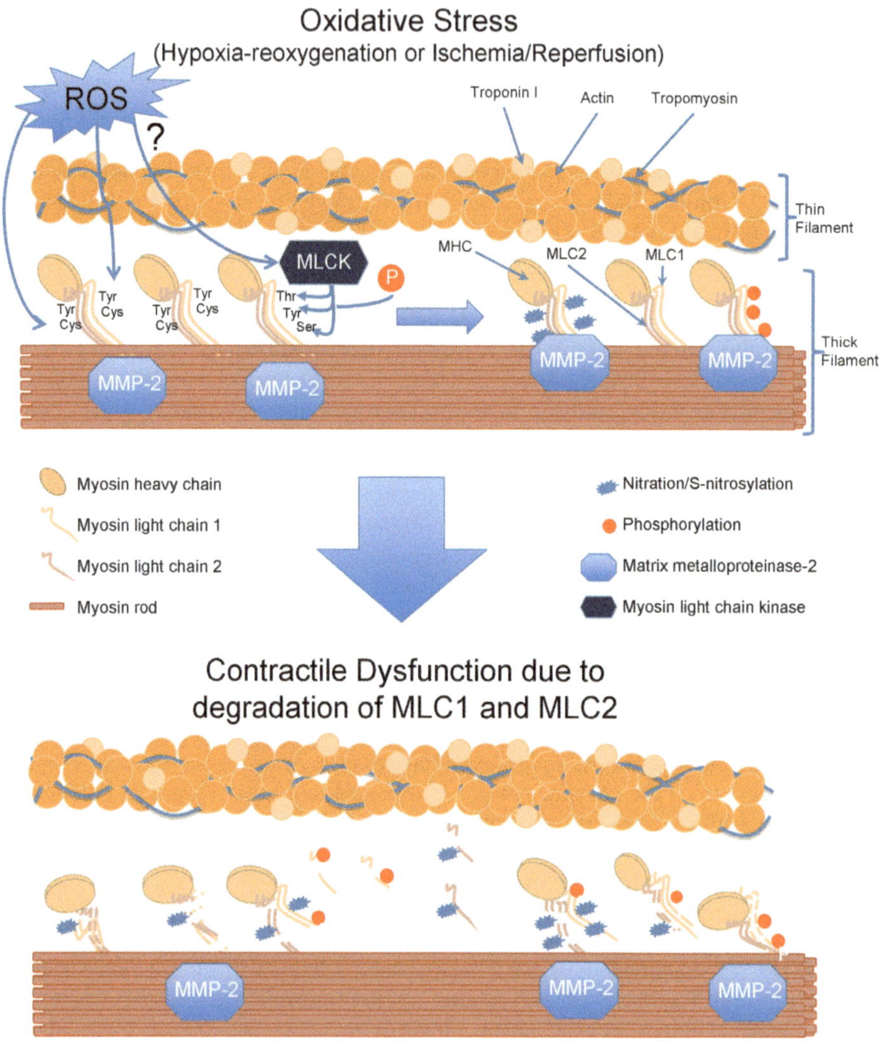

Fig. 2. Cartoon representation of our proposed model for regulation of contractile protein fate by posttranslational modifications. Reactive oxygen species (ROS) generated during ischemia/reperfusion or hypoxya-reoxygenation can lead to the direct nitration/S-nitrosylation of tyrosine and cysteine residues of MLC1 and MLC2. Also, ROS can lead to the phosphorylation of MLC1 and MLC2.

5. Conclusion

With the development of proteomics technology over the last two decades, more and more information about protein posttranslational modifications has been gathered. The difficulty of studying posttranslational modification of proteins and their physiological and pathological consequences lies on the fact that often (if not always) a protein will exhibit more than one type of posttranslational modification at any given time or more than one posttranslational modification of the same type.

Classically, enzymatic production of a certain product, from a given substrate, was limited by the enzyme activity. Also, posttranslational modification of the enzyme, such as phosphorylation, is a valid process to increase enzyme activity. We propose a new paradigm in the regulation of enzymatic activity by modification of proteins previously resistant to degradation. Here we have described the role of nitrosylation, nitration and phosphorylation of cardiac contractile proteins, as substrates for enzymatic reaction, in models of oxidative stress which result in their increased degradation by a proteolytic enzyme (MMP-2) both *in vitro* and *in vivo* (Figure 2).

It has been described that posttranslational modification of MMP-2 triggered by oxidative stress can activate the enzyme (Viappiani et al. 2009). Although this may be the case in the *in vivo* and *ex vivo* models, the same observations were made in *in vitro* experiments in which MMP-2 is not posttranslational modified. This new paradigm, that posttranslational modification determine fate of proteins, is an important advance in the understanding of the molecular mechanisms by which oxidative stress can trigger cardiac contractile dysfunction in pathological processes such as ischemia/reperfusion and hypoxia-reoxygenation. activation of MLCK and phosphorylation of MLC1. These posttranslational modifications increase the affinity of MMP-2 for MLC1 and MLC2. MMP-2 degrades MLC1 and MLC2 leading to cardiac contractile dysfunction.

6. Acknowledgements

We would like to thank Steve Arcand for the editorial contribution to this work. Also Jolanta Sawicka for the contribution in gathering the unpublished, ongoing data on phosphorylation of MLC1.

Virgilio J. J. Cadete is funded by the James Regan Graduate Scholarship in Cardiology from the College of Medicine, University of Saskatchewan.

Grzegorz Sawicki is a scholar of the Heart and Stroke Foundation of Canada and the Canadian Institutes of Health Research.

This project was funded by grants from Canadian Institutes of Health Research and the Saskatchewan Health Research Foundation.

7. References

Anderson, L. (2005). Candidate-based proteomics in the search for biomarkers of cardiovascular disease. *J Physiol* 563, Pt 1, (Feb 15 2005), 23-60.0022-3751 (Print) 0022-3751 (Linking)

Andreev, O. A. and J. Borejdo (1999). Binding of myosin cross-bridges to thin filaments of rabbit skeletal muscle. *Biochem Biophys Res Commun* 258, 3, (May 19 1999), 628-31.0006-291X (Print) 0006-291X (Linking)

Antman, E. M., D. T. Anbe, P. W. Armstrong, E. R. Bates, L. A. Green, M. Hand, J. S. Hochman, H. M. Krumholz, F. G. Kushner, G. A. Lamas, C. J. Mullany, J. P. Ornato, D. L. Pearle, M. A. Sloan, S. C. Smith, Jr., J. S. Alpert, J. L. Anderson, D. P. Faxon, V. Fuster, R. J. Gibbons, G. Gregoratos, J. L. Halperin, L. F. Hiratzka, S. A. Hunt and A. K. Jacobs (2004). ACC/AHA guidelines for the management of patients with ST-elevation myocardial infarction: a report of the American College of Cardiology/American Heart Association Task Force on Practice Guidelines (Committee to Revise the 1999 Guidelines for the Management of Patients with Acute Myocardial Infarction). *Circulation* 110, 9, (Aug 31 2004), e82-292.1524-4539 (Electronic) 0009-7322 (Linking)

Arrell, D. K., I. Neverova, H. Fraser, E. Marban and J. E. Van Eyk (2001a). Proteomic analysis of pharmacologically preconditioned cardiomyocytes reveals novel phosphorylation of myosin light chain 1. *Circ Res* 89, 6, (Sep 14 2001a), 480-7.1524-4571 (Electronic)

Arrell, D. K., I. Neverova and J. E. Van Eyk (2001b). Cardiovascular proteomics: evolution and potential. *Circ Res* 88, 8, (Apr 27 2001b), 763-73.1524-4571 (Electronic) 0009-7330 (Linking)

Blantz, R. C. and K. Munger (2002). Role of nitric oxide in inflammatory conditions. *Nephron* 90, 4, (Apr 2002), 373-8.0028-2766 (Print) 0028-2766 (Linking)

Brindicci, C., S. A. Kharitonov, M. Ito, M. W. Elliott, J. C. Hogg, P. J. Barnes and K. Ito (2010). Nitric oxide synthase isoenzyme expression and activity in peripheral lung tissue of patients with chronic obstructive pulmonary disease. *Am J Respir Crit Care Med* 181, 1, (Jan 1 2010), 21-30.1535-4970 (Electronic) 1073-449X (Linking)

Christenson, R. H. and H. M. Azzazy (1998). Biochemical markers of the acute coronary syndromes. *Clin Chem* 44, 8 Pt 2, (Aug 1998), 1855-64.0009-9147 (Print) 0009-9147 (Linking)

Collins, J. H. (2006). Myoinformatics report: myosin regulatory light chain paralogs in the human genome. *J Muscle Res Cell Motil* 27, 1, 2006), 69-74.0142-4319 (Print) 0142-4319 (Linking)

Corbett, J. M., H. J. Why, C. H. Wheeler, P. J. Richardson, L. C. Archard, M. H. Yacoub and M. J. Dunn (1998). Cardiac protein abnormalities in dilated cardiomyopathy detected by two-dimensional polyacrylamide gel electrophoresis. *Electrophoresis* 19, 11, (Aug 1998), 2031-42.0173-0835 (Print) 0173-0835 (Linking)

Craig, R. and J. L. Woodhead (2006). Structure and function of myosin filaments. *Curr Opin Struct Biol* 16, 2, (Apr 2006), 204-12.0959-440X (Print) 0959-440X (Linking)

Dominguez, R., Y. Freyzon, K. M. Trybus and C. Cohen (1998). Crystal structure of a vertebrate smooth muscle myosin motor domain and its complex with the essential light chain: visualization of the pre-power stroke state. *Cell* 94, 5, (Sep 4 1998), 559-71.0092-8674 (Print) 0092-8674 (Linking)

Donnini, S., M. Monti, R. Roncone, L. Morbidelli, M. Rocchigiani, S. Oliviero, L. Casella, A. Giachetti, R. Schulz and M. Ziche (2008). Peroxynitrite inactivates human-tissue inhibitor of metalloproteinase-4. *FEBS Lett* 582, 7, (Apr 2 2008), 1135-40.0014-5793 (Print) 0014-5793 (Linking)

Doroszko, A., D. Polewicz, V. J. Cadete, J. Sawicka, M. Jones, D. Szczesna-Cordary, P. Y. Cheung and G. Sawicki (2010). Neonatal asphyxia induces the nitration of cardiac myosin light chain 2 that is associated with cardiac systolic dysfunction. *Shock* 34, 6, (Dec 2010), 592-600.1540-0514 (Electronic) 1073-2322 (Linking)

Doroszko, A., D. Polewicz, J. Sawicka, J. S. Richardson, P. Y. Cheung and G. Sawicki (2009). Cardiac dysfunction in an animal model of neonatal asphyxia is associated with increased degradation of MLC1 by MMP-2. *Basic Res Cardiol* 104, 6, (May 19 2009), 669-79.1435-1803 (Electronic)

Dunn, M. J. (2000). Studying heart disease using the proteomic approach. *Drug Discov Today* 5, 2, (Feb 2000), 76-84.1878-5832 (Electronic) 1359-6446 (Linking)

Efimova, N. N., D. Stepkowski, H. Nieznanska and Y. S. Borovikov (1998). The shortening of the N-terminus of myosin essential light chain A1 influences the interaction of heavy meromyosin with actin. *Biochem Mol Biol Int* 46, 6, (Dec 1998), 1101-8.1039-9712 (Print) 1039-9712 (Linking)

Evans, G., C. H. Wheeler, J. M. Corbett and M. J. Dunn (1997). Construction of HSC-2DPAGE: a two-dimensional gel electrophoresis database of heart proteins. *Electrophoresis* 18, 3-4, (Mar-Apr 1997), 471-9.0173-0835 (Print) 0173-0835 (Linking)

Foster, D. B. and J. E. Van Eyk (1999). In search of the proteins that cause myocardial stunning. *Circ Res* 85, 5, (Sep 3 1999), 470-2.0009-7330 (Print) 0009-7330 (Linking)

Giasson, B. I., J. E. Duda, I. V. Murray, Q. Chen, J. M. Souza, H. I. Hurtig, H. Ischiropoulos, J. Q. Trojanowski and V. M. Lee (2000). Oxidative damage linked to neurodegeneration by selective alpha-synuclein nitration in synucleinopathy lesions. *Science* 290, 5493, (Nov 3 2000), 985-9.0036-8075 (Print) 0036-8075 (Linking)

Goto, T., H. Takase, T. Toriyama, T. Sugiura, K. Sato, R. Ueda and Y. Dohi (2003). Circulating concentrations of cardiac proteins indicate the severity of congestive heart failure. *Heart* 89, 11, (Nov 2003), 1303-7.1468-201X (Electronic) 1355-6037 (Linking)

Hansen, M. S., E. B. Stanton, Y. Gawad, M. Packer, B. Pitt, K. Swedberg and J. L. Rouleau (2002). Relation of circulating cardiac myosin light chain 1 isoform in stable severe congestive heart failure to survival and treatment with flosequinan. *Am J Cardiol* 90, 9, (Nov 1 2002), 969-73.0002-9149 (Print) 0002-9149 (Linking)

Henry, G. D., M. A. Winstanley, D. C. Dalgarno, G. M. Scott, B. A. Levine and I. P. Trayer (1985). Characterization of the actin-binding site on the alkali light chain of myosin. *Biochim Biophys Acta* 830, 3, (Aug 23 1985), 233-43.0006-3002 (Print) 0006-3002 (Linking)

Hernandez, O. M., M. Jones, G. Guzman and D. Szczesna-Cordary (2007). Myosin essential light chain in health and disease. *Am J Physiol Heart Circ Physiol* 292, 4, (Apr 2007), H1643-54.0363-6135 (Print) 0363-6135 (Linking)

High, C. W. and J. T. Stull (1980). Phosphorylation of myosin in perfused rabbit and rat hearts. *Am J Physiol* 239, 6, (Dec 1980), H756-64.0002-9513 (Print) 0002-9513 (Linking)

Jager, D., P. R. Jungblut and U. Muller-Werdan (2002). Separation and identification of human heart proteins. *J Chromatogr B Analyt Technol Biomed Life Sci* 771, 1-2, (May 5 2002), 131-53.1570-0232 (Print) 1570-0232 (Linking)

Jiang, L., M. Tsubakihara, M. Y. Heinke, M. Yao, M. J. Dunn, W. Phillips, C. G. dos Remedios and N. J. Nosworthy (2001). Heart failure and apoptosis: electrophoretic methods support data from micro- and macro-arrays. A critical review of genomics and proteomics. *Proteomics* 1, 12, (Dec 2001), 1481-8.1615-9853 (Print) 1615-9853 (Linking)

Jones, L. E., Jr., L. Ying, A. B. Hofseth, E. Jelezcova, R. W. Sobol, S. Ambs, C. C. Harris, M. G. Espey, L. J. Hofseth and M. D. Wyatt (2009). Differential effects of reactive nitrogen species on DNA base excision repair initiated by the alkyladenine DNA glycosylase. *Carcinogenesis* 30, 12, (Dec 2009), 2123-9.1460-2180 (Electronic) 0143-3334 (Linking)

Kang, M., G. R. Ross and H. I. Akbarali (2010). The effect of tyrosine nitration of L-type Ca2+ channels on excitation-transcription coupling in colonic inflammation. *Br J Pharmacol* 159, 6, (Mar 2010), 1226-35.1476-5381 (Electronic) 0007-1188 (Linking)

Karim, S. M., A. Y. Rhee, A. M. Given, M. D. Faulx, B. D. Hoit and F. V. Brozovich (2004). Vascular reactivity in heart failure: role of myosin light chain phosphatase. *Circ Res* 95, 6, (Sep 17 2004), 612-8.1524-4571 (Electronic) 0009-7330 (Linking)

Koeck, T., J. A. Corbett, J. W. Crabb, D. J. Stuehr and K. S. Aulak (2009). Glucose-modulated tyrosine nitration in beta cells: targets and consequences. *Arch Biochem Biophys* 484, 2, (Apr 15 2009), 221-31.1096-0384 (Electronic) 0003-9861 (Linking)

Labugger, R., L. Organ, C. Collier, D. Atar and J. E. Van Eyk (2000). Extensive troponin I and T modification detected in serum from patients with acute myocardial infarction. *Circulation* 102, 11, (Sep 12 2000), 1221-6.1524-4539 (Electronic) 0009-7322 (Linking)

Lee, D. S. and R. S. Vasan (2005). Novel markers for heart failure diagnosis and prognosis. *Curr Opin Cardiol* 20, 3, (May 2005), 201-10.0268-4705 (Print) 0268-4705 (Linking)

MacMillan-Crow, L. A., J. P. Crow, J. D. Kerby, J. S. Beckman and J. A. Thompson (1996). Nitration and inactivation of manganese superoxide dismutase in chronic rejection of human renal allografts. *Proc Natl Acad Sci U S A* 93, 21, (Oct 15 1996), 11853-8.0027-8424 (Print) 0027-8424 (Linking)

Milligan, R. A., M. Whittaker and D. Safer (1990). Molecular structure of F-actin and location of surface binding sites. *Nature* 348, 6298, (Nov 15 1990), 217-21.0028-0836 (Print) 0028-0836 (Linking)

Miyanishi, T., T. Ishikawa, T. Hayashibara, T. Maita and T. Wakabayashi (2002). The two actin-binding regions on the myosin heads of cardiac muscle. *Biochemistry* 41, 17, (Apr 30 2002), 5429-38.0006-2960 (Print) 0006-2960 (Linking)

Mizuno, Y., E. Isotani, J. Huang, H. Ding, J. T. Stull and K. E. Kamm (2008). Myosin light chain kinase activation and calcium sensitization in smooth muscle in vivo. *Am J Physiol Cell Physiol* 295, 2, (Aug 2008), C358-64.0363-6143 (Print) 0363-6143 (Linking)

Morano, I., O. Ritter, A. Bonz, T. Timek, C. F. Vahl and G. Michel (1995). Myosin light chain-actin interaction regulates cardiac contractility. *Circ Res* 76, 5, (May 1995), 720-5.0009-7330 (Print) 0009-7330 (Linking)

Naito, Y., T. Takagi, H. Okada, Y. Nukigi, K. Uchiyama, M. Kuroda, O. Handa, S. Kokura, N. Yagi, Y. Kato, T. Osawa and T. Yoshikawa (2008). Expression of inducible nitric oxide synthase and nitric oxide-modified proteins in Helicobacter pylori-associated atrophic gastric mucosa. *J Gastroenterol Hepatol* 23 Suppl 2, (Dec 2008), S250-7.1440-1746 (Electronic) 0815-9319 (Linking)

Nieznanska, H., K. Nieznanski, N. Efimova, I. Kakol and D. Stepkowski (1998). Dual effect of actin on the accessibility of myosin essential light chain A1 to papain cleavage. *Biochim Biophys Acta* 1383, 1, (Mar 3 1998), 71-81.0006-3002 (Print) 0006 3002 (Linking)

Nieznanska, H., K. Nieznanski and D. Stepkowski (2002). The effects of the interaction of myosin essential light chain isoforms with actin in skeletal muscles. *Acta Biochim Pol* 49, 3, 2002), 709-19.0001-527X (Print) 0001-527X (Linking)

Nieznanski, K., H. Nieznanska, K. Skowronek, A. A. Kasprzak and D. Stepkowski (2003). Ca2+ binding to myosin regulatory light chain affects the conformation of the N-terminus of essential light chain and its binding to actin. *Arch Biochem Biophys* 417, 2, (Sep 15 2003), 153-8.0003-9861 (Print) 0003-9861 (Linking)

Pacher, P., J. S. Beckman and L. Liaudet (2007). Nitric oxide and peroxynitrite in health and disease. *Physiol Rev* 87, 1, (Jan 2007), 315-424.0031-9333 (Print)

Pandey, A. and M. Mann (2000). Proteomics to study genes and genomes. *Nature* 405, 6788, (Jun 15 2000), 837-46.0028-0836 (Print) 0028-0836 (Linking)

Pavlides, S., A. Tsirigos, I. Vera, N. Flomenberg, P. G. Frank, M. C. Casimiro, C. Wang, P. Fortina, S. Addya, R. G. Pestell, U. E. Martinez-Outschoorn, F. Sotgia and M. P. Lisanti (2010). Loss of stromal caveolin-1 leads to oxidative stress, mimics hypoxia and drives inflammation in the tumor microenvironment, conferring the "reverse Warburg effect": a transcriptional informatics analysis with validation. *Cell Cycle* 9, 11, (Jun 1 2010), 2201-19.1551-4005 (Electronic) 1551-4005 (Linking)

Pieper, G. M., I. A. Ionova, B. C. Cooley, R. Q. Migrino, A. K. Khanna, J. Whitsett and J. Vasquez-Vivar (2009). Sepiapterin decreases acute rejection and apoptosis in cardiac transplants independently of changes in nitric oxide and inducible nitric-oxide synthase dimerization. *J Pharmacol Exp Ther* 329, 3, (Jun 2009), 890-9.1521-0103 (Electronic) 0022-3565 (Linking)

Polewicz, D., V. J. Cadete, A. Doroszko, B. E. Hunter, J. Sawicka, D. Szczesna-Cordary, P. E. Light and G. Sawicki (2010). Ischemia induced peroxynitrite dependent modifications of cardiomyocyte MLC1 increases its degradation by MMP-2 leading to contractile dysfunction. *J Cell Mol Med* 15, 5, (May 26 2010), 1136-1147.1582-4934 (Electronic) 1582-1838 (Linking)

Rayment, I., H. M. Holden, M. Whittaker, C. B. Yohn, M. Lorenz, K. C. Holmes and R. A. Milligan (1993a). Structure of the actin-myosin complex and its implications for muscle contraction. *Science* 261, 5117, (Jul 2 1993a), 58-65.0036-8075 (Print) 0036-8075 (Linking)

Rayment, I., W. R. Rypniewski, K. Schmidt-Base, R. Smith, D. R. Tomchick, M. M. Benning, D. A. Winkelmann, G. Wesenberg and H. M. Holden (1993b). Three-dimensional structure of myosin subfragment-1: a molecular motor. *Science* 261, 5117, (Jul 2 1993b), 50-8.0036-8075 (Print) 0036-8075 (Linking)

Reyes, J. F., M. R. Reynolds, P. M. Horowitz, Y. Fu, A. L. Guillozet-Bongaarts, R. Berry and L. I. Binder (2008). A possible link between astrocyte activation and tau nitration in Alzheimer's disease. *Neurobiol Dis* 31, 2, (Aug 2008), 198-208.1095-953X (Electronic) 0969-9961 (Linking)

Reynolds, M. R., R. W. Berry and L. I. Binder (2005). Site-specific nitration and oxidative dityrosine bridging of the tau protein by peroxynitrite: implications for Alzheimer's disease. *Biochemistry* 44, 5, (Feb 8 2005), 1690-700.0006-2960 (Print) 0006-2960 (Linking)

Reynolds, M. R., R. W. Berry and L. I. Binder (2007). Nitration in neurodegeneration: deciphering the "Hows" "nYs". *Biochemistry* 46, 25, (Jun 26 2007), 7325-36.0006-2960 (Print) 0006-2960 (Linking)

Sato, Y., T. Kita, Y. Takatsu and T. Kimura (2004). Biochemical markers of myocyte injury in heart failure. *Heart* 90, 10, (Oct 2004), 1110-3.1468-201X (Electronic) 1355-6037 (Linking)

Sawicki, G., H. Leon, J. Sawicka, M. Sariahmetoglu, C. J. Schulze, P. G. Scott, D. Szczesna-Cordary and R. Schulz (2005). Degradation of myosin light chain in isolated rat hearts subjected to ischemia-reperfusion injury: a new intracellular target for matrix metalloproteinase-2. *Circulation* 112, 4, (Jul 26 2005), 544-52.1524-4539 (Electronic)

Schaub, M. C., M. A. Hefti, R. A. Zuellig and I. Morano (1998). Modulation of contractility in human cardiac hypertrophy by myosin essential light chain isoforms. *Cardiovasc Res* 37, 2, (Feb 1998), 381-404.0008-6363 (Print) 0008-6363 (Linking)

Scheler, C., X. P. Li, J. Salnikow, M. J. Dunn and P. R. Jungblut (1999). Comparison of two-dimensional electrophoresis patterns of heat shock protein Hsp27 species in normal and cardiomyopathic hearts. *Electrophoresis* 20, 18, (Dec 1999), 3623-8.0173-0835 (Print) 0173-0835 (Linking)

Schwertz, H., T. Langin, H. Platsch, J. Richert, S. Bomm, M. Schmidt, H. Hillen, G. Blaschke, J. Meyer, H. Darius and M. Buerke (2002). Two-dimensional analysis of myocardial protein expression following myocardial ischemia and reperfusion in rabbits. *Proteomics* 2, 8, (Aug 2002), 988-95.1615-9853 (Print) 1615-9853 (Linking)

Smith, D. J. (2009). Mitochondrial dysfunction in mouse models of Parkinson's disease revealed by transcriptomics and proteomics. *J Bioenerg Biomembr* 41, 6, (Dec 2009), 487-91.1573-6881 (Electronic) 0145-479X (Linking)

Stull, J. T., D. R. Manning, C. W. High and D. K. Blumenthal (1980). Phosphorylation of contractile proteins in heart and skeletal muscle. *Fed Proc* 39, 5, (Apr 1980), 1552-7.0014-9446 (Print) 0014-9446 (Linking)

Sweeney, H. L. and J. T. Stull (1986). Phosphorylation of myosin in permeabilized mammalian cardiac and skeletal muscle cells. *Am J Physiol* 250, 4 Pt 1, (Apr 1986), C657-60.0002-9513 (Print) 0002-9513 (Linking)

Szczesna, D. (2003). Regulatory light chains of striated muscle myosin. Structure, function and malfunction. *Curr Drug Targets Cardiovasc Haematol Disord* 3, 2, (Jun 2003), 187-97.1568-0061 (Print) 1568-0061 (Linking)

Timson, D. J., H. R. Trayer, K. J. Smith and I. P. Trayer (1999). Size and charge requirements for kinetic modulation and actin binding by alkali 1-type myosin essential light chains. *J Biol Chem* 274, 26, (Jun 25 1999), 18271-7.0021-9258 (Print) 0021-9258 (Linking)

Trayer, I. P., H. R. Trayer and B. A. Levine (1987). Evidence that the N-terminal region of A1-light chain of myosin interacts directly with the C-terminal region of actin. A proton magnetic resonance study. *Eur J Biochem* 164, 1, (Apr 1 1987), 259-66.0014-2956 (Print) 0014-2956 (Linking)

Upmacis, R. K. (2008). Atherosclerosis: A Link Between Lipid Intake and Protein Tyrosine Nitration. *Lipid Insights* 2008, 2, (Nov 11 2008), 75.1178-6353 (Electronic)

Van Eyk, J. E., F. Powers, W. Law, C. Larue, R. S. Hodges and R. J. Solaro (1998). Breakdown and release of myofilament proteins during ischemia and ischemia/reperfusion in rat hearts: identification of degradation products and effects on the pCa-force relation. *Circ Res* 82, 2, (Feb 9 1998), 261-71.0009-7330 (Print)

VanBuren, P., G. S. Waller, D. E. Harris, K. M. Trybus, D. M. Warshaw and S. Lowey (1994). The essential light chain is required for full force production by skeletal muscle myosin. *Proc Natl Acad Sci U S A* 91, 26, (Dec 20 1994), 12403-7.0027-8424 (Print) 0027-8424 (Linking)

Viappiani, S., A. C. Nicolescu, A. Holt, G. Sawicki, B. D. Crawford, H. Leon, T. van Mulligen and R. Schulz (2009). Activation and modulation of 72kDa matrix metalloproteinase-2 by peroxynitrite and glutathione. *Biochem Pharmacol* 77, 5, (Mar 1 2009), 826-34.1873-2968 (Electronic) 0006-2952 (Linking)

White, M. Y., S. J. Cordwell, H. C. McCarron, A. S. Tchen, B. D. Hambly and R. W. Jeremy (2003). Modifications of myosin-regulatory light chain correlate with function of stunned myocardium. *J Mol Cell Cardiol* 35, 7, (Jul 2003), 833-40.0022-2828 (Print) 0022-2828 (Linking)

Yakovlev, V. A. and R. B. Mikkelsen (2010). Protein tyrosine nitration in cellular signal transduction pathways. *J Recept Signal Transduct Res* 30, 6, (Dec 2010), 420-9.1532-4281 (Electronic) 1079-9893 (Linking)

Zhang, L., C. L. Chen, P. T. Kang, V. Garg, K. Hu, K. B. Green-Church and Y. R. Chen (2010). Peroxynitrite-mediated oxidative modifications of complex II: relevance in myocardial infarction. *Biochemistry* 49, 11, (Mar 23 2010), 2529-39.1520-4995 (Electronic) 0006-2960 (Linking)

Part 3

Proteomic Approaches to Dissecting Disease Processes

12

Proteomic Study of Esophageal Squamous Cell Carcinoma

Yi-Jun Qi[1] and Jen-Fu Chiu[2]
[1]*College of Medicine, Henan University*
[2]*College of Medicine, Shantou University and University of Hong Kong*
P.R. China

1. Introduction

Comprehensive profiling of genome and transcriptome has identified myriads of alternations at the level of gene and gene expression, which drive malignant development and progression in context of oncology. As a result, qualitative or quantitative changes of protein expression pattern will inevitably ensue during multi-stage of carcinogenesis. In this sense, the proteome is a functional translation of the genome and is the actual manipulator of cellular behavior. Therefore, proteomic profiling of cellular protein constituents should generate the most relevant marker of the functional state of a cell. On the other hand, lack of correlation between mRNA and protein expression have been documented for a variety of genes. Unlike the genome which is static in certain sense, the proteome of a cell is dynamic and changes over time in terms of protein pattern, protein interactions and modifications triggered by external or internal signals[Kolch et al., 2004; Kolch et al., 2005]. Only dynamic information flow through protein circuitry reflects the course of a disease and allows us to track the pathogenetic mechanisms as well as treatment response[Kolch et al., 2005]. Furthermore, examining DNA sequences and measuring mRNA expression do not specify splicing, post-translational modifications, cleavages, protein subcellular localization and complex formations[Banks et al., 2000; Chambers et al., 2000]. There exists a huge information gulf between RNA transcription and protein expression. Proteome represents a much richer source for the functional description of diseases and the biomarker discovery implicated in cancer. Moreover, most of diagnostic assays currently applied in clinical practice are protein-based immunological methods, which are well adapted to standardization and clinical implementation. Proteomic profiling during disease formation and evolution not only provides an integrated understanding of pathogenesis in context of genome and proteome but also holds greater promise to identify the biomarkers of diagnosis and therapeutic targets for diseases such as cancer.

1.1 Epidemiology and etiology of ESCC

Accounting for more than 400,000 deaths per year, esophageal cancer (EC) ranks as the sixth most common cause of cancer-related mortality worldwide[Parkin et al., 2005]. Moreover, about half of world's EC cases newly diagnosed each year occurred in China[Holmes & Vaughan, 2007]. Histologically, esophageal squamous cell carcinoma (ESCC) and esophageal adenocarcinoma (EAC) contribute to more than 90% of EC[Daly et al., 2000]. In China, ESCC is the predominant histological subtype and account for nearly 90% of all EC[Li et al., 2011]. In developed countries, in contrast, EAC has been increasingly more frequent over the past two decades and has now surpassed the previously more predominant ESCC[Brown et al., 2008; Trivers et al., 2008]. The incidence of ESCC is characterized by its striking geographical distribution across the world. In the extremely high incidence areas, e.g. northern China, the incidence of EC exceeds 100/100 000/year, while the incidence is less than 5/100 000/year in Europe and the USA[Cheng & Day, 1996]. Heavy smoking and alcohol consumption are associated with increased risk of ESCC in developed countries[Brown et al., 2008; Messmann, 2001; Morita et al., 2010], but not major contributing factors in the pathogenesis of ESCC in China, where major risk factors include nutritional deficiency, consumption of pickled vegetables, dietary contamination with nitrosamine or mycotoxin, and low socioeconomic status[Kamangar et al., 2009; Yang et al., 1984]. In light of the poor nutrition status in Linxian, one of the highest incidence areas for ESCC in the world, two large nutrition intervention studies implemented in the late 1980s reported that the combination of selenium/vitamin E/β-carotene significantly reduced total mortality, total cancer mortality and stomach cancer incidence[Blot et al., 1993; Li et al., 1993]. High baseline serum selenium concentrations showed strong protective effects on ESCC and stomach cancer in prospective studies[Mark et al., 2000]. Recently, opposing trends in incidence of EAC and ESCC, i.e. decrease of ESCC incidence and reciprocal increase of EAC incidence has been observed not only worldwide but also in high risk areas in China, pointing to the roles of economic level and lifestyle factors in EC pattern change[Devesa et al., 1998; Fan et al., 2008; Hongo et al., 2009]. In addition, familial aggregation of ESCC has been reported in high-risk areas for ESCC[Chang-Claude et al., 1997]. Taken together, these facts indicate that both genetic susceptibility and environmental risk factors contribute to the etiology of ESCC.

1.2 Current situation of clinical management of ESCC

Early detection of ESCC is formidable and the majority of ESCC patients have advanced metastatic disease at initial diagnosis. Therefore, 40-60% ESCC patients are inappropriate for curative resection, which remains the primary treatment of ESCC as it provides sustained palliation of dysphagia and the best chance of cure[Hagymasi & Tulassay, 2007; Triboulet et al., 2001]. Nonetheless, more than 50% ESCC develop recurrence within 2-3 years after surgery[Dresner & Griffin, 2000; Hulscher et al., 2000; Nakagawa et al., 2004]. Moreover, the overall 5-year survival rate is < 10% despite significant improvements in surgical techniques and adjuvant chemoradiation[Lightdale, 1999]. In contrast, the 5-year survival rate for EC patients at early stages could be as high as 90%[Hu et al., 2001]. Long-term survival correlates with stages of EC, as evidenced by 40-62% of 5-year survival rate for stage I and IIA contrasting with 18-25% for stage IIB and III of EC[Iizuka et al., 1989]. This suggests that the reasons for this disappointingly low survival rate include ineffective screening tools for high-risk population, cancer detection at an advanced stage, high-risk for recurrence, lack of targets for treatment, unreliable noninvasive tools to monitor complete response to chemoradiotherapy and so on. Clearly, identification of effective biomarkers for early detection, monitoring tumor progression and potential therapeutic targets offer the best chances to lower the morbidity and mortality of ESCC.

1.3 Molecular biology studies of ESCC and its contribution to clinical management

Extensive molecular biology studies of ESCC have identified a wealth of dysregulated molecular events involved in esophageal carcinogenesis, which cover a broad range of genes with diverse functions, such as vulnerable genes to chemicals, tumor-related genes, tumor suppressor genes, metastasis genes, apoptosis gene, proliferation genes, etc[Enzinger & Mayer, 2003; Greenawalt et al., 2007; Kwong, 2005; Lin et al., 2009]. Moreover, epigenetic alterations, chromosomal changes and transcriptional changes have also been found to play crucial roles in the pathogenesis of ESCC[Abnet et al., 2010; Greenawalt et al., 2007; Wang et al., 2010]. Although these findings improve our general understanding about the molecular biology of ESCC, the appropriate biomarkers for high-risk population screening, for clinical diagnosis and prognosis, for evaluation of treatment efficiency have not been identified yet. Therefore, it is imperative to search more effective biomarkers for such purposes.

2. ESCC analysis by proteomics

2.1 Advantages of proteomics compared with genomics

The completion of human genome sequence did not ensure panacea solutions to all problems related to biological deregulation. In fact, human proteome is far more complex and dynamic than genome sequence. It is estimated that the human genome contains about 32 000 protein coding genes, which code for 100 000 to 10 million proteins due to alternative RNA splicing, overlapping of transcription units, post-translational processing and modifications[Lander et al., 2001; Venter et al., 2001]. Thus, a big disparity between genome and proteome exists, which indicates that the combinatorial diversification of regulatory networks lead to functional evolution of proteins. Through detecting the functioning units, proteomic studies generate a protein fingerprint, which reflects both the intrinsic genetic programme of the cell and the impact of its immediate environment. Therefore, proteomics is valuable for biomarker discovery since its application provides higher opportunity to identify genuine determinants or causal factors involved in biological functions or the pathogenesis of disease.

2.2 Two-dimensional electrophoresis-based proteomic findings of ESCC

Two-dimensional electrophoresis (2DE) has been used for over 30 years now due to its high resolution for the separation of complex protein mixtures. In combination with mass spectrometry, 2DE has been so far the most commonly used method for analyzing protein expression and identity. Our laboratory used 2DE to profile the proteome from ESCC tumors and matched adjacent non-cancer mucosa, and proteome from immortalized esophageal cell line and cancer cell lines. Comparative analysis and MS for protein identification showed that the over-expressions of four proteins were common in ESCC tissues and cancer cell lines, which include tropomyosin isoform 4 (TPM4), prohibitin, peroxiredoxin (PRX1) and manganese superoxide dismutase (MnSOD); the expressions of another three proteins, i.e. stratifin, prohibitin, squamous cell carcinoma antigen 1 (SCCA1), were correlated inversely with dedifferentiation of ESCC[Qi et al., 2005; Qi et al., 2008]. Immunohistochemistry (IHC) analysis showed that loss of expressions of annexin A2 and stratifin were 45% and 64% in ESCC, respectively[Qi et al., 2007a; Qi et al., 2007b; Ren et al., 2010]. Differential expressions of ten proteins including TPM1, SCCA1, stratifin, peroxiredoxin 2 isoform a, alpha B-crystalline, annexin A2, heterogeneous nuclear ribonucleoprotein L (hnRNP L), triosephosphate isomerase1 (TPI), laminA/C, and cyclophilin A (CypA) can be observed as well. Our findings may suggest that these differential proteins contribute to the multistage process of carcinogenesis, tumor progression, and invasiveness of ESCC. Published in the same issue, Zhou et al found 28 proteins aberrantly expressed in ESCC cancer cells with at least three-fold difference between ESCC and normal epithelial cells[Zhou et al., 2005]. The overlap between these two studies was quite small. Only expression of SCCA1 was commonly down-expressed in ESCC, but transgelin showed increased expression in tumor in our study and decreased expression in Zhou's study. The disparity of proteins identified between these two studies may be due to different sample source, different methods used by these two groups, such as laser capture microdissection vs. bulk tissues, 2D-DIGE vs. silver staining. Later, five groups reported proteomic signatures associated with ESCC using ESCC samples collected from different regions of China, including high risk areas for ESCC such as Linzhou, Xinjiang and low risk areas like Beijing and Guangdong, but only four reports displayed details of identified proteins. Interestingly, more overlap of the identified proteins came from Fu's study and ours, both of which used ESCC samples from Linzhou, one of the highest areas for ESCC adjacent to Taihang Mountain[Fu et al., 2007]. The commonly identified proteins with the same change direction included alpha enolase, TPM, tubulin, prohibitin and PRX2. Although the prevalence of ESCC in Xinjiang is comparable to Linzhou, the protein signatures were unique to sample origin, indicative of more important roles of environmental, ethnic or hereditary factors in the carcinogenesis of ESCC[Liu et al., 2011]. It seems that hsp27 was a general molecular events involved in ESCC since four out of five studies observed down-expression in ESCC except ours. Only one among seven studies performed survival assay after identifying the candidate proteins by ESCC proteomic profiling. Du et al. reported that over-expression of calreticulin and GRP78 could predicate poor prognosis of ESCC[Du et al., 2007]. Although 2DE is indeed a very useful method for biomarker discovery, more examinations of the biological functions and the clinical relevance of biomarker candidates involved in ESCC are necessary to verify its clinical value.

Two reports described the proteomic signatures of ESCC with samples from Japan. Nishimori et al. used the agarose IEF gel in the first dimension, which not only allows for large-scale quantitative comparisons of protein expression but also is able to resolve high molecular mass proteins larger than 150 kDa[Nishimori et al., 2006]. As a result, a different protein pattern was revealed, including a few protein candidates with MW > 70 kDa. Western blot and IHC verified the different expression of a 195 kDa protein, periplakin, between cancer and adjacent non-cancer tissues. Not only was the expression of periplakin significantly down-regulated in ESCC but also translocation of periplakin was observed, which localized at cell-cell boundaries in normal epithelium and dysplastic precursor lesions, and disappeared from cell boundaries and shifted to cell cytoplasm in early cancers. The other research group from Japan used unsupervised classification to analyze the 2D-DIGE protein spots and procured the protein signatures most relevant to clinical parameters with progression of ESCC[Hatakeyama et al., 2006]. The authors developed the largest protein database relevant to ESCC, which identified 240 proteins with expression level associated with carcinogenesis, histological differentiation and the number of lymph node metastases. A significant overlapping was observed between the proteins identified in ESCC with other different types of tumor. In addition, Jazii et al did proteomic profiling using ESCC samples from Iran, another high incidence area for ESCC like northern China, and identified six over-expressed proteins and six under-expressed proteins associated with ESCC[Jazii et al., 2006]. However, the authors only used RT-PCR to verify the loss of β-tropomyosin in ESCC. The functions of identified proteins associated with the development and progression of ESCC include cytoskeletal/structural organization, transport, chaperon, oxioreduction, proliferation, glycolysis, cell motility, transcription, signal transduction, suggesting multiple dysregulated pathways involved in ESCC. For better understanding the pathogenesis of ESCC and development of biomarkers, integrated and comprehensive studies on these protein candidates are needed.

An alternative approach to identify novel tumor biomarkers is the assessment of immune response elicited by tumor antigen since the humoral immune response to cancer in humans has been evidenced by the identification of autoantibodies to a variety of intracellular and surface antigens in cancer patients with different types of tumors[Chen et al., 2007; Disis et al., 1997; Hong et al., 2004; Soussi, 2000]. In ESCC, a number of reports have documented the presence of autoantibodies in serum against various proteins, including p53, cytokeratins, myomegalin, TRIM21, peroxiredoxin VI proteins, Hsp70, and CDC25B[Bergqvist et al., 2001; Fujita et al., 2006; Fujita et al., 2008; Liu et al., 2008; Shimada et al., 2007; Shimada et al., 2005; Veale et al., 1988]. The proteomic-based approach to identify panels of tumor antigens and related autoantibodies was introduced by Brichory et al. in 2001, which identified anti-annexin I and II antibodies in sera from patients with lung cancer[Brichory et al., 2001]. There have been four articles published by two research groups, which reported the existence of autoantibodies in sera of ESCC patients. The first report was published by Fujita et al from Japan, who used 2DE to resolve protein extracts from ESCC cell line TE-2 as tumor antigens and then probed the blot with sera of ESCC patients, healthy controls and patients with other cancers[Fujita et al., 2006]. One positive spot was identified as PRX VI by MALDI TOF/TOF MS. The frequency of autoantibody against PRX VI was 50% (15/30) in ESCC, only 6.6% (2/30) in health controls and 3.3% (1/30) in colon cancer. Two years later, the same research group discovered augmented concentration of Hsp70 autoantibody in the serum of ESCC patients, which was significantly higher in ESCC patients than gastric and colon cancer, healthy controls[Fujita et al., 2008]. On the other hand, Liu et al. used ESCC tissue protein extracts and autologous sera to search for autoantibodies in ESCC patients and identified autoantibody CDC25B[Liu et al., 2008]. Furthermore, CDC25B expression was significantly higher in ESCC tissues with positive autoantibody CDC25B and significantly correlated with tumor stage. The sensitivity and specificity of autoantibody CDC25B for ESCC detection was 56.7% and 91%, respectively[Dong et al., 2010]. The autoantibody-driven research is indeed a promising approach for the identification of novel serum biomarkers present in ESCC and for the tumor antigen itself, which may aid the diagnosis of ESCC and development of more effective immunotherapies.

Similar to other cancers, development of multiple drug resistance in ESCC is one of major causes of failure to chemotherapy treatment. Furthermore, recent studies have shown that there exists intrinsic sensitivity and resistance to chemotherapy and/or radiotherapy in malignant cells of ESCC, which may predict clinical outcome of ESCC patients receiving neoadjuvant chemotherapy. Prior stratification of ESCC patients according to reliable biomarkers could not only save patients unnecessary adverse effects of chemotherapeutic agents but also render patients more chance to access to alternative curative treatment options. Therefore, it is imperative to define new diagnostic indicators that can reliably predict response to chemotherapy and radiotherapy in advance. A recent study compared the 2DE gels of parental esophageal cancer cell line EC109 and its resistant sub-cell line EC109/CDDP to determine the different proteins spots and identified 44 proteins with potential contribution to chemotherapy resistance[Wen et al., 2010]. In another study, radioactive 2DE proteomic comparative analysis was performed using protein extracts of biopsies from 34 patients with locally advanced EAC receiving neoadjuvant chemotherapy.

The identified proteins with different expression between responders and non-responders were classified into two major families, cytoskeleton proteins and molecular chaperon proteins. Further validation by IHC and RT-PCR showed that weak expression of HSP27 at protein level and mRNA level were associated with non-response to platin-based chemotherapy[Langer et al., 2008]. As serum represents a rich source for biomarker discovery, proteomic spectra were examined using 27 and 12 serum samples of responders and non-responders, respectively, to preoperative chemoradiotherapy in a training set by surface-enhanced laser desorption and ionization coupled with mass spectrometry analysis. A proteomic classifier comprising four mass peaks, at 7 420, 9 112, 17 123 and 12 867 m/z was identified with 93.3% predicative accuracy in the validation set[Hayashida et al., 2005]. Since chemotherapy resistance is a complex and multi-factorial event, proteomic-based studies enable comprehensive characterization of resistance phenotype of malignant cancers, which may lead to identification of potential distinguishing biomarkers between responders and non-responders and lay foundation for further molecular mechanism studies.

In addition of 2DE gel for proteomic studies, surface enhanced laser desorption/ionization time-of-flight mass spectrometry (SELDI-TOF-MS) is an alternative proteomic tool to profile the serum or other body fluids and define potential protein pattern with diagnostic potential. By profiling of the serum proteome with SELDI-TOF-MS combined with bioinformatics tools, a number of highly sensitive and specific potential diagnosis markers have been revealed in various types of cancers. Wang et al. used weak cation exchange (WCX2) protein chips and SELDI-TOF-MS to profile 130 symptom-free serum samples collected from high-incidence area of ESCC in northern China, Linzhou, which included 63 subjects with normal esophageal mucosa, 40 subjects with basal cell hyperplasia, 27 subjects with dysplasia and 30 ESCC patients. Biomarker pattern's software identified four protein features at m/z of 9 306.61, 13 765.9, 2 942.15 and 15 953.4, which could distinguish normal esophageal epithelium, basal cell hyperplasia, dysplasia and ESCC with satisfactory diagnostic accuracy[Wang et al., 2006]. Xinjiang is one of the high-incidence areas for ESCC and comprise different ethnic peoples including Han decent. Using CM10 protein chips to capture targets from serum, SELDI-TOF-MS and bioinformatics analysis resulted in identification of six protein peaks (m/z 5667, 5790, 5876, 5979, 6043 and 6102) with diagnostic power with sensitivity and specificity of 91.43% and 88.89%, respectively[Xu et al., 2009]. In the case of ESCC profiled by SELDI-TOF-MS, further purification and identification of discriminatory peaks is necessary for development of simple methods for wider clinical application, and to enhance our understanding of the molecular mechanisms of esophageal carcinogenesis as well.

2.3 SILAC-based proteomic findings of ESCC

Quantitative proteomics is one of the hot research fields in post-genomic era, which has been used extensively in oncology to identify biomarkers with diagnostic and therapeutic potential, thereby avoiding proteins without biological importance. In traditional 2DE, quantitative information of protein spots on 2DE gels is represented by staining intensity. Although 2DE is a versatile tool for visualization of thousands of proteins, detection of post-translational modified isoforms and targeting of protein expression alternations, it has inherent limitations, such as limited resolution of membrane or extreme pI proteins, low sensitivity and throughput, poor reproducibility, etc., which result in only part of proteome uncovered[Ong & Mann, 2005]. In this context, two classes of MS-based quantitative

Protein name	T/N ratio	Functions	References
Annexin A2	↑or ↓	Calcium-dependent phospholipid binding calcium ion binding	[Du et al., 2007; *Liu et al., 2011*]
Annexin A8	↓		[Nishimori et al., 2006]
Annexin I	↓or↑		[Du et al., 2007; Jazii et al., 2006; Liu et al., 2011; Nishimori et al., 2006; Zhou et al., 2005; *Zhu et al., 2010*]
Annexin V	↑		[Du et al., 2007]
Annexin VI	↓		[Nishimori et al., 2006]
Reticulocalbin	↑		[Zhou et al., 2005]
S100 A9	↓		[Zhou et al., 2005]
Syntaxin binding protein	↑	calcium ion binding	[Liu et al., 2011]
Translationally controlled tumor protein	↑		[Zhu et al., 2010]
Zinc finger protein 410	↑	Zink/DNA binding	[Du et al., 2007]
Mutuant hemoglobin beta chain	↓	Heme binding	[Du et al., 2007]
Myoglobin	↓		[Zhu et al., 2010]
TPM-4-ALK fusion oncoprotein type 2	↑	NA	[Du et al., 2007; Jazii et al., 2006]
TPM	↓	Cytoskeleton constituent	[Fu et al., 2007; Liu et al., 2011; Nishimori et al., 2006; Zhou et al., 2005]
TPM2	↓		[Jazii et al., 2006; Nishimori et al., 2006; Zhu et al., 2010]
TPM1	↓		[Qi et al., 2005]
TPM3	↑or ↓		[Fu et al., 2007; *Zhu et al., 2010*]
TPM4	↑		[Qi et al., 2005]
TPM isoform	↑		[Fu et al., 2007; Qi et al., 2005]
Vinculin	↓		[Nishimori et al., 2006]
Capping protein, gelsolin-like	↓		[Fu et al., 2007]
Smooth muscle myosin heavy chain 11 isoform SM1	↓		[Nishimori et al., 2006]
Smooth muscle protein	↓		[Liu et al., 2011]
Apha-actinin 4	↑		[Fu et al., 2007]
Tubulin alpha-6, ubiquitous	↑		[Fu et al., 2007]
Tubulin beta-5 chain	↑		[Fu et al., 2007; Qi et al., 2005]
Gamma-actin	↑		[Qi et al., 2005]
Beta-actin	↑		[Fu et al., 2007]
ACTB protein	↑		[Liu et al., 2011]
Profilin-1	↑		[Zhu et al., 2010]
Periplakin	↓		[Nishimori et al., 2006]
Calreticulin	↑	Stress response and immunity	[Du et al., 2007; Jazii et al., 2006]
Calreticulin precursor	↑		[Nishimori et al., 2006]
Keratin 6A	↑	Intermediate filament	[Du et al., 2007]
Keratin 1	↑	Intermediate filament	[Jazii et al., 2006; Zhou et al., 2005]
Keratin 6	↑		[Nishimori et al., 2006]
Keratin 8	↓		[Zhou et al., 2005]
Keratin 13	↓		[Nishimori et al., 2006; Zhou et al., 2005]
Desmin	↓		[Nishimori et al., 2006; Zhou et al., 2005]
Vimentin	↑		[Nishimori et al., 2006]
MnSOD	↑	Superoxide dismutase activity	[Du et al., 2007; Qi et al., 2005]
Proliferation cell nuclear antigen (PCNA)	↑	DNA polymerase activity	[Du et al., 2007; Zhou et al., 2005]
PRO1708	↑	Stress response and chaperone binding	[Du et al., 2007]
Dank-type molecular chaperone HSPAIL	↑ or ↓		[Du et al., 2007; *Nishimori et al., 2006*]
DnaJ(Hsp40) homolog	↑		[Nishimori et al., 2006]

Protein name	T/N ratio	Functions	References
Heat shock protein 27 kDa	↓ or ↑		[Du et al., 2007; Fu et al., 2007; *Liu et al., 2011*; Zhou et al., 2005]
Similar to heat shock congnate 71-kDa protein	↑		[Du et al., 2007]
Heat shock 70kDa protein 8	↓		[Nishimori et al., 2006]
Heat shock protein 70 kDa	↑		[Jazii et al., 2006]
gp96	↑		[Zhou et al., 2005]
GRP78	↑		[Du et al., 2007]
Alpha-B-Crystalline	↓		[Qi et al., 2005; Zhu et al., 2010]
Fibrin beta	↓		[Liu et al., 2011]
Crystal structure of huma recombinant procathepsin B	↑	NA	[Du et al., 2007]
M2-type pyruvate kinase	↑or ↑		[Du et al., 2007; Fu et al., 2007; Liu et al., 2011]
Mutant beta-actin(Q6F5I1)	↑		[Du et al., 2007]
Phosphoglycerate kinase 1	↑		[Du et al., 2007; Nishimori et al., 2006]
Alpha enolase	↑	Energy metabolism	[Du et al., 2007; Fu et al., 2007; Nishimori et al., 2006; Qi et al., 2005]
Beat-enolase	↑		[Fu et al., 2007]
Triosephosphate isomerase	↑		[Zhu et al., 2010]
GAPDH	↑		[Qi et al., 2005]
Aldolase A	↓		[Nishimori et al., 2006]
Fructose-bisphosphate aldolase A	↓		[Zhu et al., 2010]
RNA binding motif protein 8A	↑	mRNA/nucleotide/protei n binding	[Zhou et al., 2005]
Translation initiation factor Eif-1A	↑	Translation	[Zhou et al., 2005]
Transmembrane protein 4	↑		[Zhou et al., 2005]
Transgelin	↓or ↑	Protein binding	[Liu et al., 2011; Qi et al., 2005; Zhou et al., 2005; Zhu et al., 2010]
COMT protein	↑		[Liu et al., 2011]
Early endosome antigen 1	↓		[Liu et al., 2011]
Crystal structure of recombinant human fibrinogen fragment	↑	Protein binding	[Nishimori et al., 2006]
Similar to ubiquitin -conjugating enzyme E2 variant 1 isoform	↓		[Du et al., 2007]
Ubiquitin C-terminal esterase	↑	Protein degradation	[Zhou et al., 2005]
Ubiquinol-cytochrome C reductase complex core protein2	↑		[Nishimori et al., 2006]
Proteosome	↑		[Liu et al., 2011]
Galectin-7	↓	Interactionof cells and cell-matrix	[Zhou et al., 2005; Zhu et al., 2010]
Fatty acid-binding protein	↓	Lipid metabolism	[Zhou et al., 2005]
TGase	↓	Protein modification	[Zhou et al., 2005]
Fascin	↑	actin cross-lining	[Zhou et al., 2005]
SCCA1	↓	Cysteine proteinase inhibitor	[Qi et al., 2005; Zhou et al., 2005]
Proteinase inhibitor, Clade B	↓	Neutrophil elastase inhibitor	[Zhou et al., 2005]
Thioredoxin perosidase	↑		[Zhou et al., 2005; Zhu et al., 2010]
Peroxiredoxin 1	↑or ↓	Redox homeostasis	[*Fu et al., 2007*; Qi et al., 2005]
Peroxiredoxin 2	↓		[Jazii et al., 2006; Qi et al., 2005]
ARK family 1	↑	Carcinogen metabolism	[Zhou et al., 2005]
GST M_2	↑	glutathione transferase activity	[Zhou et al., 2005]
Proteasome subunit βtype 4	↑		[Zhou et al., 2005]
Proteasome subunit βtype 9	↓	Protein degradation	[Zhou et al., 2005]
Prosomal protein p30-33k	↑		[Zhou et al., 2005]
Elongation factor Tu	↑	Translation	[Qi et al., 2005]
(NADP) cytoplasmic	↑	NAD binding	[Qi et al., 2005]

Protein name	T/N ratio	Functions	References
Prohibitin	↑or ↓	Transcription regulation	[*Fu et al., 2007*; Qi et al., 2005]
Neuronal protein	↑	Neuronal growth	[Qi et al., 2005]
Nuclear autoantigenic sperm protein isoform 1	↑	Hsp90 protein binding	[Nishimori et al., 2006]
Myosin heavy chain nonmuscle form A	↓	Actin binding or	[Nishimori et al., 2006]
Caldesmon 1 isoform 1	↓	calmodulin binding	[Nishimori et al., 2006]
Myosin regulatory light chain 2	↓	Ventricular/cardiac muscle isoform	[Jazii et al., 2006; Zhu et al., 2010]
Myosin light chain 2	↓	Regulatory light chain of	[Jazii et al., 2006]
Myosin light chain 1	↓	myosin	[Zhu et al., 2010]
Heterogeneous nuclear ribonucleoprotein A2/B1:B1	↑	RNA binding and	[Nishimori et al., 2006]
Heterogeneous nuclear ribonucleoprotein A2/B1:A2	↑	processing	[Nishimori et al., 2006]
Myosin light chain 3	↓	Regulatory light chain	[Zhu et al., 2010]
Myosin light polypeptide 6	↑		[Jazii et al., 2006]
Myosin light chain 6B	↓	Regulatory light chain	[Zhu et al., 2010]
Similar to alpha-fetoprotein	↓	NA	[Nishimori et al., 2006]
Trnasferrin	↓	ferric iron binding	[Nishimori et al., 2006]
Alpha-1-antitrypsin precursor	↓	Proteinase inhibitor	[Nishimori et al., 2006]
Alpha-1-antitrypsin	↑		[Fu et al., 2007]
Procollagen-proline	↓	Oxidoreductase activity	[Nishimori et al., 2006]
Calponin 1, basic	↓	actin binding ; calmodulin binding	[Nishimori et al., 2006]
DNA directed RNA polymerase B (ropB)	↑	Transcription	[Jazii et al., 2006]
GH16431P	↑	NA	[Jazii et al., 2006]
OPTN protein	↓	Protein C-terminus binding	[Fu et al., 2007]
67 kDa laminin receptor	↑		[Fu et al., 2007]
TNF receptor associated factor 7	↑	Signal transduction	[Liu et al., 2011]
Stratifin	↓		[Du et al., 2007; Qi et al., 2005]
Cathepsin D	↑	Aspartyl proteinase activity	[Liu et al., 2011]
Chromosome1 open reading frame 8	↑	NA	[Liu et al., 2011]
Cdc42	↑	GTPase activator activity	[Liu et al., 2011]
LLDBP	↑	NA	[Liu et al., 2011]
Adenylate kinase 1	↓	Adenylate kinase activity	[Liu et al., 2011]
General transcription factor IIH	↓	Transcription	[Liu et al., 2011]
Serpin B5 precursor	↑	serine proteinase inhibitor	[Zhu et al., 2010]
Serpin B3	↑		[Zhu et al., 2010]
Transthyretin [Precursor]	↑	Thyroid hormone-binding protein	[Zhu et al., 2010]
Apolipoprotein A-I [Precursor]	↑	lipid metabolism	[Zhu et al., 2010]
Peptidyl-prolyl cis-trans isomerase A	↑	Peptidyl-prolyl cis-trans isomerase activity	[Zhu et al., 2010]
Cystatin-B	↑	Cysteine-type endopeptidase inhibitor activity	[Zhu et al., 2010]
Serum amyloid P-component [Precursor]	↓	Protein binding	[Zhu et al., 2010]
Phosphatidylethanolamine-binding protein1	↓	Serine-type endopeptidase inhibitor	[Zhu et al., 2010]
Carbonic anhydrase 1	↓	Carbonate dehydratase	[Zhu et al., 2010]
Carbonic anhydrase 3	↓	activity	[Zhu et al., 2010]
Creatine kinase M-type	↓	Creatine kinase activity	[Zhu et al., 2010]

Table 1. Reported differential proteins in esophageal cancer tissues

proteomics methods have been developed, which include extracted ion current (XIC)-based label-free quantification and stable isotope labeling quantification. Stable isotope labeling by amino acids in cell culture (SILAC) is an in vivo metabolic labeling method in which stable isotope-labeled amino acids (Heavy vs. Light amino acids) replace the natural amino acids of preexisting proteome[Ong & Mann, 2006]. We used SILAC medium to label immortalized cells (NE3 and NE6) with heavy stable isotope [U-$^{13}C_6$]-H-Lysine and [U-$^{13}C_6$]-H-Arginine and cancer cells (EC1, EC109, EC9706) with light stable isotope [$^{12}C_6$]-L-Lysine and [$^{12}C_6$]-L-Arginine, respectively. After complete labeling of the cellular proteome, equal quantity of proteins from immortalized cells and cancer cells were mixed and then subjected to SDS-PAGE separation, in-gel trypsin digestion and high performance liquid chromatography on-line with electrospray ionization-MS/MS analysis (HPLC-ESI-MS/MS). Forty-seven candidate proteins with differential expression were identified with our arbitrary criteria, which contains ratio change > 1.5 folds, ≥ 2 peptides for quantification and coefficient of variation < 50%. Then, we characterized the cellular protein expression pattern and secretome derived from cisplatin-resistant sub-cell line EC9706 and its parental sensitive cell line EC9706. By SILAC labeling and MS-based quantification, we successfully identified 74 proteins of cellular origin and 57 proteins of secretome with altered expression levels. Similar to our approach, Kashyap et al. used a SILAC-based quantitative proteomic approach to compare the secretome of ESCC cells with that of non-neoplastic esophageal squamous epithelial cells and identified 120 up-regulated proteins with >2-fold difference in the ESCC secretome[Kashyap et al., 2010]. In addition of previously known increased ESCC biomarkers, i.e. matrix metalloproteinase 1, transferrin receptor, and transforming growth factor beta-induced 68 kDa, a number of novel proteins showed distinct expression pattern, among which protein disulfide isomerase family a member 3 (PDIA3), GDP dissociation inhibitor 2 (GDI2), and lectin galactoside binding soluble 3 binding protein (LGALS3BP) were further validated by immunoblot analysis and immunohistochemical labeling using tissue microarrays. These identified proteins participate in multiple biological functions, including molecular chaperones, cytoskeletal proteins, and members of protein inhibitors family, reducing protein, etc., suggesting multiple dysregulated pathways involving in ESCC.

2.4 Clinical relevance of potential protein biomarkers in ESCC

To answer clinical questions, the protein biomarkers identified by proteomic techniques with potential diagnosis and therapeutic targets for ESCC need to be translated into clinical scenario, which is realized by using clinical samples, such as biopsy samples, resected tissue samples, plasma or serum samples, urine samples, saliva samples, etc. The methods used for validation generally comprise Western blot, IHC and ELISA at protein level, and RT-PCR at transcription level. Using 2DE- and SILAC-based quantitative proteomic approaches, we have identified a total of 78 non-redundant proteins with aberrant expression associated with ESCC, suggesting that these proteins may play functional roles in carcinogenesis of ESCC and may have clinical values. Afterwards, Western blot analysis verified the decreased expressions of three proteins, i.e. SCCA1, TPM1 and αB-Cryst in cancer, in accordance with 2DE quantitative results. At transcription level, SCCA1 mRNA was down-regulated in tumor as well. More importantly, the expression of SCCA1 decreased step by step as a function of precancer lesions progression, which suggests that SCCA1 may take part in the multi-stage transformation of ESCC, even in the earliest stages[Qi et al., 2005]. In the 2DE-based comparative proteomic study using immortalized and cancer cell model, we

Accession no.	Protein name	MW/PI	Scores	Ratio (T/N)	Matched peptides	Functions
TPM3 HUMAN	Tropomyosin alpha-3 chain	32.80/4.53	330.06	0.47	2	Actin binding
TPM4 HUMAN	Tropomyosin alpha-4 chain	28.50/4.52	199.64	0.37	2	
K2C8 HUMAN	Keratin, type II cytoskeletal 8	53.67/5.38	907.48	0.51	4	
FSCN1 HUMAN	Fascin	54.50/7.02	296.56	0.45	2	
LEG1 HUMAN	Galectin-1	14.71/5.18	424.98	0.49	3	
CLIC1 HUMAN	Chloride channel ABP	26.91/4.94	447.94	0.63	4	Signal transduction
1433E HUMAN	14-3-3 protein epsilon	29.16/4.48	400.71	0.66	3	
PRDX1 HUMAN	Peroxiredoxin-1	22.10/9.22	689.77	0.55	7	
PRDX2 HUMAN	Peroxiredoxin-2	21.88/5.59	238.11	0.65	5	
PRDX4 HUMAN	Peroxiredoxin-4	30.52/5.85	367.60	0.34	2	Redox homeostasis
PRDX5 HUMAN	Peroxiredoxin-5	22.01/9.93	522.84	0.60	2	
CBR1 HUMAN	Carbonyl reductase [NADPH]1	30.36/9.53	467.30	0.59	2	
KCRB HUMAN	Creatine kinase B-type	42.62/5.25	711.33	1.67	4	
GSTP1 HUMAN	Glutathione S-transferase P	23.34/5.32	1140.8	0.45	6	
GDIB HUMAN	Rab GDI beat	50.63/6.08	614.67	0.47	2	
DHSA HUMAN	Favoprotein subunit complex II	72.65/7.31	207.55	0.5	2	Metabolic process
ACBP HUMAN	Acyl-CoA-binding protein	10.04/6.16	135.03	0.64	2	
PHS HUMAN	PHS 2	11.99/6.33	170.64	0.43	3	
RL27A HUMAN	60S ribosomal protein L27a	16.55/11.78	233.25	0.59	2	
RSSA HUMAN	40S ribosomal protein SA	32.83/4.64	298.67	0.58	2	Translation
IF4G1_HUMAN	eIF-4-gamma 1	175.4/5.1	650.5	2.15	14	
NPM HUMAN	Nucleophosmin	32.55/4.49	444.46	0.52	2	DNA binding
GRP78 HUMAN	GRP78	72.29/4.92	1869.09	0.50	14	Chaperone binding
CH10 HUMAN	Hsp 10	10.92/9.44	219.29	0.40	3	
G6PI HUMAN	Glucose-6-phosphate isomerase	63.11/9.10	510.30	0.48	5	
UGDH HUMAN	UDP-glucose 6-dehydrogenase	54.99/6.89	604.20	0.53	2	
PPIA HUMAN	Peptidyl-prolyl isomerase A	18.00/9.05	770.25	0.59	9	
ALDOA HUMAN	Fructose-bisphosphate aldolase A	39.40/9.18	386.91	0.59	2	
PGK1 HUMAN	Phosphoglycerate kinase 1	44.59/9.22	1020.8	0.50	6	Energy metabolism
G3P HUMAN	GAPDH	36.03/9.26	1127.9	0.52	8	
IPYR HUMAN	Inorganic pyrophosphatase	32.64/5.47	485.51	0.45	3	
ENOA HUMAN	Alpha-enolase	47.14/7.71	1998.1	0.55	15	
CYTB HUMAN	Cystatin-B	11.13/7.85	144.98	0.43	2	
CPSM HUMAN	Carbamoyl-phosphate synthase 1	164.83/6.30	3115.1	0.24	6	
PHB2 HUMAN	Prohibitin-2	33.28/10.21	546.79	0.47	2	Transcription regulation
CAND1_HUMAN	TBP-interacting protein 120A	136.3/5.4	617.2	1.8	15	
PSME2 HUMAN	Proteasome activator complex subunit2	27.34/5.33	367.19	0.48	2	Cell cycle
MCM7_HUMAN	DNA replication licensing factor MCM7	81.3/6.1	510.8	1.97	13	

Accession no.	Protein name	MW/PI	Scores	Ratio (T/N)	Matched peptides	Functions
ACADV HUMAN	VLCAD	70.35/9.63	841.39	0.35	2	Lipid metabolism
ATPA HUMAN	ATP5A1	59.71/9.61	963.07	0.47	5	
THIL HUMAN	Acetoacetyl-CoA thiolase	45.17/9.63	330.39	0.45	2	
MIF HUMAN	Macrophage migration inhibitory factor	12.47/9.12	267.01	0.61	3	Cytokine activity
ATPB HUMAN	ATPB-3	56.52/5.14	1704.2	0.40	5	Ion transport
VDAC1 HUMAN	VDAC-1	30.75/9.22	548.36	2.32	2	Anion transport
VPS35_HUMAN	hVPS35	91.6/5.2	602.6	1.67	12	Protein transport
HYOU1 HUMAN	Hypoxia up-regulated protein 1	111.27/5.02	1206.8	0.56	2	ATP binding
SMD3 HUMAN	Small nuclear ribonucleoprotein 3	13.91/11.07	330.93	0.49	2	mRNA processing

Table 2. Differential proteins between immortalized and cancer cell lines derived from ESCC identified by SILAC-based proteomics

selected Annexin A2 for validation by Western blot and IHC. Stepwise decrease in annexin A2 protein expression was observed when epithelial cell was transformed malignantly. In poorly-differentiated squamous carcinoma, 46% (5/11) of cancer tissue sample lost annexin A2 protein and 36% (4/11) expressed at weak intensity[Qi et al., 2007b]. In a separate study, IHC was used to determine 14-3-3σ in 60 cases of ESCC, nearby matched normal esophageal epithelium and a variety of ESCC precursor lesions. High level of 14-3-3σ expression was found ubiquitously in normal esophageal epithelium with an immuonstaining score of 8.22 in expression. Protein 14-3-3σ was down-regulated stepwise during the multi-stage development of ESCC. Sixty-four percent of poorly-differentiated squamous cancer lost 14-3-3σ expression with a score of 0.45[Qi et al., 2007a]. In agreement with our results, Ren et al. documented that the level of 14-3-3σ in terms of mRNA and protein was markedly down-regulated in ESCC compared with nearby matched non-cancer tissues. Furthermore, decrease of 14-3-3σ expression was correlated with tumor infiltration depth, lymph node metastasis, distant metastasis and lymphovascular invasion and shorter 5-year survival rate[Ren et al., 2010]. Among the different proteins identified by SILAC-based quantitative analysis using immortal cell and cancer cell model, the clinical values of MIF in tumorigenesis of ESCC was determined as well. Not only the increased expression of MIF was detected in cellular protein but also in the conditioned medium of esophageal cancer cell lines EC1, EC109 and EC9706 compared with immortal cell lines NE3 and NE6. Low frequency and very weak expression of MIF was detected predominantly in basal cells in normal esophageal epithelium, with an immunostaining score of 1.13. Pronouncedly up-regulated expression of MIF occurred in severe dysplasia compared with weak immunostaining in mild and moderate dysplasia. In ESCC, high frequency of intense expression of MIF was observed with a score of 5.46. Furthermore, high expression of MIF was significantly correlated with advanced clinical stages. ELISA tests revealed that there was an increase trend in serum level of MIF in clinically advanced stage IV compared to stage I-III. Functional studies on MIF indicated that MIF knockdown resulted in decrease in proliferation, clonogenicity, non-adherent growth and invasive potential. Our findings indicate that MIF may play crucial roles in malignant transformation of pathogenesis of EC and MIF could become a potential biomarker for high-risk population screening, assessment of therapeutic efficiency, prognostic evaluation, and molecular targets of developing novel therapeutic regimen as well. In addition of our proteomic results in ESCC, several other reports have looked at the clinical value of potential biomarkers, including cytokeratin 14, Annexin I, SCCA1/2, calgulanulin B and HSP 60, alpha-actinin 4 and 67 kDa laminin receptor, cathepsin D and PKM2, periplakin, calreticulin and GRP78, galectin-7, anti-CD25B antibody[Dong et al., 2010; Du et al., 2007; Fu et al., 2007; Hatakeyama et al., 2006; Liu et al., 2011; Nishimori et al., 2006; Zhu et al., 2010]. Nevertheless, further extensive studies are still necessary to determine the clinical utility of the identified proteins in tumorigenesis and progression of ESCC.

3. Conclusions

Nowadays, the dilemma for cancer control and management is not due to lack of efficient treatment options but diagnosis at late stages. In the case of ESCC in China, five-year survival rate for early stage tumor reaches around 90%[Hu et al., 2001]. Obviously, to detect tumor as early as possible is the key for reducing the mortality and morbidity of ESCC. It is believed that development of ESCC from normal esophageal epithelium takes at least about 10 years, during which diseased epithelium manifests as basal cell hyperproliferation, dysplasia, carcinoma in situ in terms of morphology and finally evolves to malignant neoplasms. As such, carcinogenesis of ESCC is a multi-stage and dynamic process which accumulates ongoing changes at the level of both gene and protein expression.

Proteomic studies from various research groups worldwide have identified distinct dysregulated protein expression pattern associated with ESCC. The discrepancy might reflect the different etiology, different stages of disease and diverse pathways involved, which makes identification of biomarkers for ESCC difficult. In light of a wealth of potential biomarkers associated with ESCC identified so far in the exploratory phase, future large-scale validation studies involving symptom-free patients with precursor lesions in high-incidence area and ESCC patients compared with controls are essential toward clinical application. Therefore, ultimate translation from laboratory into bedside for ESCC biomarkers will require close collaboration and cooperation between researchers and clinicians to look into the clinical utility in diagnosis at early stage, prognosis and monitoring treatment efficiency for ESCC.

4. Acknowledgement

This work was supported in part by National Natural Science Founding of China (No. 30700366 and No. 81072039) and Cancer Research UK (to Yi-Jun Qi).

5. References

Abnet, C. C., Freedman, N. D., Hu, N., et al. (2010). A shared susceptibility locus in PLCE1 at 10q23 for gastric adenocarcinoma and esophageal squamous cell carcinoma. *Nat Genet,* Vol.42, No.9, (Sep), pp: 764-767, ISSN 1546-1718

Banks, R. E., Dunn, M. J., Hochstrasser, D. F., et al. (2000). Proteomics: new perspectives, new biomedical opportunities. *Lancet,* Vol.356, No.9243, (Nov 18), pp: 1749-1756, ISSN 0140-6736

Bergqvist, A. S., Bergqvist, M., Brattstrom, D., et al. (2001). Serum p53 autoantibodies as prognostic marker in patients with oesophageal carcinoma. *Anticancer Res*, Vol.21, No.6A, (Nov-Dec), pp: 4141-4145, ISSN 0250-7005

Blot, W. J., Li, J. Y., Taylor, P. R., et al. (1993). Nutrition intervention trials in Linxian, China: supplementation with specific vitamin/mineral combinations, cancer incidence, and disease-specific mortality in the general population. *J Natl Cancer Inst*, Vol.85, No.18, (Sep 15), pp: 1483-1492, ISSN 0027-8874

Brichory, F. M., Misek, D. E., Yim, A. M., et al. (2001). An immune response manifested by the common occurrence of annexins I and II autoantibodies and high circulating levels of IL-6 in lung cancer. *Proc Natl Acad Sci U S A*, Vol.98, No.17, (Aug 14), pp: 9824-9829, ISSN 0027-8424

Brown, L. M., Devesa, S. S. & Chow, W. H. (2008). Incidence of adenocarcinoma of the esophagus among white Americans by sex, stage, and age. *J Natl Cancer Inst*, Vol.100, No.16, (Aug 20), pp: 1184-1187, ISSN 1460-2105

Chambers, G., Lawrie, L., Cash, P., et al. (2000). Proteomics: a new approach to the study of disease. *J Pathol*, Vol.192, No.3, (Nov), pp: 280-288, ISSN 0022-3417

Chang-Claude, J., Becher, H., Blettner, M., et al. (1997). Familial aggregation of oesophageal cancer in a high incidence area in China. *Int J Epidemiol*, Vol.26, No.6, (Dec), pp: 1159-1165, ISSN 0300-5771

Chen, G., Wang, X., Yu, J., et al. (2007). Autoantibody profiles reveal ubiquilin 1 as a humoral immune response target in lung adenocarcinoma. *Cancer Res*, Vol.67, No.7, (Apr 1), pp: 3461-3467, ISSN 0008-5472

Cheng, K. K. & Day, N. E. (1996). Nutrition and esophageal cancer. *Cancer Causes and Control*, Vol.7, No.1, pp: 33-40, 0957-5243

Daly, J. M., Fry, W. A., Little, A. G., et al. (2000). Esophageal cancer: results of an American College of Surgeons Patient Care Evaluation Study. *J Am Coll Surg*, Vol.190, No.5, (May), pp: 562-572; discussion 572-563, ISSN 1072-7515

Devesa, S. S., Blot, W. J. & Fraumeni, J. F., Jr. (1998). Changing patterns in the incidence of esophageal and gastric carcinoma in the United States. *Cancer*, Vol.83, No.10, (Nov 15), pp: 2049-2053, ISSN 0008-543X

Disis, M. L., Pupa, S. M., Gralow, J. R., et al. (1997). High-titer HER-2/neu protein-specific antibody can be detected in patients with early-stage breast cancer. *J Clin Oncol*, Vol.15, No.11, (Nov), pp: 3363-3367, ISSN 0732-183X

Dong, J., Zeng, B. H., Xu, L. H., et al. (2010). Anti-CDC25B autoantibody predicts poor prognosis in patients with advanced esophageal squamous cell carcinoma. *J Transl Med*, Vol.8, (Sep 3), pp: 81, ISSN 1479-5876

Dresner, S. M. & Griffin, S. M. (2000). Pattern of recurrence following radical oesophagectomy with two-field lymphadenectomy. *Br J Surg*, Vol.87, No.10, (Oct), pp: 1426-1433, ISSN 0007-1323

Du, X. L., Hu, H., Lin, D. C., et al. (2007). Proteomic profiling of proteins dysregulted in Chinese esophageal squamous cell carcinoma. *J Mol Med (Berl)*, Vol.85, No.8, (Aug), pp: 863-875, ISSN 0946-2716

Enzinger, P. C. & Mayer, R. J. (2003). Esophageal cancer. *N Engl J Med*, Vol.349, No.23, (Dec 4), pp: 2241-2252, ISSN 1533-4406

Fan, Y. J., Song, X., Li, J. L., et al. (2008). Esophageal and gastric cardia cancers on 4238 Chinese patients residing in municipal and rural regions: a histopathological comparison during 24-year period. *World J Surg,* Vol.32, No.9, (Sep), pp: 1980-1988, ISSN 0364-2313

Fu, L., Qin, Y. R., Xie, D., et al. (2007). Identification of alpha-actinin 4 and 67 kDa laminin receptor as stage-specific markers in esophageal cancer via proteomic approaches. *Cancer,* Vol.110, No.12, (Dec 15), pp: 2672-2681, ISSN 0008-543X

Fujita, Y., Nakanishi, T., Hiramatsu, M., et al. (2006). Proteomics-based approach identifying autoantibody against peroxiredoxin VI as a novel serum marker in esophageal squamous cell carcinoma. *Clin Cancer Res,* Vol.12, No.21, (Nov 1), pp: 6415-6420, ISSN 1078-0432

Fujita, Y., Nakanishi, T., Miyamoto, Y., et al. (2008). Proteomics-based identification of autoantibody against heat shock protein 70 as a diagnostic marker in esophageal squamous cell carcinoma. *Cancer Lett,* Vol.263, No.2, (May 18), pp: 280-290, ISSN 0304-3835

Greenawalt, D. M., Duong, C., Smyth, G. K., et al. (2007). Gene expression profiling of esophageal cancer: comparative analysis of Barrett's esophagus, adenocarcinoma, and squamous cell carcinoma. *Int J Cancer,* Vol.120, No.9, (May 1), pp: 1914-1921, ISSN 0020-7136

Hagymasi, K. & Tulassay, Z. (2007). [Genetic background of esophageal squamous cell carcinoma]. *Orv Hetil,* Vol.148, No.38, (Sep 23), pp: 1795-1800, ISSN 0030-6002

Hatakeyama, H., Kondo, T., Fujii, K., et al. (2006). Protein clusters associated with carcinogenesis, histological differentiation and nodal metastasis in esophageal cancer. *Proteomics,* Vol.6, No.23, (Dec), pp: 6300-6316, ISSN 1615-9853

Hayashida, Y., Honda, K., Osaka, Y., et al. (2005). Possible prediction of chemoradiosensitivity of esophageal cancer by serum protein profiling. *Clin Cancer Res,* Vol.11, No.22, (Nov 15), pp: 8042-8047, ISSN 1078-0432

Holmes, R. S. & Vaughan, T. L. (2007). Epidemiology and pathogenesis of esophageal cancer. *Semin Radiat Oncol,* Vol.17, No.1, (Jan), pp: 2-9, ISSN 1053-4296

Hong, S. H., Misek, D. E., Wang, H., et al. (2004). An autoantibody-mediated immune response to calreticulin isoforms in pancreatic cancer. *Cancer Res,* Vol.64, No.15, (Aug 1), pp: 5504-5510, ISSN 0008-5472

Hongo, M., Nagasaki, Y. & Shoji, T. (2009). Epidemiology of esophageal cancer: Orient to Occident. Effects of chronology, geography and ethnicity. *J Gastroenterol Hepatol,* Vol.24, No.5, (May), pp: 729-735, ISSN 1440-1746

Hu, Y. C., Lam, K. Y., Law, S., et al. (2001). Identification of differentially expressed genes in esophageal squamous cell carcinoma (ESCC) by cDNA expression array: overexpression of Fra-1, Neogenin, Id-1, and CDC25B genes in ESCC. *Clin Cancer Res,* Vol.7, No.8, (Aug), pp: 2213-2221, ISSN 1078-0432

Hulscher, J. B., van Sandick, J. W., Tijssen, J. G., et al. (2000). The recurrence pattern of esophageal carcinoma after transhiatal resection. *J Am Coll Surg,* Vol.191, No.2, (Aug), pp: 143-148, ISSN 1072-7515

Iizuka, T., Isono, K., Kakegawa, T., et al. (1989). Parameters linked to ten-year survival in Japan of resected esophageal carcinoma. Japanese Committee for Registration of Esophageal Carcinoma Cases. *Chest,* Vol.96, No.5, (Nov), pp: 1005-1011, ISSN 0012-3692

Jazii, F. R., Najafi, Z., Malekzadeh, R., et al. (2006). Identification of squamous cell carcinoma associated proteins by proteomics and loss of beta tropomyosin expression in esophageal cancer. *World J Gastroenterol,* Vol.12, No.44, (Nov 28), pp: 7104-7112, ISSN 1007-9327

Kamangar, F., Chow, W. H., Abnet, C. C., et al. (2009). Environmental causes of esophageal cancer. *Gastroenterol Clin North Am,* Vol.38, No.1, (Mar), pp: 27-57, vii, ISSN 1558-1942

Kashyap, M. K., Harsha, H. C., Renuse, S., et al. (2010). SILAC-based quantitative proteomic approach to identify potential biomarkers from the esophageal squamous cell carcinoma secretome. *Cancer Biol Ther,* Vol.10, No.8, (Oct 15), pp: 796-810, ISSN 1555-8576

Kolch, W., Mischak, H., Chalmers, M. J., et al. (2004). Clinical proteomics: a question of technology. *Rapid Commun Mass Spectrom,* Vol.18, No.19, pp: 2365-2366, ISSN 0951-4198

Kolch, W., Mischak, H. & Pitt, A. R. (2005). The molecular make-up of a tumour: proteomics in cancer research. *Clin Sci (Lond),* Vol.108, No.5, (May), pp: 369-383, ISSN 0143-5221

Kwong, K. F. (2005). Molecular biology of esophageal cancer in the genomics era. *Surg Clin North Am,* Vol.85, No.3, (Jun), pp: 539-553, ISSN 0039-6109

Lander, E. S., Linton, L. M., Birren, B., et al. (2001). Initial sequencing and analysis of the human genome. *Nature,* Vol.409, No.6822, (Feb 15), pp: 860-921, ISSN 0028-0836

Langer, R., Ott, K., Specht, K., et al. (2008). Protein expression profiling in esophageal adenocarcinoma patients indicates association of heat-shock protein 27 expression and chemotherapy response. *Clin Cancer Res,* Vol.14, No.24, (Dec 15), pp: 8279-8287, ISSN 1078-0432

Li, B., Taylor, P. R., Li, J. Y., et al. (1993). Linxian nutrition intervention trials. Design, methods, participant characteristics, and compliance. *Ann Epidemiol,* Vol.3, No.6, (Nov), pp: 577-585, ISSN 1047-2797

Li, L. W., Li, Y. Y., Li, X. Y., et al. (2011). A novel tumor suppressor gene ECRG4 interacts directly with TMPRSS11A (ECRG1) to inhibit cancer cell growth in esophageal carcinoma. *BMC Cancer,* Vol.11, (Feb 3), pp: 52, ISSN 1471-2407

Lightdale, C. J. (1999). Esophageal cancer. American College of Gastroenterology. *Am J Gastroenterol,* Vol.94, No.1, (Jan), pp: 20-29, ISSN 0002-9270

Lin, D. C., Du, X. L. & Wang, M. R. (2009). Protein alterations in ESCC and clinical implications: a review. *Dis Esophagus,* Vol.22, No.1, pp: 9-20, ISSN 1442-2050

Liu, W. L., Zhang, G., Wang, J. Y., et al. (2008). Proteomics-based identification of autoantibody against CDC25B as a novel serum marker in esophageal squamous cell carcinoma. *Biochem Biophys Res Commun,* Vol.375, No.3, (Oct 24), pp: 440-445, ISSN 1090-2104

Liu, Z., Feng, J. G., Tuersun, A., et al. (2011). Proteomic identification of differentially-expressed proteins in esophageal cancer in three ethnic groups in Xinjiang. *Mol Biol Rep,* Vol.38, No.5, (Jun), pp: 3261-3269, ISSN 1573-4978

Mark, S. D., Qiao, Y. L., Dawsey, S. M., et al. (2000). Prospective study of serum selenium levels and incident esophageal and gastric cancers. *J Natl Cancer Inst,* Vol.92, No.21, (Nov 1), pp: 1753-1763, ISSN 0027-8874

Messmann, H. (2001). Squamous cell cancer of the oesophagus. *Best Pract Res Clin Gastroenterol,* Vol.15, No.2, (Apr), pp: 249-265, ISSN 1521-6918

Morita, M., Kumashiro, R., Kubo, N., et al. (2010). Alcohol drinking, cigarette smoking, and the development of squamous cell carcinoma of the esophagus: epidemiology, clinical findings, and prevention. *Int J Clin Oncol,* Vol.15, No.2, (Apr), pp: 126-134, ISSN 2547-7772

Nakagawa, S., Kanda, T., Kosugi, S., et al. (2004). Recurrence pattern of squamous cell carcinoma of the thoracic esophagus after extended radical esophagectomy with three-field lymphadenectomy. *J Am Coll Surg,* Vol.198, No.2, (Feb), pp: 205-211, ISSN 1072-7515

Nishimori, T., Tomonaga, T., Matsushita, K., et al. (2006). Proteomic analysis of primary esophageal squamous cell carcinoma reveals downregulation of a cell adhesion protein, periplakin. *Proteomics,* Vol.6, No.3, (Feb), pp: 1011-1018, ISSN 1615-9853

Ong, S. E. & Mann, M. (2005). Mass spectrometry-based proteomics turns quantitative. *Nat Chem Biol,* Vol.1, No.5, (Oct), pp: 252-262, ISSN 1552-4450

(2006). A practical recipe for stable isotope labeling by amino acids in cell culture (SILAC). *Nat Protoc,* Vol.1, No.6, pp: 2650-2660, ISSN 1750-2799

Parkin, D. M., Bray, F., Ferlay, J., et al. (2005). Global cancer statistics, 2002. *CA Cancer J Clin,* Vol.55, No.2, (Mar-Apr), pp: 74-108, ISSN 0007-9235

Qi, Y., Chiu, J. F., Wang, L., et al. (2005). Comparative proteomic analysis of esophageal squamous cell carcinoma. *Proteomics,* Vol.5, No.11, (Jul), pp: 2960-2971, ISSN 1615-9853

Qi, Y. J., He, Q. Y., Ma, Y. F., et al. (2008). Proteomic identification of malignant transformation-related proteins in esophageal squamous cell carcinoma. *J Cell Biochem,* Vol.104, No.5, (Aug 1), pp: 1625-1635, ISSN 1097-4644

Qi, Y. J., Ma, Y. F., Du, Y. W., et al. (2007a). Character ization and correlation of 14-3-3σ and P53 protein expressions in multi-stage carcinogenesis of esophageal squamous cell carcinoma. *J Fourth Mil Med Univ,* Vol.28, No.20, (June 15), pp: 1834-1837, ISSN 1000-5404

Qi, Y. J., Wang, L. D., Jiao, X. Y., et al. (2007b). [Dysregulation of Annexin II expression in esophageal squamous cell cancer and adjacent tissues from a high-incidence area for esophageal cancer in Henan province]. *Ai Zheng,* Vol.26, No.7, (Jul), pp: 730-736, ISSN 1000-467X

Ren, H. Z., Pan, G. Q., Wang, J. S., et al. (2010). Reduced stratifin expression can serve as an independent prognostic factor for poor survival in patients with esophageal squamous cell carcinoma. *Dig Dis Sci,* Vol.55, No.9, (Sep), pp: 2552-2560, ISSN 1573-2568

Shimada, H., Kuboshima, M., Shiratori, T., et al. (2007). Serum anti-myomegalin antibodies in patients with esophageal squamous cell carcinoma. *Int J Oncol,* Vol.30, No.1, (Jan), pp: 97-103, ISSN 1019-6439

Shimada, H., Nakashima, K., Ochiai, T., et al. (2005). Serological identification of tumor antigens of esophageal squamous cell carcinoma. *Int J Oncol,* Vol.26, No.1, (Jan), pp: 77-86, ISSN 1019-6439

Soussi, T. (2000). p53 Antibodies in the sera of patients with various types of cancer: a review. *Cancer Res,* Vol.60, No.7, (Apr 1), pp: 1777-1788, ISSN 0008-5472

Triboulet, J. P., Mariette, C., Chevalier, D., et al. (2001). Surgical management of carcinoma of the hypopharynx and cervical esophagus: analysis of 209 cases. *Arch Surg,* Vol.136, No.10, (Oct), pp: 1164-1170, ISSN 0004-0010

Trivers, K. F., Sabatino, S. A. & Stewart, S. L. (2008). Trends in esophageal cancer incidence by histology, United States, 1998-2003. *Int J Cancer,* Vol.123, No.6, (Sep 15), pp: 1422-1428, ISSN 1097-0215

Veale, R. B., Thornley, A. L., Scott, E., et al. (1988). Quantitation of autoantibodies to cytokeratins in sera from patients with squamous cell carcinoma of the oesophagus. *Br J Cancer,* Vol.58, No.6, (Dec), pp: 767-772, ISSN 0007-0920

Venter, J. C., Adams, M. D., Myers, E. W., et al. (2001). The sequence of the human genome. *Science,* Vol.291, No.5507, (Feb 16), pp: 1304-1351, ISSN 0036-8075

Wang, L. D., Wang, D. C., Zheng, S., et al. (2006). [Serum proteomic profiles of the subjects with esophageal precancerous and cancerous lesions from Linzhou, an area with high incidence of esophageal cancer in Henan Province, Northern China]. *Ai Zheng,* Vol.25, No.5, (May), pp: 549-554, ISSN 1000-467X

Wang, L. D., Zhou, F. Y., Li, X. M., et al. (2010). Genome-wide association study of esophageal squamous cell carcinoma in Chinese subjects identifies susceptibility loci at PLCE1 and C20orf54. *Nat Genet,* Vol.42, No.9, (Sep), pp: 759-763, ISSN1546-1718

Wen, J., Zheng, B., Hu, Y., et al. (2010). Comparative proteomic analysis of the esophageal squamous carcinoma cell line EC109 and its multi-drug resistant subline EC109/CDDP. *Int J Oncol,* Vol.36, No.1, (Jan), pp: 265-274, ISSN 1791-2423

Xu, S. Y., Liu, Z., Ma, W. J., et al. (2009). New potential biomarkers in the diagnosis of esophageal squamous cell carcinoma. *Biomarkers,* Vol.14, No.5, (Aug), pp: 340-346, ISSN 1366-5804

Yang, C. S., Sun, Y., Yang, Q. U., et al. (1984). Vitamin A and other deficiencies in Linxian, a high esophageal cancer incidence area in northern China. *J Natl Cancer Inst,* Vol.73, No.6, (Dec), pp: 1449-1453, ISSN 0027-8874

Zhou, G., Li, H., Gong, Y., et al. (2005). Proteomic analysis of global alteration of protein expression in squamous cell carcinoma of the esophagus. *Proteomics,* Vol.5, No.14, (Sep), pp: 3814-3821, ISSN 1615-9853

Zhu, X., Ding, M., Yu, M. L., et al. (2010). Identification of galectin-7 as a potential biomarker for esophageal squamous cell carcinoma by proteomic analysis. *BMC Cancer,* Vol.10, (Jun 15), pp: 290, ISSN 1471-2407

13

The Microtubule-Dissociating Tau in Neurological Disorders

Francisco José Fernández-Gómez,
Susanna Schraen-Maschke and Luc Buée
*Inserm UMR837 - Alzheimer & Tauopathies -
Jean-Pierre Aubert Reserch Center,
Université de Lille Droit & Santé, Lille
France*

1. Introduction

Around 24 million of people worldwide have some kind of dementia, and most of them are diagnosed to suffer from Alzheimer's disease (AD). In fact, every seven second a new case of dementia is identified, arriving to the rate of 4,6 new million cases per year. It is expected that by 2040 over 80 million of people will be affected. Neurological diseases are therefore a major public health problem due to the rise in the aging population, only in Europe these disorders cover approximately 35% of the burden of all diseases. In economical terms, brain diseases in Europe cost a total of 386 billion of euros per year, with an average of 829€ per inhabitant. AD and other dementias represent the second-leading cause of brain disorders after affective ones and equal with addiction diseases (Wittchen and Jacobi, 2005). Altogether dementias, and in particular AD represent a huge socio-economical impact, not only regarding the cost from the pharmacological point of view but also familiar cares which increase in an alarming rate in the last stages of the disease. Worthy to mention is the role of the family during the progression of this kind of diseases, relatives have to watch the patient every moment above all during the first lapses of memory and some of them need psychological help to assume the situation and the change in their lifestyle.
The incidence and prevalence of this group of diseases explain the need to understand mechanisms underlying dementia to uncover early and discriminative diagnostic markers as well as new therapeutic targets in order to improve the quality of life of these patients and the efficacy of the treatements. For these reasons research in AD is currently considered as a priority. At this time, the pharmacological treatments available aim to enhance the cognitive impairments once the disease is diagnosed, only cholinesterase inhibitors and one NMDA receptor antagonist are commercialized. Despite these products can alleviate the symptomatology, they are far away to constitute an effective remedy to cure or prevent the deleterious effect of the disease. In line of these observations, methods for improving diagnosis are needed, the search of biomarkers and neuroimaging techniques might help to support clinical diagnosis and detect the disease in the earliest stages. The identification of potential genetic and environmental risk factors as well as protective ones may provide a new window of action even if interventions at this level are more complex and controversial (Ballard C et al., 2011).

Despite AD covers between 60 to 80% of the causes of dementia, there are many other causes: vascular dementia, mixed dementia, dementia with Lewy bodies, Parkinson's disease, frontotemporal dementia, Creutzfeldt-Jakob disease, Huntington's disease and Wernicke-Korsakoff syndrome are some of them (http://www.alz.org). Current available diagnosis of AD is based mainly on the severity of cognitive impairments. However, even with the help of several neuroimaging techniques it is not simple to discriminate among AD and other age-related cognitive impairments. Unfortunately only an accurate diagnosis of AD can be reached after autopsy examination. Nonetheless, it is necessary and desirable to incorporate new biomarkers that are more sentitive, specific and may facilitate the diagnosis not only among the different disorders but also to discern the clinical progression (Seshadri S et al., 2011).

As it is described along this chapter the field of proteomics provides a powerful tool, which might enable to identify new proteins for early diagnostic and potentially therapeutic targets in AD. It is also remarkable the mandatory use of animal models in order to elucidate new pathways involved in the pathogenesis. Transgenic mouse models provide biochemical modulable approches where in a dependent or independent way several parameters can be studied (Sowell RA et al., 2009).

2. Historical input of proteomics to Alzheimer´s disease and other neurological disorders

AD is a progressive neurodegenerative disorder that leads to dementia. This pathology is characterized by two histopathological features: senile plaques and neurofibrillary degeneration (NFD) (Alzheimer A et al., 1907). Senile plaques are an extracellular accumulation of amyloid deposits formed by Aβ peptide. Aβ is a small 39 to 43 amino acid peptide produced by the complex catabolism of a type I transmembrane glycoprotein precursor named amyloid precursor protein (APP). Despite in AD only 1% of the cases have a familial history or inherited, most of the mutations described are related to APP, presenilin 1 (PSEN1), PSEN2 and SORL1 genes. Indeed the amyloid hypothesis of AD is considered almost like a dogma regarding the number of therapeutical research focused on this event (Hardy J and Selkoe DJ 2002). NFD has been consistently found in many neurodegenerative diseases among which the most prevalent is AD. Others include corticobasal degeneration (CBD), dementia pugilistica, fronto-temporal dementia with parkinsonism linked to chromosome 17 (FTDP-17), head trauma, Down syndrome, postencephalic parkinsonism, progressive supranuclear palsy (PSP), myotonic dystrophy (DM) and in Pick´s disease (Buee L et al, 2000). Nonetheless, the vast majority of studies have been performed in AD.

At the molecular level NFD corresponds to the aggregation of hyper- and abnormally phophorylated Tau proteins into filaments referred to paired helical filaments (PHFs) (Brion JP et al., 1985; Ihara Y et al., 1986). The spatiotemporal distribution of NFD in the diseased human nervous system is well correlated with the clinical expression of cognitive deficits (Delacourte A et al., 1999). However, there is a long and clinically silent period during which the lesions slowly developed and progress in several brain areas and are yet clinically silent. Neuropathological studies show that NFD is already detected in locus coeruleus of some people under 30. Moreover, the entorhinal cortex of non-demented individuals aged over 50 years, and the hippocampus are also often affected. During the earliest stages of AD with cognitive functions impairment, NFD is quite specific, spreading from the hippocampal formation to the anterior, inferior, and mid temporal cortex. NFD follows a stereotyped, sequential and hierarchical pathway. The progression is categorized into ten stages according to the brain regions affected: transentorhinal cortex (S1), entorhinal (S2), hippocampus (S3), anterior temporal cortex (S4), inferior temporal cortex (S5), medium temporal cortex (S6), polymodal-association areas (prefrontal, parietal inferior and temporal superior) (S7), unimodal areas (S8), primary motor (S9a) or sensory (S9b, S9c) areas and all neocortical areas (S10). Up to stage 6, the disease can be asymptomatic (Figure 1).

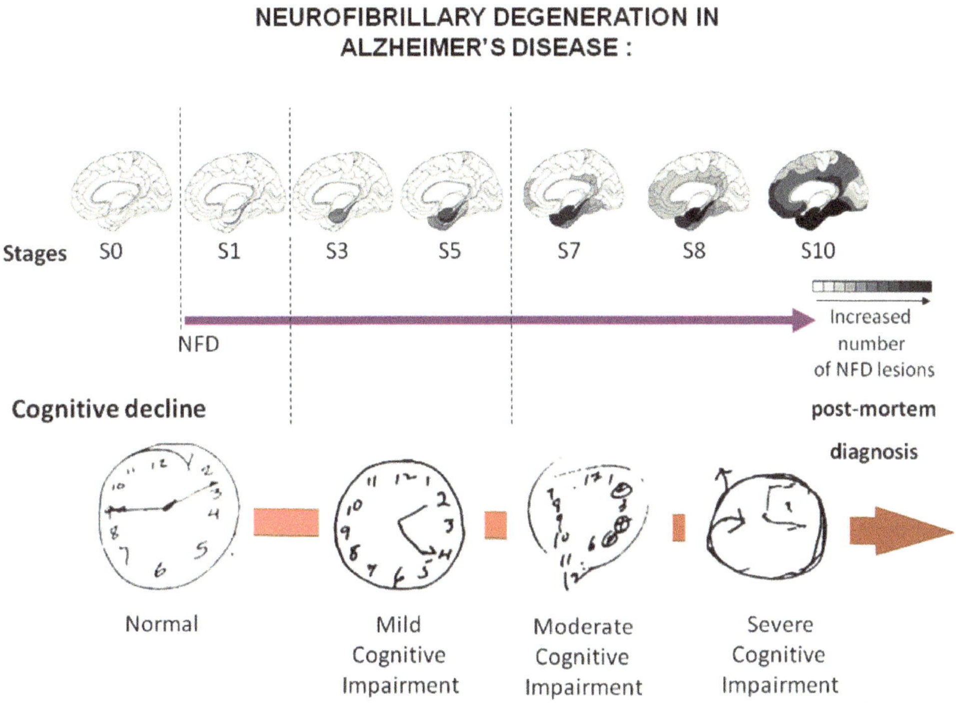

Fig. 1. NFD evolution in AD and cognitive decline. Watches represent the perception of the objects depending on the stage of the disease.

Despite tau proteins are heat stable, acid stable and very soluble in its native unfolded form (Cleveland DW et al., 1997), numerous methods have been used in order to dissect tau aggregates. First, PHFs in AD were initially observed by electron microscopy in 1963 (Kidd M. 1963). Then, in chronological order, Selkoe and collaborators described in 1982 a partial purification of PHFs from human brain tissue. PHFs showed a small solubility in urea, guanidine and detergents as sodium dodecyl sulphate (SDS), representing an example in neurons of a rigid intracellular polymer maybe as a consequence of covalent bonds that avoid a molecular separation by gel electrophoresis (Selkoe DJ et al., 1982). The first commonly used PHF preparation is that described by Nukina N and Ihara Y in 1985 and consists to have PHF in Sarkosyl insoluble fractions. Further purification of Sarkosyl pellets was described by Hasegawa and collaborators in 1992. Pellets were suspended in a small volume of 50 mM Tris-HCl (pH 7.6), and dissolved with 6 M guanidine HCl for further purification. The guanidine HCl suspension was centrifuged at 500,000 X g for 30 min on a TL100.3 microcentrifuge (Heckman). The supernatants were treated with iodoacetate after reduction and fractionated on a TSK gel G-3000 SW column (7.8 X 600 mm, Tosoh) equilibrated with 6 M guanidine HCI in 10 mM phosphate buffer (pH 6.0), at a flow rate of 1.0 ml/min. The TSK fractions contain full-length tau with unusually slow mobilities in SDS-PAGE. The second commonly used preparation is that of Greenberg and Davies: about 50% of PHF immunoreactivity can be obtained in 27,200 x g supernatants following homogenization in buffers containing 0.8 M NaCl. Further enrichment was made by taking advantage of PHF insolubility in the presence of zwitterionic detergents and 2-mercaptoethanol, then removal of aggregates by filtration through 0.45-microns filters, and sucrose density centrifugation. PHF-enriched fractions contained proteins of 57-68 kDa that displayed the same antigenic properties as PHFs. The next stept was to develop an amino acid sequencing technique for PHFs combining a purification and solubilization procedure. After electrophoresis the insoluble fraction presented identical amino acid composition despite successive electrophoresis. Electron microscopy confirmed no changes in PHFs structures for the insoluble fraction even after electrophoresis. Moreover, this insoluble fraction displayed immunoreactivity against purified PHFs antibodies. Almost totally solubilization for the insoluble part was achieved by increasing the time of electrophoresis till almost 35 h showing one predominant band at 66 kDa and three additional bands between 50 and 70 kDa (Vogelsang GD et al., 1990).

Further studies based on the soluble and insoluble fractions after sucrose density gradient showed tau amino-terminal epitopes were more abundant in the soluble part and almost nonexistent in the insoluble one, in the other way around carboxy-terminal epitopes were observed in both fractions. These last observations pointed out the proteolytic degradation involved tau amino-terminal region and not in the carboxy-terminal part in the formation of PHFs in NFD (Ksiezak-Reding H et al., 1994).

Apart from characterization of PHFs from the solubility point of view, the development of additional approaches as electronic microscopy has definitely contributed to elucidate their ultrastructure. For instance, scanning transmission electron microscopy (STEM) provides accurate measurements of samples purified from human tissue and allows quantitave comparison between aggregated and dispersed population (Ksiezak-Reding H et al., 2005). Information regarding the filamentous conformation contributes to uncover the phosphorylation role in their formation. PHFs display ultrastructural different characteristics in AD and other neurological disorders. One possible classification is according to the straight or twisted filaments, based on the width of them along the length. Particularly twisted filaments are more abundant in AD and straight ones in PSP and both can be easily differentiated in CBD.

Along this section it has been described the main attempts to solubilize PHFs in order to clarify their composition, structure and their role in the aetiology in neurodegenerative disorders, mainly focused on AD. It can be considered that these were the first proteomics contribution to uncover the NFD progress involved in the cognitive impairments and loss of memory. In the next section we will discuss about the more modern and current proteomics methods and their application in the field of neurodegeneration.

3. Proteomic methods

Proteomics is the study of proteome, which are the whole set of proteins expressed by a genome of a cell, tissue or organism. So the analysis of a proteome is any study directed to level expression, degradation or post-translational modifications of proteins. Proteomics methods enable the identification and composition of these proteins from diverse biological samples.

Proteomics field may be divided into two main areas: protein profiling and functional proteomics. Profiling proteomics provides all the proteins of a sample, level of expression and global profile. At a functional level proteomics afford a lot of new and challenge pathways that may be related to disease aetiology and development of the symptoms. Identification of theses pathways and protein changes in expression or post-translational modifications might lead to a novel window of therapeutical targets. A better knowledge of the evolution in these proteins during the pathological process may also increase the accuracy for an early clinical diagnosis. In that sense, the most challenging discovery would be to find characteristic biomarkers of each disease and their modifications concerning the worsening of the symptoms during the progress of the illness. The study of the human brain proteome is one of the most challenging aspects in science during the last decades. Brain functions and their involvement in process like memory, behavior, and emotions in physiological as well as in pathological orchestration remain far from understood.

Independently where samples come from tissue, cells or body fluids as cerebrospinal fluid (CSF), the extraction of proteins is the *caput anguli* in all experiments. It is mandatory to establish the brain area, neuronal population or affected region, which is object of study. Moreover, thanks to the enormous protocols available for protein isolation, it is possible to achieve material enough from subcellular regions such as mitochondria or lipid rafts. Nowadays it is very useful and worldwide use the microdissection that enables to select a homogenous tissue or neuronal population, using a laser-dissecting microscope. Noteworthy that proteome analysis is not always reliable, not only because of changes in the expression profile as a consequence of genomic modifications, but also due to variability in extraction protocols and the quality of the sample after autopsy.

Proteomics analyses include two key steps, on one hand the separation and isolation of the protein to study and on the other hand the identification of proteins by mass spectrometry. In addition to separation and identification methods, there are also many well characterized technology to quantify protein as 2D differential gel electrophoresis (2D-DIGE), iTRAQ-Isobaric Tags for Relative and Absolute Quantification or SILAC-Stable Isotope Labeling by Amino Acids. Proteomics and bioinformatic developing technologies run in pararell since it is not possible to achieve hight standards in protein quantification and reliable identification if softwares do not allow discriminating among the possible variants and erasing the background that all the experimental conditions generate. Filters and integrators constitutes a general paradigm for signal detection in biology (Ideker T et al., 2011). In any case the researcher owns the most powerful weapon that is the capacity to assume the feasibility of a biological data, it means how the system is constructed and the functions carried out. Software enables to have update database easily accessible on internet including genome, transcriptome, metabolome, interactome and of course proteome (Brewis IA and Brennan P, 2010). There are several databases available for the research community dedicated to the analysis of protein sequences and structures, some of them are NCBI Peptidome, Expert Protein Analysis System (ExPASy), PeptideAtlas, the PRoteomics IDEntifications database (PRIDE) and Global Proteome Machine Database (GPMDB) (Vizcaíno JA et al., 2010).

3.1 Identification methods

Mass spectrometry (MS) is one of the most widespread developed analytical technique in biological sciences. Analysis of the amino acid sequence, tridimensional structure and characterization of post-translational modifications has allowed elucidating protein functions. Despite it is not the aim of this chapter it is useful to say that MS is also used in

DNA studies (Murray KK, 1996). MS is nowadays used in a large number of fields including from biochemistry to genome studies (Pandey A and Mann M, 2000). In combination with separation techniques, MS due to its sensitivity and speed may have an important role in identifying and monitoring biomarkers in physiological fluids as well as in drug discovery. This approach enables to identify therapeutic targets present at low concentrations in complex biological samples.

From the theorical point of view MS is not a measure of the mass, indeed it is a mass-to-charge (m/z) ratio of gas-phase ion. The values should be represented in terms of Daltons (Da) per unit of charge and the unit in the International System are Kilograms per Columb. In spite of the information obtained with this analysis is directly associated with the molecular weight and amount of protein, the results offered the possibility to acquire additional information as structural disposition (Zellner M et al., 2009).

MS are composed by three different parts: an ionization source, a mass analyser and a detector. The development of this technique is strengthly linked to the introduction of new and more sensitive components in these equipments.

Ionization source

Ionization can be defined as any process by which electrically neutral compounds are converted into ions (electrically charged atoms or molecules). Samples must be ionised and transferred to the gas phase, as a consequence of this step sample is destroyed. Classically ionization takes places in two separate steps, one in which the sample is volatilized and another one where it is ionized. The improvement in ionization methods permits to ionise large, non-volatile and thermally labile biomolecules and convert them into a gas phase without dissociation (Chait BT and Kent SB, 1992). The importance of these improvements was awarded in 2002 by the Nobel Prize in Chemistry "for the development of methods for identification and structure analyses of biological macromolecules" with one half jointly to John B. Fenn and Koichi Tanaka "for their development of soft desorption ionisation methods for mass spectrometric analyses of biological macromolecules" and the other half to Kurt Wüthrich "for his development of nuclear magnetic resonance spectroscopy for determining the three-dimensional structure of biological macromolecules in solution". Electrospray ionization (ESI) and matrix-assisted laser desorption/ionization (MALDI) are the most worldwide ionization sources used nowadays.

In ESI the ion transfer from the solution to the gas phase ocurrs at atmospheric pressure (Zellner M et al., 2009). It is a process by which an aerosol is generated between two electrodes through a capillary held at a high potential (classically 3–4 kV), ions are separated of the solvent and get into the mass analyser. This method does not present a limit of size of the molecule to ionize and it can be easily coupled to MS and liquid separation techniques. Another variation of ESI is nanospray that owns a higher ionisation efficacy and it is less sensible to salt contamination. ESI might be the technique of choice for the design and development of quenchers against α,β-unsaturated aldehydes that are strongly associated with the oxidative stress (Beretta G et al., 2008), it has been used for instance to identify a human T-cell activation RhoGTPase-activating protein in a high frequency electromagnetic field irradiation model to induce AD features (Chang IF and Hsiao HY, 2005), to identify phosphorylation sites on tau (Reynolds CH et al., 2008) and analysis of phospholipids in CSF of AD patients (Kosicek M et al., 2010).

MALDI is maybe the most common ionization source used at the present time in proteomics era. Above all because it can be easily coupled to time-of-flight (TOF) mass analysers.

MALDI was introduced by Hillenkamp and Karas and currently is like ESI a suitable technique to the study of complex biological samples (Hillenkamp F and Karas M, 1990). MALDI produces mostly singly charged ions by a pulsed-laser irradiation. Moreover, MALDI owns a really high sensibility with almost no sample wasting and no desalting process is necessary since it works at physiological concentration of salts. In addition, MALDI requires relatively cheap equipment and quite easy to handle. MALDI TOF mass spectrometry is the technique of choice for protein identification separated by two-dimensional gel electrophoresis. MALDI TOF is widely used in the study of AD in different cellular compartment as synaptosomes proteins (Yang H et al., 2011), Aβ isoforms and their effect on tau phosphorylation in transgenic mouse model overexpressing Aβ1-40 and Aβ1-42 (Mustafiz T et al., 2011), evalutation of a vaccine specifically targeting the pathological amino-truncated species of Aβ42 that induces the production of specific antibodies against pathological Aβ products (Sergeant N et al., 2003), the possible role of heavy metal as copper (II) in the formation of PHFs (Zhou LX et al., 2007), identification of lipids containing in the PHFs from human brain as phosphatidylcholine, cholesterol, galactocerebrosides and sphingomyelin (Gellermann GP, et al 2006), identification of post-translational changes of proteins involved in AD as JNK-interacting protein 1 that is hyperphosphorylated following activation of stress-activated and MAP kinases (D'Ambrosio C et al., 2006), enrichment of more truncated glycans in PHFs (Sato Y et al., 2001) and decrease in the expression of M2 acetylcholine receptor (Zuchner T et al., 2005) are some examples.

Mass analyser

Once ions have been originated they are transported to the mass analyser region and separated according to their *m/z*. The election of one o the type of analyser will depend on their resolution, when more resolutive high capacity to defferentiate two close signals. Mass analysers available in the market are electric- and magnetic-field, depending on the way to separate the ions. The choise among them will depend on the application needed and the budget since each analyzer type has its strengths and weaknesses. Mass analysers systems are Quadrupoles, Sectors, Fourier transform cyclotrons and TOF. Quadrupole analysers are normally coupled to ESI ion sources and TOF analysers are often used with MALDI ion sources. Anyway, hybrid systems are also employed as ESI-TOF and MALDI-QTOF.

TOF spectrometer separates ions based on their velocity with a theorical mass gap unlimitated. TOF consists basically of a flight tube in high vacuum where ions are accelerated with equal energies and fly along the tube with different velocities. The flight time is related to the m/z values of the ions. The combination of high m/z range and compatibility with pulsed-ionization methods has made TOF the most commonly used analyser for MALDI experiments.

In Peptide Mass Fingerprinting approach gel-separated proteins are digested in the gel with a site-specific proteinase as trypsin (Hellman U et al., 1995). Then MS measurement of the cleavaged proteins is performed generally by MALDI TOF equipment. Finally Fingerprint peptides are compared to databases in which protein sequences have been already digested with the same proteinase. This is the method of choise for highthroughput identification of numerous samples. Moreover, robotic systems launched onto the market make possible the automation from detection spot in the gel till MS identification (Henzel WJ et al., 1993).

Tandem Mass Spectrometry (MS/MS) is another identification method predominantly suitable for analysing complex samples and a routine method used in research. This technique permits the identification of unkown proteins by sequencing their peptides.

MS/MS involved two steps of MS. In the first analyser ions with a desired m/z are separated (product ions) from the rest of the ions coming from the ionization source, and in the second type of analyser the mass spectrum is measured. Furthermore, MS/MS experiments improve the ratio signal/noise facilitating the resolution.

The product ions can be used to find out the primary structure of the peptide but nowadays most efforts are directed towards identification of post-translational modifications. In the case of tau protein is particulary special, since phosphorylation provides an additional negative charge to the sample. This fact complicates the analysis by MS because of detection of phosphopeptides is highly dependant on the equipment used as well as the software applied to analyze the spectra. Moreover, the existence of several adjacent serine or threonine residues allows MS/MS not to attribute the exact position of a phophate group as a result of the fragmentation of the peptide data.

The team of Hasegawa performed the earliest application for identification of Tau into PHFs. They used different fractions: purified PHF-tau, AD-soluble tau, or normal tau treated or not with alkaline phosphatase. The digests were applied to a Superspher Select B column (2.1 X 125 mm, Merck) and eluted with a linear gradient of 4-48% acetonitrile in 0.1% trifluoroacetic acid in 20 min at a flow rate of 0.2 ml/min. Amino Acid Sequence and Mass Spectrometric Analyses of the API Peptides-Fractionated peptides were sequenced on an Applied Biosystems 477A Protein Sequencer equipped with an on-line 120A PTH Analyzer or on an Applied Biosystems 473A Protein Sequencer. Mass spectral analysis was performed on a PE-SCIEX API 111 Hiomolecular Mass Analyzer (triple-stage quadrupole mass spectrometer) equipped with a standard atmospheric pressure ion source. Detailed comparison of peptide maps of PHF-tau and normal tau before and after dephosphorylation pointed to three anomalously eluted peaks which contained abnormally phosphorylated peptides, residues 191-225,226-240,260-267, and 386-438, according to the numbering of the longest tau isoform. Protein sequence and mass spectrometric analyses localized Thr-231 and ser-235 as the abnormal phosphorylation sites and further indicated that each tau 1 site (residues 191-225) and the most carboxyl-terminal portion of the protein (residues 386-438) carries more than two abnormal phosphates. Ser-262 was also phosphorylated in a fraction of PHF-tau. Modifications other than phosphorylation, removal of the initiator methionine, and Nu-acetylation at the amino terminus and deamidation at 2 asparaginyl residues were found in PHF-tau, but these modifications were also present in normal tau (Hasegawa et al., 1992).

NMR spectroscopy is an alternative to MS and it has been used to uncover physiological and pathological roles of tau protein. However, this is challenging since tau protein has 441 amino acids and an unfavorable amino acid composition. Quantification of phosphorylated tau samples is complex and studies are being performed in vitro using recombinant kisases (Landrieu I et al., 2010).

3.2 Separation methods

Analysis of a sample is always a challenge, it depends on the origin and of the aim of the experiment. Separation of the components of a sample offers the possiblility to establish a pre-selection and to perform a study concerning parameters as molecular weight (MW) and isoelectric point (pI). The separation methods available today have the enormous advantage that they can be coupled to other quantification techniques, including in this way not only the identification of the protein of interest, but also it relative amount compared to the control conditions. During this section we will converse abouth two separation approaches such as bidimensional electrophoresis and liquid chromatography.

3.2.1 Two-dimensional gel electrophoresis in AD brain

Two-dimensional gel electrophoresis (2D) is one of the most often-used separation methods in proteomics since first description by O´Farrell PH in 1975. This approach combines two electrophoretic methods: in the first dimension proteins are separated on an immobilized pH gradient strip with isoelectric focusing and migrate to the point on the strip at which their net charge is zero or pI, and in the second dimension or SDS-PAGE, proteins are separated according to their MW and thus isolating isoforms and isovariants of a certain protein.

This approache provides two kinds of information depending on the aim of the study. On one hand it can offer the global proteome profile with a high resolution containing nearly one thousand protein spots. However, the main limitation of the 2D is that several replicates of the same gel should be performed in order to reach statistically differences. The lack of a loading control makes complicated to rule out between differences in protein expression and loading variability among gels (Molloy MP et al., 2003). In addition, absence of an internal control for loading makes this approche very hand variable. On the other hand, this method is quite indicated if qualitative analysis is pointed out, ie if post-translational modifications are searched, the performance of a 2D western blot for two different conditions may supply changes in pI and /or MW. More specifically in the case of the tau protein, this method might give interesting data about the acidification or alkalinization as a consequence of phosphorylation process, which is the most common post-translational modification. For instance in figure 2 is shown 2D western blots for human total tau and phospho dependent AD2 antibodies in AD brain sample. Remarkably in the acidic part of the membrane it can be observed the characteristic triplet of phosphorylated tau (2A) in AD (60,64,69 kDa), while in the basic region all the tau isovariants dephosphorylated with postmorten delay are revealed (2B). Interestingly, in a recent study of our group it has been shown that the use of 2D may provide evidence that tau mutations dysregulate tau phosphorylation status. This event could be one of the first steps in the NFD cascade (Bretteville A et al., 2009).

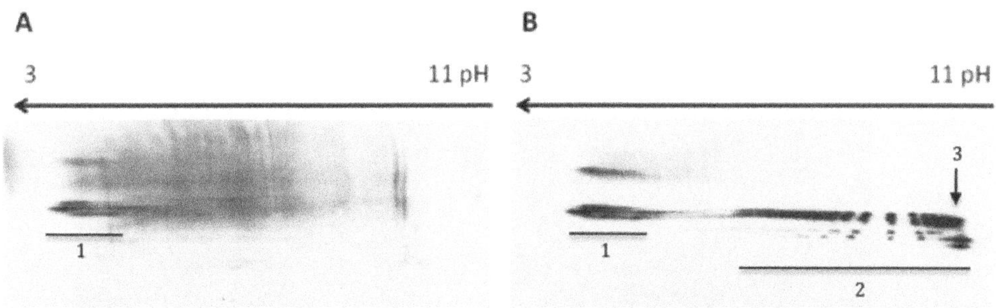

Fig. 2. 2D profiles of phospho-tau (A) and total tau (B) antibodies. Number 1 represents the hyperphosphorylated isovariants of tau while number 2 shows the low phosphorylated ones. Number 3 displays the native form of tau (Fernandez-Gomez FJ et al., personal unpublished data).

3.2.2 Quantitative proteomics by Two-Dimensional Differential Gel Electrophoresis (2D-DIGE)

2D-DIGE method is based on the same principle as "classical" 2D. The main differences rely on the fact that proteins are labeled with fluorescent dyes and all the samples are separated at the same time in the same gel reducing spot pattern variability and the number of gels in an experiment. The reduction in number of gels during the manipulation increases the cost effectiveness and accurate spot matching. 2D-DIGE presents also the advantage that it is a quantitative approche since each protein spot has its own internal standard (IS), which ensure that the differences found are real and not due to a gel-to gel variation. Moreover, 2D-DIGE is a very sensitive technique with a detection threshold of around 1 femtomole of protein (Gong L et al., 2004). In the minimal labeling proteins are stained by cyanines, these dyes has a N-hydroxysuccinimidyl ester reactive group which forms a covalent bond with the epsilon amino group of the lysine in proteins via an amide connection. The single positive charge of the cyanine replaces the single positive charge of the lysine and the pI of the protein is not altered. This labeling reaction is minimal since only affects between 1-3% of the lysine residues. Using different cyanines dyes as Cy2, Cy3 and Cy5 covalently coupled to one protein sample each, then they can be mixed and loaded in the same gel (Viswanathan S et al., 2006) as it is shown in figure 3. A pool of all the samples is labeled with Cy2 and in this way the loading variability among gel is reduced to about 7% (Tannu NS et al., 2006). Differences will be observed after measurement of the intensity of the fluorescence for each cyanine. The 2D analysis software using the IS achieves a fast detection of less than 10% of differences between samples with more than 95% of statistical confidence (Gharbi S et al., 2002).

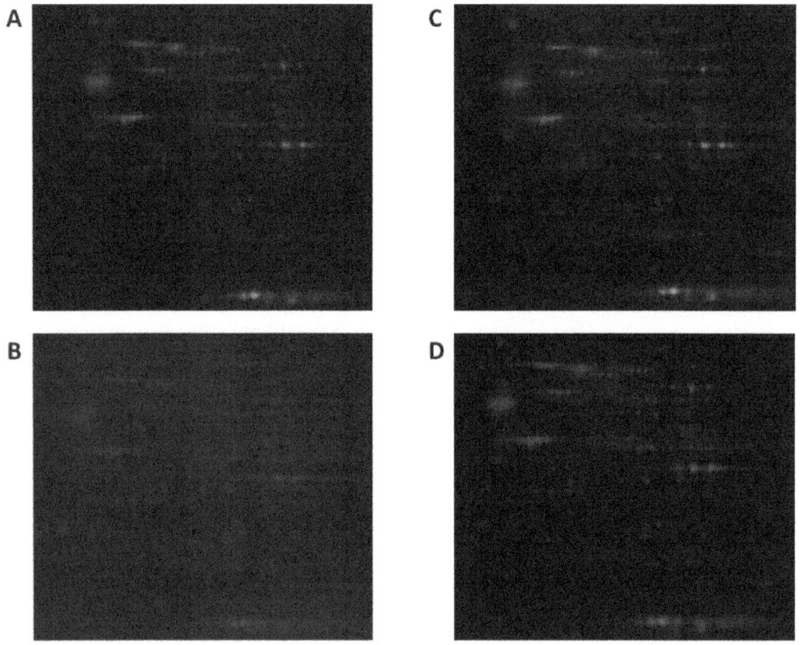

Fig. 3. Cy2, Cy3 and Cy5 merged (A) Cy2 labels IS (B) Cy3 pool of control (C) and Cy5 pool of AD samples (D). The software overlaps Cy2, Cy3 and Cy5 in order to establish the statistical differences among the replicates of the gels for each spot (Fernandez-Gomez FJ et al., personal unpublished data).

Despite the fact that it is far less used, there is in the market another 2D-DIGE method called saturation labeling where only two cyanines are used. Cy3 is the pool of samples and it constitute the IS and Cy5 is the sample object of study. In this technique saturation dyes have a maleimide reactive group, which is designed to form a covalent bond with the thiol group of cysteine residues on proteins via a thioether linkage, and a high dye-to-protein labeling ratio is required. This type of labeling approach tries to label all available cysteines on every protein. This method has the main inconvenient that only one sample can be loaded in a gel apart from the IS and not two sample like in the minimal labelling. The big adventage is that cyanines offer great sensitivity with detection over 5 orders of magnitude (Shaw J et al., 2003).

The main limitation inherent to 2D method is that the gap of separation is among pH 3-10. As a consequence of this, poor solubilisation of highly acidic and basic proteins is reached. Proteins strongly attached to the biological membranes and samples with high concentration of salt own difficulty to be separated by isoelectric focusing, for this reason it is strong recommended to perform a purification step previous to the first dimension.

2D-DIGE application accomplishes one of the new perpectives in the medical research. This approach is been widely used for many studys in neurodegenerative disorders including AD. 2D-DIGE has been utilized in the search for biomarkers in CSF in amyotrophic lateral sclerosis (Brettschneider J et al., 2008), in Creutzfeldt-Jakob disease (Brechlin P et al., 2008) in AD patients (Maarouf CL et al., 2009), in frontal cortex brain samples of AD (Müller T et al., 2008) and in animal models.

3.2.3 Quantitative proteomics by Liquid Chromatography linked to Mass Spectrometry (LC-MS)

Liquid chromatography (LC) consist in separating proteins eluted from a LC column after the peptides are enzimatically digested, then they can be measured by MS. LC separation takes place when the sample components interact to a different extent with a mobile or stationary phase and elute at different times from this system. Normally several chromatographic systems are used in order to achieve a high resolution separation since only one system may not separate the complex mixture of peptides successfully. Then eluted fractions are undertaken to MS. The biggest adventage of LC coupled with MS is that this system presents a high-speed identification of the sample in an automatically way avoiding interindividual variability (Zellner et al., 2009). LC-MS is not a quantitative method *per se*, the peptide products coming from the proteolytic cleavage may alter the intensity of the signal in MS analysis due to their physicochemical characteristics. In order to discard this problem the use of stable isotopes has had a wide acceptance in the science community to achive accurancy in the quantification. The approach is based on the idea that a stable isotope-labeled peptide is chemically identical to its native counterpart and behaves identically during fractionation, digestion, chromatographic and MS analysis, but is distinguishable in a MS due to the mass diference. The ratio of signal intensities for the labeled and unlabeled peptide pairs provides an accurate measure of relative abundance of peptides from different samples. Stable isotopic tags can be introduced onto selective sites on peptides via metabolically, chemically, enzymatically, or provided by adding synthetic peptide standards to the sample. Strategies for isotope-based quantitative proteomics can be divided into two groups, depending on whether the isotopic tag is incorporated *in vitro* during sample preparation (iTRAQ, ICAT) or *in vivo* (SILAC) (Colucci-D´Amato et al., 2011).

Isotope Coded Affinity Tagging (ICAT) reagents consist of an affinity biotin tag for selective purification, a linker that incorporates stable isotopes and an iodoacetamide group that specifically reacts with free thiol of cysteines. Proteins from two different samples are labeled with either light or heavy ICAT reagents obtaining a distinctive mass (eight or nine Da). To minimise the error, the labeled mixture of protein samples are combined, digested with protease to peptides and fractionated by multidimensional chromatography and analysed by LC-MS. The ratios of signal intensities of differentially mass-tagged peptide pairs are quantified to determine the relative levels of proteins in the two samples. An interesting application of this technique is for the redox proteomic since ICAT labels cysteine residues (Sethuraman M et al., 2004). However, this method is not suitable for quantifying proteins that do not contain enough residues of cysteine and it presents the limitation that only two samples can be done at once (Shiio Y and Aebersold R, R 2006). For this reason this approach is limited for studying of post-translational modifications and splice isoforms.

Another amino group-based isotope labeling approach is isobaric tagging for relative and absolute protein quantification (iTRAQ). Unlike ICAT this method allows identification and quantification as well as comparison of up to eight conditions at the same time. This strategy has been developed in order to overcome the limitations of the previous one, so this method targets the peptide N-terminus of the residues (Ross PL et al., 2004). The iTRAQ reagent consists of a reporter group that is a tag with a specific mass in each individual reagent and a balance group to ensure that the reporter and balanced groups remain invariant without changing the mass. After collision-induced dissociation reporter ions spectra is correlating with the protein-sequence database and relative quantification of proteins with high accuracy is reached (Gevaert K et al., 2008).

Stable Isotope Labeling by Amino Acids (SILAC) is a metabolic stable isotope labeling during cell growth and division in bacteria and afterwards was adapted to amino acids in cell cultures (Ong SE et al., 2002). SILAC is a simple procedure in which natural variants of essential amino acids are replaced by deuterated, carbon-13 or more currently by nitrogen-15. Using nitrogen-15 the number of incorporate labels is defined and not dependent of the number of carbons that constitute the peptide sequence, this facilitates the analysis of the results. The advantage of this method relies on it accurate quantification since stable isotopes are incorporated very early in the sample. The main inconvenient of this technique is that isotopes can only be incorporated during protein synthesis. This is a huge limitation for the study of CSF and human brain tissue taking into account that neurons are post-mitotic cells (Bantscheff M et al., 2007). Despite this handicap SILAC is a powerful tool to study cellular pathways as polyubiquitin involment in the aetiology of AD (Dammer EB et al., 2011), neuroinflamation (McGeer EG and McGeer PL, 2010), reactive microglia (Klegeris A et al., 2008), neurotrophin signaling (Zhang G et al., 2011), oxidative stress (Akude E et al., 2011), TDP-43 proteinopathy in frontotemporal lobar degeneration and amyotrophic lateral sclerosis (Seyfried NT et al., 2010) mitochondrial alterations in dopaminergic cells (Jin J et al., 2007) and modulation of ion channels by phosphorylation (Park KS et al., 2006).

Other methods for protein quantification are multiple reaction monitoring (MRM) that has been successfully used for low abundant proteins in plasma (Anderson L and Hunter CL, 2006) and phosphopeptides quantification (Lange V et al., 2008). The absolute quantification of proteins (AQUA) technology uses a known quantity of heavy isotope labeled peptides as IS added as soon as possible in the analytical process (Kettenbach AN et al., 2011).

3.2.4 Surface-enhanced laser desorption/ionization mass spectrometry

Surface-enhanced laser desorption/ionization mass spectrometry (SELDI) method combines retention chromatography with MS detection, and it can be used in biological samples such as cancer cells, CSF and tissue lysates. A few microliters of a sample of interest are deposited on the chromatographic surface. The protein chip arrays are incubated and then washed with a suitable buffer. SELDI protein chip surfaces are uniquely designed to retain proteins from complex mixtures according to their specific properties using chromatographic-based selectivity. The proteins of interest are captured on the chromatographic surface by adsorption, partition, electrostatic interaction or affinity chromatography depending on their properties, and analyzed by MS. SELDI is frequently coupled to MALDI-TOF and possess the significative advantage that minimal amount of sample is consuming and consequently not destroyed.

The main application of this technique is in the search of biomarker in cancer as well as in neurodegenerative disorders. In the field of AD, SELDI has been used to find significantly higher levels of amyloid-beta peptides monomer and dimer in the blood of AD subjects compare to controls (Villemagne VL et al., 2010) and in CSF the enrichment in Aβ10-40 paralleled by depletion of the fragment Aβ1-42 seems to be a common event in familial AD (Ghidoni R et al., 2009).

4. Contribution of proteomics to Tauopathies classification

Classification and characterization of neurodegenerative disorders have been one of the biggest achievements in proteomic field. Proteomics enable to separate, identify and study protein-protein interactions within the different pathologies. Nowadays the term tauopathies includes more than twenty well-characterized diseases. The high resolution separations of tau proteins in electrophoretic profiles as well as the immunoreactivity with a wide range of antibodies provide substantial information to discriminate among the different diseases. Major post-translational modification in tau proteins is phophorylation. For this reason vast of studies are focused on the role of this modification in the structure, function, pI and signalling pathways of tau proteins during the progression of the diseases.

4.1 Tau proteins

Tau (tubulin associated unit) is the major component of PHFs. Weingarten MD et al. described this protein for the first time in 1975 as an essential factor for the organization, stabilization, and dynamics of microtubules (Weingarten MD et al., 1975). Tau is essentially a neuronal phosphoprotein located within the axonal compartment (Butler M and Shelanski ML, 1986). Tau is prone to modulate the axonal transport and neuronal plasticity (Sergeant N et al., 2005). Recently, it has been established that tau regulates the motility of dynein and kinesin motors proteins by an isoform-dependent mechanism. Indeed, the shortest tau isoform lacking exon 2, 3 and 10 impedes the motility of both kinesin and dynein whereas the longest tau isoforms with all exons less affects motor protein motility (Dixit R et al., 2008). Therefore, a modified pattern of tau isoform expression/ratio, due to tau aggregation for instance, may profoundly affect the axonal transport and could possibly lead to neurodegeneration (Crosby AH, 2003). Besides its known role as a microtubule-stabilizer and organizer, tau may exert several other functions as signalling pathway in neurons (Ittner LM et al., 2010 and Leugers CJ, 2010) and DNA protection under stress stimuli (Sultan A et al., 2011).

A unique human tau (MAPT) gene is located on chromosome 17 at the band position 17q21. The restriction analysis and sequencing of the gene shows that it contains two CpG islands, one associated with the promoter region and the other with the exon 9 (Andriadis A et al., 1992). The human tau primary transcript contains 16 exons and in the adult human brain,

alternative splicing of exons 2, 3 and 10 gives rise to six tau isoforms where exon 3 never appears independently of exon 2. Alternative splicing is regulated during development and differentially between tissues. A single isoform lacking the 3 alternative exons 2, 3 and 10 is expressed in the foetal brain. Exon 10 encodes an additional microtubule-binding motif numbered R1 to R4. Half of tau proteins contain three microtubule-binding motifs and the other halves have four microtubule-binding motifs (figure 4A). Constitutive exons are 1, 4, 5, 7, 9, 11, 12 and 13 and the start codon is located in exon 1. There are two alternate stop codons located either following exon 13 or inside exon 14 (Andreadis A, 2005 and Sergeant N et al., 2008). Human brain tau isoforms have a range from 352 to 441 amino acids and a molecular weigth between 45 to 65 kDa in polyacrylamide gel electrophoresis (figure 4B).
Primary sequence analysis of tau protein shows that it can be subdivided in four structural regions. The amino-terminal region is acidic and variable, depending on the presence or absence of exons 2/3 and a proline-rich domain follows it. The latter is followed by 3 or 4 imperfect repeat motifs (R1 to R4; see figure 4A) - depending on the presence or absence of exon 10 - and corresponding to the microtubule-binding domain of tau. Finally, a short carboxy-terminal region is found and it is the basic region of the protein (figure 4C).

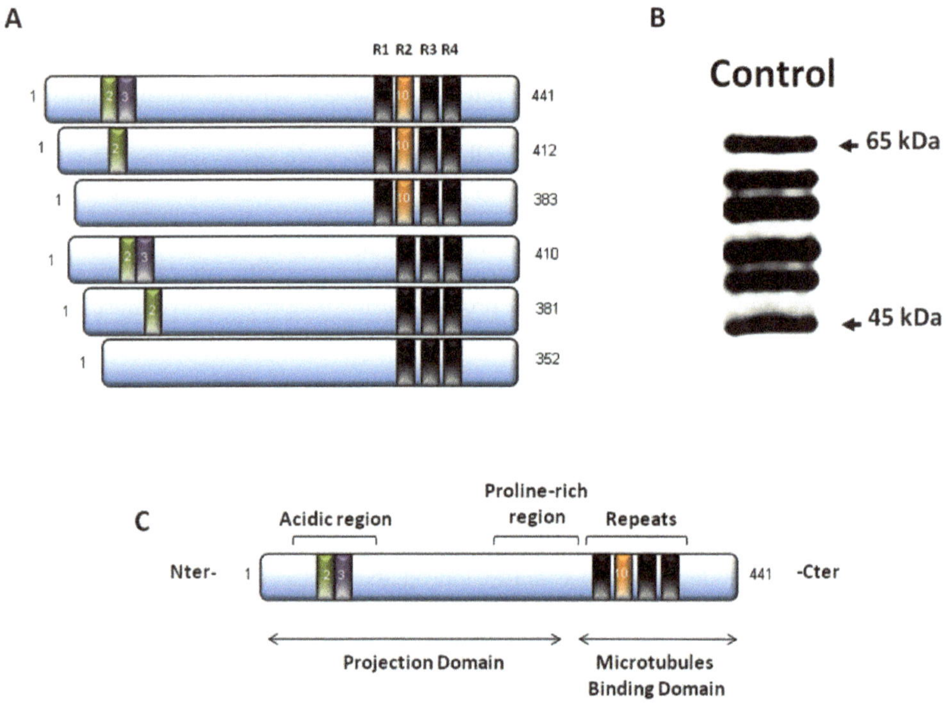

Fig. 4. Six tau isoforms are presented in human brain. These isoforms differ by the absence or presence of one or two 29 amino acids inserts encoded by exon 2 (green box) and 3 (violet box) in the amino-terminal part. Exon 3 is always incorporated with exon 2. R2 corresponds to the presence of exon 10 (orange box) that encodes an additional microtubule-binding motif numbered R1 to R4 in the carboxy-terminal part and they are represented as black boxes. (A). Molecular weight in mono-dimensional electrophoresis for the six isoforms of tau (B) and tau protein regions corresponding to the full-length isoform (C).

The amino-terminal region together with the proline-rich domain is referred to as the "projection domain". This unstructured and negatively charged region detaches from the surface microtubules (Hirokawa N et al., 1988) and can interact with the plasma membrane or cytoskeletal proteins (Brandt R et al., 1995). Tau may therefore contribute to spacing in between microtubule lattice and to the parallel ordered organization of microtubules in axons (Chen J et al., 1992). Amino-terminal region of tau also interacts with a growing panel of polypeptides including motor proteins such as kinesin-1 (Utton MA et al., 2005) and dynactin/dynein complex (Magnani E et al., 2007). All interacting polypeptides constitute the interactome of tau and indicate the functions in which tau may be implicated. The application of 2D gel electrophoresis method has been used to study tau (Janke C et al., 1996). The six main isoforms of tau are separated as several isovariants with isoelectric points comprised between 9.5 and 6.5 due to the alternative splicing and to post-translational modifications. The amino-terminal region has a pI of 3.8, proline domain has a pI of 11.4 and carboxy-terminal has a pI of 10.8. Regarding to the primary structure, the polypeptide sequences encoded by exons 2/3 add to tau acidity, whereas exon 10 encodes a positively charged sequence that adds to the basic character of tau. Thus tau is rather a dipole with two domains with opposite charge modulated either by post-translational modifications or tau proteolysis (Wischik CM et al., 1988).

Tau stabilizes oligomers of tubulins, it is partially folded while interacting with microtubules and it was shown to link laterally protofilaments made of tubulin (Santarella RA et al., 2004). NMR investigations showed that residues between Val226 to Glu372 are binding to microtubule surface involving the all four repeat binding motifs showing that amino- and carboxy-terminal domains do not participate in the binding properties of tau to microtubules (Sillen A et al., 2007). Tau mutations like in FTDP may impair the binding of tau to microtubules (Delobel P et al., 2002). Regarding the physic-chemical properties of tau protein it has been addressed that tau protein owns pro-aggregative motifs called PHF6 and PHF6* in its carboxi-terminal region at the level of R2 and R3. The amino acids sequence of these motifs (306)VQIVYK(311) and (275)VQIINK(280) are prone to promote aggregation by the formation of beta-structure (von Bergen M et al., 2001). This aggregation and accumulation of misfolded proteins might have a common cause and pathological pathway in several neurodegenerative disorders resulting in neuronal loss (Tyedmers J et al., 2010). Several studies have revealed that truncated tau drive NFD *in vivo* (Zilka N et al., 2006) and caspase activation lead to tangles formation (de Calignon et al., 2010).

4.2 Post-translational changes of Tau proteins

Phosphorylation of tau is instrumental to NFD and it is the main post-translational modification in tau isovariants as it was shown by 2D immunoblots (Butler M and Shelanski ML, 1986). These data shed light to the impact of tau protein for tau biology. There are 85 potential phosphorylation sites on the longest brain tau isoform. Phosphorylation sites were identified with proteomic approaches as MS, NMR, phospho-peptide mapping and the use of site-specific phosphorylation dependent tau antibodies (Hanger et al., 2007). Among them around 71 correspond to putative phosphorylation sites in physiological and pathological conditions. It is worthy to remark that most of the phosphorylation sites surround the microtubule-binding domains in the proline-rich region and carboxi-terminal region of tau. Phosphorylation regulates several functions of tau such as its binding to microtubules, the axonal transport of tau as well as its interactions with amino-terminal partners' particularly

SH3-containing proteins (Rosenberg KJ et al., 2008). For instance, tau transport along the axon is negatively regulated by its phosphorylation by GSK3β leading to a reduced binding to kinesin-1 (Cuchillo-Ibanez I et al., 2008). By phosphorylating amino-terminal serines 212 and 217, GSK3β also reduces the binding of SH3-containing proteins, such as Fyn, PLC-γ1, p85α (Reynolds CH et al., 2008). Once tau proteins are phosphorylated they cannot polymerize tubulin into microtubules and do not stabilize the latter.

Tau phosphorylation is mainly regulated through kinases and phosphatases, but other enzymes are also involved, such as Pin1 isomerase (Buee L et al., 2000). A total of more than 20 protein kinases can phosphorylate tau proteins (Sergeant N et al., 2008). This includes four groups of protein kinases. (a) Proline-directed protein kinases (PDPKs), which phosphorylate tau on serines or threonines that are followed by a proline residue. This group includes CDK1 and 5 (Hamdane M et al., 2003), MAPK and several SAPKs (Ferrer I et al., 2005). (b) The non-PDPK group includes tau-tubulin kinases 1 and 2, casein kinases 1 and 2, DYRK1A (dual-specificity tyrosine-phosphorylated and -regulated kinase 1A), phosphorylase kinase, Rho kinase, PKA, PKB/Akt, PKC and PKN (Sergeant N 2005). (c) The third group includes protein kinases that phosphorylate tau on serine or threonine residues followed or not by a proline. GSK (glycogen synthase kinase) 3α and GSK3β and AGC kinases (such as MSK1 (mitogen- and stressactivated protein kinase) belong to this group and have recognition motifs SXXXS or SXXXD/E and RXRXXS/T respectively (Buée L et al., 2010). (d) The fourth group corresponds to tyrosine protein kinases such as Src kinases, c-Abl and c-Met (http://cnr.iop.kcl.ac.uk/hangerlab/tautable). The principal role of tau phosphorylation is related to microtubule binding. However, phosphorylation or dephosphorylation of tau may also contribute to the cell localization of tau. For instance, phosphorylation of tau by GSK3β regulates its axonal transport by reducing its interaction with kinesin. In sharp contrast, dephosphorylated tau is located to the cell nucleus and is suggested to contribute to nucleolar organization and/or contribute to chromosome stability. Mutations in TAU gene lead to a change in the affinity of kinases that phosphorylate tau near the site of the mutation. Some mutations like R406W may reduce the phosphorylation of tau at Ser404, which is necessary for GSK3-β to phosphorylate tau at Ser396 afterwards (Tatebayashi Y et al., 2006). However, this priming putative phosphorylation site is not a prerequisite for JNK3 to phosphorylate tau at Ser396. These data provide evidence that tau mutations may potentially modify the global phophorylation state of tau.

Abnormal phospho sites on PHF-tau were identified on constitutive exons, such as Ser212–214 together and Ser422. These three new sites were identified on the alternative sequence encoded by exon 2. As tau isoforms expression may be different in subneuronal populations, these phospho epitopes would be of interest in identifying such subneuronal populations or the laminar distribution of NDF in AD (Delacourte A et al., 1996).

In normal brains the phospho-epitopes are rapidly dephosphorylate during postmorten delay, this effect may be due to the drop in ATP and inactivation of phophatases. However, in AD brains this dephosphorylatyon does not occur. Some of the hypotheses are that aggregation of tau proteins into filaments render them inaccessible to phosphatases, phosphatases are not activated any more or their activity is suddenly decreased.

Other post-translational modification of tau proteins is O-glycosylation. O-glycosylation results from the attachment of a sugar on the hydroxyl radical of serine or threonine residue in the vicinity of the proline-rich domain. Glycosylation decreases tau phosphorylation by CDK5, PKA and and GSKβ, probably due to a competition between phosphorylation and

glycosylation for the same sites. In fact, tau proteins from AD brains present abnormally glycosylation in comparison with controls. Using a recombinant O-GlcNAc modified tau, MS has mapped O-GlcNAc on tau at Thr-123, Ser-400 sites and a third one on either Ser-409, Ser-412, or Ser-413 (Yuzwa SA et al., 2011). The identification of these sites may provide evidence to elucidate the role of glycosylation in tau function.
The microtubule-associated protein tau is known to be post-translationally modified also by acetylayion. Recent studies reported that tau is acetylated and this acetylation avoids its degradation. Tau acetylation impares tau-microtubules interactions and facilitates tau aggregation. In fact, specific antibodies for acetylated tau showed an increase in acetylation in several Braak stages with the involment of histone acetyltransferase p300 and the deacetylase SIRT1 (Min SW et al., 2010). MS provides specific lysines within the microtubule-binding domain including lysine 280 (K280) that are main sites of tau acetylation. One model shows that K280 is exclusively acetylated in pathological conditions (Cohen TJ et al., 2011).

4.3 Tau as a bar code for neurodegenerative diseases

The most obvious pathological event in tauopathies is the presence of aggregates of tau isoforms into intraneuronal filamentous inclusions. The evolution in the proteomics era allows to establish different physiological and pathological electrophoretical patterns to distinguish among the diversity of tauopathies. Comparative biochemistry of tau aggregates differs in both isoform phosphorylation and content, which enables a molecular classification of tauopathies. In postmorten brain tissue tau proteins are resolved as six bands (figure 4B) whereas more acidic hyperphosphorylated isoforms present four bands between 60 and 74 kDa depending on the disorder (figure 5). The classification presented here is composed by five classes of tauopathies, depending on the type of tau aggregates that constitute the bar code for neurodegenerative diseases (Sergeant et al., 2005).

Class 0: frontal lobe degeneration non-Alzheimer non-Pick

Frontal lobe degeneration is the second more common presinile disorder that leads to dementia after AD. This class is genetically linked to mutations in the progranulin gene (Baker M et al., 2006 and Cruts M et al., 2006). Frontal lobe degeneration presents no specific neuropathological hallmarks, no tau aggregation and a loss of expression in tau proteins. The transactive response (TAR)-DNA-binding protein with a molecular weight of 43 kDa (TDP-43), encoded by the TARDBP gene, has been recently identified as a major pathological protein of frontotemporal lobar degeneration with ubiquitin-positive and tau-negative inclusions. It is the most common underlying pathology in frontotemporal dementias with and without motor neuron disease. In fact TDP-43 pathology is identified till the 50% of AD cases and it is the main component in the amyotrophic lateral sclerosis (Wilson AC et al., 2011). This pathology from the clinical point of view is quite similar to Pick´s disease. It is characterized by a frontal distribution of morphologic changes involves neuronal cell loss, spongliosis and gliosis mainly in the superficial cortical layers of the frontal and temporal cortex (Delacourte A et al., 1977).

Class I: all brain Tau isoforms are aggregated

Class I is characterized by a pathological tau quartet at 60, 64 and 69 kDa, and a minor pathological tau at 72/74 kDa (figure 5). This pathological tau quartet corresponds to the aggregation of the six tau isoforms (Sergeant N et al., 1997b and Goedert M et al., 1992). The pathological tau 60 is composed of the shortest tau isoform (2-3-10-). The pathological tau 64 and 69 are each composed of two tau isoforms: tau isoforms with either the exon 2 or exon 10 alone compose the pathological tau 64, while the pathological tau 69 is made of tau isoforms with either exon 2 + 10 or 2 + 3. The longest tau isoform containing exons 2, 3 and 10 (2 + 3 + 10) constitutes the 72/74-kDa pathological component, as determined by 2D gel electrophoresis coupled to western blotting using exon-specific tau antibodies (Sergeant N et al., 1997a). This typical tau profile was first characterized in AD, but now includes nine additional neurological disorders AD as cerebral aging (over 75 years), ALS/parkinsonism–dementia complex of Guam, Parkinson with dementia of Guadeloupe, Niemann-Pick disease type C, Postencephalitic parkinsonism, Familial British dementia, Dementia pugilisticia, Down's syndrome and FTDP-17. Using histochemistry, aggregates of this class can be observed with AD2 and antibodies against exon 2 and exon 10 (Buee L et al., 2000 and Sergeant N et al., 2008).

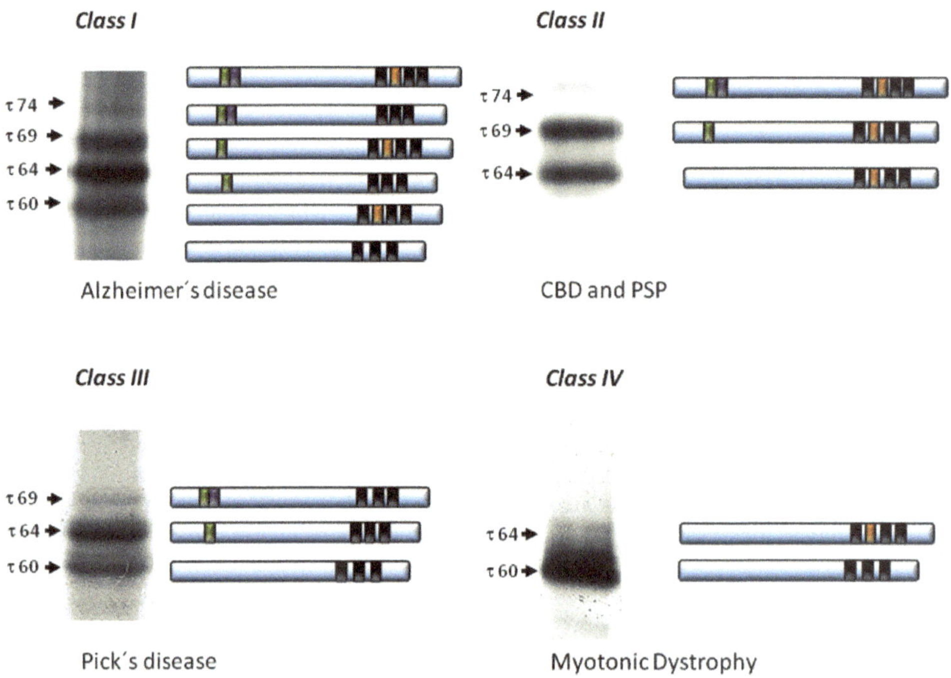

Fig. 5. Bar Code for neurodegenerative diseases. Schematic representation of the modifications leading to tau proteins aggregation in Tauopathies. Native tau proteins are detected as a triplet of bands ranging between 60 and 74 kDa by numerous phosphorylation-dependent antibodies. Tau proteins are shown by western blotting as three major bands between 60 and 69 kDa, and a minor band at 74 kDa. AD pattern is also found in Down's syndrome, post-encephalitic parkinsonism, ALS/parkinsonism–dementia complex of Guam among others (class I). The doublet tau 64, 69 represent the aggregation of hyperphosphorylated tau isoforms with exon 10 (orange box) typical for CBP and CBD (class II), the exclusion of exon 10 (only black boxes) in hyperphosphorylated tau aggregation lead to tau 60, 64 doublet characteristic for Pick's disease (class III). The aggregation of Tau isoforms lacking exons 2 (green box) and 3 (violet box) is found in myotonic dystrophy (class IV).

Class II: Tau isoforms containing the exon 10 encoding sequence aggregate

Aggregation of tau proteins with four microtubule-binding domains is the characteristic of class II (figure 5). This pathological tau profile is observed in CBD, argyrophilic grain dementia, PSP and FTDP-17 due to tau gene mutations (Sergeant N et al., 1999 and Tolnay M et al., 2002). PSP, CBD and argyrophilic grain dementia are rare atypical parkinsonism disorders.

Class III: Tau isoforms lacking the exon 10 encoding sequence aggregate

This class of tauopathies includes Pick's disease and autosomal dominant inherited FDTP-17 (figure 5). Pick's disease is a rare form of neurodegenerative disorder characterized by a progressive dementing process. Early in the clinical course, patients show signs of frontal disinhibition. Neuropathologically, Pick's disease is characterized by the presence of typical spheroid inclusions in the soma of neurons called Pick bodies. Pick bodies are labeled by tau antibodies, with a higher density in neurons of the dentate gyrus of the hippocampal formation than in the temporal and frontal cortices. The pathological tau profile of Pick's disease contrasts with that of class II tauopathies, with the pathological tau isoforms consisting essentially of the 3R tau isoforms.
Immunohistologic staining of these aggregates is positive for AD2 and exon 2 antibodies but negative for exon 10 antibodies. In addition, aggregated tau proteins in Pick's disease are not detected by the monoclonal antibody 12E8 raised against the phosphorylated residue Ser262/Ser356, whereas this phosphorylation site is detected in other neurodegenerative disorders. The lack of phosphorylation at Ser262 and Ser356 sites is likely to be related to either a kinase is not active in neurons that degenerate in Pick's disease or those neurons do not constitutively express these kinases within degenerating neurons (Mailliot C et al., 1998).

Class IV: Tau isoform lacking exon 2, 3 and 10 principally aggregate

This group is represented by a single neurological disorder: myotonic dystrophy (DM) of types I and II (figure 5). DM is the commonest form of adult-onset muscular dystrophy. Genetically it is an inherited autosomal dominant disorder caused by a single gene mutation consisting of expansion of a CTG trinucleotide motif in the 3V untranslated of the myotonic dystrophy protein kinase gene (DMPK), located on chromosome 19q. It is a multisystemic disease affecting many systems as the central nervous system (cognitive and neuropsychiatric impairments), the heart, the genital tract, the eyes, the ears, gastrointestinal tract, endocrine system, thus leading to a wide and variable complex panel of symptoms (Meola G, 2000). Cognitive impairments, as memory, visuo-spatial recall and verbal scale, cortical atrophy essentially of the frontal and the temporal lobe and white matter lesions are often described in both DM1 and DM2 (Sansone V et al., 2007).
Neuropathological lesions, as neurofibrillary tangles (NFTs), have been observed in adult DM1 individuals aged over 50 years. The pathological tau profile of DM1 is characterized by a strong pathological tau band at 60 kDa and, to a lesser extent, a pathological tau component at 64 and 69 kDa. This typical pathological tau profile is reflected by a reduced number of tau isoforms expressed in the brain of individuals with DM1, both at the protein and mRNA levels (Sergeant N et al., 2001). In addition, tau protein expression is also demonstrated to be altered in transgenic mice with human DM1 locus (Gomes-Pereira M et al., 2007). Using specific immunological probes against exon 2 and exon 3 corresponding amino acid sequences, the neurofibrillary lesions were shown to be devoid of tau isoforms with amino-terminal inserts (Maurage CA et al., 2005). An altered splicing of tau

characterized by a reduced expression of tau isoforms containing the amino-terminal inserts characterizes both DM1 and DM2. Overall, it demonstrates that the central nervous system is affected and that DMs are real tauopathies (Dhaenens CM et al., 2011). The direct relationship between the altered splicing of tau and NFD in DM remains to be established. Indeed, such an altered splicing of tau is commonly observed in FTDP- 17 and considered as reminiscent to NFD and tauopathies.

5. Use of proteomics to investigate the mechanisms leading to Tauopathies

Induction of tau fibrillization in cells remain unsatisfactory, this is a limiting factor since NFD cannot be totally reproduced *in vitro* (Sibille N et al., 2006). The development of *in vivo* models has provided an important tool to precise sequence of molecular events leading to tau aggregation. The use of proteomics in these transgenic animals has permitted to go further in the uncovering of the cellular and molecular pathways involved in NFD spreading within the brain and its relationship with the clinical expression of neurological disorders. In this section we will focus on the overexpresion either several isoforms of tau protein or mutated forms in animal models.

5.1 Tau models

Several animal models have been created to recapitulate the two main hallmarks of AD, refearing as amyloid plaques and PHFs. Despite the numerous models existing to mimic the features of this disease, none of them cover all the neuropathological, biochemical and behaviour alterations so far. There are models focus on overexpression of APP and/or presenilin containing one or more mutations linked to familial AD but they do not present NFD. Inspite tau mutations have not been described in AD patients, mutations in tau result in NFTs in an inherited form of FTDP and this dysfunction can lead to neurodegeneration and dementia. Taking into account that AD is a complex disorder and the perfect model does not exist, the large number of tau transgenic models with their strengths and weaknesses may allow for both understanding tau pathology and developing innovative therapeutic strategies. Nowadays there are several transgenic models which own combination of mutant APP, presenilin and tau (Chin J 2011). However, this triple model presents the "limitation" that tau pathology cannot be studied independently of the amyloid effects (Sergeant N and Buée L 2011).

5.1.1 *Caenorhabditis elegans*

The nematode *Caenorhabditis elegans* is widely being used to study neurodegenerative disorders despite the evolutionary difference. *C. elegans* has a short lifespan and it is easy to manipulate genetically. Modelling tauopathies is achieved through pan-neuronal overexpression either wild-type or mutated tau leading to a progressive uncoordinated locomotion which is directly correlated with the nervous system alterations in worms. This model is very useful to identify new genetic targets (Wolozin B et al., 2011). Recent data point out that tau pathology may lead to specific interference with intracellular mechanisms of axonal outgrowth and pathfinding (Brandt R et al., 2009).

5.1.2 *Drosophila melanogaster*

Another model used is the fruitfly *Drosophila melanogaster*. Regarding tauopathies, many groups developed fruitfly models by overexpressing wild-type and mutant forms of human tau. Transgenic fruitflies showed key features of tauopathies as tissue- and temporal-specific effects as adult onset, progressive neurodegeneration, early death, enhanced toxicity of mutant tau, accumulation of abnormal tau and relative anatomic selectivity coupled with differential effects of distinct tau isoforms (Papanikolopoulou K and Skoulakis EM, 2011).

5.1.3 Zebrafish

The novel use of the vertebrate zebrafish as a model system for AD research offers a powerful platform for genetic and chemical screens as well as developmental studies (Tomasiewicz HG et al., 2002). The transgenic expression of the human tau mutation P301L in zebrafish neurons by Gal4/UAS-based vector system recapitulates most pathological features of tauopathies as abnormally phosphorylated reactivity with the epitopes AT180, AT270, 12E8, PHF1, 422, and AT8 in spinal cord neurons, aggregation and behavioral impairments (Paquet D et al., 2010). Application of inhibitors of human GSK3β reduced tau phosphorylation showing that zebrafish kinases are sufficiently conserved with respect to their human orthologues. Current evidence point out that zebrafish tau models recapitulate pathological and biochemical events that occur in tauopathies and therefore may be useful tools for further studies in the aetiology of dementia (Bai Q and Burton EA, 2011).

5.1.4 Tau knock out mice and transgenic mice with wild-type human Tau

Tau mouse models where tau expression is suppressed by MAPT deletion or invalidation present no major changes and animals are physiologically normal (Harada A et al., 1994). It seems other microtubule-associated proteins such as MAP1A probably compensate tau deficiency. Among the mice models available with wild-type human tau it is remarkable to note that overexpression of 3R tau isoforms lead to an accumulation of hyperphosphorylated tau proteins in spinal cord neurons and axonal degeneration as well as a reduction in axonal transport (Brion JP et al., 1999). Similar data were observed in transgenic mice expressing the longest human brain tau isoform under the control of the human Thy-1 promoter. Hyperphosphorylated human tau protein was present in nerve cell bodies, axons and dendrites (Gotz J et al., 1995). Furthermore, recent studies in transgenic mouse models that express the entire human MAPT gene in the presence and absence of the mouse Mapt gene show differences between mouse and human tau in the regulation of exon 10 inclusion during development and in the young adult. In addition, it was observed species-specific variations in the expression of 3R- and 4R-tau within the frontal cortex and hippocampus during the development as well as in cell distribution of the isoforms (McMillan P et al., 2008).

5.1.5 Transgenic mice with mutated human Tau

Mutated tau transgenes have been used under various promoters (2′,3′-cyclic nucleotide 3′-phosphodiesterase, CaMKII, PDGF, Prion, or Thy1.2) with or without inducible systems. The most common phenotype of transgene tau animal is the motor alterations. Tau transgenic mice rTg4510 present P301L mutation in an inductible way and develop NFTs, neuronal loss and behavioural impairments (Santacruz K et al., 2005). Nonetheless the suppression of the expression of this mutated tau revers behavioural impairements despite the NFTs formation keeps on, indeed it seems soluble tau rather than NFTs may be deleterious. These observations are in agreement with a recent report in which brain extract injection from mutant P301S tau expressing mice into brain of transgenic wild-type tau-expressing animals induces assembly of wild-type human tau into filaments and spreading of pathology from the site of injection to neighbouring brain regions (Clavaguera et al., 2009).

Another transgenic mice model is TauRD/ΔK280 that expresses only the 4R tau domains and carry the ΔK280 mutation with a deletion of the amino- and carboxy terminal regions of tau protein. This mutation leads to tau aggregation followed by astrogliosis and neuronal loss. When the transgene is switched off the aggregation of the exogenous tau disappears within around one month and a haf and only aggregated murine tau proteins remain acting as a nucleation factor for tau aggregation (Mocanu MM et al., 2008). Other study suggest a "prion -like" propagation since aggregation continues even if the original tau species have disappeared (Sydow A and Mandelkov EM, 2010).

The K3 transgenic mouse strain expresses human tau carrying the K369I mutation under the Thy1 promoter (Ittner LM et al., 2008). This tau mutation was found in a family of patients presenting with Pick's disease without parkinsonism and amyotrophy (Neumann M et al., 2001). The transgenic mice present early-onset memory impairment and amyotrophy in the absence of overt neurodegeneration. Tau transgene is mainly expressed in the substantia nigra and such expression leads to an early-onset parkinsonism phenotype. Interestingly, motor performance of young, but not old K3 mice improves upon L-dopa treatment. Amyotrophy is probable to be related to tau expression in the sciatic nerve in the same way as in Tg30tau model where pathogenic mutations (P301S and G272V) are expressed in the forebrain and the spinal cord showing progressive motor impairment with neurogenic muscle atrophy besides the hippocampal atrophy (Leroy K et al., 2007). Moreover, transgenic mouse model overexpressing human 1N4R double-mutant tau (P301S and G272V) and invalidated endogenous TAU gene show an accelerated human mutant tau aggregation (Ando K et al., 2011) suggesting that murine tau proteins may act as inhibitors of tau aggregation.

Thy-Tau22 mouse transgenic line exhibits progressive neuron-specific AD-like tau pathology devoid of any motor deficits (Schindowski K et al., 2006). In addition to neurofibrillary tangle-like inclusions and mild astrogliosis, this model shows hyper- and abnormally phosphorylated tau on several Alzheimer's disease-relevant tau epitopes that accumulates within the somato-dendritic area in the hippocampus (Schindowski K et al., 2008). A progressive development of NFTs is observed in the hippocampus and amygdala, which parallels behavioural impairments as well as electrophysiological alterations (Van der Jeugd et al., 2011). These latter changes are observed despite any striking loss of neuronal/synaptic markers until 12 months of age in the hippocampus. Interestingly, at that time point, THY-Tau22 mice exhibit septo-hippocampal tau pathology accompanied by altered retrograde transport from hippocampus to medial septum (Belarbi K et al., 2009) with an accumulation of the nerve growth factor (NGF) levels in the hippocampus consistent with a decrease of its uptake or retrograde transport by cholinergic terminals (Belarbi K et al., in press). Recent data indicate that voluntary exercise prevented memory alterations in these transgenic mice and increased mRNA levels of genes involved in cholesterol trafficking such as NPC1 and NPC2 (Belarbi K et al., 2011).

6. Tau proteins as biomarkers of Tauopathies

Searching for biomarkers is one of the most challenges in current medicine. Biomarkers must be not only specific for a single pathology but also indicative of its progression

(Mayeux R et al., 2011). This is extremely complex in diseases concerning elderly since many symptoms are common and indistinguishable among them as the dementia sign. It is compulsory to find proteins and their post-translational modifications that may provide accuracy on the early diagnosis of the disease and eventually could serve as a therapeutic target. Successfully the development in neuroimaging techniques enables to facilitate and establish a preliminary diagnosis of different neurodegenerative disorders.

Focusing on tauopathies, the presence of tau in CSF was first described in 1993. In AD, tau inclusions in the brain associated with neuronal damages lead to the leakage of abnormal forms of tau in the CSF resulting in quantitative and qualitative changes in CSF-tau composition. Numerous studies demonstrated increased CSF total tau and phosphorylated tau levels in AD, with mean levels 2-3 times higher compared to healthy controls. Tau is now a validated biomarker for AD, it improves the clinical diagnostic accuracy and its assessment for AD diagnosis is now proposed (Dubois B et al., 2010). As the brain lesions develop very early during the disease course even before the first clinical symptoms appear, CSF tau is not only a useful diagnostic marker in the advanced stages of the disease but also a usefull predictive marker in the earliest stages when clinical expression is weak (Hertze J et al., 2010). However, for differential diagnosis of dementia, the actually available tests measuring tau and phosphorylated tau levels in CSF are not sufficient and the identification of more specific postranslational modifications of tau in AD by proteomic approaches is needed. In the future, for the use of tau as biomarker in large clinical trials or in clinical practice, one important goal will be to develop sensitive methods to detect the very low concentration of tau in the blood (<1 pMol). Therefore, sample pre-treatment and handling will be crucial in developing a reliable tau assay in blood/plasma.

7. Conclusion

Tau is a neuronal protein that promotes neuronal survival, it is essentially located within the axonal and indispensable for the organization, stabilization, and dynamics of microtubules. The interaction between tau and microtubules is regulated by phosphorylation. It is widely reported that abnormally and hyperphosphorylated tau proteins lead to insoluble aggregates. The presence of these aggregates is clinically correlated with cognitive decline in a process called NFD; this event common to more than twenty diseases is referred as tauopathies.

The development of the proteomics era has achieved to go further in the characterization of tauopathies and shed light to the mechanism involved in their aetiology. Proteomics approaches as chromatography, mono- and bi-dimensional gel electrophoresis have reached to separate proteins with a quite high resolution after fractioning precedures, selecting a concrete population of cells or organelle isolation. The use of additional reagents to the extraction buffer such as detergents and the evolution of concomitant technologies as microscopy have provided a broad spectrum to characterize the structure and size of a large number of biological complex samples. The combination of protein separation methods with fluorescence dyes and radioactive isotopes (ICAT, iTRAQ, SILAC) makes possible not only more sensitive and reproducible results but also provides a quantitative analysis among samples (2D-DIGE, LC-MS, SELDI).

The previous hallmark is extremely linked to the identification of the separated or isolated proteins. MS has provided the composition of the molecules and also their post-translational modifications since changes in amino acid residues may be identified and characterized by

MS/MS, Peptide Mass Fingerprinting and NMR. The utilization of the current available ionization sources as ESI and MALDI coupled to mass analysers mainly TOF allows almost any compound to be analysed by MS at low levels in complex mixtures. Furthermore, there are a large number of software tools dedicated to facilitate raw data processing, database-dependent search, statistical evaluation of the search result, quantitative algorithms and statistical analysis of quantitative data.

The generation of animal models helps to elucidate the genetic and proteomics aspects involved during the origin and development of tauopathies. Only by the knowledge of the different components of the disease and their contribution, it will be possible to proceed in the right way.

In summary, numerous proteomics approaches are available in order to accomplish new perspectives in the neurodegenerative disorders field. At the moment there are many studies focused on finding out the functions of tau protein thoughtout proteomics approaches. Proteomics methods allow to uncover the different signaling pathways involved in tau biology, proteomics data are intimately related to the protein state: post-translational modifications, cleavage, conformation, synthesis, degradation and activity (if it is known). The selection of the different techniques depends on the aim of the research: protein identification, de novo peptide sequencing, and identification of post-translational modifications or determination of protein-protein interactions. Understanding the human proteome and its variations in physiological and pathological conditions will be intimately related to uncover cellular and molecular pathways involved in the aetiology and progression of the tauopathies as well as to identify potential targets for drug design.

8. Acknowledgment

The authors thank Dr. Nicolas Sergeant, Dr Malika Hamdane and Dr. David Blum for careful reading and comments on the manuscript. This work was supported by Inserm and Lille2 University (France). F.J.F-G has a post-doctoral contract from the French National Research Agency (ANR).

9. References

Akude, E.; Zherebitskaya, E.; Chowdhury, SK.; Smith, DR.; Dobrowsky, RT. & Fernyhough, P. (2011). Diminished superoxide generation is associated with respiratory chain dysfunction and changes in the mitochondrial proteome of sensory neurons from diabetic rats. *Diabetes*, Vol. 60(1), pp. 288-297.

Alzheimer, A. (1907). Über eine eigenartige Erkrankung der Hirnrinde. *Allg Zeitschr Psychiatr*, Vol. 64, pp. 146-148.

Anderson, L. & Hunter, CL. (2006). Quantitative mass spectrometric multiple reaction monitoring assays for major plasma proteins. *Mol Cell Proteomics*, Vol. 5(4), pp. 573-588.

Ando, K.; Leroy, K.; Héraud, C.; Yilmaz, Z.; Authelet, M.; Suain, V.; De Decker, R. & Brion, JP. (2011). Accelerated human mutant tau aggregation by knocking out murine tau in a transgenic mouse model. *Am J Pathol*, Vol. 178(2), pp. 803-816.

Andreadis, A. (2005). Tau gene alternative splicing: expression patterns, regulation and modulation of function in normal brain and neurodegenerative diseases. *Biochim Biophys Acta*, Vol. 1739(2-3), pp. 91-103.

Andreadis, A.; Brown, WM. & Kosik, KS. (1992). Structure and novel exons of the human tau gene. *Biochemistry*, Vol. 31(43), pp. 10626-10633.

Bai, Q. & Burton, EA. (2011). Zebrafish models of Tauopathy. *Biochim Biophys Acta*, Vol. 1812(3), pp. 353-363.

Baker, M.; Mackenzie, IR.; Pickering-Brown, SM.; Gass, J.; Rademakers, R.; Lindholm, C.; Snowden, J.; Adamson, J.; Sadovnick, AD.; Rollinson, S.; Cannon, A.; Dwosh, E.; Neary, D.; Melquist, S.; Richardson, A.; Dickson, D.; Berger, Z.; Eriksen, J.; Robinson, T.; Zehr, C.; Dickey, CA.; Crook, R.; McGowan, E.; Mann, D.; Boeve, B.; Feldman, H. & Hutton, M. (2006). Mutations in progranulin cause tau-negative frontotemporal dementia linked to chromosome 17. *Nature*, Vol. 442(7105), pp. 916-919.

Ballard, C.; Gauthier, S.; Corbett, A.; Brayne, C.; Aarsland, D. & Jones, E. Alzheimer's disease. *Lancet*. 2011; Vol. 377(9770), pp. 1019-1031.

Bantscheff, M.; Schirle, M.; Sweetman, G.; Rick, J. & Kuster, B. (2007). Quantitative mass spectrometry in proteomics: a critical review. *Anal Bioanal Chem*, Vol. 389(4), pp. 1017-1031.

Belarbi, K.; Burnouf, S.; Fernandez-Gomez, FJ.; Desmercières, J.; Troquier, L.; Brouillette, J.; Tsambou, L.; Grosjean, ME.; Caillierez, R.; Demeyer, D.; Hamdane, M.; Schindowski, K.; Blum, D. & Buée, L. (2011). Loss of Medial Septum Cholinergic Neurons in THY-Tau22 Mouse Model: What Links with Tau Pathology? *Curr Alzheimer Res*, May 23. Vol. 8(6), pp. 633-638.

Belarbi, K.; Burnouf, S.; Fernandez-Gomez, FJ.; Laurent, C.; Lestavel, S.; Figeac, M.; Sultan, A.; Troquier, L.; Leboucher, A.; Caillierez, R.; Grosjean, ME.; Demeyer, D.; Obriot, H.; Brion, I.; Barbot, B.; Galas, MC.; Staels, B.; Humez, S.; Sergeant, N.; Schraen-Maschke, S.; Muhr-Tailleux, A.; Hamdane, M.; Buée, L. & Blum, D. (2011). Beneficial effects of exercise in a transgenic mouse model of Alzheimer's disease-like Tau pathology. *Neurobiol Dis*, Vol. 43(2), pp. 486-494.

Belarbi, K.; Schindowski, K.; Burnouf, S.; Caillierez, R.; Grosjean, ME.; Demeyer, D.; Hamdane, M.; Sergeant, N.; Blum, D. & Buée, L. (2009). Early Tau pathology involving the septo-hippocampal pathway in a Tau transgenic model: relevance to Alzheimer's disease. *Curr Alzheimer Res*, Vol. 6(2), pp. 152-157.

Beretta, G.; Arlandini, E.; Artali, R.; Anton, JM. & Maffei Facino, R. (2008). Acrolein sequestering ability of the endogenous tripeptide glycyl-histidyl-lysine (GHK): characterization of conjugation products by ESI-MSn and theoretical calculations. *J Pharm Biomed Anal*, Vol. 47(3), pp. 596-602.

Brandt, R.; Gergou, A.; Wacker, I.; Fath, T. & Hutter, H. (2009). A Caenorhabditis elegans model of tau hyperphosphorylation: induction of developmental defects by transgenic overexpression of Alzheimer's disease-like modified tau. *Neurobiol Aging*, Vol. 30(1), pp. 22-33.

Brandt, R.; Léger, J. & Lee, G. (1995).Interaction of tau with the neural plasma membrane mediated by tau's amino-terminal projection domain. *J Cell Biol*, Vol. 131(5), pp. 1327-1340.

Brechlin, P.; Jahn, O.; Steinacker, P.; Cepek, L.; Kratzin, H.; Lehnert, S.; Jesse, S.; Mollenhauer, B.; Kretzschmar, HA.; Wiltfang, J. & Otto, M. (2008). Cerebrospinal fluid-optimized two-dimensional difference gel electrophoresis (2-D DIGE) facilitates the differential diagnosis of Creutzfeldt-Jakob disease. *Proteomics*, Vol. 8(20), pp. 4357-4366.

Bretteville, A.; Ando, K.; Ghestem, A.; Loyens, A.; Bégard, S.; Beauvillain, JC.; Sergeant, N.; Hamdane, M. & Buée, L. (2009). Two-dimensional electrophoresis of tau mutants reveals specific phosphorylation pattern likely linked to early tau conformational changes. *PLoS One*, Vol. 4(3), pp. e4843.

Brettschneider, J.; Mogel, H.; Lehmensiek, V.; Ahlert, T.; Süssmuth, S.; Ludolph, AC. & Tumani, H. (2008). Proteome analysis of cerebrospinal fluid in amyotrophic lateral sclerosis (ALS). *Neurochem Res*, Vol. 33(11), pp. 2358-2363.

Brewis, IA. & Brennan, P. (2010). Proteomics technologies for the global identification and quantification of proteins. *Adv Protein Chem Struct Biol*, Vol. 80, pp. 1-44.

Brion, JP.; Couck, AM.; Passareiro, E. & Flament-Durand, J. (1985). Neurofibrillary tangles of Alzheimer's disease: an immunohistochemical study. *J Submicrosc Cytol*, Vol. 17(1), pp. 89-96.

Brion, JP.; Tremp, G. & Octave, JN. (1999). Transgenic expression of the shortest human tau affects its compartmentalization and its phosphorylation as in the pretangle stage of Alzheimer's disease. *Am J Pathol*, Vol. 154(1), pp. 255-270.

Buée, L.; Bussière, T.; Buée-Scherrer, V.; Delacourte, A. & Hof, PR. (2000). Tau protein isoforms, phosphorylation and role in neurodegenerative disorders. *Brain Res Rev*, Vol. 33(1), pp. 95-130.

Buée, L.; Troquier, L.; Burnouf, S.; Belarbi, K.; Van der Jeugd, A.; Ahmed, T.; Fernandez-Gomez, F.; Caillierez, R.; Grosjean, ME.; Begard, S.; Barbot, B.; Demeyer, D.; Obriot, H.; Brion, I.; Buée-Scherrer, V.; Maurage, CA.; Balschun, D.; D'hooge, R.; Hamdane, M.; Blum, D. & Sergeant N. (2010). From tau phosphorylation to tau aggregation: what about neuronal death? *Biochem Soc Trans*, Vol. 38(4), pp. 967-972.

Butler, M. & Shelanski, ML. (1986). Microheterogeneity of microtubule-associated tau proteins is due to differences in phosphorylation. *J Neurochem*, Vol. 47(5), pp. 1517-1522.

Chait, BT. & Kent, SB. (1992). Weighing naked proteins: practical, high-accuracy mass measurement of peptides and proteins. *Science*, Vol. 257(5078), pp. 1885-1894.

Chang, IF. & Hsiao, HY. (2005). Induction of RhoGAP and pathological changes characteristic of Alzheimer's disease by UAHFEMF discharge in rat brain. *Curr Alzheimer Res*, Vol. 2(5), pp. 559-569.

Chen, J.; Kanai, Y.; Cowan, NJ. & Hirokawa, N. (1992). Projection domains of MAP2 and tau determine spacings between microtubules in dendrites and axons. *Nature*, Vol. 360(6405), pp. 674-677.

Chin J. (2011). Selecting a mouse model of Alzheimer's disease. *Methods Mol Bio*, Vol. 670, pp. 169-189.

Clavaguera, F.; Bolmont, T.; Crowther, RA.; Abramowski, D.; Frank, S.; Probst, A.; Fraser, G.; Stalder, AK.; Beibel, M.; Staufenbiel, M.; Jucker, M.; Goedert, M. & Tolnay, M. (2009). Transmission and spreading of tauopathy in transgenic mouse brain. *Nat Cell Biol*, Vol. 11(7), pp. 909-913.

Cleveland, DW.; Hwo, SY. & Kirschner, MW. (1977). Physical and chemical properties of purified tau factor and the role of tau in microtubule assembly. *J Mol Biol*, Vol. 116(2), pp. 227-247.

Cohen, TJ.; Guo, JL.; Hurtado, DE.; Kwong, LK.; Mills, IP.; Trojanowski, JQ. & Lee, VM. (2011). The acetylation of tau inhibits its function and promotes pathological tau aggregation. *Nat Commun*, Vol. 2:252. doi:10.1038/ncomms1255.

Colucci-D'Amato, L.; Farina, A.; Vissers, JP. & Chambery, A. (2011). Quantitative neuroproteomics: classical and novel tools for studying neural differentiation and function. *Stem Cell Rev*, Vol. 7(1), pp. 77-93.

Crosby, AH. (2003). Disruption of cellular transport: a common cause of neurodegeneration? *Lancet Neurol*, Vol. 2(5), pp. 311-316.

Cruts, M.; Gijselinck, I.; van der Zee, J.; Engelborghs, S.; Wils, H.; Pirici, D.; Rademakers, R.; Vandenberghe, R.; Dermaut, B.; Martin, JJ.; van Duijn, C.; Peeters, K.; Sciot, R.; Santens, P.; De Pooter, T.; Mattheijssens, M.; Van den Broeck, M.; Cuijt, I.; Vennekens, K.; De Deyn, PP.; Kumar-Singh, S. & Van Broeckhoven, C. (2006). Null mutations in progranulin cause ubiquitin-positive frontotemporal dementia linked to chromosome 17q21. *Nature*, Vol. 442(7105), pp. 920-924.

Cuchillo-Ibanez, I.; Seereeram, A.; Byers, HL.; Leung, KY.; Ward, MA.; Anderton, BH. & Hanger, DP. (2008). Phosphorylation of tau regulates its axonal transport by controlling its binding to kinesin. *FASEB J*, Vol. 22(9), pp. 3186-3195.

D'Ambrosio, C.; Arena, S.; Fulcoli, G.; Scheinfeld, MH.; Zhou, D.; D'Adamio, L. & Scaloni, A. (2006). Hyperphosphorylation of JNK-interacting protein 1, a protein associated with Alzheimer disease. *Mol Cell Proteomics*, Vol. 5(1), pp. 97-113.

Dammer, EB.; Na, CH.; Xu, P.; Seyfried, NT.; Duong, DM.; Cheng, D.; Gearing, M.; Rees, H.; Lah, JJ.; Levey, AI.; Rush, J. & Peng, J. (2011). Polyubiquitin linkage profiles in three models of proteolytic stress suggest the etiology of Alzheimer disease. *J Biol Chem*, Vol. 286(12), pp. 10457-10465.

de Calignon, A.; Fox, LM.; Pitstick, R.; Carlson, GA.; Bacskai, BJ.; Spires-Jones, TL. & Hyman BT. (2010). Caspase activation precedes and leads to tangles. *Nature*, Vol. 464(7292), pp. 1201-1204.

Delacourte, A. & Buée, L. (1997). Normal and pathological Tau proteins as factors for microtubule assembly. *Int Rev Cytol*, Vol. 171, pp. 167-224.

Delacourte, A.; David, JP.; Sergeant, N.; Buée, L.; Wattez, A.; Vermersch, P.; Ghozali, F.; Fallet-Bianco, C.; Pasquier, F.; Lebert, F.; Petit, H. & Di Menza, C. (1999). The biochemical pathway of neurofibrillary degeneration in aging and Alzheimer's disease. *Neurology*, Vol. 52(6), pp. 1158-1165.

Delacourte, A.; Robitaille, Y.; Sergeant, N.; Buée, L.; Hof, PR.; Wattez, A.; Laroche-Cholette, A.; Mathieu, J.; Chagnon, P. & Gauvreau, D. (1996). Specific pathological Tau protein variants characterize Pick's disease. *J Neuropathol Exp Neurol*, Vol. 55(2), pp. 159-168.

Delobel, P.; Flament, S.; Hamdane, M.; Jakes, R.; Rousseau, A.; Delacourte, A.; Vilain, JP.; Goedert, M. & Buée, L. (2002). Functional characterization of FTDP-17 tau gene mutations through their effects on Xenopus oocyte maturation. *J Biol Chem*, Vol. 277(11), pp. 9199-9205.

Dhaenens, CM.; Tran, H.; Frandemiche, ML.; Carpentier, C.; Schraen-Maschke, S.; Sistiaga, A.; Goicoechea, M.; Eddarkaoui, S.; Van Brussels, E.; Obriot, H.; Labudeck, A.; Gevaert, MH.; Fernandez-Gomez, F.; Charlet-Berguerand, N.; Deramecourt, V.; Maurage, CA.; Buée, L.; de Munain, AL.; Sablonnière, B.; Caillet-Boudin, ML. & Sergeant, N. (2011). Mis-splicing of Tau exon 10 in myotonic dystrophy type 1 is reproduced by overexpression of CELF2 but not by MBNL1 silencing. *Biochim Biophys Acta*, Vol. 1812(7), pp. 732-742.

Dixit, R.; Ross, JL.; Goldman, YE. & Holzbaur, EL. (2008). Differential regulation of dynein and kinesin motor proteins by tau. *Science*, Vol. 319(5866), pp. 1086-1089.

Dubois, B.; Feldman, HH.; Jacova, C.; Cummings, JL.; Dekosky, ST.; Barberger-Gateau, P.; Delacourte, A.; Frisoni, G.; Fox, NC.; Galasko, D.; Gauthier, S.; Hampel, H.; Jicha, GA.; Meguro, K.; O'Brien, J.; Pasquier, F.; Robert, P.; Rossor, M.; Salloway, S.; Sarazin, M.; de Souza, LC.; Stern, Y.; Visser, PJ. & Scheltens, P. (2010). Revising the definition of Alzheimer's disease: a new lexicon. *Lancet Neurol*, Vol. 9(11), pp. 1118-1127.

Ferrer, I.; Gomez-Isla, T.; Puig, B.; Freixes, M.; Ribé, E.; Dalfó, E. & Avila, J. (2005).Current advances on different kinases involved in tau phosphorylation, and implications in Alzheimer's disease and tauopathies. *Curr Alzheimer Res*, Vol. 2(1), pp. 3-18.

Gellermann, GP.; Appel, TR.; Davies, P. & Diekmann, S. (2006). Paired helical filaments contain small amounts of cholesterol, phosphatidylcholine and sphingolipids. *Biol Chem*, Vol. 387(9), pp. 1267-1274.

Gevaert, K.; Impens, F.; Ghesquière, B.; Van Damme, P.; Lambrechts, A. & Vandekerckhove, J. (2008). Stable isotopic labeling in proteomics. *Proteomics*, Vol. 8(23-24), pp. 4873-4885.

Gharbi, S.; Gaffney, P.; Yang, A.; Zvelebil, MJ.; Cramer, R.; Waterfield, MD. & Timms, JF. (2002). Evaluation of two-dimensional differential gel electrophoresis for proteomic expression analysis of a model breast cancer cell system. *Mol Cell Proteomics*, Vol. 1(2), pp. 91-98.

Ghidoni, R.; Albertini, V.; Squitti, R.; Paterlini, A.; Bruno, A.; Bernardini, S.; Cassetta, E.; Rossini, PM.; Squitieri, F.; Benussi, L. & Binetti, G. (2009). Novel T719P AbetaPP mutation unbalances the relative proportion of amyloid-beta peptides. *J Alzheimers Dis*, Vol. 18(2), pp. 295-303.

Goedert, M.; Spillantini, MG.; Cairns, NJ. & Crowther, RA. (1992). Tau proteins of Alzheimer paired helical filaments: abnormal phosphorylation of all six brain isoforms. *Neuron*, Vol. 8(1), pp. 159-168.

Gomes-Pereira, M.; Foiry, L.; Nicole, A.; Huguet, A.; Junien, C.; Munnich, A. & Gourdon, G. (2007). CTG trinucleotide repeat "big jumps": large expansions, small mice. *PLoS Genet*, Vol. 3(4), pp. e52.

Gong, L.; Puri, M.; Unlü, M.; Young, M.; Robertson, K.; Viswanathan, S.; Krishnaswamy, A.; Dowd, SR. & Minden, JS. (2004). Drosophila ventral furrow morphogenesis: a proteomic analysis. *Development*, Vol. 131(3), pp. 643-656.

Götz, J.; Probst, A.; Spillantini, MG.; Schäfer, T.; Jakes, R.; Bürki, K. & Goedert, M. (1995). Somatodendritic localization and hyperphosphorylation of tau protein in transgenic mice expressing the longest human brain tau isoform. *EMBO J*, Vol. 14(7), pp. 1304-1313.

Greenberg, SG. & Davies, P. (1990). A preparation of Alzheimer paired helical filaments that displays distinct tau proteins by polyacrylamide gel electrophoresis. *Proc Natl Acad Sci U S A*, Vol. 87(15), pp. 5827-5831.

Hamdane, M.; Delobel, P.; Sambo, AV.; Smet, C.; Bégard, S.; Violleau, A.; Landrieu, I.; Delacourte, A.; Lippens, G.; Flament, S. & Buée, L. (2003). Neurofibrillary degeneration of the Alzheimer-type: an alternate pathway to neuronal apoptosis? *Biochem Pharmacol*, Vol. 66(8), pp. 1619-1625.

Hanger, DP.; Byers, HL.; Wray, S.; Leung, KY.; Saxton, MJ.; Seereeram, A.; Reynolds, CH.; Ward, MA. & Anderton, BH. (2007). Novel phosphorylation sites in tau from Alzheimer brain support a role for casein kinase 1 in disease pathogenesis. *J Biol Chem*, Vol. 282(32), pp. 23645-23654.

Harada, A.; Oguchi, K.; Okabe, S.; Kuno, J.; Terada, S.; Ohshima, T.; Sato-Yoshitake, R.; Takei, Y.; Noda, T. & Hirokawa, N. (1994). Altered microtubule organization in small-calibre axons of mice lacking tau protein. *Nature*, Vol. 369(6480), pp. 488-491.

Hardy, J. & Selkoe, DJ. (2002). The amyloid hypothesis of Alzheimer's disease: progress and problems on the road to therapeutics. *Science*, Vol. 297(5580), pp. 353-356.

Hasegawa, M.; Morishima-Kawashima, M.; Takio, K.; Suzuki, M; Titani, K. & Ihara, Y. (1992). Protein sequence and mass spectrometric analyses of tau in the Alzheimer's disease brain. *J Biol Chem*, Vol. 267(24), pp. 17047-17054.

Hellman, U.; Wernstedt, C.; Góñez, J. & Heldin, CH. (1995). Improvement of an "In-Gel" digestion procedure for the micropreparation of internal protein fragments for amino acid sequencing. *Anal Biochem*, Vol. 224(1), pp. 451-455.

Henzel, WJ.; Billeci, TM.; Stults, JT.; Wong, SC.; Grimley, C. & Watanabe, C. (1993). Identifying proteins from two-dimensional gels by molecular mass searching of peptide fragments in protein sequence databases. *Proc Natl Acad Sci U S* , Vol. 90(11), pp. 5011-5015.

Hertze, J.; Minthon, L.; Zetterberg, H.; Vanmechelen, E.; Blennow, K. & Hansson, O. (2010). Evaluation of CSF biomarkers as predictors of Alzheimer's disease: a clinical follow-up study of 4.7 years.*J Alzheimers Dis*, Vol. 21(4), pp. 1119-1128.

Hillenkamp, F. & Karas, M. (1990). Mass spectrometry of peptides and proteins by matrix-assisted ultraviolet laser desorption/ionization. *Methods Enzymol*, Vol. 193, pp. 280-295.

Hirokawa, N. Shiomura, Y. & Okabe, S. (1988). Tau proteins: the molecular structure and mode of binding on microtubules. *J Cell Biol*, Vol. 107(4), pp. 1449-1459.

Ideker, T.; Dutkowskis, J. & Hood, L. (2011). Boosting signal-to-noise in complex biology: prior knowledge is power. *Cell*, Vol. 144(6), pp. 860-863.

Ihara, Y.; Nukina, N.; Miura, R. & Ogawara, M. (1986). Phosphorylated tau protein is integrated into paired helical filaments in Alzheimer's disease. *J Biochem*, Vol. 99(6), pp. 1807-1810.

Ittner, LM.; Fath, T.; Ke, YD.; Bi, M.; van Eersel, J.; Li, KM.; Gunning, P. & Götz, J. (2008). Parkinsonism and impaired axonal transport in a mouse model of frontotemporal dementia. *Proc Natl Acad Sci U S A*, Vol. 105(41), pp. 15997-16002.

Ittner, LM.; Ke, YD.; Delerue, F.; Bi, M.; Gladbach, A.; van Eersel, J.; Wölfing, H.; Chieng, BC.; Christie, MJ.; Napier, IA.; Eckert, A.; Staufenbiel, M.; Hardeman, E. & Götz, J. (2010). Dendritic function of tau mediates amyloid-beta toxicity in Alzheimer's disease mouse models. *Cell*, Vol. 142(3), pp. 387-397.

Janke, C.; Holzer, M.; Klose, J. & Arendt, T. (1996). Distribution of isoforms of the microtubule-associated protein tau in grey and white matter areas of human brain: a two-dimensional gelelectrophoretic analysis. *FEBS Lett*, Vol. 379(3), pp. 222-226.

Jin, J.; Davis, J.; Zhu, D.; Kashima, DT.; Leroueil, M.; Pan, C.; Montine, KS. & Zhang, J. (2007). Identification of novel proteins affected by rotenone in mitochondria of dopaminergic cells. *BMC Neurosci*, Vol. 8, pp. 67.

Kettenbach, AN.; Rush, J. & Gerber, SA. (2011). Absolute quantification of protein and post-translational modification abundance with stable isotope-labeled synthetic peptides. *Nat Protoc*, Vol. 6(2), pp. 175-186.

Kidd, M. (1963). Paired helical filaments in electron microscopy of Alzheimer's disease. *Nature*, Vol. 197, pp. 192-193.

Klegeris, A.; Li, J.; Bammler, TK.; Jin, J.; Zhu, D.; Kashima, DT.; Pan, S.; Hashioka, S.; Maguire, J.; McGeer, PL. & Zhang, J. (2008). Prolyl endopeptidase is revealed following SILAC analysis to be a novel mediator of human microglial and THP-1 cell neurotoxicity. *Glia*, Vol. 56(6), pp. 675-685.

Kosicek, M.; Kirsch, S.; Bene, R.; Trkanjec, Z.; Titlic, M.; Bindila, L.; Peter-Katalinic, J. & Hecimovic, S. (2010). Nano-HPLC-MS analysis of phospholipids in cerebrospinal fluid of Alzheimer's disease patients--a pilot study. *Anal Bioanal Chem*, Vol. 398(7-8), pp. 2929-2937.

Ksiezak-Reding, H. & Wall, JS. (2005). Characterization of paired helical filaments by scanning transmission electron microscopy. *Microsc Res Tech*, Vol. 67(3-4), pp. 126-140.

Ksiezak-Reding, H.; Morgan, K. & Dickson, DW. (1994). Tau immunoreactivity and SDS solubility of two populations of paired helical filaments that differ in morphology. *Brain Res*, Vol. 649(1-2), pp. 185-196.

Landrieu, I.; Leroy, A.; Smet-Nocca, C.; Huven,t I.; Amniai, L.; Hamdane, M.; Sibille, N.; Buée, L.; Wieruszeski, JM. & Lippens, G. (2010). NMR spectroscopy of the neuronal tau protein: normal function and implication in Alzheimer's disease. *Biochem Soc Trans*, Vol. 38(4), pp. 1006-1011.

Lange, V.; Malmström, JA.; Didion, J.; King, NL.; Johansson, BP.; Schäfer, J.; Rameseder, J.; Wong, CH.; Deutsch, EW.; Brusniak, MY.; Bühlmann, P.; Björck, L.; Domon, B. & Aebersold R. (2008). Targeted quantitative analysis of Streptococcus pyogenes virulence factors by multiple reaction monitoring. *Mol Cell Proteomics*, Vol. 7(8), pp. 1489-1500.

Leroy, K.; Bretteville, A.; Schindowski, K.; Gilissen, E.; Authelet, M.; De Decker, R.; Yilmaz, Z.; Buée, L. & Brion JP. (2007). Early axonopathy preceding neurofibrillary tangles in mutant tau transgenic mice. *Am J Pathol*, Vol. 171(3), pp. 976-992.

Leugers, CJ. & Lee, G. (2010). Tau potentiates nerve growth factor-induced mitogen-activated protein kinase signaling and neurite initiation without a requirement for microtubule binding. *J Biol Chem*, Vol. 285(25), pp. 19125-19134.

Maarouf, CL.; Andacht, TM.; Kokjohn, TA.; Castaño, EM.; Sue, LI.; Beach, TG. & Roher, AE. (2009). Proteomic analysis of Alzheimer's disease cerebrospinal fluid from neuropathologically diagnosed subjects. *Curr Alzheimer Res* Vol. 6(4), pp. 399-406.

Magnani, E.; Fan, J.; Gasparini, L.; Golding, M.; Williams, M.; Schiavo, G.; Goedert, M.; Amos, LA. & Spillantini, MG. (2007). Interaction of tau protein with the dynactin complex. *EMBO J*, Vol. 26(21), pp. 4546-4554.

Mailliot, C.; Sergeant, N.; Bussière, T.; Caillet-Boudin, ML.; Delacourte, A. & Buée, L. (1998). Phosphorylation of specific sets of tau isoforms reflects different neurofibrillary degeneration processes. *FEBS Lett*, Vol. 433(3), pp. 201-204.

Maurage, CA.; Udd, B.; Ruchoux, MM.; Vermersch, P.; Kalimo, H.; Krahe, R.; Delacourte, A. & Sergeant, N. (2005). Similar brain tau pathology in DM2/PROMM and DM1/Steinert disease. *Neurology*, Vol. 65(10), pp. 1636-1638.

Mayeux, R.; Reitz, C.; Brickman, AM.; Haan, MN.; Manly, JJ.; Glymour, MM.; Weiss, CC.; Yaffe, K.; Middleton, L.; Hendrie, HC.; Warren, LH.; Hayden, KM.; Welsh-Bohmer, KA.; Breitner, JC. & Morris, JC. (2011). Operationalizing diagnostic criteria for Alzheimer's disease and other age-related cognitive impairment-Part 1. *Alzheimers Dement*, Vol. 7(1), pp. 15-34.

McGeer, EG. & McGeer, PL. (2010). Neuroinflammation in Alzheimer's disease and mild cognitive impairment: a field in its infancy. *J Alzheimers Dis*, Vol. 19(1), pp. 355-361.

McMillan, P.; Korvatska, E.; Poorkaj, P.; Evstafjeva, Z.; Robinson, L.; Greenup, L.; Leverenz, J.; Schellenberg, GD. & D'Souza, I. (2008). Tau isoform regulation is region- and cell-specific in mouse brain. *J Comp Neurol*, Vol. 511(6), pp. 788-803.

Meola, G. (2000). Clinical and genetic heterogeneity in myotonic dystrophies. *Muscle Nerve*, Vol. 23(12), pp. 1789-1799.

Min, SW.; Cho, SH.; Zhou, Y.; Schroeder, S.; Haroutunian, V.; Seeley, WW.; Huang, EJ.; Shen, Y.; Masliah, E.; Mukherjee, C.; Meyers, D.; Cole, PA.; Ott, M. & Gan, L. (2010). Acetylation of tau inhibits its degradation and contributes to tauopathy. *Neuron*, Vol. 67(6), pp. 953-966.

Mocanu, MM.; Nissen, A.; Eckermann, K.; Khlistunova, I.; Biernat, J.; Drexler, D.; Petrova, O.; Schönig, K.; Bujard, H.; Mandelkow, E.; Zhou, L.; Rune G. & Mandelkow, EM. (2008). The potential for beta-structure in the repeat domain of tau protein determines aggregation, synaptic decay, neuronal loss, and coassembly with endogenous Tau in inducible mouse models of tauopathy. *J Neurosci*, Vol. 28(3), pp. 737-748.

Molloy, MP.; Brzezinski, EE.; Hang, J.; McDowell, MT. & VanBogelen, RA. (2003). Overcoming technical variation and biological variation in quantitative proteomics. *Proteomics*, Vol. 3(10), pp. 1912-1919.

Müller, T.; Jung, K.; Ullrich, A.; Schrötter, A.; Meyer, HE.; Stephan, C.; Egensperger, R. & Marcus, K. (2008). Disease state, age, sex, and post-mortem time-dependent expression of proteins in AD vs. control frontal cortex brain samples. *Curr Alzheimer Res*,Vol. 5(6), pp. 562-571.

Murray, KK. (1996). DNA sequencing by mass spectrometry. *J Mass Spectrom*, Vol. 31(11), pp. 1203-1215.

Mustafiz, T.; Portelius, E.; Gustavsson, MK.; Hölttä, M.; Zetterberg, H.; Blennow, K.; Nordberg, A.; Unger. & Lithner, C. (2011). Characterization of the Brain β-Amyloid Isoform Pattern at Different Ages of Tg2576 Mice. *Neurodegener Dis*, Vol. 8(5), pp. 352-363.

Neumann, M.; Schulz-Schaeffer, W.; Crowther, RA.; Smith, MJ.; Spillantini, MG.; Goedert, M. & Kretzschmar, HA. (2001). Pick's disease associated with the novel Tau gene mutation K369I. *Ann Neurol*, Vol. 50(4), pp. 503-513.

Nukina, N. & Ihara Y. (1985). Proteolytic fragments of Alzheimer's paired helical filaments. *J Biochem*, Vol. 98(6), pp. 1715-1718.

O'Farrell, PH. (1975). High resolution two-dimensional electrophoresis of proteins. *J Biol Chem*, Vol. 250(10), pp. 4007-4021.

Ong, SE.; Blagoev, B.; Kratchmarova, I.; Kristensen, DB.; Steen, H.; Pandey, A. & Mann, M. (2002). Stable isotope labeling by amino acids in cell culture, SILAC, as a simple and accurate approach to expression proteomics. *Mol Cell Proteomics*, Vol. 1(5), pp. 376-386.

Pandey, A. & Mann, M. (2000). Proteomics to study genes and genomes. *Nature*, Vol. 405(6788), pp. 837-846.

Papanikolopoulou, K. & Skoulakis, EM. (2011). The Power and Richness of Modelling Tauopathies in Drosophila. *Mol Neurobiol*, Vol. 44(1), pp. 122-133.

Paquet, D.; Schmid, B. & Haass, C. Transgenic zebrafish as a novel animal model to study tauopathies and other neurodegenerative disorders in vivo. *Neurodegener Dis*, Vol. 7(1-3), pp. 99-102.

Park, KS.; Mohapatra, DP.; Misonou, H. & Trimmer, JS. (2006). Graded regulation of the Kv2.1 potassium channel by variable phosphorylation. *Science*, Vol. 313(5789), pp. 976-979.

Reynolds, CH.; Betts, JC.; Blackstock, WP.; Nebreda, AR. & Anderton, BH. (2000). Phosphorylation sites on tau identified by nanoelectrospray mass spectrometry: differences in vitro between the mitogen-activated protein kinases ERK2, c-Jun N-terminal kinase and P38, and glycogen synthase kinase-3beta. *J Neurochem*, Vol. 74(4), pp. 1587-1595.

Reynolds, CH.; Garwood, CJ.; Wray, S.; Price, C.; Kellie, S.; Perera, T.; Zvelebil, M.; Yang, A.; Sheppard, PW.; Varndell, IM.; Hanger, DP. & Anderton, BH. (2008). Phosphorylation regulates tau interactions with Src homology 3 domains of phosphatidylinositol 3-kinase, phospholipase Cgamma1, Grb2, and Src family kinases. *J Biol Chem*, Vol. 283(26), pp. 18177-18186.

Rosenberg, KJ.; Ross, JL.; Feinstein, HE.; Feinstein, SC. & Israelachvili, J. (2008). Complementary dimerization of microtubule-associated tau protein: Implications for microtubule bundling and tau-mediated pathogenesis. *Proc Natl Acad Sci U S A*, Vol. 105(21), pp. 7445-7450.

Ross, PL.; Huang, YN.; Marchese, JN.; Williamson, B.; Parker, K.; Hattan, S.; Khainovski, N.; Pillai, S.; Dey, S.; Daniels, S.; Purkayastha, S.; Juhasz, P.; Martin, S.; Bartlet-Jones, M.; He, F.; Jacobson, A. & Pappin, DJ. (2004). Multiplexed protein quantitation in Saccharomyces cerevisiae using amine-reactive isobaric tagging reagents. *Mol Cell Proteomics*, Vol. 3(12), pp. 1154-1169.

Sansone, V.; Gandossini, S.; Cotelli, M.; Calabria, M.; Zanetti, O. & Meola, G. (2007). Cognitive impairment in adult myotonic dystrophies: a longitudinal study. *Neurol Sci*, Vol. 28(1), pp. 9-15.

Santacruz, K.; Lewis, J.; Spires, T.; Paulson, J.; Kotilinek, L.; Ingelsson, M.; Guimaraes, A.; DeTure, M.; Ramsden, M.; McGowan, E.; Forster, C.; Yue, M.; Orne, J.; Janus, C.; Mariash, A.; Kuskowski, M.; Hyman, B.; Hutton, M. & Ashe, KH. (2005). Tau suppression in a neurodegenerative mouse model improves memory function. *Science*, Vol. 309(5733), pp. 476-481.

Santarella, RA.; Skiniotis, G.; Goldie, KN.; Tittmann, P.; Gross, H.; Mandelkow, EM.; Mandelkow, E. & Hoenger, A. (2004). Surface-decoration of microtubules by human tau. *J Mol Biol*, Vol. 339(3), pp. 539-553.

Sato, Y.; Naito, Y.; Grundke-Iqbal, I.; Iqbal, K. & Endo, T. (2001). Analysis of N-glycans of pathological tau: possible occurrence of aberrant processing of tau in Alzheimer's disease. *FEBS Lett*, Vol. 496(2-3), pp. 152-160.

Schindowski, K.; Belarbi, K.; Bretteville, A.; Ando, K. & Buée, L. (2008). Neurogenesis and cell cycle-reactivated neuronal death during pathogenic tau aggregation. *Genes Brain Behav*, Vol. 7 Suppl 1, pp. 92-100.

Schindowski, K.; Bretteville, A.; Leroy, K.; Bégard, S.; Brion, JP.; Hamdane, M. & Buée, L. (2006). Alzheimer's disease-like tau neuropathology leads to memory deficits and loss of functional synapses in a novel mutated tau transgenic mouse without any motor deficits. *Am J Pathol*, Vol. 169(2), pp. 599-616.

Selkoe, DJ.; Ihara, Y. & Salazar, FJ. (1982). Alzheimer's disease: insolubility of partially purified paired helical filaments in sodium dodecyl sulfate and urea. *Science*, Vol. 215(4537), pp. 1243-1245.

Sergeant, N. & Buée L. (2011). Tau models. In: *Animal model of Dementia*, Deyn P.P., Dam D, pp. 449-468, SpringerLink, ISBN: 978-160761897-3.

Sergeant, N.; Bombois, S.; Ghestem, A.; Drobecq, H.; Kostanjevecki, V.; Missiaen, C.; Wattez, A.; David, JP.; Vanmechelen, E.; Sergheraert, C. & Delacourte, A. (2003). Truncated beta-amyloid peptide species in pre-clinical Alzheimer's disease as new targets for the vaccination approach. *J Neurochem*, Vol. 85(6), pp. 1581-1591.

Sergeant, N.; Bretteville, A.; Hamdane, M.; Caillet-Boudin, ML.; Grognet, P.; Bombois, S.; Blum, D.; Delacourte, A.; Pasquier, F.; Vanmechelen, E.; Schraen-Maschke, S. & Buée, L. (2008). Biochemistry of Tau in Alzheimer's disease and related neurological disorders. *Expert Rev Proteomics*, Vol. 5(2), pp. 207-224.

Sergeant, N.; David, JP.; Goedert, M.; Jakes, R.; Vermersch, P.; Buée, L.; Lefranc, D.; Wattez, A. & Delacourte, A. (1997). Two-dimensional characterization of paired helical filament-tau from Alzheimer's disease: demonstration of an additional 74-kDa component and age-related biochemical modifications. *J Neurochem*, Vol. 69(2), pp. 834-844.

Sergeant, N.; David, JP.; Lefranc, D.; Vermersch, P.; Wattez, A. & Delacourte, A. (1997). Different distribution of phosphorylated tau protein isoforms in Alzheimer's and Pick's diseases. *FEBS Lett*, Vol. 412(3), pp. 578-582.

Sergeant, N.; Delacourte, A. & Buée, L. (2005). Tau protein as a differential biomarker of tauopathies. *Biochim Biophys Acta*, Vol. 1739(2-3), pp. 179-197.

Sergeant, N.; Sablonnière, B.; Schraen-Maschke, S.; Ghestem, A.; Maurage, CA.; Wattez, A.; Vermersch, P. & Delacourte, A. (2001). Dysregulation of human brain microtubule-associated tau mRNA maturation in myotonic dystrophy type 1. *Hum Mol Genet*, Vol. 10(19), pp. 2143-2155.

Sergeant, N.; Wattez, A. & Delacourte, A. (1999). Neurofibrillary degeneration in progressive supranuclear palsy and corticobasal degeneration: tau pathologies with exclusively "exon 10" isoforms. *J Neurochem*, Vol. 72(3), pp. 1243-1249.

Seshadri, S.; Beiser, A.; Au, R.; Wolf, PA.; Evans, DA.; Wilson, RS.; Petersen, RC.; Knopman, DS.; Rocca, WA.; Kawas, CH.; Corrada, MM.; Plassman, BL.; Langa, KM. & Chui, HC. (2011). Operationalizing diagnostic criteria for Alzheimer's disease and other age-related cognitive impairment-Part 2. *Alzheimers Dement*, Vol. 7(1), pp. 35-52.

Sethuraman, M.; McComb, ME.; Huang, H.; Huang, S.; Heibeck, T.; Costello, CE. & Cohen, RA. (2004). Isotope-coded affinity tag (ICAT) approach to redox proteomics:

identification and quantitation of oxidant-sensitive cysteine thiols in complex protein mixtures. *J Proteome Res*, Vol. 3(6), pp. 1228-1233.

Seyfried, NT.; Gozal, YM.; Dammer, EB.; Xia, Q.; Duong, DM.; Cheng, D.; Lah, JJ.; Levey, AI. & Peng, J. (2010). Multiplex SILAC analysis of a cellular TDP-43 proteinopathy model reveals protein inclusions associated with SUMOylation and diverse polyubiquitin chains. *Mol Cell Proteomics*, Vol. 9(4), pp. 705-718.

Shaw, J.; Rowlinson, R.; Nickson, J.; Stone, T.; Sweet, A.; Williams, K. & Tonge, R. (2003). Evaluation of saturation labelling two-dimensional difference gel electrophoresis fluorescent dyes. *Proteomics*, Vol. 3(7), pp. 1181-1195.

Shiio, Y. & Aebersold, R. (2006). Quantitative proteome analysis using isotope-coded affinity tags and mass spectrometry. *Nat Protoc* Vol. 1(1), pp. 139-145.

Sibille, N.; Sillen, A.; Leroy, A.; Wieruszeski, JM.; Mulloy, B.; Landrieu, I. & Lippens, G. (2006). Structural impact of heparin binding to full-length Tau as studied by NMR spectroscopy. *Biochemistry*, Vol. 45(41), pp. 12560-12572.

Sillen, A.; Barbier, P.; Landrieu, I.; Lefebvre, S.; Wieruszeski, JM.; Leroy, A.; Peyrot, V. & Lippens, G. (2007). NMR investigation of the interaction between the neuronal protein tau and the microtubules. *Biochemistry*, Vol. 46(11), pp. 3055-3064.

Sowell, RA.; Owen, JB. & Butterfield, DA. (2009). Proteomics in animal models of Alzheimer's and Parkinson's diseases. *Ageing Res Rev*, Vol. 8(1), pp. 1-17.

Sultan, A.; Nesslany, F.; Violet, M.; Bégard, S.; Loyens, A.; Talahari, S.; Mansuroglu, Z.; Marzin, D.; Sergeant, N.; Humez, S.; Colin, M.; Bonnefoy, E.; Buée, L. & Galas, MC. (2011). Nuclear tau, a key player in neuronal DNA protection. *J Biol Chem*, Vol. 286(6), pp. 4566-4575.

Sydow, A. & Mandelkow, EM. (2010). 'Prion-like' propagation of mouse and human tau aggregates in an inducible mouse model of tauopathy. *Neurodegener Dis*, Vol. 7(1-3), pp. 28-31.

Tannu, NS. & Hemby, SE. (2006). Two-dimensional fluorescence difference gel electrophoresis for comparative proteomics profiling. *Nat Protoc*, Vol. 1(4), pp. 1732-1742.

Tatebayashi, Y.; Planel, E.; Chui, DH.; Sato, S.; Miyasaka, T.; Sahara, N.; Murayama, M.; Kikuchi, N.; Yoshioka, K.; Rivka, R. & Takashima, A. (2006). c-jun N-terminal kinase hyperphosphorylates R406W tau at the PHF-1 site during mitosis. *FASEB J*, Vol. 20(6), pp. 762-764.

Tolnay, M.; Sergeant, N.; Ghestem, A.; Chalbot, S.; De Vos, RA.; Jansen Steur, EN.; Probst, A. & Delacourte, A. (2002). Argyrophilic grain disease and Alzheimer's disease are distinguished by their different distribution of tau protein isoforms. *Acta Neuropathol*, Vol. 104(4), pp. 425-434.

Tomasiewicz, HG.; Flaherty, DB.; Soria, JP. & Wood, JG. (2002). Transgenic zebrafish model of neurodegeneration. *J Neurosci Res*, Vol. 70(6), pp. 734-745.

Tyedmers, J.; Mogk, A. & Bukau, B. (2010). Cellular strategies for controlling protein aggregation. *Nat Rev Mol Cell Biol*, Vol. 11(11), pp. 777-788.

Utton, MA.; Noble, WJ.; Hill, JE.; Anderton, BH. & Hanger, DP. (2005). Molecular motors implicated in the axonal transport of tau and alpha-synuclein. *J Cell Sci*, Vol. 118(Pt 20), pp. 4645-4654.

Van der Jeugd, A.; Ahmed, T.; Burnouf, S.; Belarbi, K.; Hamdame, M.; Grosjean, ME.; Humez, S.; Balschun, D.; Blum, D.; Buée, L. & D'Hooge, R. (2011). Hippocampal tauopathy in tau transgenic mice coincides with impaired hippocampus-dependent learning and memory, and attenuated late-phase long-term depression of synaptic transmission. *Neurobiol Learn Mem*, Vol. 95(3), pp. 296-304.

Villemagne, VL.; Perez, KA.; Pike, KE.; Kok, WM.; Rowe, CC.; White, AR.; Bourgeat, P.; Salvado, O.; Bedo, J.; Hutton, CA.; Faux, NG.; Masters, CL. & Barnham, KJ. (2010). Blood-borne amyloid-beta dimer correlates with clinical markers of Alzheimer's disease. *J Neurosci*, Vol. 30(18), pp. 6315-6322.

Viswanathan, S.; Unlü, M.; & Minden, JS. (2006). Two-dimensional difference gel electrophoresis. *Nat Protoc*, Vol. 1(3), pp. 1351-1358.

Vizcaíno, JA.; Foster, JM. & Martens, L. (2010). Proteomics data repositories: providing a safe haven for your data and acting as a springboard for further research. *J Proteomics*, Vol. 73(11), pp. 2136-2146.

Vogelsang, GD.; Zemlan, FP. & Dean, GE. (1990). Purification and solubilization of paired helical filaments from Alzheimer brains. *J Neurochem*, Vol. 54(1), pp. 148-155.

von Bergen, M.; Barghorn, S.; Li, L.; Marx, A.; Biernat,J.; Mandelkow, EM. & Mandelkow, E. (2001). Mutations of tau protein in frontotemporal dementia promote aggregation of paired helical filaments by enhancing local beta-structure. *J Biol Chem*, Vol. 276(51), pp. 48165-48174.

Weingarten, MD.; Lockwood, AH.; Hwo, SY. & Kirschner, MW. (1975). A protein factor essential for microtubule assembly. *Proc Natl Acad Sci U S A*, Vol. 72(5), pp. 1858-1862.

Wilson, AC.; Dugger, BN.; Dickson, DW. & Wang, DS. (2011). TDP-43 in aging and Alzheimer's disease - a review. *Int J Clin Exp Pathol*, Vol. 4(2), pp. 147-155.

Wischik, CM.; Novak, M.; Thøgersen, HC.; Edwards, PC.; Runswick, MJ.; Jakes, R.; Walker, JE.; Milstein, C.; Roth, M. & Klug, A. (1988). Isolation of a fragment of tau derived from the core of the paired helical filament of Alzheimer disease. *Proc Natl Acad Sci U S A*, Vol. 85(12), pp. 4506-4510.

Wittchen, HU. & Jacobi, F. (2005). Size and burden of mental disorders in Europe--a critical review and appraisal of 27 studies. *Eur Neuropsychopharmacol*, Vol. 15(4), pp. 357-376.

Wolozin, B.; Gabel, C.; Ferree, A.; Guillily, M. & Ebata, A. (2011). Watching worms whither: modeling neurodegeneration in C. elegans. *Prog Mol Biol Transl Sci*, Vol. 100, pp. 499-514.

Yang, H.; Qiao, H. & Tian, X. (2011). Proteomic analysis of cerebral synaptosomes isolated from rat model of alzheimer's disease. *Indian J Exp Biol*, Vol. 49(2), pp. 118-124.

Yuzwa, SA.; Yadav, AK.; Skorobogatko, Y.; Clark, T.; Vosseller, K. & Vocadlo, DJ. (2011). Mapping O-GlcNAc modification sites on tau and generation of a site-specific O-GlcNAc tau antibody. *Amino Acids*, Vol. 40(3), pp. 857-868.

Zellner, M.; Veitinger, M. & Umlauf, E. (2009). The role of proteomics in dementia and Alzheimer's disease. *Acta Neuropathol*, Vol. 118(1), pp. 181-195.

Zhang, G.; Deinhardt, K.; Chao, MV. & Neubert, TA. (2011). Study of neurotrophin-3 signaling in primary cultured neurons using multiplex stable isotope labeling with amino acids in cell culture. *J Proteome Res*, Vol. 10(5), pp. 2546-2554.

Zhou, LX.; Du, JT.; Zeng, ZY.; Wu, WH.; Zhao, YF.; Kanazawa, K.; Ishizuka, Y.; Nemoto, T.; Nakanishi, H. & Li, YM. (2007). Copper (II) modulates in vitro aggregation of a tau peptide. *Peptides*, Vol. 28(11), pp. 2229-2234.

Zilka, N.; Filipcik, P.; Koson, P.; Fialova, L.; Skrabana, R.; Zilkova, M.; Rolkova, G.; Kontsekova, E. & Novak, M. (2006). Truncated tau from sporadic Alzheimer's disease suffices to drive neurofibrillary degeneration in vivo. *FEBS Lett*, Vol. 580(15), pp. 3582-3588.

Zuchner, T.; Schliebs, R. & Perez-Polo, JR. (2005). Down-regulation of muscarinic acetylcholine receptor M2 adversely affects the expression of Alzheimer's disease-relevant genes and proteins. *J Neurochem*, Vol. 95(1), pp. 20-32.

Alzheimer's Association. Copyright © 2011 Alzheimer's Association®. All rights reserved. http://www.alz.org

Diane Hanger, MRC Centre for Neurodegeneration Research, King's College London, UK http://cnr.iop.kcl.ac.uk/hangerlab/tautable

14

Multidimensional Proteomics for the Identification of Endothelial Post Mortem Signals of Importance in Vascular Remodeling

Isabelle Sirois, Alexey V. Pshezhetsky and Marie-Josée Hébert
Université de Montréal
Canada

1. Introduction

1.1 Endothelial apoptosis and vascular remodeling

Atherosclerotic diseases (AD) and immune-mediated vasculopathy of the transplanted organ (referred to as transplant vasculopathy (TV)) are both characterized by vessel wall thickening and fibrotic changes that lead to progressive vascular obliteration (Al-Lamki et al., 2008; Cailhier et al., 2006; Cornell et al., 2008; Mitchell, 2009; Rahmani et al., 2006; Valantine, 2003). The endothelium, positioned at the interface of blood flow and the vessel wall, serves as a physiological barrier and sensor of environmental stress. The "response to injury hypothesis" proposed by Russell Ross in the 70's suggested that endothelial injury prompts vascular smooth muscle cell (VSMC) migration and proliferation, therefore initiating neointima formation (Ross et al., 1977; Ross and Glomset, 1976). Initially, vascular remodeling is beneficial but repeated cycles of injury, proliferation and repair lead to maladaptive remodeling and lumen narrowing. To date, *in vitro* and *in vivo* studies in animals and humans confirmed that endothelial apoptosis is a key determinant in the development of AD and TV (Rossig et al., 2001). Various immune and non-immune factors, such as cytotoxic T-cells, donor-specific antibodies, high cholesterol and hyperglycemia account for increased endothelial apoptosis (Cailhier et al., 2006). In turn, migration and accumulation of VSMC, surviving and accumulating within a hostile environment through acquisition of an anti-apoptotic phenotype, form the initial neointima. Histological and biochemical features characterizing AD and TV include 1) extracellular matrix (ECM) degradation that likely facilitate VSMC migration; 2) acquisition of a synthetic and anti-apoptotic phenotype by neointimal cells (VSMC), mesenchymal stem cells (MSC) and fibroblasts associated with Bcl-xl overexpression (Gennaro et al., 2004; Hirata et al., 2000; Pollman et al., 1998) and 3) differentiation of fibroblasts into myofibroblasts of importance in fibrogenic vascular changes (Tomasek et al., 2002) (Figure 1). The molecular interplay regulating intercellular communication between apoptotic endothelial cells (EC) and neointimal cells are only beginning to be unraveled.

1.2 Proteomics for studying Post Mortem Signals (PMS) exported by apoptotic EC

Apoptotic programmed cell death is classically considered a silent process. The first clues suggesting that apoptotic endothelial cells may not "go quietly" stems from pharmacological

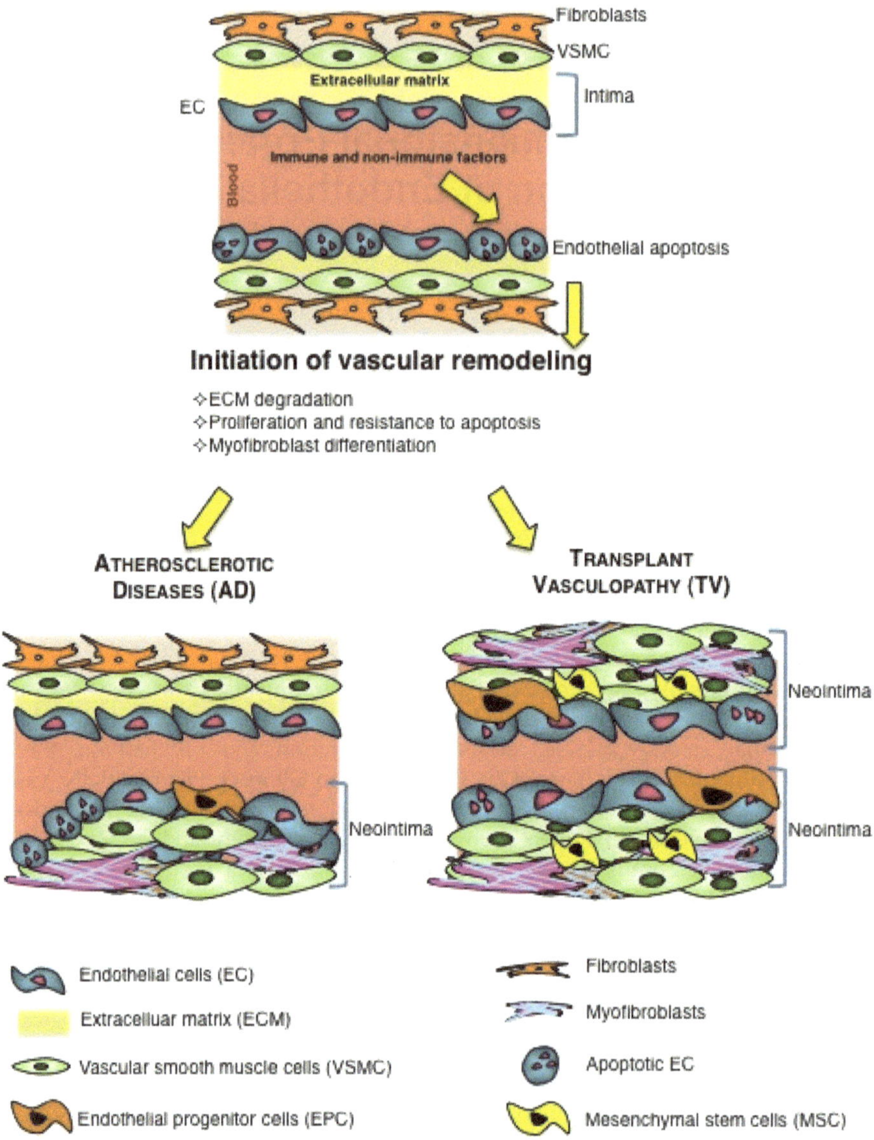

Fig. 1. Schematic diagram of the initiation of vascular remodeling characteristic of AD and TV. Immune and non-immune factors induce endothelial apoptosis. Endothelial apoptosis precedes neo-intima formation. The latter is accompanied by ECM degradation and proliferation and resistance to apoptosis of neo-intimal cells (VSMC, MSC, EPC, fibroblasts and myofibroblasts). Homing of MSC and EPC as well as myofibroblast differentiation contribute to fibrogenic changes observed with vascular remodeling.

or genetic approaches aimed at inhibiting endothelial apoptosis in models of AD or TV. Inhibition of endothelial apoptosis was shown to block the development of vascular remodeling, suggesting a paracrine role for the apoptotic endothelium in triggering pathways of importance in neointima formation (Cailhier et al., 2006; Choy et al., 2004a; Choy et al., 2004b; Shimizu et al., 2000a; Shimizu et al., 2000b, 2002a, b). Cell biology approaches supported this contention and showed that medium conditioned by apoptotic EC regulates the survival and differentiation of major cellular constituents of the vessel wall (Cailhier et al., 2006; Laplante et al., 2005; Raymond et al., 2004; Soulez et al., 2010). Execution of the apoptotic program relies mainly on post-translational modifications, such as protein-protein interactions, protein translocation and proteolysis that will set in motion the molecular pathways regulating the various phases of apoptosis (Thiede and Rudel, 2004;Wang and Chen, 2011; Mahrus et al., 2008). The caspase family of cysteine proteases is central to the regulation of the various phases of apoptosis. Their activation in association with mitochondrial destabilization or extracellular death receptor activation leads to modifications in the architecture of intracellular organelles and fragmentation of the cytoskeleton, the ER and the nucleus (Taylor et al., 2008). Apoptosis triggers changes in the cell membrane including blebbing and extracellular exposure of PS of importance as a phagocyte recognition signal (Leroyer et al., 2008; Martinez et al., 2005; Pober and Sessa, 2007; Verhoven et al., 1995). In addition, mounting evidence suggests that the apoptotic program also regulates the extracellular export of a finely regulated set of signals of importance in leukocyte trafficking, phagocytosis and coagulation (Bournazou et al., 2009; Lauber et al., 2003; Truman et al., 2008).

The complete set of mediators released by a cell at a given time, defined as a secretome, can be decrypted through high-throughput methods based on mass-spectrometry. Use of technology focusing on post-transcriptional events bears special importance in dying cells where the various levels of molecular regulation depend on protein degradation, translocation and specific protein-protein interactions rather than gene transcription. Proteomics was instrumental in characterizing the complex mixture of several secretomes composed of both soluble and vesicular mediators including microparticles and exosomes (Mathivanan and Simpson, 2009). As illustrated by the following reports, large-scale mass-spectrometry also eased the identification of paracrine signals (lipids, proteins and microparticles) specifically enriched within the secretome of apoptotic cells. For example, apoptotic Burkitt lymphoma cells release lysophosphatidylcholine (LPC) through activated caspase-3 dependent mechanisms, which in turn favors recruitment of macrophages and clearance of apoptotic bodies (Lauber et al., 2003). Apoptotic MCF7 epithelial cells secrete lactoferrin as a means of promoting migration of mononuclear leukocytes while inhibiting migration of polymorphonuclear leukocytes (Bournazou et al., 2009). Apoptotic EC shed microparticles with potent immunogenic and pro-coagulant abilities (Smalley and Ley, 2008; Smalley et al., 2007). In sum, these proteomic-based reports suggested that a paracrine response embedded within the apoptotic program and herein referred to as post mortem signals (PMS), controls a finely orchestrated network of intercellular communication.

In the following sections, we will highlight the advantage of different proteomic strategies for characterization of PMS released by apoptotic cells. The systematic analysis of the secretome of apoptotic EC is central to gain insights into novel mechanisms of intercellular communication of importance in TV and AD. Also, the characterization of endothelial apoptotic secretome represents a unique opportunity to identify biomarkers of the initial stage of vascular remodeling.

2. Studying the secretome of apoptotic EC: Methodological aspects

2.1 In vitro experimental systems aimed at studying endothelial apoptosis

Two major pathways, the intrinsic and extrinsic pathways, regulate the initiation of apoptosis. The intrinsic pathway is activated by metabolic disturbances, such as nutrient deprivation and oxidative stress, leading to mitochondrial permeabilization, release of cytochrome C and activation of caspase-9. The extrinsic pathway is activated by death receptors that, upon ligand-mediated activation, recruit an initiator caspase (ex. caspase-8). The effector phase of apoptosis responsible for cleavage of key substrates that bring about the morphological changes of apoptosis is controlled by a common phase regulated by effector caspases (-3, -6, -7) (Taylor et al., 2008). Serum starvation (SS) is a classical inducer of the intrinsic apoptotic pathway in EC and offers several advantages for the characterization of an apoptotic secretome. First, four hours of SS in cultured EC induces sequentially mitochondrial permeabilization, activation of caspases -9 and -3, PARP cleavage and chromatin condensation characteristic of apoptotic cell death. The functional importance of caspase activation in SS-induced apoptosis was validated with caspase inhibitors (the pan-caspase inhibitor (ZVAD-FMK) and caspase-3 inhibitor (DEVD-FMK)) as well as small interfering RNA (siRNA) targeting caspase-3 (Sirois et al., 2011). Second, apoptosis induced by brief SS does not induce necrotic features and cell membrane permeabilization, as assessed by fluorescence microscopy with propidium iodide and evaluation of lactacte dehydrogenase (LDH) activity in medium conditioned by serum-starved EC (Laplante et al., 2010; Sirois et al., 2011). The absence of necrosis in this system is an asset for studying secretory events in absence of uncontrolled leakage secondary to cell membrane damage. Finally, SS circumvents contamination of the secretome by residual components of culture medium (such as albumin) that could interfere with the identification of less abundant proteins specifically released by apoptotic EC downstream of caspase activation.

2.2 Identification of endothelial PMS by multidimensional proteomics

A comparative and multidimensional proteomic analysis was undertaken to characterize the secretome of apoptotic EC (Sirois et al., 2011) (Figure 2). Proteins specifically released by apoptotic EC were identified through comparison of the secretomes generated by equal numbers of serum-starved apoptotic EC (SSC-apo) and serum-starved EC in which apoptosis was blocked by the irreversible pan-caspase inhibitor ZVAD-fmk (SSC-no-apo). Cell media were cleared of cell debris and apoptotic blebs prior to proteomic analysis (Cailhier et al., 2008; Laplante et al., 2010; Sirois et al., 2011; Soulez et al., 2010). An equivalent amount of proteins were fractionated either by SDS-PAGE or by HPLC anion exchange chromatography followed by protein identification by MS/MS (Pshezhetsky et al., 2007). The two comparative strategies were complemented by a functional approach aimed at identifying proteins with an anti-apoptotic activity on VSMC, therefore recapitulating induction of the neointimal anti-apoptotic phenotype (Raymond et al., 2004). Proteins present in SSC-apo were fractionated by ultrafiltration followed by ion-exchange FPLC. Eluted fractions were individually tested *in vitro* for their ability to inhibit apoptosis of VSMC and the fraction displaying a significant anti-apoptotic activity was further fractionated by SDS-PAGE followed by protein identification by LC-MS/MS. Computational analysis of the peptides identified by mass-spectrometry generated three lists built by the functional and the two semi-quantitative comparative approaches.

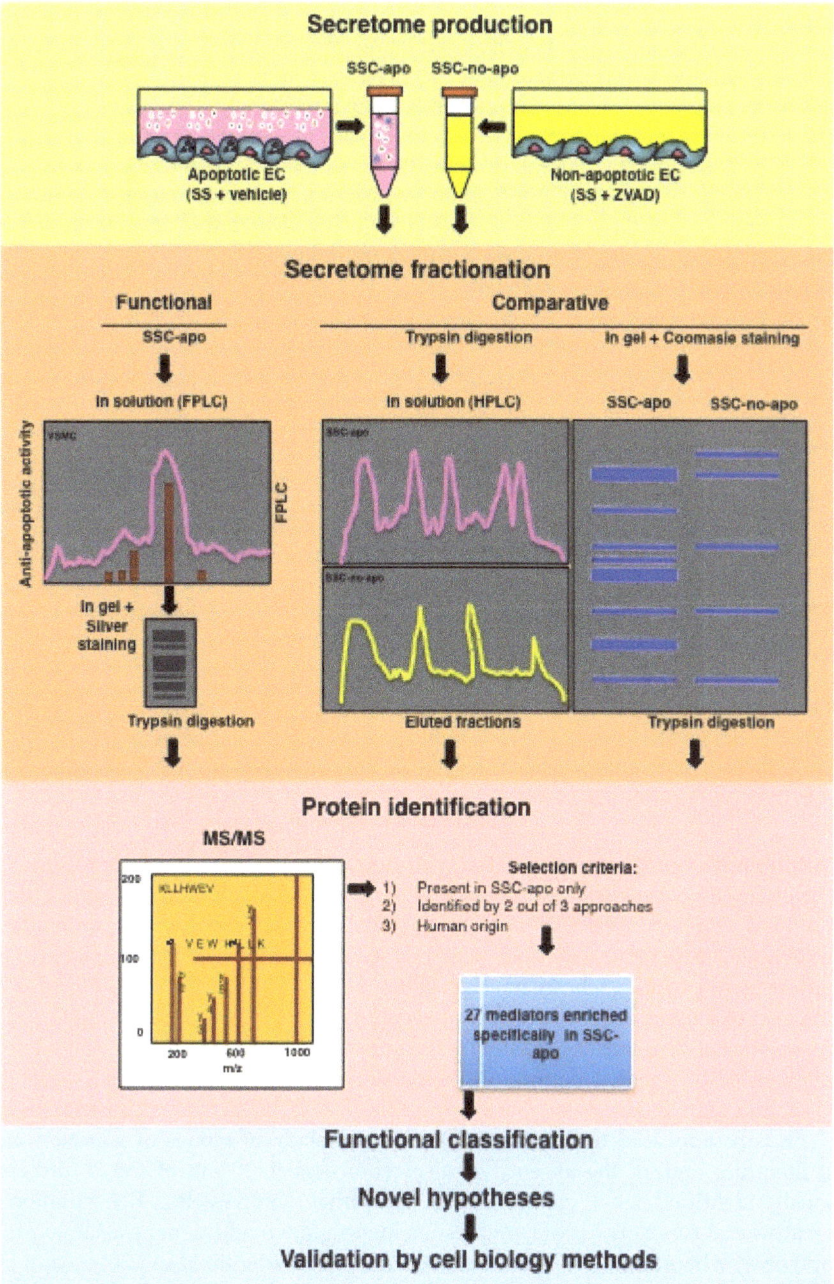

Fig. 2. Schematic representation of the experimental strategy for generating serum-free media (conditioned by equal EC numbers in equal volumes of serum-free media for 4 hours) by apoptotic (SSC-Apo) and non-apoptotic EC (SSC-No-Apo). Secretomes were collected

and depleted of cell debris and apoptotic blebs prior to fractionation. Multidimensional proteomics of the secretomes was performed using one functional and two comparative approaches. SSC-apo was fractionated by FPLC and each eluted fraction was tested for its anti-apoptotic activity in serum-starved VSMC. The fraction with the most significant activity was further separated by SDS-PAGE followed by silver staining and in-gel trypsin digestion. SSC-apo and SSC-no-apo proteins were also compared and fractionated by HPLC or SDS-PAGE prior to protein identification by mass-spectrometry analysis. Identification of specific components of the SSC-apo was achieved using stringent selection criteria. To be considered a specific component of the apoptotic secretome, the protein had to meet the following criteria: protein present in SSC-apo only; protein identified by 2 out of the 3 proteomic approaches; protein of human origin. 27 proteins were identified and classified according to their mode of secretion and the presence of signal peptide, generating novel hypotheses that were further validated by cell biology methods.

3. The caspase-specific endothelial secretome

A targeted screening strategy was developed to focus on the proteins with the highest likelihood of representing caspase-specific secretome components of importance in vascular remodeling. 1300 proteins were identified by LC- MS/MS analysis, 2385 were detected by SDS-PAGE-MS/MS and 28 proteins were identified by the functional approach. To be considered a specific component of the secretome of apoptotic EC, identified proteins had to meet concomitantly the following criteria: 1) they had to be identified by at least 2 out of the 3 different MS/MS approaches, 2) they had to be found exclusively in SSC-Apo, and 3) they had to be of human origin. According to these criteria, 27 proteins were classified as specific components of endothelial apoptotic secretome (Table 1) (Sirois et al., 2011). In the following section we will describe some of the observed changes and discuss the potential function of this apoptotic secretome.

3.1 Enrichment of proteins associated with non-classical modes of secretion

Most proteins that are directed to the cell surface or the extracellular space through a conventional secretory pathway contain a signal peptide (Nickel and Rabouille, 2009). Recent evidence suggests alternative modes of secretion for leaderless proteins, i.e. proteins without a signal peptide (Schotman et al., 2008) (Nickel and Rabouille, 2009). To define the contribution of classical and non-classical secretory pathways during apoptotic cell death, the 27 specific constituents of the endothelial apoptotic secretome were classified according to the presence of a signal peptide in their primary amino acid sequence, their mode of secretion, and their intracellular distribution (Table 1). This analysis showed that 25 out of the 27 proteins appeared to be associated with non-classical modes of secretion, based on recent literature and/or the absence of a secretion signal. 13 out of the 27 proteins were previously identified as a component of exosomal nanovesicles. Reevaluation of the comparative and functional proteomic results identified ten additional exosomal proteins in SSC-apo only, whereas only two exosomal proteins were identified in SSC-no-apo (Sirois et al., 2011). Finally, 4 proteins (Table 1 group 2) were annotated as potential components of exosome-like nanovesicles in other cell types. In total, 31 proteins associated with exosome-like nanovesicles were considered to be specific components of the secretome of apoptotic EC.

TYPE OF SECRETION (CLASSICAL OR NON-CLASSICAL)	GENE NAME	SIGNAL PEPTIDE	SECRETION MECHANISM	REF.	CELLULAR LOCALIZATION				
					Mem.	V.E.	C	N	Ext.
Group 1: Non-classical associated to the exosome pathway (13 proteins)	ALDH1A1	NO	Exosome	(Gonzales et al., 2009)			♦		♦
	EIF4G1	NO	Exosome	(Gonzalez-Begne et al., 2009)			♦		♦
	HSPA1L	NO	Exosome	(Thery, et al., 2001)			♦		♦
	TPT1	NO	Exosome	(Yu et al., 2006) (Lespagnol et al., 2008)		♦	♦		♦
	NAPA	NO	Exosome	(Pisitkun et al., 2004)	♦	♦			♦
	HLA-DQA1	YES	Exosome	(Wubbolts et al., 2003)	♦	♦			♦
	LRP2	YES	Exosome	(Pisitkun et al., 2004)	♦	♦			♦
	IGFR2	YES	Exosome	(Pisitkun et al., 2004)	♦	♦			♦
	PLA2G2D	YES	Exosome	(Subra et al., 2010) (Bette-Bobillo and Vidal, 1995)	♦	♦			♦
	TGFBR3	YES	Exosome**	(Pisitkun et al., 2004) (Lopez-Casillas et al., 1994)	♦				♦
	EGF	YES	Exosome**	(Pisitkun et al., 2004) (Le Gall et al., 2003)	♦	♦			♦
	L1CAM	YES	Exosome**	(Gutwein et al., 2005; Looze et al., 2009; Mechtersheimer et al., 2001)	♦	♦			♦
	LRP1	YES	Exosome **	(Nguyen et al., 2004)	♦	♦	♦	♦	♦
Group 2: Non-classical potentially associated to the exosome pathway (4 proteins)	BRCA2	NO	Exosome (potential)	N.D.		Sec. Gran .		♦	N.D.
	ABCC2	NO	Exosome (potential)	N.D.	♦				N.D.
	ATPA4	NO	Tubulovesicles and apical membrane Exosome (potential)	(Wang et al., 2004)	♦				♦
	ITGA10	YES	Grasp-dépendant Exosome (potential)	(Schotman et al., 2008)	♦				♦
Group 3: Non-classical (8 proteins)	ANLN	NO	P2 particles prominin-1 $^{+ve}$	(Dubreuil et al., 2007)			♦	♦	♦
	ASH1L	NO	ER et microsome	(Aronov et al., 2007)					♦
	NOS2A	NO	N.D.	N.D.			♦	♦	N.D.
	GVIN1	NO	N.D.	N.D.			♦	♦	N.D.
	MTPN	NO	N.D.	N.D.			♦		N.D.
	COQ4	NO	N.D.	N.D.	Mito		♦		N.D.
	SPIN2A	NO	N.D.	N.D.			♦		N.D.
	GOLGA2	NO	N.D.	N.D.	Golgi				N.D.
Group 4: Classical (2 proteins)	ADAMTS4	YES	Trans golgi	(Wang et al., 2004)					♦
	TPA	YES	WPBs	(Knipe et al., 2010)					♦

Abbreviations: Mem: Membranne; V.E.: endocytic pathway including endosomes, MVB and lysosomes; C: cytoplasmic; N: nuclear, Ext.: Identified in the extracellular milieu; N.D.: information non available; Mito: mitochondria; WPBs: Weibel Palade Bodies; **: shedding; Sec. Gran. : Secretory granules

Table 1. Specific components of the apoptotic secretome (SSC-apo) regrouping 27 mediators selected according to stringent criteria (see Figure 2 and the text). Proteins were listed according to their mode of secretion, the presence of a signal peptide and their intracellular localization. Classical type of secretion was defined as a protein containing a signal peptide with secretion mechanism described in the literature. Non-classical type of secretion was defined by the absence of a signal peptide or by reports describing their non-classical secretion.

Initially characterized by Rose Johnstone in the 80's, exosomes are now recognized as important intercellular carrier devices detected in most biological liquids including plasma and urine as well as in the media of cultured mammalian cells (Mathivanan et al., 2010; Pan and Johnstone, 1983; Pan et al., 1985). These nanovesicles with a diameter ranging for 50-100 nm are generated from inward budding of multivesicular bodies (MVB). Exosomes contain proteins of the MVB machinery including TSG101 and Alix, both considered classical exosome markers (Keller et al., 2006; Thery et al., 2002). Exosomes express MHC class I and II associated proteins and play important role in the innate immune system and in antigen presentation (Thery et al., 2009). They also contain different cargos including proteins, lipids, microRNAs and mRNA (Valadi et al., 2007). Their extracellular release stems from the fusion of MVB with the cell membrane but the molecular regulation of MVB exocytosis remains ill defined. A wide diversity of cell types have been shown to secrete exosomes but their protein composition appears to be cell specific and/or dependent on the metabolic state of the cell.
Guided by the proteomic results, we hypothesized that apoptotic cells release nanovesicle-associated mediators and that this process was triggered by caspase activation. This hypothesis was further validated by several biochemical techniques, cell biology approaches and electron microscopy (Sirois et al., 2011). Apoptotic nanovesicles were shown to express classical constituents of exosomes. Electron microscopy with morphometry analysis demonstrated that secreted nanovesicles are structurally and functionally distinct from apoptotic bodies and represent a novel entity of potential significance in vascular remodeling.

3.1.1 Nanovesicular PMS as novel anti-apoptotic factors exported by apoptotic EC

Translationally Controlled Tumour Protein (TCTP) was identified by both functional and comparative proteomics in SSC-apo (Table 1, group 1). TCTP is an evolutionarily conserved protein of crucial importance during development (Chen et al., 2007) and for intracellular inhibition of apoptosis (Telerman and Amson, 2009). TCTP does not contain a secretion peptide signal and its extracellular export depends on the exosomal pathway (Amzallag et al., 2004; Lespagnol et al., 2008). Using electron microscopy in association with immunogold labeling we showed that TCTP was present on the outer surface of endothelial apoptotic nanovesicles (Sirois et al., 2011). Caspase-activated apoptotic VSMC and fibroblasts also released TCTP-positive nanovesicles in association with apoptosis, suggesting that this pathway is active in various cellular components of the vessel wall. TCTP was found to play a central role in the activation of an anti-apoptotic phenotype in neointimal cells. VSMC exposed to TCTP(+) apoptotic nanovesicles mounted a robust anti-apoptotic response whereas VSMC exposed to nanovesicles generated by TCTP-silenced EC failed to develop an anti-apoptotic phenotype. Collectively these results suggest that TCTP released by apoptotic nanovesicles is a novel and central inducer of resistance to apoptosis in VSMC and a biomarker of apoptotic endothelial nanovesicles.

3.2 PMS characterized as biological mediators of vascular remodeling

We further addressed the relevance of the secretome released by apoptotic EC in vascular remodeling. Since development of AD and TV depends initially on ECM degradation and phenotypical changes within neointimal cells (i.e. anti-apoptotic and fibrogenic), the list of proteins generated by the multidimensional proteomic strategy was screened for the presence of mediators sharing these biological functions. Functional studies on EC, VSMC, MSC and fibroblasts highlighted a multifunctional and biochemically complex paracrine activity of the endothelial apoptotic secretome (Cailhier et al., 2008; Laplante et al., 2006; Raymond et al., 2004; Raymond et al., 2002; Sirois et al., 2011; Soulez et al., 2010).

3.2.1 Anti-apoptotic PMS

The importance of ECM proteolysis in association with endothelial apoptosis was highlighted by the identification of the C-terminal perlecan fragment referred to as LG3 by MS/MS and validated by western blot analysis (Raymond et al., 2004). This fragment induces a significant anti-apoptotic activity on MSC through alpha-integrin-dependent activation of the ERK1-2 pathway leading to Bcl-xl overexpression (Soulez et al., 2010). LG3 also interacts with beta-integrins on fibroblasts to induce an anti-apoptotic response but the intermediate signaling component differs (Laplante et al., 2006). LG3–integrin interactions in fibroblasts leads to sequential activation of Src family kinases with downstream phosphatidylinositol 3-kinase (PI3K)-dependent induction of Bcl-xl (Laplante et al., 2006). In support of a functionally important role for LG3 in TV, increased LG3 urinary levels were reported in renal allograft recipients with chronic rejection (Goligorsky et al., 2007).
Comparative and functional proteomics of media conditioned by apoptotic and non-apoptotic EC also revealed the presence of proteases, including ADAM17, ADMTS4, SPUVE, tPA and cathepsin L of potential importance in ECM proteolysis (Cailhier et al., 2008). The extracellular export of cathepsin L, which was validated by WB analysis and functional studies, was found to occur through caspase-3 dependent pathways and to play a central role in cleavage of perlecan and generation of the bioactive LG3 anti-apoptotic fragment (Cailhier et al., 2008). Apoptotic EC export a complex array of soluble and vesicular transport-assisted mediators sharing a common anti-apoptotic activity. Interestingly, these mediators target differentially the cellular components of the vascular wall through non-redundant signaling mechanisms, adding specificity to the secreted signals.

3.2.2 Fibrogenic PMS

Vascular remodeling is associated with fibrogenic changes characterized by the accumulation of myofibroblasts within the vessel wall. Myofibroblasts represent a differentiated and activated subset of fibroblasts characterized by *de novo* expression of contractile stress fibers and alpha-smooth-muscle actin (α-SMA) and enhanced production of collagen I and II. The accumulation of myofibroblasts plays an important role in myointimal thickening and vascular stiffness characteristic of AD and TV. The fibrogenic mediator Connective Tissue Growth Factor (CTGF) was identified with an abundance ratio of 2.5 in medium conditioned by apoptotic EC as compared with medium conditioned by non-apoptotic EC (Laplante et al., 2010). Western blotting confirmed that caspase activation significantly increased the release of CTGF by EC during apoptosis. The central importance of CTGF in the fibrogenic response triggered by the endothelial secretome was highlighted by injecting mice sub-cutaneously with medium conditioned by apoptotic or non-apoptotic EC. A significant fibrogenic response with increased skin thickness and enhanced production of collagen I developed in mice injected with medium conditioned by apoptotic EC. Also, CTGF immunodepletion abrogated the fibrogenic activity of medium conditioned by apoptotic EC.

3.2.3 PMS with potential biological activity on vascular repair

Besides PMS characterized and described above, other components of the secretome released by apoptotic EC are potential regulators of vascular remodeling. PLA2G2D was enriched in the secretome of apoptotic EC (Table 1, Group 1) and recent evidence suggests that it could participate in vascular remodeling. PLA2G2D belongs to a family of secreted phospholipases ($sPLA_2$), which catalyze hydrolysis of membrane glycerophospholipids to release fatty acids and lysophospholipids (Murakami et al., 2010). PLA2G2D secreted through the exosomal pathway favors intercellular transfer of inflammatory molecules, including prostaglandins (Subra et al., 2010). Tissue plasminogen activator (tPA) was also identified in the secretome of apoptotic EC (Table 1, Group 4) (Cailhier et al., 2008). Recent studies suggest that extracellular release of tPA fosters the development of fibrogenic changes (Edgtton et al., 2004; Hu et al., 2008b; Zhang et al., 2007). Convincing evidence also suggests a predominant role for tPA in atherosclerotic diseases (Gramling and Church, 2010). In fibroblasts and myofibroblasts, tPA favors myofibroblast differentiation and induces anti-apoptotic phenotypes through phosphorylation of Bad and the inhibition of the intrinsic apoptotic pathway (Hu et al., 2008a).

4. Conclusion

Characterizing secretomes released by apoptotic cells implies inherent experimental challenges. Cell death is regulated by post-transcriptional events based on protein translocation and cleavage. Failure to take into consideration the importance of proteolysis, protein translocation and activation of non-classical secretion pathways during apoptosis will undermine the experimental strategy. The type of initiating apoptotic signal and the phase of apoptosis to be studied should also guide the design of the proteomic strategy. Creative data mining based on a combination of technical and functional criteria is necessary to gain novel insights into the modes of intercellular communication associated with cell death. The use of a multidimensional proteomics was instrumental in characterizing the importance of caspase activation as a novel regulator of non-classical modes of secretion. It allowed us to demonstrate that apoptotic cells release apoptotic nanovesicles, a novel type of membrane vesicle distinct from apoptotic bodies and reminiscent of exosomes. Mediators of importance in vascular remodeling and of potential use as biomarkers of endothelial injury, such as TCTP, LG3, CTGF, cathepsin L, EGF, PLA2GD2 and tPA were also identified. Further analysis of the complex secretome of apoptotic cells, including biochemical and functional characterization of apoptotic blebs and nanovesicles, should provide further insights into the mechanisms of intercellular communication between dying cells and the local microenvironment.

5. Acknowledgment

This work was supported by research grants from the Canadian Institutes of Health Research (CIHR) (MOP-15447 and MOP-89869) and Fonds de la recherche en santé du Québec (FRSQ) to MJH. MJH is the holder of the Shire Chair in Nephrology, Transplantation and Renal Regeneration of Université de Montréal. We thank the J.-L. Lévesque Foundation for renewed support.

6. References

Al-Lamki, R.S., Bradley, J.R., and Pober, J.S. (2008). Endothelial cells in allograft rejection. Transplantation *86*, 1340-1348.

Amzallag, N., Passer, B.J., Allanic, D., Segura, E., Thery, C., Goud, B., Amson, R., and Telerman, A. (2004). TSAP6 facilitates the secretion of translationally controlled tumor protein/histamine-releasing factor via a nonclassical pathway. J Biol Chem *279*, 46104-46112.

Aronov, S., Gelin-Licht, R., Zipor, G., Haim, L., Safran, E., and Gerst, J.E. (2007). mRNAs encoding polarity and exocytosis factors are cotransported with the cortical endoplasmic reticulum to the incipient bud in Saccharomyces cerevisiae. Mol Cell Biol *27*, 3441-3455.

Bette-Bobillo, P., and Vidal, M. (1995). Characterization of phospholipase A2 activity in reticulocyte endocytic vesicles. Eur J Biochem *228*, 199-205.

Bournazou, I., Pound, J.D., Duffin, R., Bournazos, S., Melville, L.A., Brown, S.B., Rossi, A.G., and Gregory, C.D. (2009). Apoptotic human cells inhibit migration of granulocytes via release of lactoferrin. J Clin Invest *119*, 20-32.

Cailhier, J.F., Laplante, P., and Hebert, M.J. (2006). Endothelial apoptosis and chronic transplant vasculopathy: recent results, novel mechanisms. Am J Transplant *6*, 247-253.

Cailhier, J.F., Sirois, I., Laplante, P., Lepage, S., Raymond, M.A., Brassard, N., Prat, A., Iozzo, R.V., Pshezhetsky, A.V., and Hebert, M.J. (2008). Caspase-3 activation triggers extracellular cathepsin L release and endorepellin proteolysis. J Biol Chem *283*, 27220-27229.

Chen, S.H., Wu, P.S., Chou, C.H., Yan, Y.T., Liu, H., Weng, S.Y., and Yang-Yen, H.F. (2007). A knockout mouse approach reveals that TCTP functions as an essential factor for cell proliferation and survival in a tissue- or cell type-specific manner. Mol Biol Cell *18*, 2525-2532.

Choy, J.C., Hung, V.H., Hunter, A.L., Cheung, P.K., Motyka, B., Goping, I.S., Sawchuk, T., Bleackley, R.C., Podor, T.J., McManus, B.M., *et al.* (2004a). Granzyme B induces smooth muscle cell apoptosis in the absence of perforin: involvement of extracellular matrix degradation. Arterioscler Thromb Vasc Biol *24*, 2245-2250.

Choy, J.C., Kerjner, A., Wong, B.W., McManus, B.M., and Granville, D.J. (2004b). Perforin mediates endothelial cell death and resultant transplant vascular disease in cardiac allografts. Am J Pathol *165*, 127-133.

Consortium, U. (2010). The Universal Protein Resource (UniProt) in 2010. Nucleic Acids Res *38*, D142-148.

Cornell, L.D., Smith, R.N., and Colvin, R.B. (2008). Kidney transplantation: mechanisms of rejection and acceptance. Annu Rev Pathol *3*, 189-220.

Dubreuil, V., Marzesco, A.M., Corbeil, D., Huttner, W.B., and Wilsch-Brauninger, M. (2007). Midbody and primary cilium of neural progenitors release extracellular membrane particles enriched in the stem cell marker prominin-1. J Cell Biol *176*, 483-495.

Edgtton, K.L., Gow, R.M., Kelly, D.J., Carmeliet, P., and Kitching, A.R. (2004). Plasmin is not protective in experimental renal interstitial fibrosis. Kidney Int *66*, 68-76.

Gennaro, G., Menard, C., Michaud, S.E., Deblois, D., and Rivard, A. (2004). Inhibition of vascular smooth muscle cell proliferation and neointimal formation in injured arteries by a novel, oral mitogen-activated protein kinase/extracellular signal-regulated kinase inhibitor. Circulation *110*, 3367-3371.

Goligorsky, M.S., Addabbo, F., and O'Riordan, E. (2007). Diagnostic potential of urine proteome: a broken mirror of renal diseases. J Am Soc Nephrol *18*, 2233-2239.

Gonzalez-Begne, M., Lu, B., Han, X., Hagen, F.K., Hand, A.R., Melvin, J.E., and Yates, J.R. (2009). Proteomic analysis of human parotid gland exosomes by multidimensional protein identification technology (MudPIT). J Proteome Res *8*, 1304-1314.

Gramling, M.W., and Church, F.C. (2010). Plasminogen activator inhibitor-1 is an aggregate response factor with pleiotropic effects on cell signaling in vascular disease and the tumor microenvironment. Thromb Res *125*, 377-381.

Gutwein, P., Stoeck, A., Riedle, S., Gast, D., Runz, S., Condon, T.P., Marme, A., Phong, M.C., Linderkamp, O., Skorokhod, A., *et al.* (2005). Cleavage of L1 in exosomes and apoptotic membrane vesicles released from ovarian carcinoma cells. Clin Cancer Res *11*, 2492-2501.

Hirata, A., Igarashi, M., Yamaguchi, H., Suwabe, A., Daimon, M., Kato, T., and Tominaga, M. (2000). Nifedipine suppresses neointimal thickening by its inhibitory effect on vascular smooth muscle cell growth via a MEK-ERK pathway coupling with Pyk2. Br J Pharmacol *131*, 1521-1530.

Hu, K., Lin, L., Tan, X., Yang, J., Bu, G., Mars, W.M., and Liu, Y. (2008a). tPA protects renal interstitial fibroblasts and myofibroblasts from apoptosis. J Am Soc Nephrol *19*, 503-514.

Hu, K., Mars, W.M., and Liu, Y. (2008b). Novel actions of tissue-type plasminogen activator in chronic kidney disease. Front Biosci *13*, 5174-5186.

Keller, S., Sanderson, M.P., Stoeck, A., and Altevogt, P. (2006). Exosomes: from biogenesis and secretion to biological function. Immunol Lett *107*, 102-108.

Knipe, L., Meli, A., Hewlett, L., Bierings, R., Dempster, J., Skehel, P., Hannah, M.J., and Carter, T. (2010). A revised model for the secretion of tPA and cytokines from cultured endothelial cells. Blood *116*, 2183-2191.

Laplante, P., Raymond, M.A., Gagnon, G., Vigneault, N., Sasseville, A.M., Langelier, Y., Bernard, M., Raymond, Y., and Hebert, M.J. (2005). Novel fibrogenic pathways are activated in response to endothelial apoptosis: implications in the pathophysiology of systemic sclerosis. J Immunol *174*, 5740-5749.

Laplante, P., Raymond, M.A., Labelle, A., Abe, J., Iozzo, R.V., and Hebert, M.J. (2006). Perlecan proteolysis induces an alpha2beta1 integrin- and Src family kinase-dependent anti-apoptotic pathway in fibroblasts in the absence of focal adhesion kinase activation. J Biol Chem *281*, 30383-30392.

Laplante, P., Sirois, I., Raymond, M.A., Kokta, V., Beliveau, A., Prat, A., Pshezhetsky, A.V., and Hebert, M.J. (2010). Caspase-3-mediated secretion of connective tissue growth factor by apoptotic endothelial cells promotes fibrosis. Cell Death Differ *17*, 291-303.

Lauber, K., Bohn, E., Krober, S.M., Xiao, Y.J., Blumenthal, S.G., Lindemann, R.K., Marini, P., Wiedig, C., Zobywalski, A., Baksh, S., *et al.* (2003). Apoptotic cells induce migration of phagocytes via caspase-3-mediated release of a lipid attraction signal. Cell *113*, 717-730.

Le Gall, S.M., Auger, R., Dreux, C., and Mauduit, P. (2003). Regulated cell surface pro-EGF ectodomain shedding is a zinc metalloprotease-dependent process. J Biol Chem *278*, 45255-45268.

Leroyer, A.S., Tedgui, A., and Boulanger, C.M. (2008). Role of microparticles in atherothrombosis. J Intern Med *263*, 528-537.

Lespagnol, A., Duflaut, D., Beekman, C., Blanc, L., Fiucci, G., Marine, J.C., Vidal, M., Amson, R., and Telerman, A. (2008). Exosome secretion, including the DNA damage-induced p53-dependent secretory pathway, is severely compromised in TSAP6/Steap3-null mice. Cell Death Differ *15*, 1723-1733.

Looze, C., Yui, D., Leung, L., Ingham, M., Kaler, M., Yao, X., Wu, W.W., Shen, R.F., Daniels, M.P., and Levine, S.J. (2009). Proteomic profiling of human plasma exosomes identifies PPARgamma as an exosome-associated protein. Biochem Biophys Res Commun *378*, 433-438.

Lopez-Casillas, F., Payne, H.M., Andres, J.L., and Massague, J. (1994). Betaglycan can act as a dual modulator of TGF-beta access to signaling receptors: mapping of ligand binding and GAG attachment sites. J Cell Biol *124*, 557-568.

Mahrus, S., Trinidad, J.C., Barkan, D.T., Sali, A., Burlingame, A.L., and Wells, J.A. (2008). Global sequencing of proteolytic cleavage sites in apoptosis by specific labeling of protein N termini. Cell *134*, 866-876.

Martinez, M.C., Tesse, A., Zobairi, F., and Andriantsitohaina, R. (2005). Shed membrane microparticles from circulating and vascular cells in regulating vascular function. Am J Physiol Heart Circ Physiol *288*, H1004-1009.

Mathivanan, S., Ji, H., and Simpson, R.J. (2010). Exosomes: extracellular organelles important in intercellular communication. J Proteomics *73*, 1907-1920.

Mathivanan, S., and Simpson, R.J. (2009). ExoCarta: A compendium of exosomal proteins and RNA. Proteomics *9*, 4997-5000.

Mechtersheimer, S., Gutwein, P., Agmon-Levin, N., Stoeck, A., Oleszewski, M., Riedle, S., Postina, R., Fahrenholz, F., Fogel, M., Lemmon, V., *et al.* (2001). Ectodomain shedding of L1 adhesion molecule promotes cell migration by autocrine binding to integrins. J Cell Biol *155*, 661-673.

Mitchell, R.N. (2009). Graft vascular disease: immune response meets the vessel wall. Annu Rev Pathol *4*, 19-47.

Murakami, M., Taketomi, Y., Girard, C., Yamamoto, K., and Lambeau, G. (2010). Emerging roles of secreted phospholipase A2 enzymes: Lessons from transgenic and knockout mice. Biochimie *92*, 561-582.

Nguyen, N.V., Gleeson, P.A., Courtois-Coutry, N., Caplan, M.J., and Van Driel, I.R. (2004). Gastric parietal cell acid secretion in mice can be regulated independently of H/K ATPase endocytosis. Gastroenterology *127*, 145-154.

Nickel, W., and Rabouille, C. (2009). Mechanisms of regulated unconventional protein secretion. Nat Rev Mol Cell Biol *10*, 148-155.

Pan, B.T., and Johnstone, R.M. (1983). Fate of the transferrin receptor during maturation of sheep reticulocytes in vitro: selective externalization of the receptor. Cell *33*, 967-978.

Pan, B.T., Teng, K., Wu, C., Adam, M., and Johnstone, R.M. (1985). Electron microscopic evidence for externalization of the transferrin receptor in vesicular form in sheep reticulocytes. J Cell Biol *101*, 942-948.

Pisitkun, T., Shen, R.F., and Knepper, M.A. (2004). Identification and proteomic profiling of exosomes in human urine. Proc Natl Acad Sci U S A *101*, 13368-13373.

Pober, J.S., and Sessa, W.C. (2007). Evolving functions of endothelial cells in inflammation. Nat Rev Immunol *7*, 803-815.

Pollman, M.J., Hall, J.L., Mann, M.J., Zhang, L., and Gibbons, G.H. (1998). Inhibition of neointimal cell bcl-x expression induces apoptosis and regression of vascular disease. Nat Med *4*, 222-227.

Pshezhetsky, A.V., Fedjaev, M., Ashmarina, L., Mazur, A., Budman, L., Sinnett, D., Labuda, D., Beaulieu, J.F., Menard, D., Nifant'ev, I., *et al.* (2007). Subcellular proteomics of cell differentiation: Quantitative analysis of the plasma membrane proteome of Caco-2 cells. Proteomics *7*, 2201-2215.

Rahmani, M., Cruz, R.P., Granville, D.J., and McManus, B.M. (2006). Allograft vasculopathy versus atherosclerosis. Circ Res *99*, 801-815.

Raymond, M.A., Desormeaux, A., Laplante, P., Vigneault, N., Filep, J.G., Landry, K., Pshezhetsky, A.V., and Hebert, M.J. (2004). Apoptosis of endothelial cells triggers a caspase-dependent anti-apoptotic paracrine loop active on VSMC. Faseb J *18*, 705-707.

Raymond, M.A., Vigneault, N., Luyckx, V., and Hebert, M.J. (2002). Paracrine repercussions of preconditioning on angiogenesis and apoptosis of endothelial cells. Biochem Biophys Res Commun *291*, 261-269.

Ross, R., Glomset, J., and Harker, L. (1977). Response to injury and atherogenesis. Am J Pathol *86*, 675-684.

Ross, R., and Glomset, J.A. (1976). The pathogenesis of atherosclerosis (first of two parts). N Engl J Med *295*, 369-377.

Rossig, L., Dimmeler, S., and Zeiher, A.M. (2001). Apoptosis in the vascular wall and atherosclerosis. Basic Res Cardiol *96*, 11-22.

Schotman, H., Karhinen, L., and Rabouille, C. (2008). dGRASP-mediated noncanonical integrin secretion is required for Drosophila epithelial remodeling. Dev Cell *14*, 171-182.

Shimizu, A., Yamada, K., Meehan, S.M., Sachs, D.H., and Colvin, R.B. (2000a). Acceptance reaction: intragraft events associated with tolerance to renal allografts in miniature swine. J Am Soc Nephrol *11*, 2371-2380.

Shimizu, A., Yamada, K., Sachs, D.H., and Colvin, R.B. (2000b). Intragraft events preceding chronic renal allograft rejection in a modified tolerance protocol. Kidney Int *58*, 2546-2558.

Shimizu, A., Yamada, K., Sachs, D.H., and Colvin, R.B. (2002a). Mechanisms of chronic renal allograft rejection. II. Progressive allograft glomerulopathy in miniature swine. Lab Invest *82*, 673-686.

Shimizu, A., Yamada, K., Sachs, D.H., and Colvin, R.B. (2002b). Persistent rejection of peritubular capillaries and tubules is associated with progressive interstitial fibrosis. Kidney Int *61*, 1867-1879.

Sirois, I., Raymond, M.A., Brassard, N., Cailhier, J.F., Fedjaev, M., Hamelin, K., Londono, I., Bendayan, M., Pshezhetsky, A.V., and Hebert, M.J. (2011). Caspase-3-dependent export of TCTP: a novel pathway for antiapoptotic intercellular communication. Cell Death Differ *18*, 549-562.

Smalley, D.M., and Ley, K. (2008). Plasma-derived microparticles for biomarker discovery. Clin Lab *54*, 67-79.

Smalley, D.M., Root, K.E., Cho, H., Ross, M.M., and Ley, K. (2007). Proteomic discovery of 21 proteins expressed in human plasma-derived but not platelet-derived microparticles. Thromb Haemost *97*, 67-80.

Soulez, M., Sirois, I., Brassard, N., Raymond, M.A., Nicodeme, F., Noiseux, N., Durocher, Y., Pshezhetsky, A.V., and Hebert, M.J. (2010). Epidermal growth factor and perlecan fragments produced by apoptotic endothelial cells co-ordinately activate ERK1/2-dependent antiapoptotic pathways in mesenchymal stem cells. Stem Cells *28*, 810-820.

Subra, C., Grand, D., Laulagnier, K., Stella, A., Lambeau, G., Paillasse, M., De Medina, P., Monsarrat, B., Perret, B., Silvente-Poirot, S., *et al.* (2010). Exosomes account for vesicle-mediated transcellular transport of activatable phospholipases and prostaglandins. J Lipid Res *51*, 2105-2120.

Taylor, R.C., Cullen, S.P., and Martin, S.J. (2008). Apoptosis: controlled demolition at the cellular level. Nat Rev Mol Cell Biol *9*, 231-241.

Telerman, A., and Amson, R. (2009). The molecular programme of tumour reversion: the steps beyond malignant transformation. Nat Rev Cancer *9*, 206-216.

Thery, C., Boussac, M., Veron, P., Ricciardi-Castagnoli, P., Raposo, G., Garin, J., and Amigorena, S. (2001). Proteomic analysis of dendritic cell-derived exosomes: a secreted subcellular compartment distinct from apoptotic vesicles. J Immunol *166*, 7309-7318.

Thery, C., Ostrowski, M., and Segura, E. (2009). Membrane vesicles as conveyors of immune responses. Nat Rev Immunol *9*, 581-593.

Thery, C., Zitvogel, L., and Amigorena, S. (2002). Exosomes: composition, biogenesis and function. Nat Rev Immunol *2*, 569-579.

Thiede, B., and Rudel, T. (2004). Proteome analysis of apoptotic cells. Mass Spectrom Rev *23*, 333-349.

Tomasek, J.J., Gabbiani, G., Hinz, B., Chaponnier, C., and Brown, R.A. (2002). Myofibroblasts and mechano-regulation of connective tissue remodelling. Nat Rev Mol Cell Biol *3*, 349-363.

Truman, L.A., Ford, C.A., Pasikowska, M., Pound, J.D., Wilkinson, S.J., Dumitriu, I.E., Melville, L., Melrose, L.A., Ogden, C.A., Nibbs, R., *et al.* (2008). CX3CL1/fractalkine is released from apoptotic lymphocytes to stimulate macrophage chemotaxis. Blood *112*, 5026-5036.

Valadi, H., Ekstrom, K., Bossios, A., Sjostrand, M., Lee, J.J., and Lotvall, J.O. (2007). Exosome-mediated transfer of mRNAs and microRNAs is a novel mechanism of genetic exchange between cells. Nat Cell Biol *9*, 654-659.

Valantine, H.A. (2003). Cardiac allograft vasculopathy: central role of endothelial injury leading to transplant "atheroma". Transplantation *76*, 891-899.

Verhoven, B., Schlegel, R.A., and Williamson, P. (1995). Mechanisms of phosphatidylserine exposure, a phagocyte recognition signal, on apoptotic T lymphocytes. J Exp Med *182*, 1597-1601.

Wang, L., and Chen, G. (2011). Current advances in the application of proteomics in apoptosis research. Sci China Life Sci *54*, 209-219.

Wang, P., Tortorella, M., England, K., Malfait, A.M., Thomas, G., Arner, E.C., and Pei, D. (2004). Proprotein convertase furin interacts with and cleaves pro-ADAMTS4 (Aggrecanase-1) in the trans-Golgi network. J Biol Chem *279*, 15434-15440.

Wubbolts, R., Leckie, R.S., Veenhuizen, P.T., Schwarzmann, G., Mobius, W., Hoernschemeyer, J., Slot, J.W., Geuze, H.J., and Stoorvogel, W. (2003). Proteomic and biochemical analyses of human B cell-derived exosomes. Potential implications for their function and multivesicular body formation. J Biol Chem *278*, 10963-10972.

Yu, X., Harris, S.L., and Levine, A.J. (2006). The regulation of exosome secretion: a novel function of the p53 protein. Cancer Res *66*, 4795-4801.

Zhang, G., Kernan, K.A., Collins, S.J., Cai, X., Lopez-Guisa, J.M., Degen, J.L., Shvil, Y., and Eddy, A.A. (2007). Plasmin(ogen) promotes renal interstitial fibrosis by promoting epithelial-to-mesenchymal transition: role of plasmin-activated signals. J Am Soc Nephrol *18*, 846-859.

15

Identification of Factors Involved in Neurogenesis Recovery After Irradiation of the Adult Mouse Subventricular Zone: A Preliminary Study

François Chevalier[1*], Alexandra Chicheportiche[2,3,4,5*], Mathieu Daynac[2,3,4,5], Jordane Depagne[1], Pascale Bertrand[1], François D. Boussin[2,3,4,5] and Marc-André Mouthon[2,3,4,5]

[1]*CEA DSV iRCM, Plateforme de Protéomique, F-92265 Fontenay-aux-Roses*

[2]*CEA DSV iRCM SCSR, Laboratoire de Radiopathologie, F-92265 Fontenay-aux-Roses*

[3]*INSERM, U967, F-92265 Fontenay-aux-Roses*

[4]*Université Paris Diderot, Sorbonne Paris Cité, UMR 967, F-92265 Fontenay-aux-Roses*

[5]*Université Paris Sud, UMR 967, F-92265 Fontenay-aux-Roses, Institut de Radiobiologie Cellulaire et Moléculaire, Fontenay-aux-Roses*

France

1. Introduction

Neurogenesis insures the production of functional neurons throughout life and occurs in two narrow regions of the adult mammalian brain, the subventricular zone (SVZ) lining the lateral ventricles and the subgranular zone in the hippocampus (Alvarez-Buylla&Lim,2004). The adult SVZ, which is separated from the lateral ventricle by a layer of epithelial cells known as ependymal cell, contains three main populations of neural progenitors: neural stem cells (NSCs), transit-amplifying cells (TAPs) and neuroblasts. NSCs are undifferentiated cells generally characterized by their functional capacities to both self-renew and to generate a large number of differentiated progeny cells (Song, et al.,2011). Adult NSCs have an astrocyte-like phenotype (type B cells) and represent only 0.2-0.4 % of the SVZ cells, they are relatively quiescent and divide very slowly *in vivo* with a cell cycle length of 14 days (Morshead, et al.,1994). These cells are the precursors of rapidly dividing TAPs, or type C cells, which have the capacity to differentiate into neuroblasts (type A). Neuroblasts are organized as migratory chains along the rostral migratory stream (RMS) and integrate the Olfactory bulb (OB) to become interneurons (Fig. 1).
The highly organised cytoarchitecture of the SVZ constitutes a niche for NSCs (Ihrie&Alvarez-Buylla, 2011). Cells localized in this specific microenvironment secrete a variety of factors involved in NSC proliferation, migration and/or differentiation

---

* Contributed equally to this work

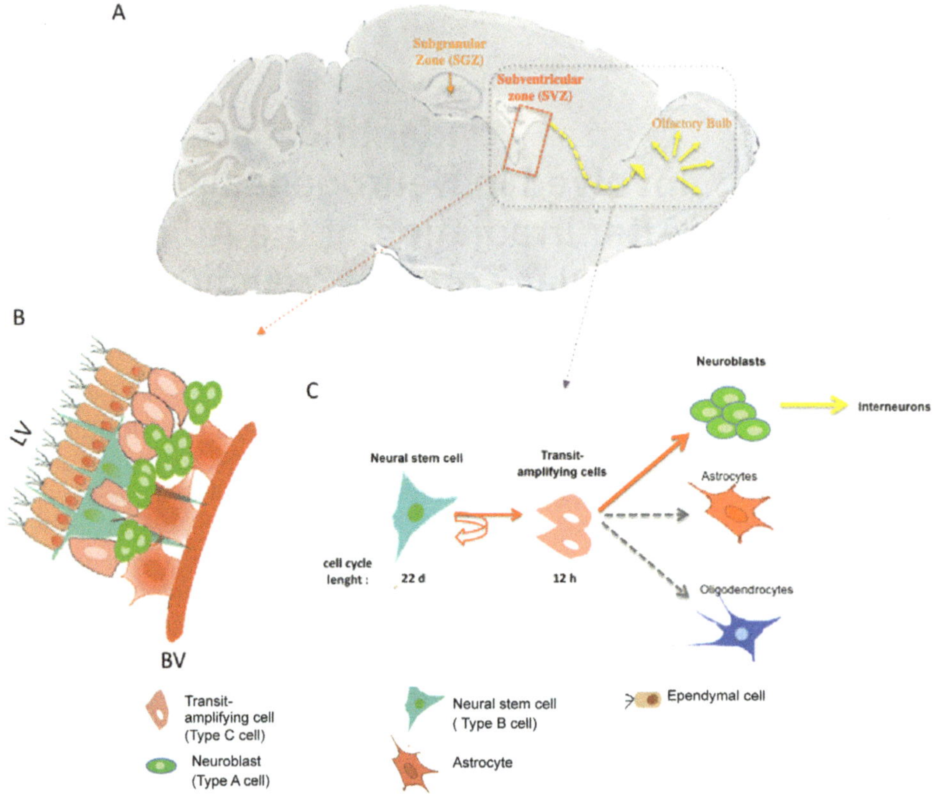

(A) In adult mouse brain, neurons are continuously produced in two restricted regions: the subgranular zone (SGZ) of the dentate gyrus in the hippocampus and the subventricular zone (SVZ) lining the lateral ventricles (LV). The former produces neurons that functionally integrate into the granular cell layer of the hippocampus, whereas the SVZ produces neuroblasts, which migrate along the rostral migratory stream (RMS) to integrate the olfactory bulbs (OB) and differentiate into interneurons.
(B) The SVZ is an highly organized neurogenic area which contains three cell types of neural cells: neural stem cells (NSCs), transit-amplifying progenitors (TAPs) and neuroblasts. Ependymal cells that contact the NSCs are organized as a single layer of epithelial cells separating the SVZ from the ventricles.
(C) NSCs are defined as slow dividing cells having capacities to self-renew and to generate multiple cell types (neurons, astrocytes and oligodendrocytes). NSCs give rise to highly proliferating TAPs, which differentiate mostly in neuroblasts. NSCs are also able to produce oligodendrocytes and astrocytes according to development stages, in response to brain injury or *in vitro* conditions. The length of the cell cycle for NSCs and TAPs lasts 22 days and 12 h, respectively (Doetsch, et al.,1999, Morshead, et al.,1994). BV (blood vessel).

Fig. 1. Neurogenesis in the adult mouse brain

(Doetsch,2003). For example, GABA released from neuroblasts provides a feedback mechanism to control proliferation of NSCs in the SVZ (Liu, et al.,2005). Bone morphogenetic proteins signalling can direct neural progenitors to glial fate in the adult brain (Lim, et al.,2000), whereas the secretion by ependymal cells of Noggin, a polypeptide antagonist of bone morphogenetic proteins, antagonizes Bone morphogenetic protein signalling and stimulates neurogenesis (Lim, et al.,2000). Brain endothelial cells are thought to be crucial for the NSC niche because they lie in close proximity to NSCs (Tavazoie, et al.,2008), where they probably regulate self-renewal of NSCs and their differentiation into neurons (Ramirez-Castillejo, et al.,2006). Brain endothelial cells may also balance proliferation/quiescence of NSCs by secreting Bone morphogenetic proteins (Mathieu, et al.,2008).

A number of studies indicate that brain injury can induced SVZ cells to migrate towards non-OB areas especially towards lesions and participate in neuronal and glial repair (Alonso,1999, Cayre, et al.,2006, Goings, et al.,2004, Jankovski, et al.,1998, Macas, et al.,2006, Picard-Riera, et al.,2002, Yamashita, et al.,2006). Adult NSCs may therefore promise hopes in the repair of damaged central nervous system (Dubois-Dalcq,2005).

Adult NSCs survive anti-mitotic cytosine arabinoside treatment *in vivo* unlike actively dividing TAPs and neuroblasts, which rapidly disappear. This assay has been used by Doetsch et al. to demonstrate that quiescent NSCs are able regenerate to the neurogenic SVZ niches (Doetsch, et al.,1999). Exposition of the brain to ionizing radiation induces apoptosis of proliferating cells in the SVZ (Shinohara, et al.,1997). For high doses of irradiation an incomplete repopulation of the SVZ occurred and neurogenesis is collapsed for long term (Tada, et al., 1999).

However, exposition to low doses allows SVZ to be replenished. A recovery of proliferating cells is observed starting 3 days after radiation and peaking at day 7 (Hopewell and Cavanagh 1972; Tada, et al.,1999).

In light of the recovery capacity of SVZ, we developed a model of low dose irradiation (2 Gy) of adult mouse brain, which provokes a transient collapse of neurogenesis followed by a rapid recovery of the SVZ. The repopulation of the SVZ was most probably due to the stimulation of relatively quiescent NSCs and their proliferation (Morshead, et al.,1994, Pastrana, et al.,2009).

Seek for factors involved in the stimulation of neurogenesis and production of new neurons remains a challenging task. We assume that our *in vivo* irradiation model will be helpful to identify proteins coinciding with SVZ reconstitution, i.e. those involved in NSC proliferation.

Only few global proteomic analyses on rodent brains have been reported, attempting to identify proteins that are involved in brain injury such as middle cerebral artery occlusion ischemia (Sung, et al. 2010), or to gain further insight into the molecular mechanisms of neurodegenerative diseases (Broadwater, et al., Castegna, et al.,2002). Others proteomic studies aimed to identify crucial proteins by comparison between different brain developmental stages and during brain aging (Shoemaker, et al. 2010, Yang, et al.,2008). Therefore, we performed a global proteomic analysis based on 2 dimensional-gels and identification by mass spectroscopy in our SVZ reconstitution model. We decided to work with proteins extracted from SVZ, instead of cells isolated using a specific marker. Indeed, with all SVZ extract, including NSC, progenitor cells and the SVZ extracellular matrix, it was possible to search for protein and secreted factors potentially involved in NSC proliferation, migration and/or differentiation.

In this preliminary study, an accurate analysis of 2D-gel revealed that several proteins from SVZ appeared as modulated following brain radiation. Important issues of this study are the identification of candidates possibly involved in the stimulation of quiescent NSCs.

2. Material and methods

2.1 Mouse irradiation

We used eight-week old male C57BL/6J mice (Janvier, Le Genest-Saint-Isle, France). All experimental procedures complied with the European Communities Council Directive of 24 November 1986 (86/609/EEC) and European Union guidelines.

Mice were irradiated with a medical Alcyon irradiator (γ-rays ^{60}Co) (Fig. 2). Prior to radiation, mice were anesthetized with ketamine (75 mg/kg, Merial, Lyon, France) and medetomidine (1 mg/kg, Pfizer, Paris, France) by intraperitoneal (i.p.) route. Immobilized mice were placed under a lead shield in order to expose the head and to protect the rest of the body. A total dose of 2 Gy was delivered with a dose rate of 1 Gy/mn. After exposure, mice were woken up by i.p. injection of antipamezole (1 mg/kg, Pfizer, Paris, France).

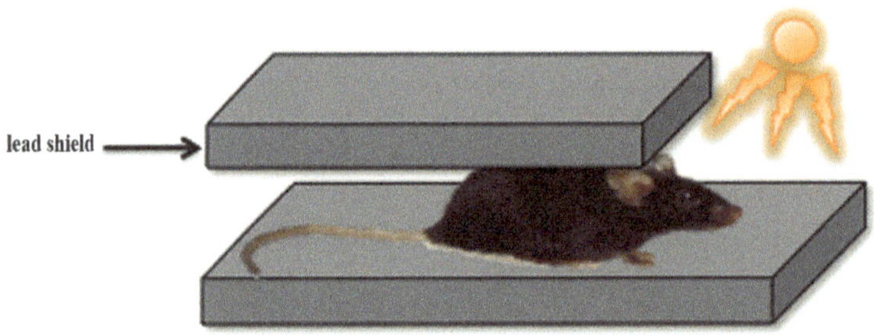

Irradiation was performed with a medical irradiator (Alcyon, ^{60}Co source). Irradiation window was focused at the level of the head of the anesthetized mouse. The rest of the body was protected by a lead shield.

Fig. 2. Schematic representation of brain irradiation

2.2 Micro-dissection of the brain

At different time points after radiation, mice were euthanatized and SVZ and striatum (STR) were micro-dissected (Fig. 3). The micro-dissection method used to isolate SVZ is very tricky since SVZ is a very tiny part of brain tissue. Briefly, skull was cut with scissors at the midline and carefully removed with forceps. The brain was transferred into a Petri dish containing phosphate buffered saline and 6g/L of glucose. OBs were removed and a coronal cut was made at the optical chiasma. Then, under a stereomicroscope, septum was removed from the fore part of the brain with small forceps. Lateral walls of ventricle, containing the SVZ, were microdissected using small forceps and cleared out of contaminating corpus callosum and STR. A piece of STR adjacent to SVZ was taken. Tissue pieces were immediately frozen in liquid nitrogen.

2.3 Protein extraction

Proteins were extracted from SVZ and STR of control (Ctr) and irradiated mice. Tissues were homogenized in buffer containing 9M urea, 4% CHAPS, 0.05% Triton X100, 65 mM DTT and a protease inhibitor cocktail (Roche) with a small Teflon pestle and cell debris were removed by ultra-centrifugation at 100 000g for 1 hour (TL100, Beckman). The protein

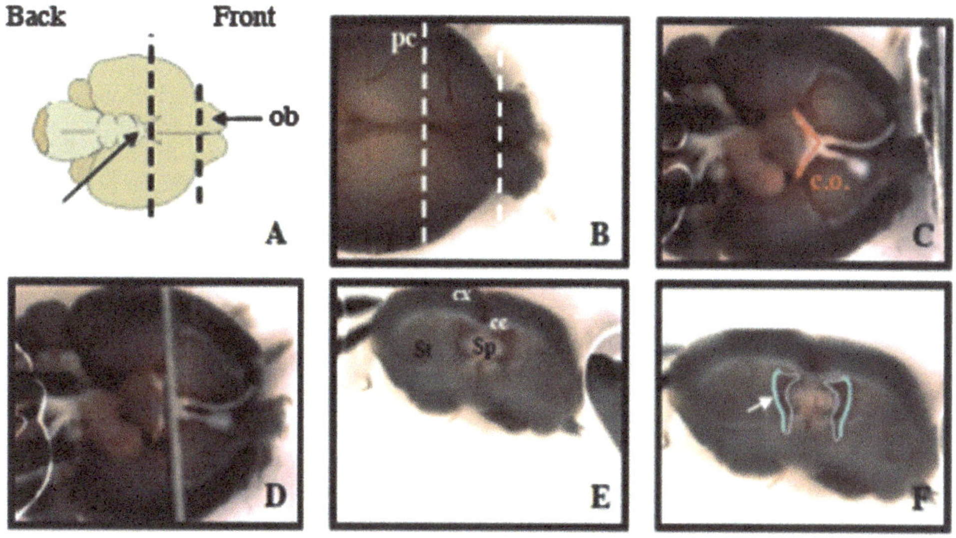

(A) A schematic representation of ventral face of the brain with the two cuts: one at the front just behind the OB and one at the level of optic chiasma. (B) Representative photographs of dorsal face and (C, D) ventral face of the mouse brain. (E, F) Coronal views of brain slices after cuts. (E) Lateral ventricles are visible from each part the septum. The ventricular walls to be dissected out containing the SVZ are indicated by arrow and light blue lines.
Cx: cortex; cc: corpus callosum; St: striatum; Sp: septum.

Fig. 3. Process for micro-dissection of the SVZ

content was estimated in the supernatant using the Bradford assay. To limit variability, tissue pieces from mice with the same treatment were mixed together in proteomic sample buffer.

2.4 Two-dimensional electrophoresis

Two-dimensional electrophoresis was performed with at least 5 technical replicates. Briefly, precast 18 cm strips, pH range 3-10 NL (GE), were rehydrated in the presence of 100 µg of protein extract. Isoelectric focusing was carried out using a Protean IEF Cell (Bio-Rad, Hercules, CA, USA) isoelectric focusing system until 80 KV h-1. The strips were then incubated in the first equilibration solution (50 mM Tris–HCl pH 8.8, 6 M urea, 30% (v/v) glycerol, 2% (w/v) SDS) with 130 mM DTT and then in the second equilibration solution (50 mM Tris–HCl pH 8.8, 6 M urea, 30% (v/v) glycerol, 2% (w/v) SDS) with 130 mM iodoacetamide. Strips were then embedded using 1% (w/v) low-melting agarose on the top of the acrylamide gel. SDS-PAGE was carried out on a 12% acrylamide SDS-polyacrylamide gel, using the Dodeca Cell electrophoresis unit (Bio-Rad).
Gels were stained with Sypro-Ruby and scanned to images, which were digitized with a Typhoon 9400 fluorescent scanner (Typhoon 9400 GE) using the 532 nm excitation laser and the 610BP emission filter. Image were acquired at a 100 µm resolution with a 550 voltage applied to the photomultiplier tube.

2.5 Image analysis

Images from stained gels were analyzed using the Samespots software v4.1 (Non-linear Dynamics, UK). All pictures were first aligned and gel replicates were then grouped to create a global analysis with all conditions. Spots of each sample were compared between control and irradiated conditions. A multivariate statistic analysis was performed using the statistic mode of the Samespots software v4.1 (Non-linear Dynamics, UK). Spots with significant differences between control and irradiated cells (Anova t-test $p<0.05$) were first extracted. Then, only spots with a P value < 0.05 and a power > 0.8 were finally selected. Spots of interest were selected for subsequent protein identification by mass spectrometry analysis.

2.6 Two-D gel reproductibility

Using gel-based proteomics analysis, it is important to estimate the contribution of biological and technical variations. We assessed the degree of biological variation inherent to the 2-DE process. SVZ were extracted separately from 9 mice. For each mouse, about 150 µg proteins were extracted in buffer containing 9M urea, 4% CHAPS, 0.05% Triton X100, 65 mM DTT and a protease inhibitor cocktail (Roche) then were used to produce a corresponding 2D-gel. Protein spot volume was determined for all spots matched in an experimental set using the Samespots software packages with default settings, as used for all the study. Coefficients of variation (CV) were calculated for each protein sample, or as a function of spot intensity. CV was calculated as a percentage of standard variation as related to mean: (SD/mean) x100 (Anderson, et al., 1985).

The SVZ of each animal were used to perform a single 2-D gel. All spots of the corresponding 9 gels were compared as biological replicates (Fig. 4 A).

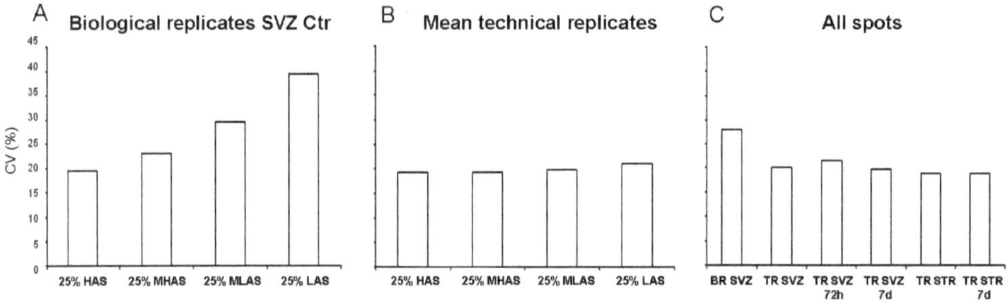

(A) coefficient of variation of SVZ Ctr samples between 9 biological replicates, as a function of spot intensity (HAS: high abundant spots; MHAS: medium high abundant spots; MLAS: medium low abundant spots; LAS: low abundant spots).
(B) coefficient of variation of all technical replicates, as a function of spot intensity.
(C) comparison between coefficients of variation of biological replicates (BR) and technical replicates (TR) of SVZ and STR samples.

Fig. 4. Biological and technical variability of proteomes as measured by 2-D gel electrophoresis.

Coefficient of variation grew up from 20% for high abundant spots to about 40% for low abundant spots. As a comparison, the degree of technical variation inherent to the 2-DE process was estimated for each SVZ and STR samples. Biological samples corresponding to the same treatment were mixed and the resulting protein samples were used to perform technical 2-D gel replicates (Fig. 4 B). In this case, a constant coefficient of variation was observed (about 20%) whatever spot abundance (Fig. 4 B) and sample treatment (Fig. 4 C). This analysis of 2-D gel reproducibility clearly showed the advantage to perform technical replicates with mixed biological samples.

2.7 MALDI-TOF MS analysis

Spots were excised from preparative two-dimensional electrophoresis gels by hand, and processed using a Packard Multiprobe II liquid-handling robot (Perkin Elmer, Courtaboeuf, France). After washing successively with water, 25 mM ammonium bicarbonate, acetonitrile / 25 mM ammonium bicarbonate (1:1, v/v) and acetonitrile, gel fragments were dried at 37°C. Protein digestion was carried out at 37°C for 5 hours following addition of 0.125 µg trypsin (sequencing grade, modified, Promega, Charbonières, France), and resulting fragments were extracted twice with 50 µL acetonitrile / water (1:1, v/v) containing 0.1 % trifluoroacetic acid for 15 min. Pooled supernatants were concentrated with a speedvac to a final volume of 20 µL. Peptides were simultaneously desalted and concentrated with C18 Zip-Tip micro-columns to a final volume of 3 µL, an aliquot of each sample was mixed (1/1) with the alpha-cyano-4- hydroxycinnamic acid matrix at half saturation in acetonitrile/water (1:1, v/v) and the mixture was immediately spotted on the MALDI target by the Multiprobe II robot. Mass spectra were recorded in the reflector mode on a UltraFlex II MALDI-TOF/TOF mass spectrometer (Bruker Daltonics, Bremen, Germany). Automatic annotation of monoisotopic masses was performed using Bruker's SNAPTM procedure. The MASCOT search engine software (Matrix Science, London, UK) was used to search the NCBInr database.
The following parameters were used: mass tolerance of 30 to 100 ppm, a minimum of five peptides matching to the protein, carbamidomethylation of cysteine as fixed modification, oxidation of methionine as variable modification, and one missed cleavage allowed.

2.8 Nano LC MS analysis

When low abundant spots could not be identified by PMF, LC-MS/MS analysis was conducted. Stained protein spots were excised manually, washed, digested with trypsin and extracted using formic acid. Protein digests were analysed using an ion trap mass spectrometer (Esquire HCT plus; Bruker, Billerica, MA, USA) coupled to a nano-chromatography system (HPLC 1200, Agilent, Santa Clara, CA, USA) interfaced with an HPLC-Chip system (Chip Cube, Agilent). MS/MS data were searched against NCBI (National center for Biotechnology information) and MSDB databases using Mascot software.

3. Results and discussion

3.1 Regeneration of the SVZ after radiation

We have developed a model of SVZ reconstitution after low dose irradiation (2 Gy) of adult mouse brain. Radiation exposure provoked a transient collapse of neurogenesis followed by a rapid recovery of the SVZ (Fig. 5).
Cell proliferation was assessed in the SVZ by injection with the thymidine analog 5-bromo-2'-deoxyuridine (BrdU). We observed a sharp decrease in BrdU incorporation 72h after radiation, however, BrdU labelling subsequently recovered within 7 days after exposure (Fig. 6A). BrdU positive cells were scarce 72h after irradiation but most of them expressed

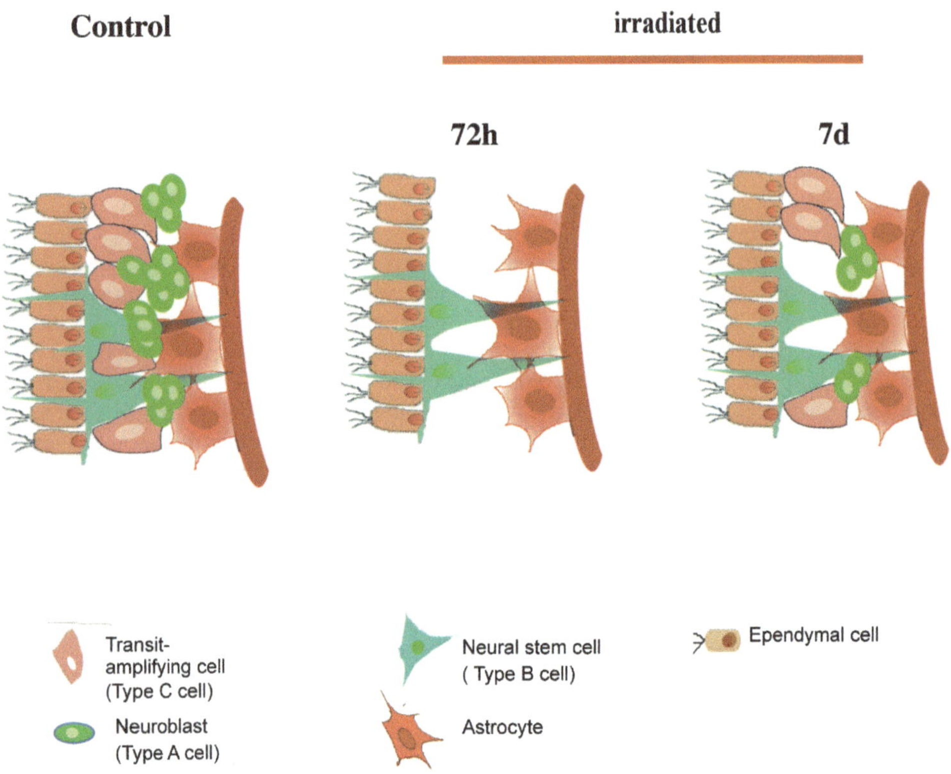

Radiation exposure of mice at 2Gy provoked a transient disappearance of progenitors of the subventricular zone (SVZ) such as transit-amplifying cells (Type C cell) and neuroblasts (Type A cell) at 72 hours. Four days later, those cells had almost completely replenished the SVZ.

Fig. 5. Schematic representation of SVZ reconstitution model after adult mouse brain irradiation.

Glial Fibrillary acidic protein (GFAP), a marker for NSCs, suggesting that quiescent NSCs are activated to re-enter cell cycle. Seven days after radiation, more numerous BrdU positive cells were observed and expressed the neuroblast marker PSA-NCAM arguing that neurogenesis recovered (Fig. 6B).

On the basis of these data and with the aim of finding proteins, such as growth factors secreted in the microenvironment involved in regeneration of the cells of the SVZ after radiation, we extracted proteins of non-irradiated SVZ and 2 Gy-irradiated SVZ at 3 and 7 days after exposure.

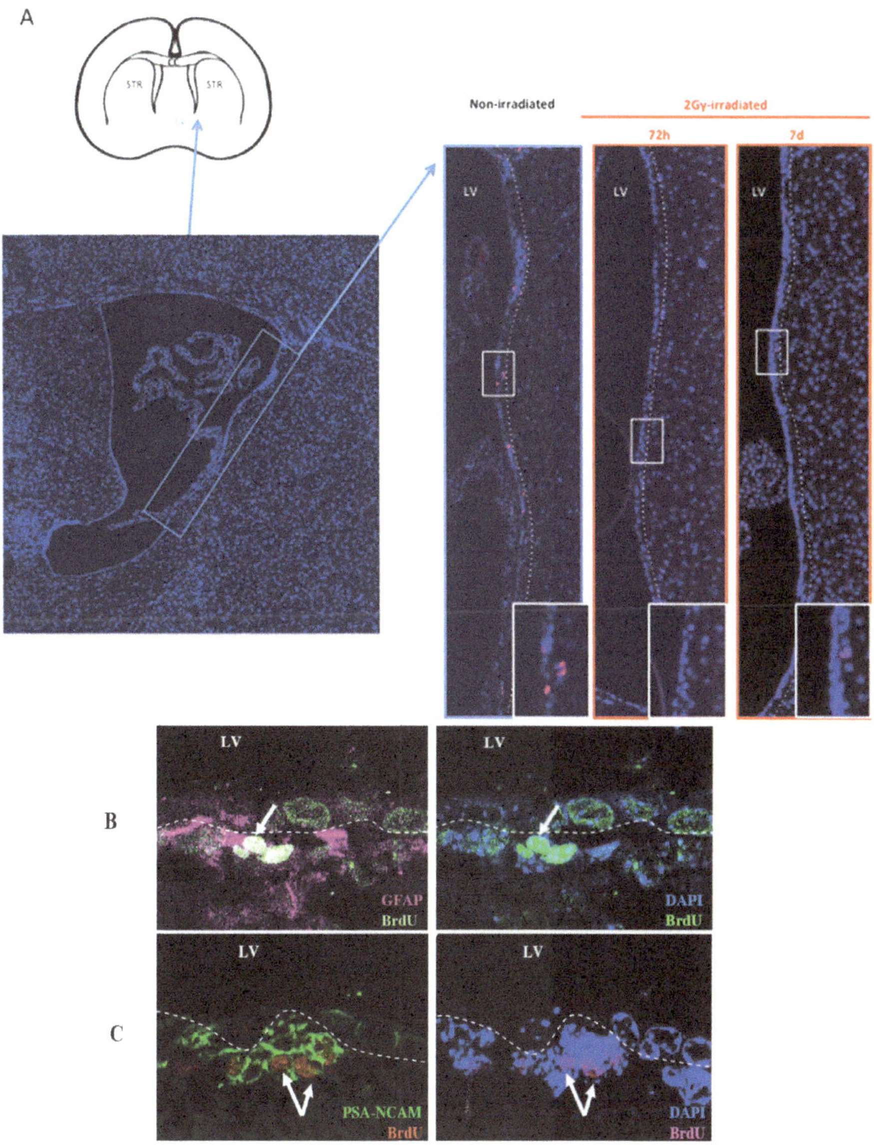

Mice were injected with BrdU 3 hours before sacrifice to label proliferating cells in control mice and after 2Gy-irradiation. Brain slices were counterstained with 4',6-diamidino-2-phenylindole (DAPI). (A) BrdU positive cells almost completely disappeared 72h post irradiation then they subsequently recovered in the SVZ niches.(B) 72 hours post-irradiation, some GFAP positive cells (pink), corresponding to candidate NSCs, have incorporated BrdU positive (green). At that time after irradiation, essentially NSCs proliferated in the SVZ niche. This result might underlie an activation of relatively quiescent NSCs 72h after irradiation. (C) 7 days after irradiation, the SVZ regeneration is evidenced by numerous neuroblasts PSA-NCAM postivie (green) and BrdU positive (red) in the SVZ.

Fig. 6. Regeneration of the SVZ after irradiation

3.2 Proteomic strategy

We combined 2D-gel electrophoresis and MS analyses of SVZ samples to determine proteins that are altered following radiation in adult neurogenic niches in comparison to a non-neurogenic brain region, i.e. STR. Protein samples were separated using two-dimensional electrophoresis in 3-10 non-linear pH gradient strips and 12% acrylamide gels.
SVZ samples obtained from irradiated mice at 3 and 7 days after radiation were compared with SVZ samples from non-irradiated control mice (Fig. 7). Along with micro-dissection procedures, SVZ can be contaminated with STR. For that reason and because the striatum is not a neurogenic zone, non-irradiated and 7 days-irradiated striatum samples were also taken.

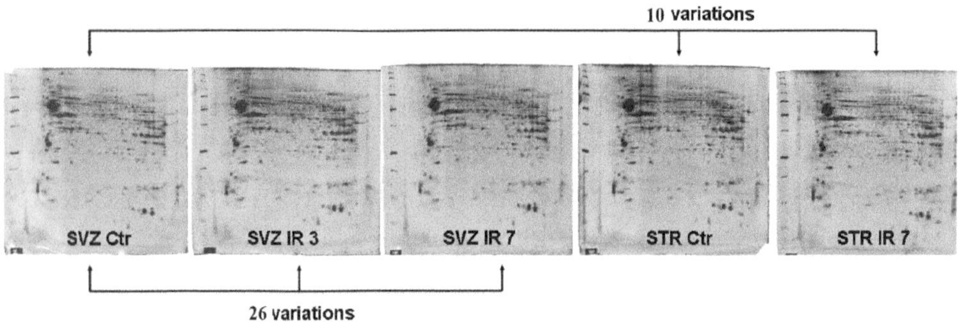

Fig. 7. Proteomic strategy of SVZ and STR samples comparison with no radiation (Ctr) and 3 days (IR 3) or 7 days (IR 7) after radiation.

3.3 Proteomic map analysis

As it can be observed in Fig. 7, pictures corresponding to the different samples analysed were very close and only minor differences can be observed, using a dedicated image analysis software.
From the 871 spots observed, a total of 36 spots were significantly modified for all the comparisons (Fig. 8). Thirty-two spots were modulated after irradiation and 4 spots were different between SVZ and STR. From these last spots, only one spot was more abundant in the SVZ than in STR suggesting a protein specifically expressed in the SVZ.
Using non-irradiated SVZ as control, 5 spots were modulated 3 days after radiation, 16 spots were modulated at 7 days (Table 1). Sixteen spots were altered at day 7 after radiation when compared with day 3. In addition, SVZ samples were also compared with STR and 4 spots appeared as modulated 7 days following radiation. The variation in spot intensity was ranged between 1.2 and 1.9 that was in agreement with previously published data using similar 2D-gel approach (Broadwater, et al. 2011, Gasperini, et al. 2011).
These spots, according to their localisation on the 2D reference map (Fig. 8), displayed an heterogeneous repartition on the gel, with a large range of iso-electric points (from 4 to 8) and of molecular weights (from 13 to 46 kDa).
Different profiles were established according to spot modifications, as illustrated in the Fig. 9.

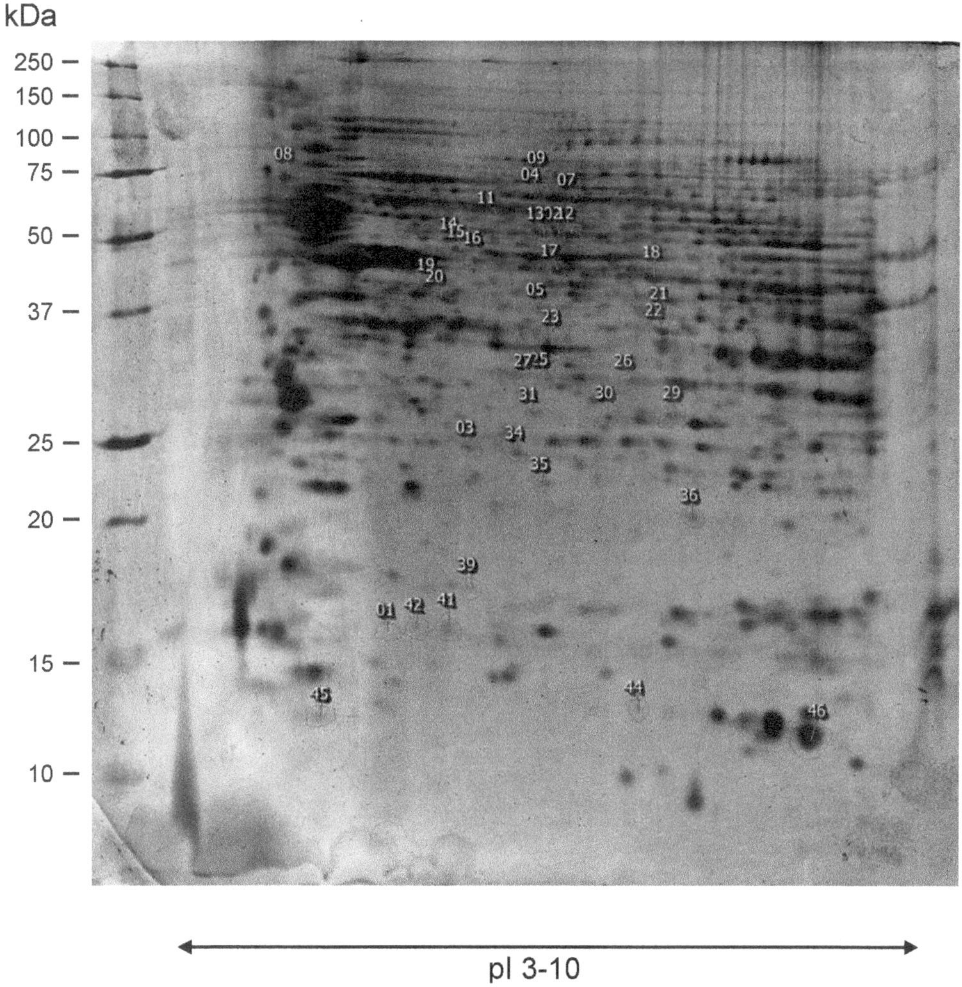

Fig. 8. Two-dimensional electrophoresis of SVZ proteins, separated under reducing conditions using 18-cm pH 3-10 strips for the first dimension, and a 12% acrylamide gel for the second dimension.

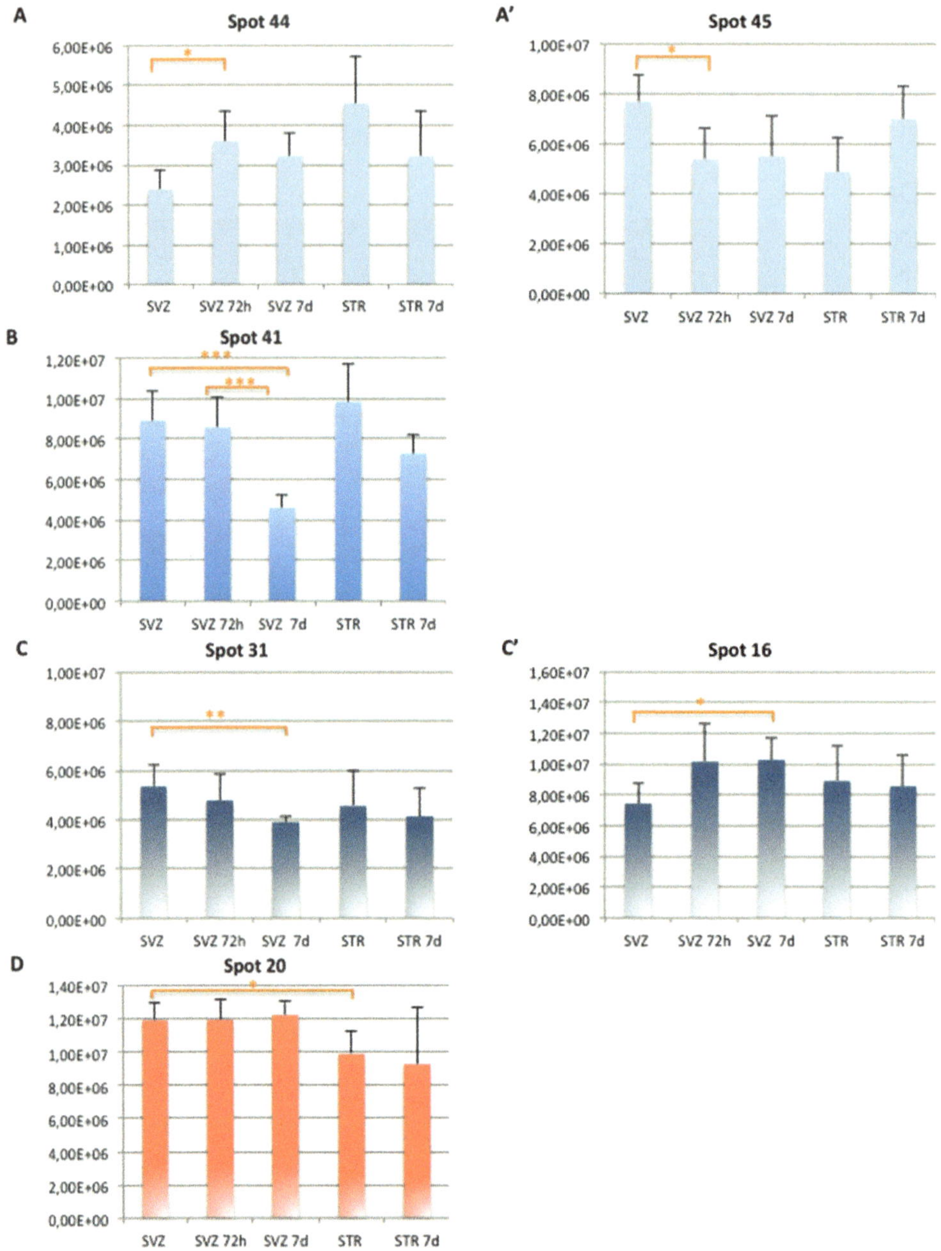

In comparison to non-irradiated SVZ: (A,A') early modified from 3 days after radiation, (B) downregulated by irradiation from 3 days to 7days or (C,C') late response to radiation at 7 days. In comparison to STR (D): no response to radiation. Numbers of spots corresponded to those listed in Fig. 3 and Table 1. Results are representative of volume intensity of the spot ± standard deviation from 5 technical replicates.

Fig. 9. Intensity profiles of spots specifically modified in the SVZ

Interestingly, 79% of the spot variations were obtained from comparison between non-irradiated SVZ and irradiated SVZ and appeared to be specific of the SVZ. Forty three percent of these spots were found modified between 3 and 7 days post-irradiation that might underlie functions of these proteins during the intense proliferation phase. Thirteen percent of them were modified 3 days after radiation as compared with control SVZ suggesting a role for the proteins in the activation of quiescent NSCs.

The rest of them (21%) corresponded to spots altered in both regions after radiation in comparison to respective region controls, suggesting a role of these proteins in the response to radiation.

Among the 32 spots identified with a significant response to radiation, we eliminated 9 abundant spots (more than 0.1% of the total volume of spots) because they might not correspond to proteins involved in proliferation processes but rather have a cytoarchitecture function in the tissue. In a first round of analysis, among the 21 remaining spots, only 15 were abundant enough and well separated in the gel to be excised allowing identification by MS (Table 1).

3.4 Biological functions of the proteins

We verified the expression of the genes corresponding to the identified proteins (Table1) using the Allen Brain Atlas database (Fig. 10). This database contained a thorough list of genes expression in the mouse brain by RNA hybridization (http://mouse.brain-map.org) (Lein, et al.,2007). We found that indeed 47% of our identified proteins have its gene expressed in the SVZ; the others being at least expressed in the adjacent regions, i.e. striatum or in the corpus callosum (**Fig. 10**).

Identified proteins were classified according to their known biological activity (Fig. 11). Surprisingly, we did not identify proteins matching with growth factors or cell cycle regulation, as they may be present in too small quantity to be identified. Otherwise, we cannot exclude that gel resolution might not be optimized for the identification of this type of proteins.

Myelin basic protein (MBP) that wraps axons has been identified in two adjacent spots (41, 42) that varied according to Pi but not in their MW indicating posttranslational modifications. Strikingly, the amount of these spots decreased after radiation, which suggested a degradation of myelin sheets by radiation. This is of importance because MBP modifications have never been reported with such a low radiation dose (Tian, et al.,2008).

Otherwise, this current proteomic analysis of SVZ demonstrates that a 2 Gy-radiation exposure affected major cellular functions such as proteasome, energy production, vesicle trafficking and cytoskeletal maintenance.

Thirteen percent of the spots belong to the proteasome system known to be involved in the degradation of unneeded or damaged proteins by proteolysis (Mcbride, et al.,2003). The intensity of these spots were decreased between 3 and 7 days (spot) 34 or only 7 days post irradiation (spot 3) that might underscore a decrease of proteasome activity that has already been reported after irradiation in a variety of cell types (Mcbride, et al.,2002, Pajonk&Mcbride,2001). This reduction of proteasome activity has been proposed to be related, at least in part, to an increased expression of proteasome inhibitors (Conconi&Friguet, 1997, Zaiss, et al., 2002).

Twenty percent of the spots corresponded to proteins having functions in metabolism pathways. Two of them (5, 44) were modified within 3 days after radiation. Another was increased 7 days after radiation and the identified protein have been implicated in

Spot	Observed pI	MW	Abundance	Variations	reference sample	ANOVA (p)
1	5.28	16	0.03899	-1.9 in SVZ IR 7 -1.8 in SVZ IR 7	SVZ CT SVZ IR 3	0.008 0.013
2	**6.53**	**49**	**0.09853**	**-1.3 in SVZ IR 7**	**SVZ IR 3**	**0.022**
3	5.95	25	0.05079	+1.3 in SVZ IR 7	SVZ CT	0.033
4	**6.4**	**62**	**0.06269**	**+1.3 in SVZ IR 7**	**SVZ IR 3**	**0.004**
5	6.41	36	0.04725	-1.3 in SVZ IR 3	SVZ CT	0.012
7	**6.68**	**60**	**0.27306**	**+1.3 in SVZ IR 7**	**SVZ IR 3**	**0.043**
8	**4.3**	**68**	**0.19432**	**+1.4 in STR CT**	**SVZ CT**	**0.05**
9	**6.44**	**68**	**0.01876**	**+1.3 in SVZ IR 7**	**SVZ IR 3**	**0.019**
11	**6.12**	**57**	**0.04227**	**-1.3 in STR IR 7**	**STR CT**	**0.031**
12	**6.61**	**49**	**0.10724**	**+1.2 in SVZ IR 7 +1.2 in SVZ IR 7**	**SVZ CT SVZ IR 3**	**0.05 0.010**
13	**6.43**	**49**	**0.06881**	**+1.2 in SVZ IR 7 +1.3 in STR CT**	**SVZ IR 3 SVZ CT**	**0.028 0.007**
14	**5.74**	**48**	**0.08356**	**+1.2 in SVZ IR 7**	**SVZ IR 3**	**0.004**
15	5.82	46	0.08980	+1.3 in SVZ IR 7	SVZ CT	0.02
16	5.98	44	0.06190	+1.4 in SVZ IR 7	SVZ CT	0.021
17	**6.53**	**43**	**0.10764**	**+1.3 in SVZ IR 7**	**SVZ IR 3**	**0.003**
18	**7.18**	**41**	**0.25750**	**+1.2 in STR CT**	**SVZ CT**	**0.018**
19	5.58	40	0.07969	-1.2 in SVZ IR 3	SVZ CT	0.012
20	5.72	37	0.09955	-1.2 in STR CT	SVZ CT	0.012
21	**7.28**	**36**	**0.03971**	**-1.4 in SVZ IR 7**	**SVZ CT**	**0.038**
22	**7.29**	**34**	**0.12789**	**+1.2 in SVZ IR 3 +1.4 in STR IR 7**	**SVZ CT STR CT**	**0.021 0.001**
23	**6.47**	**33**	**0.38047**	**+1.2 in STR CT**	**SVZ CT**	**0.011**
25	6.47	30	0.03257	-1.7 in SVZ IR 7 -1.6 in SVZ IR 7	SVZ CT SVZ IR 3	0.027 0.047
26	**7.04**	**30**	**0.05344**	**-1.5 in SVZ IR 7**	**SVZ CT**	**0.04**
27	**6.35**	**30**	**0.02708**	**-1.6 in SVZ IR 7 -1.6 in SVZ IR 7**	**SVZ CT SVZ IR 3**	**0.01 0.015**
29	**7.33**	**27**	**0.10550**	**-1.3 in SVZ IR 7 +1.4 in STR IR 7**	**SVZ IR 3 STR CT**	**0.041 0.004**
30	6.88	27	0.05109	-1.3 in SVZ IR 7	SVZ CT	0.038
31	6.37	27	0.04457	-1.4 in SVZ IR 7	SVZ CT	0.01
34	6.24	24	0.05691	-1.3 in SVZ IR 7 -1.3 in SVZ IR 7	SVZ CT SVZ IR 3	0.017 0.036
35	**6.45**	**22**	**0.03776**	**-1.4 in SVZ IR 7**	**SVZ CT**	**0.016**
36	7.49	20	0.06499	-1.6 in SVZ IR 7	SVZ IR 3	0.046
39	**5.92**	**17**	**0.02929**	**-1.4 in SVZ IR 7 -1.4 in SVZ IR 7**	**SVZ CT SVZ IR 3**	**0.015 0.018**
41	5.74	16	0.07440	-1.9 in SVZ IR 7 -1.9 in SVZ IR 7	SVZ CT SVZ IR 3	0.001 0.001
42	**5.5**	**16**	**0.04760**	**-1.6 in SVZ IR 7 -1.5 in STR IR 7**	**SVZ CT STR CT**	**0.002 0.013**
44	7.09	13	0.02003	+1.5 in SVZ IR 3	SVZ CT	0.018
45	4.63	13	0.06425	-1.4 in SVZ IR 3	SVZ CT	0.028
46	**8.48**	**12**	**0.94660**	**+1.4 in STR IR 7**	**STR CT**	**0.002**

Table 1. List of spots significantly modified in: control SVZ; 3 days following radiation SVZ, 7 days following radiation SVZ, control STR; 7 days following radiation STR. Spot number; experimental protein molecular weight and pI; variation level, under-expressed (-) or over-expressed (+) in the corresponding sample, *vs* reference sample; and ANOVA, (significant when $p<0.05$). Spots indicated in bold were excised from the gels and analysed by MS to allow the identification the proteins. The abundance corresponds to the ratio (%) of the volume one spot on the total volume of spots.

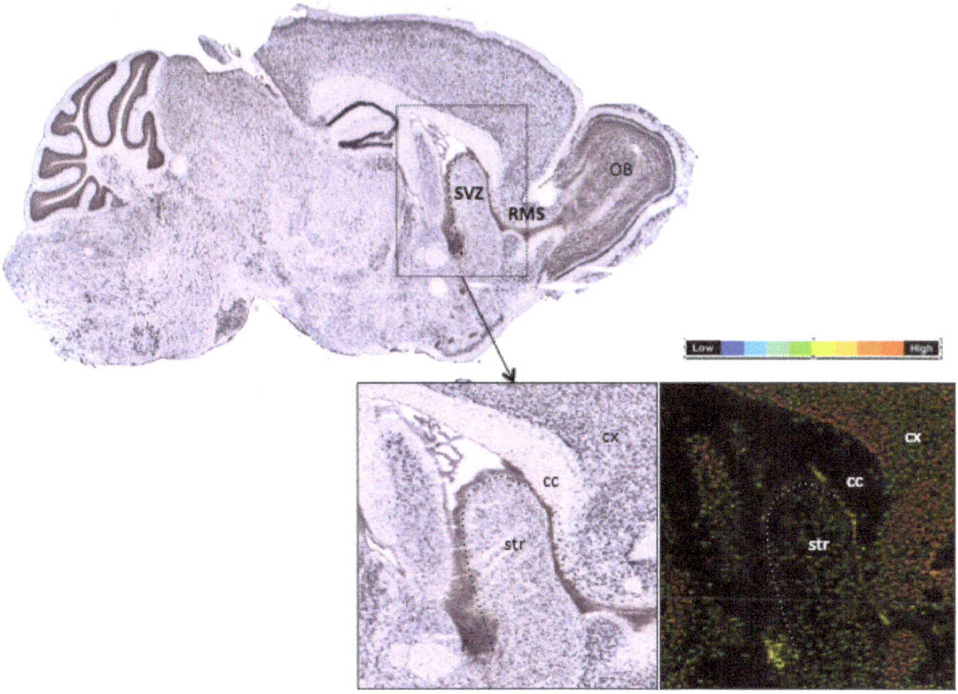

Fig. 10. An example of the expression of one gene corresponding to an identified protein using the Allen Brain Atlas database. This gene is expressed along the SVZ, a part of the RMS and also in the cortex (cx) but not in the corpus callosum (cc).

Biological functions	Spot number	Response to radiation
Mitochondrial respiratory chain	3 15 45	Late Late Early
Intracellular transport	20 30	No response Late
Proteasome	31 34	Late Mid
Metabolism	5 16 44	Early Late Early
Cytoskeleton	1 19	Mid Early
Axogenesis/myelination	25 41 42	Early Mid Late

Fig. 11. Distribution of the proteins identified by MS according to their biological function.

phospholipid biosynthesis that might correspond to proteins involved in the organisation of membrane structure during cell proliferation. In our context, these identified proteins might interfere with the proliferation wave during SVZ regeneration.

Thirteen percent of the modulated proteins (spots 34, 30, 20) are central effectors in intracellular signal transduction pathways like GTPases mediating the formation of vesicles in neural cells, a fundamental process of neurotransmitter release (De Camilli, et al.,1995).

Thirteen percent of the spots referred to cytoskeleton proteins (spots 1, 19) showing alteration from day 3 to 7. Thus, this proteomic analysis revealed that radiation exposure influence the expression of proteins involved the reorganisation of actin cytoskeleton probably associated with proliferation and/or migration.

It appeared that 20% of the modulated proteins were known for being implicated in oxidative metabolism. One of them (spot 45) decreased early after radiation that might reflect a radio-induced defect of mitochondrial metabolism. The two other spots (3, 15) were

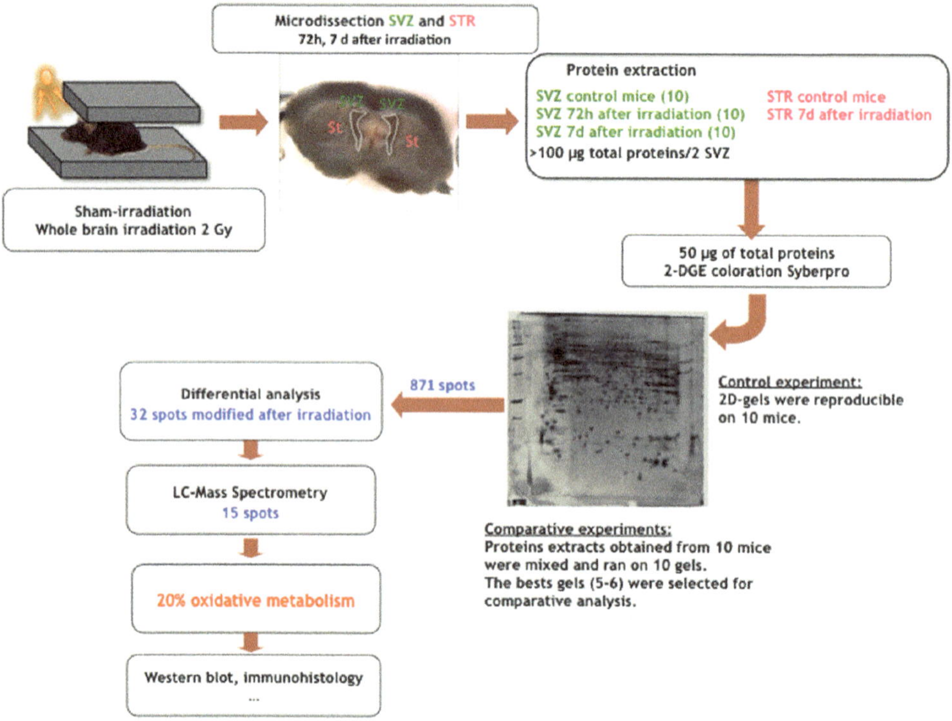

From 871 spots, 32 spots showed variations of intensity after irradiation. Among the last spots, we analysed and identified 17 spots. Twenty-six percents of the identified proteins matched with proteins already described in oxidative metabolism. The next step of this work will consist firstly, in confirming these variations of intensity by other technical approaches such as western blot and immunohistochemistry and secondly, in demonstrating their involvement in the neurogenesis stimulation after SVZ irradiation.

Fig. 12. Schematic representation of the current comparative proteomic analysis from control SVZ and 2Gy-irradiated SVZ at 3 and 7 days after exposure.

increased 7 days after radiation probably as a consequence of an increased metabolic activity of proliferating SVZ cells.
The approach of the current proteomic analysis and the main results are represented in the Fig. 12. The next step of this work will be the validation of the variation of identified proteins and a deep analysis to demonstrate their involvement in neurogenesis stimulation following SVZ radiation and their potential use to stimulate neurogenesis in aged brains and/or neurodegenerative diseases.

4. Conclusion

This preliminary study demonstrates that 2D-gel electrophoresis is an accurate global proteomic analysis to analyse modifications in very small brain regions. In our model of neurogenic niche regeneration after 2Gy irradiation, which is associated with stem cell proliferation, we have identified proteins, which have major cellular functions such as energy production, cytoskeletal maintenance and vesicle trafficking. Interestingly, identified proteins have functions known to be involved in pathways previously reported to be altered by radiation which underscores the reliability of our proteomic approach. Especially, proteins involved in mitochondrial respiratory chain have been identified in our study; they produce energy and generate reactive oxygen species. Acharya et al. have shown that human NSCs significantly increased their oxidative and nitrosative stresses after radiation (Acharya, et al. 2010). The importance of endogenous oxygen reactive species to control NSC proliferation has been reported as well (Le Belle, et al. 2010). Moreover, oxidative stress is implicated in the progression of aging and neurodegenerative disorders (Berlett&Stadtman, 1997, Butterfield, et al.,1997, Lauderback, et al.,2002, Richardson, 2009). In light of theses studies, our data concerning mitochondrial respiratory chain are very promising. This chapter describes the first part of our project, including a validation of the technical strategy, with examples of protein functions, associated with SVZ regeneration following 2Gy irradiation. The characterization of identified proteins is still under investigation, and needs further biological validations.

5. Acknowledgment

This work was supported by grants of ANR-SEST (Neurorad) and Electricité de France.

6. References

Acharya, M. M., Lan, M. L., Kan, V. H., Patel, N. H., Giedzinski, E., Tseng, B. P. & Limoli, C. L., (2010), Consequences of ionizing radiation-induced damage in human neural stem cells. Free Radic Biol Med, Vol. 49, No.12, pp. 1846-1855, 1873-4596 (Electronic)

Alonso, G., (1999). Neuronal progenitor-like cells expressing polysialylated neural cell adhesion molecule are present on the ventricular surface of the adult rat brain and spinal cord. J Comp Neurol, Vol. 414, No.2, pp. 149-166, 0021-9967 (Print)

Anderson, N. L., Nance, S. L., Tollasken S. L., Giere F. A., Anderson N. G., (1985), Quantitative reproducibility of measurements from coomassie blue-stained two-dimensional gels-analysis of mouse-liver protein-patterns and compmarison of BALC/C and C57 strains. *Electrophoresis*, Vol. 6; No12, pp. 592-599, 0173-0835 (Print).

Alvarez-Buylla, A. & Lim, D. A., (2004). For the long run: maintaining germinal niches in the adult brain. *Neuron*, Vol. 41, No.5, pp. 683-686, 0896-6273 (Print)

Berlett, B. S. & Stadtman, E. R., (1997). Protein oxidation in aging, disease, and oxidative stress. *J Biol Chem*, Vol. 272, No.33, pp. 20313-20316, 0021-9258 (Print)

Broadwater, L., Pandit, A., Clements, R., Azzam, S., Vadnal, J., Sulak, M., Yong, V. W., Freeman, E. J., Gregory, R. B. & McDonough, J., (2011), Analysis of the mitochondrial proteome in multiple sclerosis cortex. *Biochim Biophys Acta,* Vol. 1812, No.5, pp. 630-641, 0006-3002 (Print)

Butterfield, D. A., Howard, B. J., Yatin, S., Allen, K. L. & Carney, J. M., (1997). Free radical oxidation of brain proteins in accelerated senescence and its modulation by N-tert-butyl-alpha-phenylnitrone. *Proc Natl Acad Sci U S A,* Vol. 94, No.2, pp. 674-678, 0027-8424 (Print)

Castegna, A., Aksenov, M., Thongboonkerd, V., Klein, J. B., Pierce, W. M., Booze, R., Markesbery, W. R. & Butterfield, D. A., (2002). Proteomic identification of oxidatively modified proteins in Alzheimer's disease brain. Part II: dihydropyrimidinase-related protein 2, alpha-enolase and heat shock cognate 71. J *Neurochem,* Vol. 82, No.6, pp. 1524-1532, 0022-3042 (Print)

Cayre, M., Bancila, M., Virard, I., Borges, A. & Durbec, P., (2006). Migrating and myelinating potential of subventricular zone neural progenitor cells in white matter tracts of the adult rodent brain. *Mol Cell Neurosci,* Vol. 31, No.4, pp. 748-758, 1044-7431 (Print)

Conconi, M. & Friguet, B., (1997). Proteasome inactivation upon aging and on oxidation-effect of HSP 90. *Mol Biol Rep,* Vol. 24, No.1-2, pp. 45-50, 0301-4851 (Print)

De Camilli, P., Takei, K. & McPherson, P. S., (1995). The function of dynamin in endocytosis. *Curr Opin Neurobiol,* Vol. 5, No.5, pp. 559-565, 0959-4388 (Print)

Doetsch, F., (2003). A niche for adult neural stem cells Curr Opin Genet Dev, Vol. 13, No.5, pp. 543-550, 0959-437X (Print)

Doetsch, F., Garcia-Verdugo, J. M. & Alvarez-Buylla, A., (1999). Regeneration of a germinal layer in the adult mammalian brain. *Proc Natl Acad Sci U S A,* Vol. 96, No.20, pp. 11619-11624, 0027-8424 (Print)

Dubois-Dalcq, M., (2005). Development and regeneration of oligodendrocytes: therapeutic perspectives in demyelinating diseases. *Bull Mem Acad R Med Belg,* Vol. 160, No.10-12, pp. 407-415; discussion 415-406, 0377-8231 (Print)

Gasperini, L., Piubelli, C. & Carboni, L., (2011), Proteomics of rat hypothalamus, hippocampus and pre-frontal/frontal cortex after central administration of the neuropeptide PACAP, *Mol Biol Rep,* Vol. pp. 1573-4978 (Electronic)

Goings, G. E., Sahni, V. & Szele, F. G., (2004). Migration patterns of subventricular zone cells in adult mice change after cerebral cortex injury. *Brain Res,* Vol. 996, No.2, pp. 213-226, 0006-8993 (Print)

Hopewell, J. W., Cavanagh, J. B., (1972). Effects of X-irradiation on the mitotic activity of the subependymal plate of rats. *Br. J. Radiol.,* Vol. 45, pp. 461-465., 0007-1285 (Pint)

Ihrie, R. A. & Alvarez-Buylla, A., (2011), Lake-front property: a unique germinal niche by the lateral ventricles of the adult brain. *Neuron,* Vol. 70, No.4, pp. 674-686, 1097-4199 (Electronic)

Jankovski, A., Garcia, C., Soriano, E. & Sotelo, C., (1998). Proliferation, migration and differentiation of neuronal progenitor cells in the adult mouse subventricular zone surgically separated from its olfactory bulb. *Eur J Neurosci,* Vol. 10, No.12, pp. 3853-3868, 0953-816X (Print)

Lauderback, C. M., Kanski, J., Hackett, J. M., Maeda, N., Kindy, M. S. & Butterfield, D. A., (2002). Apolipoprotein E modulates Alzheimer's Abeta(1-42)-induced oxidative damage to synaptosomes in an allele-specific manner. *Brain Res,* Vol. 924, No.1, pp. 90-97, 0006-8993 (Print)

Le Belle, J. E., Orozco, N. M., Paucar, A. A., Saxe, J. P., Mottahedeh, J., Pyle, A. D., Wu, H. & Kornblum, H. I., (2011), Proliferative neural stem cells have high endogenous ROS levels that regulate self-renewal and neurogenesis in a PI3K/Akt-dependant manner. *Cell Stem Cell*, Vol. 8, No.1, pp. 59-71, 1875-9777 (Electronic)

Lein, E. S., Hawrylycz, M. J., Ao, N., Ayres, M., Bensinger, A., Bernard, A., Boe, A. F., Boguski, M. S., Brockway, K. S., Byrnes, E. J., Chen, L., Chen, T. M., Chin, M. C., Chong, J., Crook, B. E., Czaplinska, A., Dang, C. N., Datta, S., Dee, N. R., Desaki, A. L., Desta, T., Diep, E., Dolbeare, T. A., Donelan, M. J., Dong, H. W., Dougherty, J. G., Duncan, B. J., Ebbert, A. J., Eichele, G., Estin, L. K., Faber, C., Facer, B. A., Fields, R., Fischer, S. R., Fliss, T. P., Frensley, C., Gates, S. N., Glattfelder, K. J., Halverson, K. R., Hart, M. R., Hohmann, J. G., Howell, M. P., Jeung, D. P., Johnson, R. A., Karr, P. T., Kawal, R., Kidney, J. M., Knapik, R. H., Kuan, C. L., Lake, J. H., Laramee, A. R., Larsen, K. D., Lau, C., Lemon, T. A., Liang, A. J., Liu, Y., Luong, L. T., Michaels, J., Morgan, J. J., Morgan, R. J., Mortrud, M. T., Mosqueda, N. F., Ng, L. L., Ng, R., Orta, G. J., Overly, C. C., Pak, T. H., Parry, S. E., Pathak, S. D., Pearson, O. C., Puchalski, R. B., Riley, Z. L., Rockett, H. R., Rowland, S. A., Royall, J. J., Ruiz, M. J., Sarno, N. R., Schaffnit, K., Shapovalova, N. V., Sivisay, T., Slaughterbeck, C. R., Smith, S. C., Smith, K. A., Smith, B. I., Sodt, A. J., Stewart, N. N., Stumpf, K. R., Sunkin, S. M., Sutram, M., Tam, A., Teemer, C. D., Thaller, C., Thompson, C. L., Varnam, L. R., Visel, A., Whitlock, R. M., Wohnoutka, P. E., Wolkey, C. K., Wong, V. Y., Wood, M., Yaylaoglu, M. B., Young, R. C., Youngstrom, B. L., Yuan, X. F., Zhang, B., Zwingman, T. A. & Jones, A. R., (2007). Genome-wide atlas of gene expression in the adult mouse brain. *Nature*, Vol. 445, No.7124, pp. 168-176, 1476-4687 (Electronic)

Lim, D. A., Tramontin, A. D., Trevejo, J. M., Herrera, D. G., Garcia-Verdugo, J. M. & Alvarez-Buylla, A., (2000). Noggin antagonizes BMP signaling to create a niche for adult neurogenesis Neuron, Vol. 28, No.3, pp. 713-726, 0896-6273 (Print)

Liu, X., Wang, Q., Haydar, T. F. & Bordey, A., (2005). Nonsynaptic GABA signaling in postnatal subventricular zone controls proliferation of GFAP-expressing progenitors. *Nat Neurosci*, Vol. 8, No.9, pp. 1179-1187, 1097-6256 (Print)

Macas, J., Nern, C., Plate, K. H. & Momma, S., (2006). Increased generation of neuronal progenitors after ischemic injury in the aged adult human forebrain. *J Neurosci*, Vol. 26, No.50, pp. 13114-13119, 1529-2401 (Electronic)

Mathieu, C., Sii-Felice, K., Fouchet, P., Etienne, O., Haton, C., Mabondzo, A., Boussin, F. D. & Mouthon, M. A., (2008). Endothelial cell-derived bone morphogenetic proteins control proliferation of neural stem/progenitor cells. *Mol Cell Neurosci*, Vol. 38, No.4, pp. 569-577, 1095-9327 (Electronic)

McBride, W. H., Iwamoto, K. S., Syljuasen, R., Pervan, M. & Pajonk, F., (2003). The role of the ubiquitin/proteasome system in cellular responses to radiation. *Oncogene*, Vol. 22, No.37, pp. 5755-5773, 0950-9232 (Print)

McBride, W. H., Pajonk, F., Chiang, C. S. & Sun, J. R., (2002). NF-kappa B, cytokines, proteasomes, and low-dose radiation exposure. *Mil Med*, Vol. 167, No.2 Suppl, pp. 66-67, 0026-4075 (Print)

Ming, G. L., Song, H. (2011). Adult neurogenesis in the mammalian brain:significant answers and significant questions. *Neuron*, Vol. 70, No4, pp. 687-702, 1097-4199 (Electronic)

Morshead, C. M., Reynolds, B. A., Craig, C. G., McBurney, M. W., Staines, W. A., Morassutti, D., Weiss, S. & van der Kooy, D., (1994). Neural stem cells in the adult mammalian forebrain: a relatively quiescent subpopulation of subependymal cells. *Neuron*, Vol. 13, No.5, pp. 1071-1082, 0896-6273 (Print)

Pajonk, F. & McBride, W. H., (2001). Ionizing radiation affects 26s proteasome function and associated molecular responses, even at low doses. *Radiother Oncol*, Vol. 59, No.2, pp. 203-212, 0167-8140 (Print)

Pastrana, E., Cheng, L. C. & Doetsch, F., (2009). Simultaneous prospective purification of adult subventricular zone neural stem cells and their progeny. *Proc Natl Acad Sci U S A*, Vol. 106, No.15, pp. 6387-6392, 1091-6490 (Electronic)

Picard-Riera, N., Decker, L., Delarasse, C., Goude, K., Nait-Oumesmar, B., Liblau, R., Pham-Dinh, D. & Evercooren, A. B., (2002). Experimental autoimmune encephalomyelitis mobilizes neural progenitors from the subventricular zone to undergo oligodendrogenesis in adult mice. *Proc Natl Acad Sci U S A*, Vol. 99, No.20, pp. 13211-13216, 0027-8424 (Print)

Ramirez-Castillejo, C., Sanchez-Sanchez, F., Andreu-Agullo, C., Ferron, S. R., Aroca-Aguilar, J. D., Sanchez, P., Mira, H., Escribano, J. & Farinas, I., (2006). Pigment epithelium-derived factor is a niche signal for neural stem cell renewal. *Nat Neurosci*, Vol. 9, No.3, pp. 331-339, 1097-6256 (Print)

Richardson, R. B., (2009). Ionizing radiation and aging: rejuvenating an old idea Aging (Albany NY), Vol. 1, No.11, pp. 887-902, 1945-4589 (Electronic)

Romanko, M. J., Rola, R., Fike, J. R., Szele, F. G., Dizon, M. L., Felling, R. J., Brazel, C. Y. & Levison, S. W., (2004). Roles of the mammalian subventricular zone in cell replacement after brain injury. *Prog Neurobiol*, Vol. 74, No.2, pp. 77-99, 0301-0082 (Print)

Shinohara, C., Gobbel, G. T., Lamborn, K. R., Tada, E. & Fike, J. R., (1997). Apoptosis in the subependyma of young adult rats after single and fractionated doses of X-rays. *Cancer Res*, Vol. 57, No.13, pp. 2694-2702, 0008-5472 (Print)

Shoemaker, L. D., Orozco, N. M., Geschwind, D. H., Whitelegge, J. P., Faull, K. F. & Kornblum, H. I., (2010), Identification of differentially expressed proteins in murine embryonic and postnatal cortical neural progenitors. *PLoS One*, Vol. 5, No.2, pp. e9121, 1932-6203 (Electronic)

Sung, J. H., Cho, E. H., Min, W., Kim, M. J., Kim, M. O., Jung, E. J. & Koh, P. O., (2010), Identification of proteins regulated by estradiol in focal cerebral ischemic injury--a proteomics approach. *Neurosci Lett*, Vol. 477, No.2, pp. 66-71, 1872-7972 (Electronic)

Tada, E., Yang, C., Gobbel, G. T., Lamborn, K. R. & Fike, J. R., (1999). Long-term impairment of subependymal repopulation following damage by ionizing irradiation Exp Neurol, Vol. 160, No.1, pp. 66-77, 0014-4886 (Print)

Tavazoie, M., Van der Veken, L., Silva-Vargas, V., Louissaint, M., Colonna, L., Zaidi, B., Garcia-Verdugo, J. M. & Doetsch, F., (2008). A specialized vascular niche for adult neural stem cells. *Cell Stem Cell*, Vol. 3, No.3, pp. 279-288, 1875-9777 (Electronic)

Tian, Y., Shi, Z., Yang, S., Chen, Y. & Bao, S., (2008). Changes in myelin basic protein and demyelination in the rat brain within 3 months of single 2-, 10-, or 30-Gy whole-brain radiation treatments. *J Neurosurg*, Vol. 109, No.5, pp. 881-888, 0022-3085 (Print)

Yamashita, T., Ninomiya, M., Hernandez Acosta, P., Garcia-Verdugo, J. M., Sunabori, T., Sakaguchi, M., Adachi, K., Kojima, T., Hirota, Y., Kawase, T., Araki, N., Abe, K., Okano, H. & Sawamoto, K., (2006). Subventricular zone-derived neuroblasts migrate and differentiate into mature neurons in the post-stroke adult striatum. *J Neurosci*, Vol. 26, No.24, pp. 6627-6636, 1529-2401 (Electronic)

Yang, S., Liu, T., Li, S., Zhang, X., Ding, Q., Que, H., Yan, X., Wei, K. & Liu, S., (2008). Comparative proteomic analysis of brains of naturally aging mice. *Neuroscience*, Vol. 154, No.3, pp. 1107-1120, 0306-4522 (Print)

Zaiss, D. M., Standera, S., Kloetzel, P. M. & Sijts, A. J., (2002). PI31 is a modulator of proteasome formation and antigen processing. *Proc Natl Acad Sci U S A*, Vol. 99, No.22, pp. 14344-14349, 0027-8424 (Print)

Part 4

Organelles and Secretome Proteomics

16

Analysis of Organelle Dynamics by Quantitative Mass Spectrometry Based Proteomics

Florian Fröhlich, Tobias C. Walther and Romain Christiano
Yale University School of Medicine, Department of Cell Biology
USA

1. Introduction

A major goal of cell biology is to understand the dynamic interplay between different reactions in the cell. In eukaryotes, compartmentalization of the cytoplasm into organelles facilitates the coordinated execution of many cellular functions. To understand how this is achieved, it is important to know the protein composition of the different organelles, and to determine how it may change over time. In addition, the activity of many proteins is regulated by often reversible and dynamic post-translational modifications (PTMs). In recent years, proteomics has matured into a staple technique for cell biology. Modern approaches of proteomics rely on mass-spectrometry. Here, we build on several reviews (Aebersold and Mann, 2003; Choudhary and Mann, 2010; Walther and Mann, 2010) to summarize and highlight contemporary applications of MS-based proteomics to the analysis of organelle dynamics.

2. MS-based quantitative proteomics approaches for proteins and their post-translational modifications

Most proteomics studies aim to not just identify proteins but to quantitate their abundance in different samples. In the past few years, several quantitative proteomics approaches have been developed to accomplish this task.

2.1 MS-based quantitative proteomics approaches

2.1.1 Stable isotope labeling by amino acids in cell culture (SILAC)

The most commonly used method to quantitate proteins is stable isotope labeling by amino acids in cell culture (SILAC; (Ong et al., 2002)) in combination with liquid chromatography (LC) and tandem high resolution mass spectrometry (LC-MS/MS). Cells are labeled with non-radioactive heavy labeled amino acids, typically arginine and /or lysine. After cell lysis, extracts from differently labeled and differently treated cells are mixed and digested with a protease that cuts after the labeled amino acids, such as trypsin for the case of arginine/lysine. The resulting peptide mixture is fractionated by LC on a C18 column and analyzed in a high resolution mass spectrometer. The mass shift between labeled and unlabeled peptides allows the quantification of intensities of peptides, and based on that of proteins, derived from cells differentially labeled and subjected to different conditions. Since chemically identical peptides are quantitated in the same spectrum, the accuracy of this methodology is very high. In addition, mixing samples directly after lysis limits the chance for experimental errors. However, in its simplest rendition, SILAC-based proteomics is limited to samples that can be metabolic labeled, including cells and model organisms (ranging from yeast to mice) (de Godoy et al., 2008; Kruger et al., 2008). Recently developed "spike-in" approaches that use isotope labeled cell extracts as standards for analysis of samples of interests from sources that cannot be labeled, such as patient samples, are compared. In case a single cell extract does not adequately represent a particular tissue or sample, several extracts can be mixed to obtain a "super-SILAC" standard (Geiger et al., 2010). This approach of SILAC reference standards is not limited to quantitation of protein abundance but can also be applied to quantify changes in PTMs, such as phosphorylation. In an example of such an analysis, a phosphopeptide standard combining untreated or insulin treated mouse liver cell lines were spiked into samples derived from the liver of insulin treated or untreated mice. This method led to the identification of over 15,000 and quantitation of 10,000 phosphosites (Monetti et al., 2011).

2.1.2 Isobaric tags for relative and absolute quantification (iTRAQ)

Chemically labeling of proteins in different samples can also be used for their quantitation. One such technique uses **i**sobaric **t**ags for **r**elative and **a**bsolute **q**uantification (iTRAQ). In iTRAQ experiments, different chemical groups modify the primary amino group of either the N-terminus or lysine side chains of peptides in different samples (Ross et al., 2004). These differentially labeled peptides are pooled and analyzed by LC-MS/MS setup. Each of the labels has the same mass and therefore each peptide is visible in a single peak in the MS spectrum. However, fragmentation of that peak leads to formation of a low molecular mass reporter ion characteristic for each tag in the MS/MS spectrum that is used to quantify the relative amounts of the corresponding peptides and proteins. It is very important for this technique to distinguish peptides which have a similar mass and elute at the same time because this would lead to false ratios as both peptides contribute to the abundance of the same reporter ions (Ow et al., 2009; Zhang et al., 2010). In addition, it is crucial to ensure complete labeling of the sample. Moreover, side reactions of chemical labeling may be unavoidable, but can lead to false positive identifications of PTMs. For example, alkylation of a peptide mixture with iodoacetamide can produce a 2-acetamidoacetamide covalent adduct to lysine. This has the same atomic composition as a diglycine adduct of a ubiquitinated peptide after tryptic digest (Nielsen et al., 2008).

2.1.3 Label free approaches

In addition to the described labeling methods, so called "label-free" approaches that directly compare the abundance of peptides and proteins between samples are very attractive to analyze complex protein mixtures. Such approaches enable the analysis of samples which cannot be easily labeled. One type of label free quantitation approaches uses alignments of separate LC-MS/MS runs to compare peptide intensities between different samples. Recent advances in computational proteomics enable quantification of peptides from less complex samples by this approach (Mueller et al., 2008; Wong and Cagney, 2010). However, the accuracy of this approach is still somewhat lower compared to measurements from metabolic labeled samples. The analysis is particularly challenging for PTMs. Post translational modified peptides are generally of low abundance and even small changes can have important effects on the cell.

Sometimes only a few modified peptides are of interest for the question under consideration. In these cases, proteomics can be targeted to sequencing to a subset of previously identified peptides (Schmidt et al., 2009). One method to achieve this, called **m**ultiple **r**eaction **m**onitoring (MRM), is performed on so called triple quadrupole mass analyzers. In the first quadrupole, peptides of interest are isolated by their mass. The second quadrupole is a collision cell where the peptides are fragmented. The last quadrupole is set to some specific fragments that are characteristic for the peptide. The advantage of MRMs over unbiased approaches is the high sensitivity and speed (Kitteringham et al., 2009; Malmstrom et al., 2009; Wolf-Yadlin et al., 2007). However, false positive rates in these experiments can be high due to limited resolution of the quadrupole instruments compared to orbitraps. In alternative approaches using high resolution orbitrap instruments, the specific m/z of peptides of interest are written in an "inclusion list" (Jaffe et al., 2008). Whenever a peptide of this m/z is found in the MS spectrum it is selected for fragmentation and MS/MS analysis. If higher sensitivity of the instrument is required, **s**elected **i**on **m**onitoring (SIM) scans can be used to survey one or several pre-defined ranges of the m/z spectrum rather than a full spectrum during the chromatography run (Michalski et al., 2011).

2.2 Posttranslational modifications

Quantitative proteomics can detect changes of the abundance of proteins in a whole proteome from cells in different conditions. In addition biological activity of proteins varies and is often regulated by PTMs. Therefore, it is important to measure changes of PTMs spatially and temporarily. MS is ideal to study PTMs because it can detect specific mass shifts due to the modification and assign its exact position in the amino acid sequence.

2.2.1 Phosphorylation

The most studied PTM is phosphorylation of the amino acids serine, threonine or tyrosine. Phosphorylation is important for many cellular processes. Protein phosphorylation conventionally is analyzed by ^{32}P labeling, band shifts on SDS-PAGE gels or the detection of phosphorylated residues by site-specific antibodies. While these techniques yielded great insights, they focus usually on just one or a few proteins at a time. To study the complexity of signaling networks, systematic methods to study phosphorylation of many proteins at the same time are required. MS-based methods analyzing phosphorylation of proteins by detecting the phosphorylated peptides resulting from their digestion require enrichment of phosphorylated peptides to overcome their low abundance in cells. Several different methods have been established to enrich phosphorylated peptides. Antibodies specific for a specific phosphorylated amino acid, e.g., phospho-tyrosine, are used. These enrichment methods are very useful to study a specific phosphorylation species. A different enrichment method is **i**mmobilized **m**etal (e.g., Fe^{3+}) **a**ffinity **c**hromatography (IMAC) (Corthals et al., 2005; Muszynska et al., 1992). With IMAC, all phosphopeptides are enriched due to the interaction between negatively charged phosphate groups and the immobilized positive metal ions. A similar technique uses TiO_2 to complex phosphorylated peptides on a resin by their charge (Pinkse et al.,

2004). In contrast to IMAC, phosphopeptide enrichment by TiO_2 requires a competitor for the binding sites, such as dihydrobenzoic acid (DHB) or lactic acid, to exclude unphosphorylated negatively charged peptides (Larsen et al., 2005). A drawback of these competitors is possible contamination of the MS instruments by the competitor. In organisms of relatively low proteome complexity, such as *Saccharomyces cerevisiae,* this setup was sufficient to identify 5534 phosphosites (Soufi et al., 2009). However, due to the much higher complexity of the mammalian phosphoproteome, some studies use a pre-fractionation step of peptides before phosphopeptides enrichment, e.g., by strong cation exchange chromatography (SCX) (Villen and Gygi, 2008).

After enrichment of phosphorylated peptides, samples are analyzed by LC-MS/MS. To identify phosphorylated peptides and assign the localization of the phosphorylation site with high confidence, distinct fragmentation methods have been used. Collision induced dissociation (CID) fragmentation often results in a neutral loss because the phosphoester bond is relatively fragile. The resulting lost ions of 98 or 80 Da were used to scan specifically for phosphorylated peptides. However, this phenomenon often dominates the MS/MS scans (Tholey et al., 1999) and leads to reduced backbone fragmentation. For efficient identification of phosphorylated peptides in ion traps, the neutral loss signal can be isolated after MS/MS and subjected to additional CID to yield a MS^3 spectrum (Jin et al., 2004). Multistage activation virtually combines MS^2 and MS^3 by parallel excitation and fragmentation (Schroeder et al., 2004). Even with multistage activation, fragmentation of phosphopeptides can be insufficient to identify the peptide sequence or to assign the phosphorylation site correctly with high confidence. Recent technical developments allow for different fragmentation techniques. Electron capture dissociation (ECD) or electron transfer dissociation (ETD) lead to sole backbone fragmentation between N and C bonds thereby generating c and z ions (Syka et al., 2004; Zubarev et al., 2000). PTMs unstable during CID fragmentation therefore stay intact with ETD fragmentation and make site specific assignment easier. Higher collision energy dissociation (HCD) uses the same principle of CID but higher collision energies, thus efficiently fragmenting the peptide backbone even in the presence of a low energy bond to a PTM. A recent study used a LTQ OrbitrapVelos to analyze both the precursor ion and its peptide fragments after HCD with high resolution in an orbitrap. This so called "high-high" technique yielded up to 16,000 identified phosphorylation sites with high confident assignments (Nagaraj et al., 2010).

Data quality is a particularly important issue for large scale PTM studies. For example, it is possible to identify a phosphorylated peptide with high confidence (>99%), but it is sometimes impossible to assign its site with high confidence between two adjacent serines. Therefore large scale datasets should always contain a peptide identification score and a PTM localization score (Beausoleil et al., 2006; Gnad et al., 2011; Olsen et al., 2006).

2.2.2 Glycosylation

Although phosphorylation is by far the most studied PTM, MS can also be used to study other PTMs. Another example for a prominent PTM is N-glycosylation of asparagine residues occurring in the endoplasmic reticulum. N-glycosylation plays an important role in the assembly of complex organelles and is involved in many cellular processes, such as apoptosis and the immune response (Varki, 2009). Due to the complexity of sugar moieties it is very challenging to analyze N-glycosylated proteins or peptides by MS approaches. Additionally the abundance of N-glycosylated proteins is usually very low in comparison to their unmodified counterparts. Thus, N-glycosylated proteins are enriched for analysis by affinity purification using lectins (Bunkenborg et al., 2004) or by chemical linkage of the sugar moiety to a solid phase (Zhang et al., 2003).

After enrichment, samples are treated with a global deglycosylating enzyme leading to the deamidation of the asparagine residue to aspartic acid. The resulting mass increase of 0.9848 Da can be detected in the precursor scan as well as in the peptide fragments (Kuster and Mann, 1999). Previously, N-glycosylated peptides were identified with low resolution of the peptide precursor mass. A recent study, using high resolution MS instead, mapped roughly 6,400 N-glycosylation sites in different murine cell lines quantitatively (Zielinska et al., 2010).

2.2.3 Acetylation and methylation

Other common PTMs are acetylation or methylation of lysines and arginines. These are reversible PTMs that change the charge of the amino acid thereby possibly regulating protein function. The most prominent example is histone acetylation or methylation, which regulates transcription. Acetylated or methylated peptides are relatively low abundant and specific enrichment is required, similar as in the case of phosphorylation analysis. Enrichment with antibodies which recognize the modified amino acid is generally performed prior to analysis by MS. A recent study identified an unexpected large number of acetylation sites. By using high resolution MS in combination with SILAC, 3600 acetylation sites were identified on 1750 proteins. Due to the low abundance of acetylated peptides, Choudhary et al used isoelectric focusing after enrichment of acetylated peptides to further reduce sample complexity (Choudhary et al., 2009). A previous study revealed an unexpected role of acetylation in mitochondrial function (Kim et al., 2006). A method to measure methylation quantitatively is heavy methyl- SILAC. In this approach, heavy methionine serves as the sole donor for the methyl group. The mass shift of the peptide containing the heavy versus light methyl groups is detected by high resolution mass spectrometry (Ong et al., 2004).

2.2.4 Ubiquitination

Ubiquitination of proteins is another PTM amenable to MS based proteomics. The protein ubiquitin is crosslinked to lysine residues on target proteins. Ubiquitination plays an important role in proteasomal degradation and endocytosis of plasma membrane proteins. Since ubiquitin is a protein, it can be tagged for subsequent affinity enrichment. HIS tagged versions of ubiquitin can be used to isolate ubiquitinated proteins by affinity purification, leading in one example to the identification of 110 ubiquitination sites on 72 proteins in *Saccharomyces cerevisiae* (Peng et al., 2003). Instead of isolating ubiquitinated proteins, a site specific antibody that detects the diGly motif of ubiquitinated peptides, yielded 374 diglycine modified lysines on 236 ubiquitinated proteins from HEK293 cells (Xu et al., 2010). One problem analyzing ubiquitinated proteins are their very complex fragmentation spectra. In addition it is difficult to distinguish by MS analysis modification by ubiquitin or by other ubiquitin-like molecules, such as interferon-induced 17kDA protein (ISG15) that leave the same diGly tag after digestion. Furthermore, it is not possible to distinguish if a protein is mono- or polyubiquitinated by LC MS/MS since digestion of the proteins with a protease is necessary and cleaves polyubiquitin chains. For a representative analysis of post translational modified proteins see Figure 1.

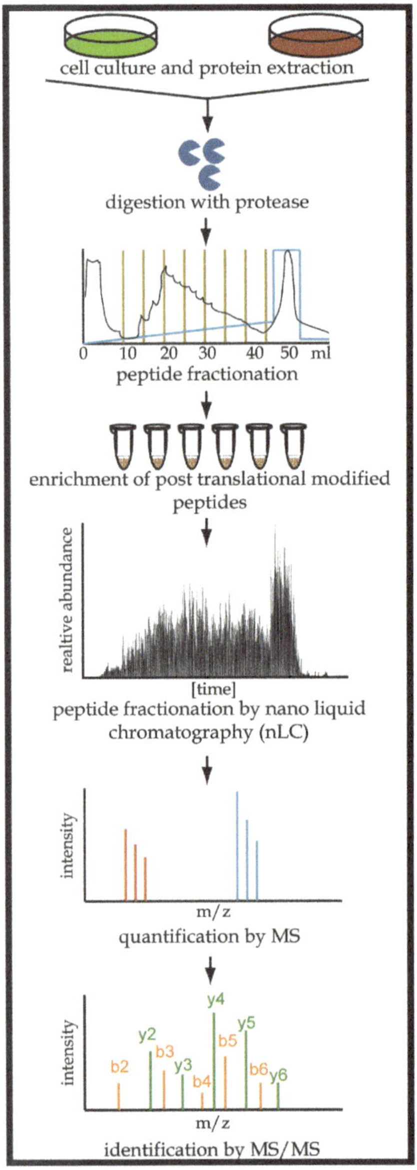

Cells are grown (label free or SILAC) and lysed for protein extraction. Extracted proteins are digested with an endoproteinase (Trypsin; LysC) and resulting peptides are fractionated (strong cation exachange (SCX) or strong anion exchange (SAX) chromatography). Peptides are enriched by their PTMs (specific antibodies, IMAC, TiO_2, lectin affinity). Enriched peptides are fractionated by nano-flow LC and directly injected by electrospray ionization into the MS. Relative abundances of peptides are quantified by the first, full-scan MS event (MS). Peptide identification and determination of the PTM is achieved by fragmentation (CID, HCD, ETD, ECD) in the second stage of MS (MS/MS).

Fig. 1. Workflow for quantitative proteomics of post translational modified proteins.

3. Spatial analysis of the cellular proteome

3.1 MS-based proteomics approaches to map protein composition of organelles

Each organelle is composed of a specific set of proteins that contribute to its function and that allow for communication with the rest of the cell. The content of organelles is highly dynamic and includes resident as well as transient proteins coming from and going to other compartments in the cell. Traditionally, to identify protein localization, cell biologists employ protein tagging by fluorescent labels or subcellular fractionation of cells in combination with detection of proteins by immunolabeling. These techniques have been successfully applied over many years and were adapted to high throughput studies, for example to tag nearly the complete proteome of budding (Huh et al., 2003) or of fission yeast (Matsuyama et al., 2006). However, technical limitations (e.g., absence of homologous recombination in many systems) and the enormous effort required for these approaches impede its application to more complex systems, such as mammalian cells. Therefore, organelle proteomics based on LS-MS was developed into a complementary approach that has made valuable contributions to the elucidation of organelles' inventory in many systems. In this approach, organelles or parts thereof, including protein complexes, are purified biochemically and analyzed by MS-based techniques.

3.1.1 MS based proteomics of purified organelle

For few compartments, such as nucleus or mitochondrion, that are rather easy to isolate with high purity, MS-based proteomics has yielded protein inventories (Andersen et al., 2002; Taylor et al., 2003). These and all other organellar proteomics experiments usually start with cell disruption under mild conditions designed to maintain organelle integrity. Organelles are then purified from crude cell extracts by differential centrifugations and are then processed for MS analysis. In this scheme, separation of organelles depends on their sedimentation velocity, a function of their size and density. Generally purification is improved by combining velocity sedimentation centrifugation with density gradient centrifugation (Michelsen and von Hagen, 2009; Wiederhold et al., 2010). Alternatively, higher purity is obtained by affinity purification using e.g., an antibody directed against a surface protein of the organelle, free flow electrophoresis (Islinger et al., 2010) or by modification of organelles density. An example for the latter is the report of phagosomes or endosomes inventories isolated after flotation gradient. In these cases, latex beads of different diameters can be internalized either by phagocytosis (Duclos and Desjardins, 2011; Jutras et al., 2008) or endocytosis (Duclos et al., 2011) and the resulting organelles are purified by a single step flotation gradient centrifugation before analysis by MS.

For some organelles, no efficient purification schemes exist based solemnly on differences of density or sedimentation. Therefore, in some instances, chemical modification is used to facilitate the purification. For example, cell surface modification by cell impermeable chemicals is commonly used to modify plasma membrane proteins from the extracellular environment. In such strategy, plasma membrane proteins are covalently linked to biotin, which in turn is used as an affinity tag for subsequent purification on a column carrying streptavidin. Cell surface modification relying on different chemical properties of proteins such as the reactivity of primary amines (N-termini of proteins and side chains of lysines, (Elia, 2008; Scheurer et al., 2005), thiols (Laragione et al., 2003) or of carbohydrates (Teckchandani et al., 2009) have been developed to analyze the proteome of plasma membranes in normal (Zhao et al., 2004) and in pathological conditions (Hubbard et al.,

2011; Yang et al., 2011) or to identify the dynamic proteome of the plasma membrane (Christiano et al., 2010).

3.1.2 Differential proteomics

Despite the remarkable success of these simple organelle proteomics approaches in some cases, formidable technical challenges to obtain pure organelles remain. Particularly in combination with highly sensitive mass spectrometers, simple purification schemes often result in the identification of large numbers of proteins. It is difficult to determine which ones among them are *bona fide* constituents of the target organelle and which ones are contaminants. One solution to overcome this limitation is the application of differential proteomics to subtract the proteins in the fraction in which the target organelle is found from a closely resembling fraction containing the most prominent contaminants. For this approach to work, the target organelle of interest should be enriched to the highest possible degree in one fraction, but be absent completely from the control fraction. This control sample could be as simple as a crude cell extract devoid of the target organelle, or better, reflect a similar purification in the absence of the organelle. After analysis of both samples, proteins that have been exclusively identified in the fraction enriched in the target organelle are considered as genuine proteins. In this approach, the accuracy of the obtained results strongly depends on the quality of two different MS analyses, as missing a protein in the control will lead its assignment to the target organelle. This point is critical considering the variability of analysis inherent to many MS approaches. For example, identification of a particular protein depends on different properties of the protein (such as abundance in the sample, ability of its peptide to be ionized in the mass spectrometer), as well as the MS methodology used. Failure to detect a protein does not necessarily mean it is absent from the sample. In differential proteomics approaches, this may lead to false negative or positive results, if a protein is randomly not detected in either the organelle enriched or the control fraction, respectively. Moreover, as sensitivity of MS analysis is improved and hence the number of identified proteins in each sample increases, the lists derived from each of the two fractions will more and more overlap, since proteins are likely to differ only in abundance and not strictly be absent from one sample. Thus, a large set of false negative proteins of the target organelle may be subtracted due to their identification in both samples.

3.1.3 Quantitative organellar MS-based proteomics

Quantitative proteomics is particularly useful in cases where sufficient enrichment for a specific organelle cannot be achieved. For example, organelles of the secretory pathway are similar to each other in their physical properties, with their content dynamically exchanging between them. Methods that only catalogue proteins in a sample cannot provide information on the dynamic behavior of proteins and are prone to detect contamination from co-purifying organelles. Intensive efforts have focused on sample preparation prior to MS. Successful strategies combine gradient profiling and quantitative MS-based proteomics. Such strategies rely on partial separation and distribution of subcellular compartments along density gradients. In **p**rotein **c**orrelation **p**rofiling (PCP) protein abundance profiles along the gradient are obtained by MS analysis and matched to profiles of known organelle markers. In this strategy, the accuracy of the quantification is a critical parameter to obtain reliable mapping of the organelle constituents. To date MS-based quantitative PCP analyses have been performed using label free (Andersen et al., 2003) and SILAC quantitation (Dengjel et al., 2010). SILAC-PCP allows determination of accurate profiles. In that case, two independent gradients are obtained from two differently labeled cells. A fraction enriched for the organelle of interest is isolated from a gradient and spiked into each fraction of the other gradient (with a ratio 1 to 1). Profiles based on SILAC ratios can be extracted from each fraction of the gradient. Genuine proteins from the organelle of interest will show the highest ratio (close to one) in the organelle fraction, but have lower fractions elsewhere in the profile. In contrast, contaminants have higher ratios in other fractions that represent the organelles that they mostly purify with (Figure 2). Such approaches rely on the reproducibility of the gradient separation. An alternate gradient-based approach, localization of proteins by isotope tagging (LOPIT) has been successfully applied to plant

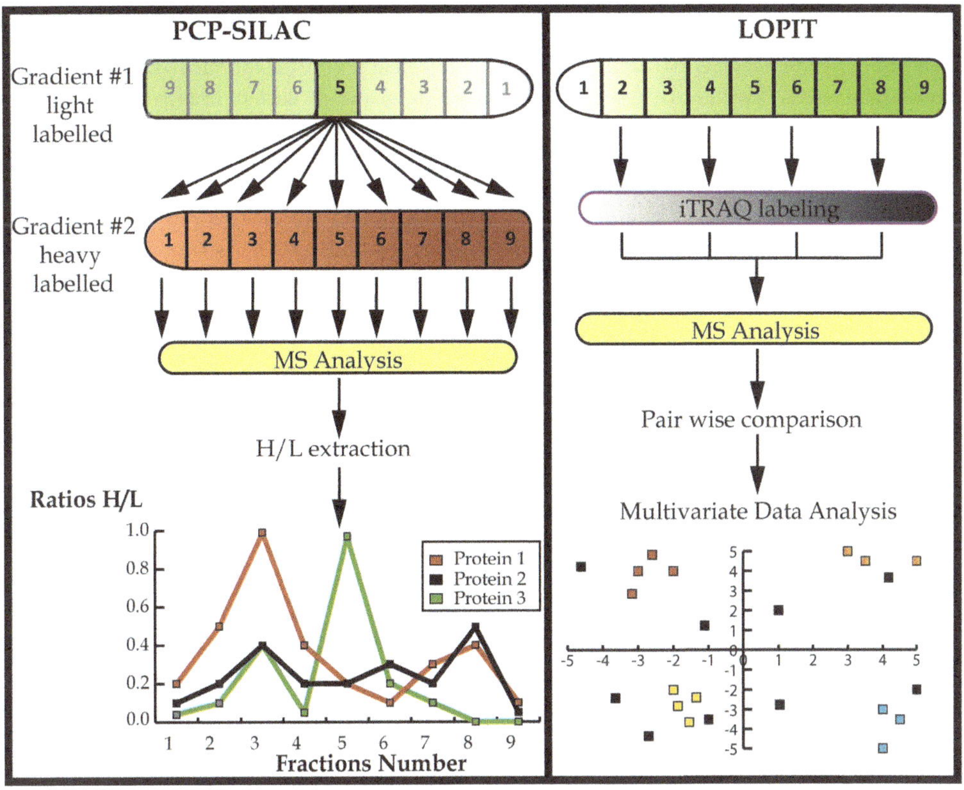

PCP-SILAC: A light labeled (L) fraction enriched in a target organelle by gradient centrifugation is spiked into each fraction of a gradient of heavy (H) labeled cells Then, each combined fraction is analyzed independently. H/L ratios are extracted for proteins in all fractions and then abundance profiles are estimated. LOPIT: Specific organelle enriched fractions from a gradient are separated and labeled separately with different iTRAQ reagents. Fractions are pooled and processed into peptides. Then, the fraction is analyzed in a single MS run. Ratios from pair wise analyses are extracted and submitted to multivariate data analyses to identify genuine proteins.

Fig. 2. Gradient Profiling based organelle proteomics.

organelles (Dunkley et al., 2004; Lilley and Dunkley, 2008). In that case, several organelle-enriched fractions from one gradient are separately labeled with different iTRAQ reagents and pooled. Ratios derived from pair-wise comparisons are analyzed by multivariate data analyses to assign organelle localization to the proteins identified. (Figure 2)

3.2 Protein complexes

Proteins interact with each other to form complexes that contribute to cellular functions. Therefore, identifying protein interactions is of critical importance to unravel mechanisms underlying cellular functions. To identify complexes, **a**ffinity **p**urification-based **MS** (AP-MS) is the method of choice: Prior to MS analysis, protein complexes are purified with affinity matrices that bind to one subunit of the complex. The confident identification of true binders to the bait protein relies on the comparison with a good control fraction of the affinity purification. The emergence of affinity tags and robust antibodies greatly contributed to the success of AP-MS.

The use of affinity tags is particularly attractive because it allows standardizing procedures that can be applicable to any system or protein. To date, a wide variety of tags has been used in AP-MS ranging from small peptides to proteins of several kDa. Fluorescent tags, such as **g**reen **f**luorescent **p**rotein (GFP), are common because they can also be used for live cell imaging. Furthermore, GFP purification allows recovery of most of the GFP-fused protein from a complex mixture in a single step. In this approach, proteins co-purifying with the bait are compared to a control condition where only the GFP protein is expressed (Figure 3 B). Nevertheless, tag insertion might affect protein functions or prevent/trigger interactions with other proteins. Moreover, expression levels of fusion protein can be significantly different compared to their native counterparts and can affect binding capacities. Therefore, when efficient and specific antibodies are available, it is preferable to rely on purification of the native protein subunits to purify complexes. In that case, the control fraction can be obtained by incubating lysates with the beads alone (Trinkle-Mulcahy et al., 2008) or by depleting the protein of interest by RNA interference (**qu**antitative **i**mmunoprecipitation **c**ombined with **k**nockdown, QUICK) (Selbach and Mann, 2006) (Figure 3 A). Recently, Hubner et al. (Hubner et al., 2010) described **qu**antitative **b**acterial artificial chromosome **i**nteractomics (QUBIC), using tagged proteins expressed under endogenous control in mammalian cells. Identification of interacting partners is achieved by robust and efficient affinity purification based on the GFP tag (Hubner and Mann, 2011; Vermeulen et al., 2010). However, most protein-protein interactions are dynamic and are hardly assessed by single AP-MS experiments. Depending on internal or external cues protein binding specificities can be modulated, e.g., by post-translational modification. This can result in their release from or recruitment to specific protein complexes thus potentially affecting their function(s) or their localization.

At steady state, different forms of a protein are present in the cell which can hinder the discrimination among its interactors. A solution to this problem can be to use exogenous baits corresponding to a specific state of the protein of interest or of a peptide to identify interactions specific to a particular state. Different strategies have been developed for the identification of genuine interactors with high confidence. Generally, single step purifications are associated with a large number of contaminants. Lower background signal is achieved using more stringent purification, for instance by sequential purification using two affinity tags (**t**andem **a**ffinity **p**urification; TAP). In TAP, two tags separated by a

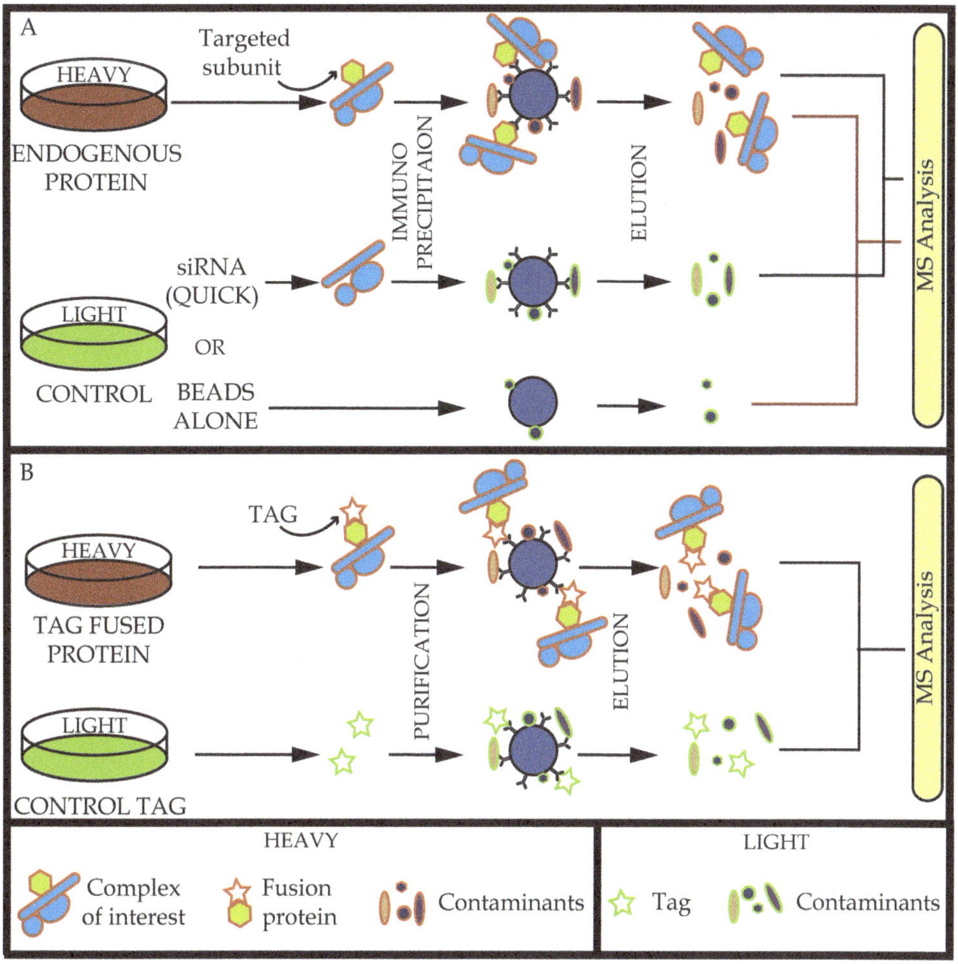

A) Immunoprecipitation of endogenous proteins. Complexes from heavy (red) and light (green, control) labeled cells are purified using antibody-conjugated beads that target a specific subunit. Then the fractions are pooled before sample preparation and subsequent MS analysis. Control fraction can be obtained by using a cell lysate devoid of the target subunit by siRNA (QUICK) or by incubating a total lysate with the beads alone. B) One step purification of tagged proteins. A tagged subunit is expressed in heavy labeled cells (red). Using affinity columns, protein complexes are affinity purified using the tag and then eluted before being pooled with the control light fraction (green). After sample preparation the combined fraction is analyzed by MS. The control light fraction is obtained by expressing the tag alone in the cells.

Fig. 3. Affinity purification based MS (AP-MS).

cleavage site are fused to the protein of interest. In a first step the complex is purified with the fusion protein using the first tag, then the protein of interest (along with its interactors) is released from the affinity matrix by specific cleavage of the tag before performing a second round of purification with the remainder of the tag. Different combinations of tags have been combined and TAP strategies have been extensively used for AP-MS purification in many model systems (Gavin et al., 2006; Krogan et al., 2006). However, one drawback is the loss of weak interactors during stringent purification. A compromise is achieved by inserting a cleavage site between a tag and the protein of interest thus reducing the number of treatments and decreasing significantly the number of non-specific binders (Aguilar et al., 2010). In case of weak interactions, complexes can be fixed by treating with cross-linking chemicals either in live cells (Stingl et al., 2008; Yong et al., 2010) or cell lysates (Sinz, 2010).

In general, quantitation greatly helps to discriminate false positive from true interactors. SILAC quantitation is more accurate and has advantages for protein complexes that are difficult to purify and where enrichment over background is smaller. As in all SILAC experiments, two differently labeled samples, here a control and a sample enriched in the target complex, are mixed and relative abundances of protein ratios are extracted from the MS spectra. In case of AP-MS, background proteins have a ratio of one as they bind as efficiently in both conditions. In contrast, true interactors have a high ratio as they are preferable purified from the labeled sample enriched in the complex of interest. Samples can be mixed either before (**p**urification **a**fter **m**ixing, PAM, (Wang and Huang, 2008)) or after purification (**m**ixed **a**fter **p**urification, MAP). The main drawback of PAM strategies is that dynamic interactions result in equilibrium between the light and heavy form during the purification, thus decreasing the observed ratio even for true interactors.

4. Temporal analysis of proteomes

4.1 Quantification of protein turnover by pulsed SILAC

Protein turnover and protein degradation are critical for numerous biological processes, including the cell cycle, signal transduction and apoptosis. Organelle proteomes change over time and can be quickly adapted to respond to changing conditions. Therefore, unraveling mechanisms that determine protein abundances is important for understanding organelle dynamics and regulation.

In general, quantitative approaches described before can be employed to gather snapshots of protein repertoires over time or in different conditions. However, such approaches quantify abundance changes of a given protein but fail to address what are the mechanisms underlying protein dynamics (decrease/increase turnover). Pulse-chase isotope tracer-based methods have been the method of choice to study protein degradation for decades. In such approaches, cells or animals are first metabolically pulse-labeled with radioisotope tracers (most commonly ^{3}H, ^{15}N, ^{35}S are used). After a chase period concomitant with the beginning of the experiment, loss of the radiolabel from the protein of interest is followed by scintillation or autoradiography as a readout of protein degradation. Such classical pulse chase experiments have been successfully translated to protein turnover analyses by MS. In MS-based turnover analyses, cells are only pulsed. For cells in culture, the most common approach is a modification of SILAC. Instead of combining two differently labeled cell populations, cells are pulsed with stable isotope containing amino acids (pSILAC). The replacement of amino-acids in proteins is followed by MS analysis over time to extract turnover rates. Similarly to results from a standard SILAC experiment, pSILAC yields two forms of the same peptide. At the time point corresponding to the half-life ($t_{1/2}$) of a specific protein, the intensities of the light and heavy peaks for a peptide pair derived from this protein are equal (Figure 4).

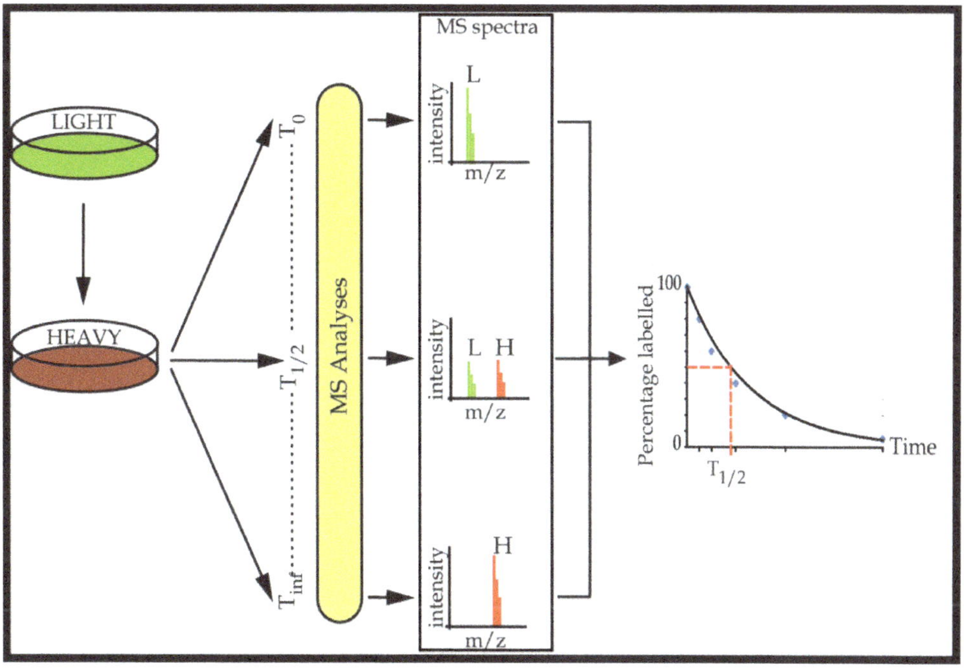

Light labeled cells (green) are pulsed with heavy amino acid containing medium (red). Cells are harvested at different time points, lysed, processed into peptides and analyzed independently. Ratios H/L are derived from intensities of heavy (H, red) and light (L, green) peptide peaks in the MS spectra. Note, at protein half life ($T_{1/2}$) intensity of light and heavy peptides are equal in the mass spectra. Then loss of light label can be calculated over time and turnover rates are extracted from non-linear curve fitting.

Fig. 4. pSILAC to analyze protein turnover.

To date, pSILAC has been mostly applied to cells in culture: *Saccharomyces cerevisiae* (Pratt et al., 2002), *Streptomyces coelicolor* (Jayapal et al., 2010) and human cells (Doherty et al., 2009; Schwanhäusser et al., 2011; Zee et al., 2010). Schwanhäusser et al. measured protein abundances and turnover of more than 5,000 proteins in HeLa cells. Combination of pSILAC with metabolic pulse labeling of mRNA in the same cells enabled comparison of proteins and mRNAs turnover at an unprecedented depth.

At steady state, protein levels are constant. Therefore synthesis and degradation rates are equal. This feature is critical when comparing proteome turnover, but this assumption may not always be fulfilled when comparing different conditions. An alternative approach overcoming this limitation is to follow synthesis and degradation independently from each other. To follow regulation of protein synthesis during changes of cellular iron, Schwannäusser et al. combined control (non-treated) and iron-treated HeLa cells that have been differently SILAC pulsed (Schwanhäusser et al., 2009). At the beginning of the experiment, cells in both conditions were identically light labeled (L). Concomitantly with iron treatment, cells were differently pulsed with medium (M) or heavy (H) amino-acids. Then cell lysates were combined and analyzed by MS. The relative abundance of newly synthesized proteins in both conditions was then extracted from intensities of the M and H peaks in the MS spectrum. As expected, most of the 1311 proteins identified in this study do not present specific synthesis regulation upon iron treatment (ratio M/H of 1). However proteins such as ferritins show up to 13 fold synthesis upregulation compared to normal conditions.

4.2 Analysis of cell signaling as an example of dynamic PTM analysis

Unbiased, quantitative proteomics enables studying signaling networks in a time resolved manner. Protein abundance is often the output of complete signaling cascades. MS can detect PTM changes as an early response to system perturbations, as well as the changed protein abundance as the output of a signaling cascade.

Combination of phosphoproteomics with quantitative approaches such as SILAC enables the temporal analysis of signaling networks. In these experiments, cells are labeled in different SILAC states and stimulated for different periods of time. Applying this methodology, Olsen et al. quantified 6,600 phosphorylation sites in HeLa cells at 5 different time points after stimulation with **e**pidermal **g**rowth **f**actor (EGF) (Olsen et al., 2006). These experiments revealed insights into the early response of cells to EGF stimulation. Interestingly, this study showed that different phosphorylation sites on the same protein can react with completely different timing to a stimulus. Such results are easiest obtained by MS because it allows for detection of phosphorylation changes at particular amino acids of the protein sequence. Effects at different sites can otherwise easily be missed with classical methods that detect total phosphorylation of a protein. Other studies used a combination of SILAC labeling and different drug treatments to analyze the proteome and phosphoproteome of HeLa cells over the complete cell cycle (Olsen et al., 2010). A similar study in *Saccharomyces cerevisiae* used a mutant of the cell cycle kinase Cdk1 that allows inhibition of the kinase with an ATP analogue (Holt et al., 2009). Another recent phosphoproteome revealed great insights into the early differentiation of embryonic stem cells after stimulation with a diacylglycerol analogue. This study yielded roughly 20,000 phosphosites with almost 50% of them responding to the stimulus (Rigbolt et al., 2011). These experiments help to dissect complex signaling networks since proteins are clustered into certain groups according to their response. In addition, the high resolution datasets serve as a great resource for the scientific community and provide data for further analyses to generate models for signaling networks.

5. Conclusion

Quantitative mass spectrometry based proteomics emerged over the last few years as a crucial technique for cell biology and biochemistry research. The exciting developments in this field discussed in this chapter have provided unexpected aspects of organelle dynamics, protein turnover and PTMs. Future developments in methodology, computation and technical developments will make these technologies accessible for a larger group of scientists. This should help to generate more high quality datasets which will serve as a reference for the larger scientific community. In addition, integration of proteomics data with data from other system-wide approaches, such as genetic screens or transcriptome analysis, will help to understand complex biological processes.

6. Acknowledgement

We thank current and former members of the Walther laboratory for discussions of this book chapter. We apologize to colleagues whose contributions have not been cited due to space limitation. Research in the Walther laboratory is supported by the German Academic Research Council (DFG).

7. References

Aebersold, R., and M. Mann. 2003. Mass spectrometry-based proteomics. *Nature*. 422:198-207.

Aguilar, P.S., F. Fröhlich, M. Rehman, M. Shales, I. Ulitsky, A. Olivera-Couto, H. Braberg, R. Shamir, P. Walter, M. Mann, C.S. Ejsing, N.J. Krogan, and T.C. Walther. 2010. A plasma-membrane E-MAP reveals links of the eisosome with sphingolipid metabolism and endosomal trafficking. *Nature structural & molecular biology*. 17:901-8.

Andersen, J.S., C.E. Lyon, A.H. Fox, A.K.L. Leung, Y.W. Lam, H. Steen, M. Mann, and A.I. Lamond. 2002. Directed proteomic analysis of the human nucleolus. *Current biology: CB*. 12:1-11.

Andersen, J.S., C.J. Wilkinson, and T. Mayor. 2003. Proteomic characterization of the human centrosome by protein correlation profiling. *Nature*. 426.

Beausoleil, S.A., J. Villen, S.A. Gerber, J. Rush, and S.P. Gygi. 2006. A probability-based approach for high-throughput protein phosphorylation analysis and site localization. *Nat Biotechnol*. 24:1285-92.

Bunkenborg, J., B.J. Pilch, A.V. Podtelejnikov, and J.R. Wisniewski. 2004. Screening for N-glycosylated proteins by liquid chromatography mass spectrometry. *Proteomics*. 4:454-65.

Choudhary, C., C. Kumar, F. Gnad, M.L. Nielsen, M. Rehman, T.C. Walther, J.V. Olsen, and M. Mann. 2009. Lysine acetylation targets protein complexes and co-regulates major cellular functions. *Science*. 325:834-40.

Choudhary, C., and M. Mann. 2010. Decoding signalling networks by mass spectrometry-based proteomics. *Nat Rev Mol Cell Biol*. 11:427-39.

Christiano, R., M. Amessou, G. Shi, M. Azoulay, A. Blanpain, H. Drobecq, O. Melnyk, J.-C. Florent, and L. Johannes. 2010. Chemistry-based protein modification strategy for endocytic pathway analysis. *Biology of the cell* 102:351-9.

Corthals, G.L., R. Aebersold, and D.R. Goodlett. 2005. Identification of phosphorylation sites using microimmobilized metal affinity chromatography. *Methods Enzymol*. 405:66-81.

de Godoy, L.M., J.V. Olsen, J. Cox, M.L. Nielsen, N.C. Hubner, F. Frohlich, T.C. Walther, and M. Mann. 2008. Comprehensive mass-spectrometry-based proteome quantification of haploid versus diploid yeast. *Nature*. 455:1251-4.

Dengjel, J., L. Jakobsen, and J.S. Andersen. 2010. Organelle proteomics by label-free and SILAC-labeled protein correlation profiling. *Methods in Molecular Biology*. 658:255-265.

Doherty, M.K., D.E. Hammond, M.J. Clague, S.J. Gaskell, and R.J. Beynon. 2009. Turnover of the human proteome: determination of protein intracellular stability by dynamic SILAC. *Journal of proteome research*. 8:104-12.

Duclos, S., G. Clavarino, G. Rousserie, G. Goyette, J. Boulais, V. Camossetto, E. Gatti, S. LaBoissière, P. Pierre, and M. Desjardins. 2011. The endosomal proteome of macrophage and dendritic cells. *Proteomics*. 11:854-64.

Duclos, S., and M. Desjardins. 2011. Gel-Free Proteomics. *Methods in Molecular Biology*. 753:117-128.

Dunkley, T.P.J., R. Watson, J.L. Griffin, P. Dupree, and K.S. Lilley. 2004. Localization of organelle proteins by isotope tagging (LOPIT). *Molecular & cellular proteomics : MCP*. 3:1128-34.

Elia, G. 2008. Biotinylation reagents for the study of cell surface proteins. *Proteomics*. 8:4012-24.

Gavin, A.-C., P. Aloy, P. Grandi, R. Krause, M. Boesche, M. Marzioch, C. Rau, L.J. Jensen, S. Bastuck, B. Dümpelfeld, A. Edelmann, M.-A. Heurtier, V. Hoffman, C. Hoefert, K. Klein, M. Hudak, A.-M. Michon, M. Schelder, M. Schirle, M. Remor, T. Rudi, S. Hooper, A. Bauer, T. Bouwmeester, G. Casari, G. Drewes, G. Neubauer, J.M. Rick, B. Kuster, P. Bork, R.B. Russell, and G. Superti-Furga. 2006. Proteome survey reveals modularity of the yeast cell machinery. *Nature*. 440:631-6.

Geiger, T., J. Cox, P. Ostasiewicz, J.R. Wisniewski, and M. Mann. 2010. Super-SILAC mix for quantitative proteomics of human tumor tissue. *Nat Methods*. 7:383-5.

Gnad, F., J. Gunawardena, and M. Mann. 2011. PHOSIDA 2011: the posttranslational modification database. *Nucleic Acids Res*. 39:D253-60.

Holt, L.J., B.B. Tuch, J. Villen, A.D. Johnson, S.P. Gygi, and D.O. Morgan. 2009. Global analysis of Cdk1 substrate phosphorylation sites provides insights into evolution. *Science*. 325:1682-6.

Hubbard, S.C., M. Boyce, C.T. McVaugh, D.M. Peehl, and C.R. Bertozzi. 2011. Cell surface glycoproteomic analysis of prostate cancer-derived PC-3 cells. *Bioorganic & medicinal chemistry letters*. 21:4945-4950.

Hubner, N.C., A.W. Bird, J. Cox, B. Splettstoesser, P. Bandilla, I. Poser, A. Hyman, and M. Mann. 2010. Quantitative proteomics combined with BAC TransgeneOmics reveals in vivo protein interactions. *The Journal of cell biology*. 189:739-54.

Hubner, N.C., and M. Mann. 2011. Extracting gene function from protein-protein interactions using Quantitative BAC InteraCtomics (QUBIC). *Methods (San Diego, Calif.)*. 53:453-9.

Huh, W.-K., J.V. Falvo, L.C. Gerke, A.S. Carroll, R.W. Howson, J.S. Weissman, and E.K. O'Shea. 2003. Global analysis of protein localization in budding yeast. *Nature*. 425:686-91.

Islinger, M., K.W. Li, M. Loos, S. Liebler, S. Angermu, C. Eckerskorn, G. Weber, A. Abdolzade, and A. Vo. 2010. Peroxisomes from the Heavy Mitochondrial Fraction : Isolation by Zonal Free Flow Electrophoresis and Quantitative Mass Spectrometrical Characterization research articles. *Journal of Proteome Research*: 113-124.

Jaffe, J.D., H. Keshishian, B. Chang, T.A. Addona, M.A. Gillette, and S.A. Carr. 2008. Accurate inclusion mass screening: a bridge from unbiased discovery to targeted assay development for biomarker verification. *Mol Cell Proteomics*. 7:1952-62.

Jayapal, K.P., S. Sui, R.J. Philp, Y.-J. Kok, M.G.S. Yap, T.J. Griffin, and W.-S. Hu. 2010. Multitagging proteomic strategy to estimate protein turnover rates in dynamic systems. *Journal of proteome research*. 9:2087-97.

Jin, W.H., J. Dai, H. Zhou, Q.C. Xia, H.F. Zou, and R. Zeng. 2004. Phosphoproteome analysis of mouse liver using immobilized metal affinity purification and linear ion trap mass spectrometry. *Rapid Commun Mass Spectrom*. 18:2169-76.

Jutras, I., M. Houde, N. Currier, J. Boulais, S. Duclos, S. LaBoissière, E. Bonneil, P. Kearney, P. Thibault, E. Paramithiotis, P. Hugo, and M. Desjardins. 2008. Modulation of the phagosome proteome by interferon-gamma. *Molecular & cellular proteomics : MCP*. 7:697-715.

Kim, S.C., R. Sprung, Y. Chen, Y. Xu, H. Ball, J. Pei, T. Cheng, Y. Kho, H. Xiao, L. Xiao, N.V. Grishin, M. White, X.J. Yang, and Y. Zhao. 2006. Substrate and functional diversity of lysine acetylation revealed by a proteomics survey. *Mol Cell*. 23:607-18.

Kitteringham, N.R., R.E. Jenkins, C.S. Lane, V.L. Elliott, and B.K. Park. 2009. Multiple reaction monitoring for quantitative biomarker analysis in proteomics and metabolomics. *J Chromatogr B Analyt Technol Biomed Life Sci*. 877:1229-39.

Krogan, N.J., G. Cagney, H. Yu, G. Zhong, X. Guo, A. Ignatchenko, J. Li, S. Pu, N. Datta, A.P. Tikuisis, T. Punna, J.M. Peregrín-Alvarez, M. Shales, X. Zhang, M. Davey, M.D. Robinson, A. Paccanaro, J.E. Bray, A. Sheung, B. Beattie, D.P. Richards, V. Canadien, A. Lalev, F. Mena, P. Wong, A. Starostine, M.M. Canete, J. Vlasblom, S. Wu, C. Orsi, S.R. Collins, S. Chandran, R. Haw, J.J. Rilstone, K. Gandi, N.J. Thompson, G. Musso, P. St Onge, S. Ghanny, M.H.Y. Lam, G. Butland, A.M. Altaf-Ul, S. Kanaya, A. Shilatifard, E. O'Shea, J.S. Weissman, C.J. Ingles, T.R. Hughes, J. Parkinson, M. Gerstein, S.J. Wodak, A. Emili, and J.F. Greenblatt. 2006. Global landscape of protein complexes in the yeast Saccharomyces cerevisiae. *Nature*. 440:637-43.

Kruger, M., M. Moser, S. Ussar, I. Thievessen, C.A. Luber, F. Forner, S. Schmidt, S. Zanivan, R. Fassler, and M. Mann. 2008. SILAC mouse for quantitative proteomics uncovers kindlin-3 as an essential factor for red blood cell function. *Cell*. 134:353-64.

Kuster, B., and M. Mann. 1999. 18O-labeling of N-glycosylation sites to improve the identification of gel-separated glycoproteins using peptide mass mapping and database searching. *Anal Chem*. 71:1431-40.

Laragione, T., V. Bonetto, F. Casoni, T. Massignan, G. Bianchi, E. Gianazza, and P. Ghezzi. 2003. Redox regulation of surface protein thiols: identification of integrin alpha-4 as a molecular target by using redox proteomics. *Proceedings of the National Academy of Sciences of the United States of America*. 100:14737-41.

Larsen, M.R., T.E. Thingholm, O.N. Jensen, P. Roepstorff, and T.J. Jorgensen. 2005. Highly selective enrichment of phosphorylated peptides from peptide mixtures using titanium dioxide microcolumns. *Mol Cell Proteomics*. 4:873-86.

Lilley, K.S., and T.P.J. Dunkley. 2008. Determination of genuine residents of plant endomembrane organelles using isotope tagging and multivariate statistics. *Methods in molecular biology (Clifton, N.J.)*. 432:373-87.

Malmstrom, J., M. Beck, A. Schmidt, V. Lange, E.W. Deutsch, and R. Aebersold. 2009. Proteome-wide cellular protein concentrations of the human pathogen Leptospira interrogans. *Nature*. 460:762-5.

Matsuyama, A., R. Arai, Y. Yashiroda, A. Shirai, A. Kamata, S. Sekido, Y. Kobayashi, A. Hashimoto, M. Hamamoto, Y. Hiraoka, S. Horinouchi, and M. Yoshida. 2006. ORFeome cloning and global analysis of protein localization in the fission yeast Schizosaccharomyces pombe. *Nature biotechnology*. 24:841-7.

Michalski, A., E. Damoc, J.P. Hauschild, O. Lange, A. Wieghaus, A. Makarov, N. Nagaraj, J. Cox, M. Mann, and S. Horning. 2011. Mass Spectrometry-based Proteomics Using Q Exactive, a High-performance Benchtop Quadrupole Orbitrap Mass Spectrometer. *Mol Cell Proteomics*. 10:M111 011015.

Michelsen, U., and J. von Hagen. 2009. Isolation of subcellular organelles and structures. *Methods in enzymology*. 463:305-28.

Monetti, M., N. Nagaraj, K. Sharma, and M. Mann. 2011. Large-scale phosphosite quantification in tissues by a spike-in SILAC method. *Nat Methods*. 8:655-8.

Mueller, L.N., M.Y. Brusniak, D.R. Mani, and R. Aebersold. 2008. An assessment of software solutions for the analysis of mass spectrometry based quantitative proteomics data. *J Proteome Res*. 7:51-61.

Muszynska, G., G. Dobrowolska, A. Medin, P. Ekman, and J.O. Porath. 1992. Model studies on iron(III) ion affinity chromatography. II. Interaction of immobilized iron(III) ions with phosphorylated amino acids, peptides and proteins. *J Chromatogr*. 604:19-28.

Nagaraj, N., R.C. D'Souza, J. Cox, J.V. Olsen, and M. Mann. 2010. Feasibility of large-scale phosphoproteomics with higher energy collisional dissociation fragmentation. *J Proteome Res*. 9:6786-94.

Nielsen, M.L., M. Vermeulen, T. Bonaldi, J. Cox, L. Moroder, and M. Mann. 2008. Iodoacetamide-induced artifact mimics ubiquitination in mass spectrometry. *Nat Methods*. 5:459-60.

Olsen, J.V., B. Blagoev, F. Gnad, B. Macek, C. Kumar, P. Mortensen, and M. Mann. 2006. Global, in vivo, and site-specific phosphorylation dynamics in signaling networks. *Cell*. 127:635-48.

Olsen, J.V., M. Vermeulen, A. Santamaria, C. Kumar, M.L. Miller, L.J. Jensen, F. Gnad, J. Cox, T.S. Jensen, E.A. Nigg, S. Brunak, and M. Mann. 2010. Quantitative phosphoproteomics reveals widespread full phosphorylation site occupancy during mitosis. *Sci Signal*. 3:ra3.

Ong, S.E., B. Blagoev, I. Kratchmarova, D.B. Kristensen, H. Steen, A. Pandey, and M. Mann. 2002. Stable isotope labeling by amino acids in cell culture, SILAC, as a simple and accurate approach to expression proteomics. *Mol Cell Proteomics*. 1:376-86.

Ong, S.E., G. Mittler, and M. Mann. 2004. Identifying and quantifying in vivo methylation sites by heavy methyl SILAC. *Nat Methods*. 1:119-26.

Ow, S.Y., M. Salim, J. Noirel, C. Evans, I. Rehman, and P.C. Wright. 2009. iTRAQ underestimation in simple and complex mixtures: "the good, the bad and the ugly". *J Proteome Res*. 8:5347-55.

Peng, J., D. Schwartz, J.E. Elias, C.C. Thoreen, D. Cheng, G. Marsischky, J. Roelofs, D. Finley, and S.P. Gygi. 2003. A proteomics approach to understanding protein ubiquitination. *Nat Biotechnol*. 21:921-6.

Pinkse, M.W.H., P.M. Uitto, M.J. Hilhorst, B. Ooms, and A.J.R. Heck. 2004. Selective Isolation at the Femtomole Level of Phosphopeptides from Proteolytic Digests Using 2D-NanoLC-ESI-MS/MS and Titanium Oxide Precolumns. *Analytical Chemistry*. 76:3935-3943.

Pratt, J.M., J. Petty, I. Riba-garcia, D.H.L. Robertson, S.J. Gaskell, S.G. Oliver, and R.J. Beynon. 2002. Dynamics of Protein Turnover , a Missing Dimension in Proteomics *. *Molecular & Cellular Proteomics*:579-591.

Rigbolt, K.T., T.A. Prokhorova, V. Akimov, J. Henningsen, P.T. Johansen, I. Kratchmarova, M. Kassem, M. Mann, J.V. Olsen, and B. Blagoev. 2011. System-wide temporal characterization of the proteome and phosphoproteome of human embryonic stem cell differentiation. *Sci Signal*. 4:rs3.

Ross, P.L., Y.N. Huang, J.N. Marchese, B. Williamson, K. Parker, S. Hattan, N. Khainovski, S. Pillai, S. Dey, S. Daniels, S. Purkayastha, P. Juhasz, S. Martin, M. Bartlet-Jones, F. He, A. Jacobson, and D.J. Pappin. 2004. Multiplexed protein quantitation in

Saccharomyces cerevisiae using amine-reactive isobaric tagging reagents. *Mol Cell Proteomics*. 3:1154-69.

Scheurer, S.B., C. Roesli, D. Neri, and G. Elia. 2005. A comparison of different biotinylation reagents, tryptic digestion procedures, and mass spectrometric techniques for 2-D peptide mapping of membrane proteins. *Proteomics*. 5:3035-9.

Schmidt, A., M. Claassen, and R. Aebersold. 2009. Directed mass spectrometry: towards hypothesis-driven proteomics. *Curr Opin Chem Biol*. 13:510-7.

Schroeder, M.J., J. Shabanowitz, J.C. Schwartz, D.F. Hunt, and J.J. Coon. 2004. A neutral loss activation method for improved phosphopeptide sequence analysis by quadrupole ion trap mass spectrometry. *Anal Chem*. 76:3590-8.

Schwanhäusser, B., D. Busse, N. Li, G. Dittmar, J. Schuchhardt, J. Wolf, W. Chen, and M. Selbach. 2011. Global quantification of mammalian gene expression control. *Nature*. 473:337-42.

Schwanhäusser, B., M. Gossen, G. Dittmar, and M. Selbach. 2009. Global analysis of cellular protein translation by pulsed SILAC. *Proteomics*. 9:205-9.

Selbach, M., and M. Mann. 2006. Protein interaction screening by quantitative immunoprecipitation combined with. *Nature Methods*. 3:981-983.

Sinz, A. 2010. Investigation of protein-protein interactions in living cells by chemical crosslinking and mass spectrometry. *Analytical and bioanalytical chemistry*. 397:3433-40.

Soufi, B., C.D. Kelstrup, G. Stoehr, F. Frohlich, T.C. Walther, and J.V. Olsen. 2009. Global analysis of the yeast osmotic stress response by quantitative proteomics. *Mol Biosyst*. 5:1337-46.

Stingl, K., K. Schauer, C. Ecobichon, A. Labigne, P. Lenormand, J.-C. Rousselle, A. Namane, and H. de Reuse. 2008. In vivo interactome of Helicobacter pylori urease revealed by tandem affinity purification. *Molecular & cellular proteomics : MCP*. 7:2429-41.

Syka, J.E., J.J. Coon, M.J. Schroeder, J. Shabanowitz, and D.F. Hunt. 2004. Peptide and protein sequence analysis by electron transfer dissociation mass spectrometry. *Proc Natl Acad Sci U S A*. 101:9528-33.

Taylor, S.W., E. Fahy, B. Zhang, G.M. Glenn, D.E. Warnock, S. Wiley, A.N. Murphy, S.P. Gaucher, R.a. Capaldi, B.W. Gibson, and S.S. Ghosh. 2003. Characterization of the human heart mitochondrial proteome. *Nature biotechnology*. 21:281-6.

Teckchandani, A., N. Toida, J. Goodchild, C. Henderson, J. Watts, B. Wollscheid, and J.a. Cooper. 2009. Quantitative proteomics identifies a Dab2/integrin module regulating cell migration. *The Journal of cell biology*. 186:99-111.

Tholey, A., J. Reed, and W.D. Lehmann. 1999. Electrospray tandem mass spectrometric studies of phosphopeptides and phosphopeptide analogues. *J Mass Spectrom*. 34:117-23.

Trinkle-Mulcahy, L., S. Boulon, Y.W. Lam, R. Urcia, F.-M. Boisvert, F. Vandermoere, N.a. Morrice, S. Swift, U. Rothbauer, H. Leonhardt, and A. Lamond. 2008. Identifying specific protein interaction partners using quantitative mass spectrometry and bead proteomes. *The Journal of cell biology*. 183:223-39.

Varki, A. 2009. Essentials of glycobiology. Cold Spring Harbor Laboratory Press, Cold Spring Harbor, N.Y. xxix, 784 p. pp.

Vermeulen, M., H.C. Eberl, F. Matarese, H. Marks, S. Denissov, F. Butter, K.K. Lee, J.V. Olsen, A.A. Hyman, H.G. Stunnenberg, and M. Mann. 2010. Quantitative interaction proteomics and genome-wide profiling of epigenetic histone marks and their readers. *Cell*. 142:967-80.

Villen, J., and S.P. Gygi. 2008. The SCX/IMAC enrichment approach for global phosphorylation analysis by mass spectrometry. *Nat Protoc*. 3:1630-8.

Walther, T.C., and M. Mann. 2010. Mass spectrometry–based proteomics in cell biology. *Cell*.

Wang, X., and L. Huang. 2008. Identifying dynamic interactors of protein complexes by quantitative mass spectrometry. *Molecular & cellular proteomics : MCP*. 7:46-57.

Wiederhold, E., L.M. Veenhoff, B. Poolman, and D.J. Slotboom. 2010. Proteomics of Saccharomyces cerevisiae Organelles. *Molecular & cellular proteomics : MCP*. 9:431-45.

Wolf-Yadlin, A., S. Hautaniemi, D.A. Lauffenburger, and F.M. White. 2007. Multiple reaction monitoring for robust quantitative proteomic analysis of cellular signaling networks. *Proc Natl Acad Sci U S A*. 104:5860-5.

Wong, J.W., and G. Cagney. 2010. An overview of label-free quantitation methods in proteomics by mass spectrometry. *Methods Mol Biol*. 604:273-83.

Xu, G., J.S. Paige, and S.R. Jaffrey. 2010. Global analysis of lysine ubiquitination by ubiquitin remnant immunoaffinity profiling. *Nature biotechnology*. 28:868-73.

Yang, L., J.O. Nyalwidhe, S. Guo, R.R. Drake, and O.J. Semmes. 2011. Targeted Identification of Metastasis-associated Cell-surface Sialoglycoproteins in Prostate Cancer. *Molecular & cellular proteomics : MCP*. 10:M110.007294.

Yong, J., M. Kasim, J.L. Bachorik, L. Wan, and G. Dreyfuss. 2010. Gemin5 delivers snRNA precursors to the SMN complex for snRNP biogenesis. *Molecular cell*. 38:551-62.

Zee, B.M., R.S. Levin, P.A. Dimaggio, and B.A. Garcia. 2010. Global turnover of histone post-translational modifications and variants in human cells. *Epigenetics & Chromatin*. 3:22.

Zhang, H., X.J. Li, D.B. Martin, and R. Aebersold. 2003. Identification and quantification of N-linked glycoproteins using hydrazide chemistry, stable isotope labeling and mass spectrometry. *Nat Biotechnol*. 21:660-6.

Zhang, Y., M. Askenazi, J. Jiang, C.J. Luckey, J.D. Griffin, and J.A. Marto. 2010. A robust error model for iTRAQ quantification reveals divergent signaling between oncogenic FLT3 mutants in acute myeloid leukemia. *Mol Cell Proteomics*. 9:780-90.

Zhao, Y., W. Zhang, Y. Kho, and Y. Zhao. 2004. Proteomic analysis of integral plasma membrane proteins. *Analytical chemistry*. 76:1817-23.

Zielinska, D.F., F. Gnad, J.R. Wisniewski, and M. Mann. 2010. Precision mapping of an in vivo N-glycoproteome reveals rigid topological and sequence constraints. *Cell*. 141:897-907.

Zubarev, R.A., D.M. Horn, E.K. Fridriksson, N.L. Kelleher, N.A. Kruger, M.A. Lewis, B.K. Carpenter, and F.W. McLafferty. 2000. Electron capture dissociation for structural characterization of multiply charged protein cations. *Anal Chem*. 72:563-73.

17

Mitochondrial Proteomics: From Structure to Function

Bernardo A. Petriz, Jeeser A. Almeida, Mirna S. Freire, Luiz A. O. Rocha, Taia M. B. Rezende and Octavio L. Franco
Center of Proteomic and Biochemical Analyses, Postgraduate Program in Genomic Sciences and Biotechnology, Catholic University of Brasília, Brasília-DF Brazil

1. Introduction

Mitochondria may be considered an evolutionary product originating from the endosymbiotic process of an aerobic bacterium with a protoeukaryotic cell, which started about 2 billion years ago. This hypothesis was based on the similarities in DNA and protein synthesis machinery between prokaryotic and eukaryotic cells (Margulis, 1970). In 1890, Altmann, who termed this organelle the "bioblast", concluded that these were elementary organisms for performing vital functions (Ernster & Schatz, 1981). Furthermore, in 1898 Benda introduced the name "mitochondrion" from the Greek (*Mitos*: thread and *Chondrion*: granule). Other authors showed the appearance of these structures during spermatogenesis (Ernster & Schatz, 1981) and defined them as subcellular organelles commonly found in the cytoplasm, with essential functions of aerobic metabolism for eukaryotic cells. These organelles have a wide plasticity and mobility, allowing some modifications in shape. Mitochondrial movement into the cytosol has been associated with microtubules, which may determine organelle organization in different cell types (Yaffe, 1999). Mitochondria can form long filaments of mobile chains, as observed in cardiac muscle cells, or be fixed into a single position as studied in sperm flagella (Yaffe, 1999). The number of mitochondria per cell may also vary according to cell type, usually located in high ATP utilization regions such as cardiac muscle and liver (Frederick & Shaw, 2007; Scheffler, 2008). This organelle also occupies a considerable portion of the cytoplasmic volume, being essential for the evolution of a number of organisms.

Mitochondria are also involved in several central metabolic pathways that are important for cell function, modulation of cytosolic Ca^{+2} signaling, determination of cell death (apoptosis) (Camara et al., 2011), aging and associated diseases (Kowald & Kirkwood, 2011), autophagous embryonic development (Ong & Hausenloy, 2010), as well as being a continuous source of superoxide and reactive oxygen species (Stowe & Camara, 2009; Koopman et al., 2010). Nevertheless, the main function of mitochondria is to generate chemical energy sources (ATP) through oxidative phosphorylation (Saraste, 1999), acting as the organism's "powerhouse". Without the presence of this particular organelle, animal cells would depend on anaerobic glycolysis for their energy production, which would be completely insufficient to meet demand. Mitochondrial metabolism of sugars is considered highly efficient, producing more energy than the glycolysis pathway.

Each mitochondrion has its own DNA and RNA with a complete system of transcription and translation, which synthesizes only a few proteins (Yoon et al., 2010). The mitochondrial genome of different tissues differs in size and gene content (Gray et al., 1999). In mammals, the mitochondrial genome is composed of a circular DNA molecule that has been reduced to approximately 16.5kb in size, encoding genes for only 13 proteins, all of them indispensable for electron transport chain functioning. The human mitochondrial genome is composed of a single double-stranded DNA molecule that curiously does not have an intron, but contains 37 genes essential to the mitochondrial respiratory function (Wallace, 1999). Moreover, two ribosomal RNAs and 22 transfer RNAs are absolutely crucial for the mitochondria translation system (Yoon et al., 2010). All other genes responsible for normal mitochondrial operations are encoded in the cell nucleus (Wallace, 1999).

Mitochondria have a double membrane system and are structurally divided into four compartments: inner membrane, outer membrane, matrix and intermembrane space (Chan, 2006), as represented in Figure 1. Several porin molecules are present in the outer mitochondrial membrane. Porins are transporter proteins, which form aqueous channels through the lipid bilayer (Schirmer, 1998). Thus, the outer membrane functions as a filter, being impermeable to molecules above 5,000 kDa (Weissig et al., 2004). However, larger proteins can enter the mitochondrion through an N-terminus signal sequence connecting it to a specific protein (outer membrane translocase), located in the outer mitochondrial membrane (Herrmann & Neupert, 2000). An outer membrane disruption can lead to a

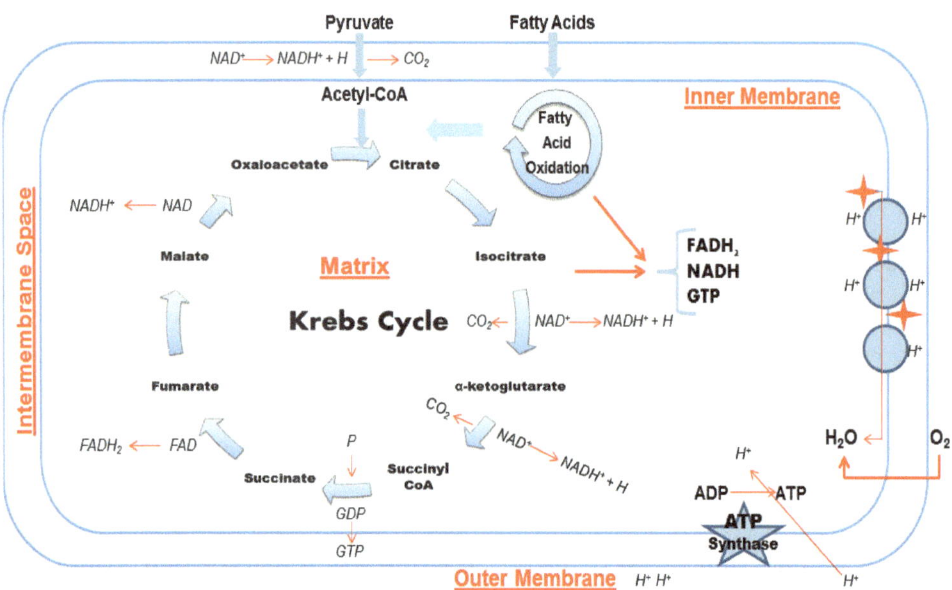

Fig. 1. Scheme of the structure and function of mitochondria by a diagrammatic representation of the Krebs cycle, electron transport chain and ATP synthesis.

diffusion of proteins into the cytosol, inducing possible cell death (Chipuk et al., 2006). The intermembrane determines the space between the outer and inner membrane. Some proteins enter the intermembrane space, but they do not show the ability to penetrate the inner membrane due to enhanced hydrophobicity (Yoon et al., 2010).

The inner membrane is characterized by a major phospholipid structure termed cardiolipin. This structure consists of four fatty acids, allowing the membrane potentially to become impervious to almost all molecules (McMillin & Dowhan, 2002). The membrane is convoluted in form, due to the presence of numerous cristae, which tend to be projected into the matrix, considerably increasing the inner membrane area. Interestingly, mitochondria from heart muscle cells have three times more cristae than those from liver cells (Alberts et al., 2002). Possibly this difference occurs due to ATP demand for different cell types. Inside the inner membrane there is a widely varying number of transporter proteins, which provide limited permeability and assist the entry and exit of ions and molecules that are required or metabolized by enzymes located in the mitochondrial matrix (Herrmann & Neupert, 2000). In summary, the inner membrane proteins have basically three categories and corresponding functions: ATP synthase which produces ATP in the matrix, carrier proteins to regulate the passage of metabolites from within the matrix to outside it, and proteins involved in oxidation reactions in the respiratory chain.

The matrix is considered the highly functional zone inside mitochondria, due to its responsibility for ATP production (Krebs, 1940). It also contains mitochondrial DNA, RNA and ribosome special carriers. The matrix contains a vast amount of the enzyme responsible for the tricarboxylic acid cycle (TAC), also known as the Krebs cycle. This produces NADH + H^+ and $FADH_2$, essential for ATP synthesis by electrons donated to the electron transport chain (Krebs, 1940). These electron pairs are transferred to an O_2 molecule to form H_2O molecules. In this way, protons are loaded from the intermembrane space to the mitochondrial matrix by ATP synthase enzyme, yielding ATP for each proton loaded (Ernster & Schatz, 1981).

2. Classic and novel techniques applied to the mitochondrial proteome

Progress in mitochondrial research has been made with a range of molecular research tools that have been used to identify and compare several compounds. Proteins are one of the major molecules of interest within mitochondria, because their disturbance is directly responsible for several biologic modulations. Proteomics is the study of all proteins at a single given moment; it involves tools to identify and elicit the entire protein composition of a single tissue, cell or organelle (Wilkins et al., 1996). Proteomic tools have developed steadily, and each has been used in its time in mitochondrial proteome research, starting with the classic combination of IEF (isoelectric focusing) and SDS-PAGE (sodium dodecyl sulfate polyacrylamide gel electrophoresis) known as 2-DE (two-dimensional electrophoresis). Next came the DIGE (Differential Gel Electrophoresis) fluorescent method, and now tools include several gel-free (MudPIT) and novel peptide labeling techniques, in addition to complementary functional analysis methods (e.g. Blue Native and Native DIGE).

The analysis of cell compartments and specific organelles has become more common among proteomics researchers, now that subcellular research has provided in-depth knowledge of specific cellular signaling and other related functions (Scheffler, 2008). Up to now, mitochondria have been one of the main organelles to be investigated with a wide range of research tools (Lopez & Melov, 2002), which have generated valuable molecular data (Scheffler, 2008). The main interest driving mitochondrial research stems from the wide spectrum of important molecular signaling that this organelle performs within the cell and also the entire organism, including its crucial role in energy production (Ernster & Schatz, 1981), calcium homeostasis (Deluca et al., 1962), programmed cell apoptosis (Liu et al., 1996) and several pathologies (Chan, 2006; Pagliarini et al., 2008). Furthermore, mitochondrial dysfunction may play a crucial role in neurological (e.g. Alzheimer's, Parkinson's) (Lovell et al., 2005; Jones, 2010), cardiovascular (e.g. Ischemia, heart failure) and muscular diseases (Kim et al., 2006; Finsterer & Stollberger, 2010), as well as in the development of cancer (Kamp et al., 2011) and aging processes (Dencher et al., 2007; O'Connell & Ohlendieck, 2009).

It is also known that the mitochondrion network within a multicellular organism may be coordinated by a proteome reservoir of thousands of polypeptides (~1500), which can be up or down-regulated and have not been fully covered until now (Meisinger et al., 2008). Therefore the cataloging of the entire organelle proteome is of inestimable value to biomedical research, and further understanding of molecular mitochondrial modulation of positive stimulus or pathological insults shows enormous pharmacological potential (Fearnley et al., 2007; Wang et al., 2009). By different proteomic methods, much progress has been made in this direction in order to target and catalogue mitochondrial proteins from different organisms, such as humans (Rabilloud et al., 1998; Lefort et al., 2009), rodents (Zhang et al., 2008; Doran et al., 2009), fungi (Grinyer et al., 2004) and plants (Taylor et al., 2011).

In addition to simple proteome cataloging, several studies have been carried out to compare mitochondrial proteomes from different tissues (Forner et al., 2006; Fang & Lee, 2009; Forner et al., 2009), as well as from organ structures (e.g. heart atria, ventricle) (Forner et al., 2009) and mitochondrial subpopulations (e.g. intermyofibrillar and subsarcolemmal) (Kavazis et al., 2009; Ferreira et al., 2010; Ferreira et al., 2010), with the aim of characterizing specific molecular profiles and functions. Using these tissues, specific proteome characterization during various biologic stimuli and disturbances, such as aging (Dencher et al., 2007; O'Connell & Ohlendieck, 2009), exercise (Kavazis et al., 2009; Egan et al., 2011) and oxidative stress (2008; Lee et al., 2008; Zhang et al., 2008) have also been investigated to attempt to answer the numerous questions concerning the disturbance and adaptation of mitochondrial homeostasis.

Concerning the delicate process of organelle isolation and some proteomic analysis limitations, much has been achieved in surveying the mitochondrial proteome, as reviewed elsewhere (Mathy & Sluse, 2008). Classic protein detection methods, such as 2-DE, have been improved. Moreover, other proteomical techniques have reached higher levels of accuracy; data collection has improved with sample labeling and gel-free analysis, such as shotgun proteomics performed by multidimensional chromatography (2D-LC-MS) directly coupled with high throughput mass spectrometry (Aebersold & Mann, 2003; Tao et al., 2009). By means of these classic and up-to-date techniques, mitochondrial proteins have also been confirmed by the functional proteomic approach using native electrophoresis (e.g. Blue Native PAGE and Native DIGE) to investigate protein-protein interactions and membrane protein complexes (Brookes et al., 2002), increasing insights into molecular expression and signaling within inner and outer mitochondrial compartments.

2.1 Proteomic gel-based techniques in mitochondrial research

The bulk of mitochondria proteome research has been performed using 2-DE associated with MS (mass spectrometry) identification. By combining IEF and protein separation by molecular mass (SDS-PAGE), after the staining process 2-DE gels may reveal up to 3000 protein spots (Lopez & Melov, 2002). The capacity to simultaneously resolve thousands of proteins and by this technique compare different proteomes is possibly the main strength of this technique, which has undergone constant improvement since its invention in the middle of the 70´s (Klose, 1975; O'Farrell, 1975). To overcome its various limitations, such as sample complexity, poor protein solubilizing (e.g. membrane proteins) and low resolution (e.g. hydrophobic and extreme acid or basic proteins) observed in 2-DE analyses, several upgrades have been developed, from sample preparation (e.g. protein extraction and solubilizing process) to gel conduction. Given the precision needed in mitochondrial proteomic analysis, these limitations represent a considerable barrier. Marty and Sluse (2008) reported that mitochondrial proteins appear mostly within the pH range of 3 to 11, and within the 15 to 100 kDa molecular mass range. Furthermore, several proteins from the electron transporter chain, which represent about 40% of inner membrane proteins (Schwerzmann et al., 1986), have high hydrophobic properties, a property that clearly makes IEF processes more difficult (Santoni et al., 2000). An incomplete proteome map may reflect a series of misconducted analyses and slightly erroneous insights, leading overall to a very poor understanding of mitochondrial processes.

Moving on from the classic gel-based technique, the limitations positively promoted a series of upgrades in proteomic methods, leading mitochondriomics research to provide more accurate, qualitative, quantitative and functional proteome data. Development of several fluorescent staining methods and protein labeling prior to 2-DE separation as performed by the Difference Gel Electrophoresis method, known as DIGE (Unlu et al., 1997), responded to specific concerns about the qualitative and quantitative limitations of protein spot detection. The DIGE method is based on the incorporation of different fluorescent cyanide dyes (Cydye3, Cydye5 and Cydye7 by GE Healthcare) into lysine residue present in the protein samples (Byrne et al., 2009). Once each sample is labeled with a distinct fluorescent dye, which includes an internal standard (a mixture of all labeled samples), samples are resolved together by the same 2-DE experiment. As the gel is scanned, fluorescent excitation from each distinct dye is captured and overlapped for spot expression comparison between the other dyes and the standard signal, enabling the results to overcome possible intra-gel variability errors (Lilley & Friedman, 2004). In comparison to classic 2-DE, the DIGE technique has been successfully used by various research groups to shed some light on the mitochondrial proteome in a wide variety of organisms and physiological modulations (Jacoby et al., 2010; Egan et al., 2011; Glancy & Balaban, 2011). Because it overcomes the problem of data reproducibility, DIGE is the ultimate gel-based method and strongly recommended when protein quantification and comparison is desirable, as has been well reviewed (Mathy & Sluse, 2008).

Most of the gel-based methods (2-DE and DIGE) started with treatments using strong solubilizing detergents (e.g. SDS, CHAPS, Sulfobetaines, Triton-X) and chaotropic agents (e.g Urea, Thiourea) as reviewed by Petriz *et al.*, (2011). The use of such agents leads to a real limitation on gel-based analysis caused by denaturing processes, which prevent any functional and protein-cross-talk analysis. However, major protein complexes present in abundance in the mitochondrial membrane may be analyzed from a functional perspective, as proposed by differential analyses, such as Blue-Native Electrophoresis (BN-PAGE) developed by Schagger and Von Jagow (1991). The main idea of BN-PAGE in mitochondrial research is first to separate membrane and other functional protein complexes by preserving enzyme activity using a non-denaturing gel. These entire complexes are then separated within a denaturating SDS-PAGE gel in order to divide protein complexes subunits by their molecular weight (Schagger & von Jagow, 1991). Brookes *et al.* (2002) have shown the great potential that this technique has demonstrated in functional proteomics for mitochondrial molecular signaling, protein-to-protein interaction and post-translational modifications, especially in respiratory chain proteins from the mitochondrial membrane. A variation of 2D BN-PAGE is the Native DIGE (Difference Gel Electrophoresis) technique (Dani & Dencher, 2008), which couples the fluorescent dyes labeling technique to the previously described BN-PAGE (Dani & Dencher, 2008). DIGE analyses use fluorescent labeling and internal standards to enhance the accuracy of analyses. Thus, non-denaturing techniques have been well used (van den Ecker et al., 2010; Phillips et al., 2011), demonstrating that these techniques may contribute extensively to greater knowledge on the part that molecular signaling plays in mitochondrial functionality.

2.2 Gel-free and proteomic straightforward methods

Up-to-date gel-free proteomic techniques, such as LC/LC-MSMS (Reinders & Sickmann, 2007; Lefort et al., 2009) have complemented gel-based experiments, leading mitochondrial molecular investigation to higher levels of data production and accuracy. It is well known that protein quantitation and low abundant protein detection have been among the major limitations on proteomic research. Fortunately, a series of gel-free methods have empowered this research by overcoming some of the main in-gel limitations and functioning as complementary tools for proteomic data mining. Gel-free methods are based on the separation of complex protein samples by liquid chromatography (e.g. reversed-phase, strong cationic exchange) followed by direct mass spectrometry analysis. When performed by more than one LC column this entire process characterizes 2D-LC analysis, known as multidimensional protein identification technology (MudPIT) (Link et al., 1999). MudPIT has been recognized as a high throughput method with enhanced ability to identify thousands of proteins within a single experiment (Motoyama & Yates, 2008). To enhance multidimensional chromatography for MS analysis, a series of chemical molecular labeling methods were developed to facilitate proteomic mining and especially quantitative proteome comparisons. Basically, different proteome samples are mixed with isobaric or stable isotope chemical tags, digested with proteolytic enzymes such as trypsin and then loaded together into MudPIT, enabling quantitative comparisons (Aebersold & Mann, 2003).

ICAT (Isotope-Coded Affinity Tags), SILAC (Stable Isotope Labeling with Amino acids in Cell culture) and iTRAQ (Isobaric Tags for Relative and Absolute Quantitation) are the main quantitative-labeling methods for gel-free methodology, permitting comparisons between different samples (2 to ~4) within the same experiment, as well as increasing the amount of quantitative proteome data that can be gathered by making the final process of peptide MS identification easier (Lovell et al., 2005; Jin et al., 2007; Meany et al., 2007). Each of these labeling techniques has its own peculiarity; for instance, the SILAC method is based on the incorporation of "light" or "heavy" isotope agents (^{2}H, ^{13}C, ^{15}N) within distinct cell cultures, which will further synthetize labeled proteins for proteomic comparisons. SILAC was first described by Ong *et al.*, (2002) to quantify protein expression differences from mammalian cells through a differentiation process. This method is also known as metabolic stable-isotope labeling and has been used to investigate thousands of mitochondrial proteins identified by a variety of studies in pathology, such as Parkinson's treatment (Jin et al., 2007), human cytomegalovirus infection (Zhang et al., 2011) and diabetic sensory neuropathy etiology (Akude et al., 2011).

Another well-established labeling method, ICAT, was first described by Gygi *et al.*, (1999) to quantify proteome modulation of yeast metabolic function under glucose-repressed stimulus. The ICAT technique labels cysteine (Cys) side chains with "light" or "heavy" isotope tags, permitting intensity pair comparison from peptide ions from distinctly labeled protein samples. This labeling technique has also been well implemented in mitochondrial analysis (Jiang et al., 2005; Lovell et al., 2005), but ICAT fails to identify non-cysteine-containing proteins, which is its major technical limitation.

A vital property of gel-free methods (2D-MSMS) is the generation of a great number of MS spectra, which may be further quantified by several peptide tagging methods (e.g. ICAT, SILAC, iTRAQ). Nevertheless, the identification and analysis of proteins from marked peptide spectra is usually time-consuming. Overcoming this limitation, the ultimate labeling method is iTRAQ, which has made the entire process less laborious. Another major improvement brought by this method is the ability to analyze up to four different protein samples in the same experiment, leading to a single MS spectrum peak (Ross et al., 2004). By labeling the peptides' N-termini iTRAQ is a successful tool in mitochondrial proteome development, principally within quantitation research design (Jullig et al., 2007; Kavazis et al., 2009; Glancy & Balaban, 2011). Gel-based and gel-free methods for mitochondrial analysis are schematically represented in Figure 2. Undoubtedly, mitochondrial proteomic research still leaves several gaps. It is clear that the classic proteomic approach alone will not be enough to fill these gaps. The two strategies together are likely to be the most complete and secure path to successful mitochondrial proteome research.

3. Proteomic tools applied to understanding mitochondria: The effects of drugs

The mitochondrion plays a key role in normal and healthy cells. However, under abnormal conditions this organelle can also be involved in cell dysfunction and death. Mitochondrial dysfunction may be implicated in a large number of diseases, such as cancer, neurodegenerative diseases (such as Alzheimer's), diabetes, ischemia-reperfusion injury and aging (Wallace, 1999). The identification of mitochondrial proteins may therefore be a beneficial tool in drug development and also to diagnose targets for such diseases. The treatment of these illnesses involves the drug-mitochondrial interaction that acts in the three main mitochondrial functions: energy production, reactive oxygen species fabrication, and cell death control via both apoptotic and necrotic pathways (Green & Reed 1998; Kristal & Brown 1999). These organelles have a superoxide radical anion source, which arises from oxidative phosphorylation and can produce reactive oxygen species and also their precursors. Although protective mechanisms are known to regulate these molecular species, reversible and irreversible oxidative damage to proteins, nucleic acids and lipids may occur. Under elevated oxidative stress conditions, such as cell aging or disease, these oxidative lesions can be accumulated and have drastic consequences for cellular function, leading ultimately to senescence, environmental

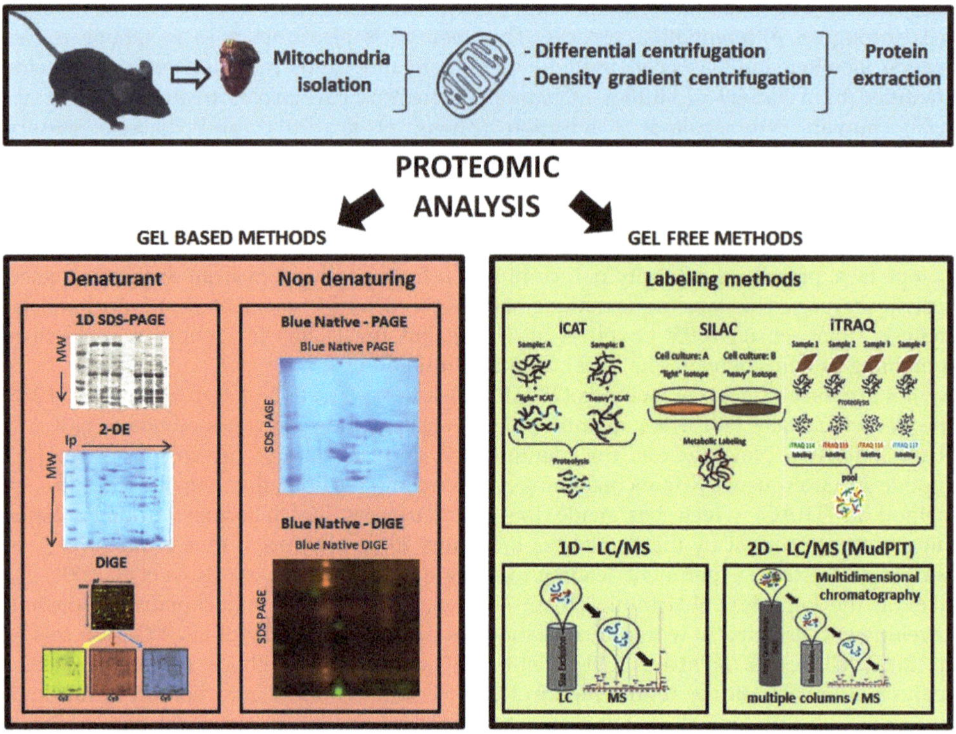

Fig. 2. Proteomic tools for mitochondrial analysis. Schematic workflow of the gel-based (red) and gel-free (green) proteomic tools used to compose the mitochondrial proteome after extraction process (blue).

modification, for example in the S-nitrosylation process or the oxidation of cysteine to sulfenic acid, and also to cell death (Gibson, 2004).

In this context, mitochondria are a pharmacological target for drugs that modulate oxidative stress (Murphy & Smith, 2000). There are various compounds that can target oxidative stress in mitochondria. Coenzyme Q and vitamin E are natural compounds that are both used as dietary supplements. MitoQ and MitoVitE are based on triphenylphosphorium modifications of coenzyme Q and vitamin E, respectively. They are more potent than their natural sources and have been suggested for treating Friedreich's ataxia, since they prevent cell death (Jauslin et al., 2003). Another pharmacological example is flupirtine, a nonopioid analgesic drug with mitochondrial antioxidant activity, which acts as a free radical scavenger (Schluter et al., 2000). Flupirtine has been shown to inhibit ischemic injury (Osborne et al., 1996) and apoptosis, and may be protective against Alzheimer's and prion disease (Perovic et al., 1998).

In spite of the role of mitochondria in different diseases and their potential target for some disease treatments, there is little information about the proteome associated with drug-mitochondrial interaction and target biomarker drugs for treatment design. Based on proteome analysis, with 2D-gel analysis followed by MALDI TOF MS or ESI MS/MS for protein identification, Arrell *et al.*, (2006) analyzed pharmacologically mimicked ischemic preconditioning. This pathology is characterized by resistance to ischemia reperfusion injury in response to previous short ischemic episodes. In this study, the authors mimicked preconditioning, treating isolated rabbit ventricular myocytes with adenosine or diazoxide. They observed a distinctive pattern of affected proteins consistent with specific perturbation of mitochondrial metabolism through changes to a selected number of mitochondrial protein complexes, with specificity and complexity of the drug response. Compared to the vehicle-treated controls, expression of 28 significantly altered proteins was observed and 19 of them were identified. The majority of these proteins are involved in mitochondrial energetics, including subunits of enzymes from the tricarboxylic acid cycle and oxidative phosphorylation complexes. Among these changed proteins, the β-subunit of ATP synthase was adenosine-phosphorylated after 60 min of treatment. These results prove that adenosine and diazoxide treatment acts in different cell parts, especially in the mitochondria (Arrell et al., 2006).

Regarding the anti-inflammatory agents that target mitochondria, the proteome-related literature has reported some data about simvastatin. Simvastatin is a 3-hydroxy-3-methylglutaryl coenzyme A reductase inhibitor that provides neuroprotection, acting against cell loss resulting from strokes (Law et al., 2003), Alzheimer's disease (Vega et al., 2003), Parkinson's disease (Rajanikant et al., 2007) and traumatic brain injury (Lu et al., 2004), all of which are pathologies that target mitochondria. In the same line, Pienaar *et al.*, (2009) compared rat mitochondrial proteins pre-treated with simvastatin for 14 days, followed or not by a unihemispheric injection of a mitochondrial complex S inhibitor. The authors identified 24 different mitochondrial proteins by mass spectroscopy, which represented many facets of mitochondrial integrity, with most of them forming part of the electron transport chain machinery (Pienaar et al., 2009). These results demonstrated that the simvastatin-mitochondrial interaction may contribute to beneficial effects, especially when associated with statin use.

Research with cancer has shown that cancer cells are adapted to fast growth and proliferation in acid pH conditions and low oxygen tension (Griffiths, 2001). Cancer cells have a mitochondrial defect in oxidative phosphorylation, and this can be reversible. Therefore, mitochondrial-drug interaction in cancer pathology should divert energy production from the anaerobic path to oxidative phosphorylation. The effect is to decrease nuclear ATP, leading to a consequent reduction in cell proliferation, so that the tumor cells begin cellular differentiation and subsequently undergo cell death and apoptosis (Harris et al., 2000).

Neoplastic drugs that target different mitochondrial proteins are already on the market for the treatment of various types of cancer. One of these, doxorubicin, also known by the trademark name Adriamycn, is an anthracycline antibiotic and extremely effective antineoplastic agent used in a wide variety of solid cancers and hematological malignancies since the early 1960's (Di Marco et al., 1969). Hammer *et al.*, (2010) analyzed proteomically the doxorubicin-induced changes in a hepatocellular carcinoma cell model, using 2D DIGE, liquid chromatography coupled with electrospray ionization and a hybrid quadrupole linear ion-trap and Fourier-transform ion-cyclotron-resonance mass spectrometry (LC-ESI-LTQ-FTICR-MS) and nano-LC coupled offline to MALDI-TOF/TOF-MS (LC-offline-MALDI-TOF-TOF-MS.) These methods identified 155 different proteins that could be assigned to a wide variety of biological processes, compared to non-treated control cells. Functional analysis revealed major influences of doxorubicin on proteins involved in protein synthesis, DNA damage control, electron transport/mitochondrial function and tumor growth.

Further, as regards mitochondrial proteins, the authors above observed that doxorubicin increases the Bax level (apoptosis regulator), which is involved in cytochrome C release from mitochondria and in turn caspase activation and decreased expression of Bcl-2. Oxidative stress induction was also shown by the enhanced levels of ferredoxin reductase and transferring receptor protein 1 and decreased levels of ERO1-like protein-α. Proteins involved in β-oxidation, such as acyl-CoA dehydrogenase, acetyl-CoA carboxylase 1 and hydroxymethylglutaryl-CoA synthase, were also increased in the doxorubicin-treated group. These results demonstrated that application of doxorubicin led to up-regulation of proteins involved in adaptation to oxidative stress and maintenance of cell integrity (Hammer et al., 2010).

Doxorubicin is widely used in drug combination strategies for non-Hodgkin lymphoma therapy (Multani et al., 2001). Jiang, Sun *et al.*, (2009) used 2D-DIGE in combination with ESI-MS/MS to analyze changes in mitochondrial protein expression in controlling Raji (lymphoblast-like cells) and doxorubicin-treated Raji cells. Defects in the mitochondrial antioxidant defense system, DNA repair, and oxidative phosphorylation may be the main mechanisms involved in the effect of doxorubicin on the mitochondria of Raji cells. Imperfections in the mitochondrial antioxidant defense system have dual effects on the anticancer mechanism and cardiac toxicity. The authors also found numerous proteins associated with significant chemo-resistance to doxorubicin, including heat shock protein (HSP) 70, prohibitin and ATP-binding cassette B6 transporter isoform. The reported results identified several biomarkers with the potential to enable prediction of anticancer therapy response (Jiang et al., 2009).

Another example of a highly potent chemotherapeutic drug that interacts with mitochondria is cisplatin, commonly used for a variety of human malignancies, such as testicular, prostate, ovarian, cervical, lung, and colon cancers (Wang & Lippard, 2005). Cisplatin cytotoxicity is primarily mediated by its ability to cause DNA damage and apoptotic cell death (Siddik, 2003). Zhang *et al.*, (2009) demonstrated, by different experimental methods, together with proteome analysis, that the induction of phospholipase A2-activating protein (PLAA) promoted cisplatin-associated apoptosis in cervical carcinoma HeLa cells by four pathways: activation of phospholipase A2 and accumulation of arachidonic acid, which causes mitochondrial damage; down-regulation of clusterin, a cytoprotective protein which promotes chemoresistance; upregulation of IL-32, which causes apoptosis in HeLa cells; and activation of JNK/c-jun signaling, which is an established inducer of Fas ligand expression and apoptosis mediated receptor (Zhang et al., 2009).

Analgesics also interact with mitochondria. The literature has reported the widely used analgesic acetaminophen and its mitochondrial interaction, including the fact that acetaminophen overdose may cause severe centrilobular hepatic necrosis in experimental animal models and humans (Davidson & Eastham, 1966). Ruepp *et al.*, (2002) explored acetaminophen overdose effects in mitochondria from animal model liver by genomic and proteomic tools. Proteomics showed that protein changes in mitochondria were present at 15 min post injection, thus preceding most of the gene regulations. The decrease in ATP synthase subunits and β-oxidation pathway proteins indicated a loss of energy production. Since mitochondrial morphology was also affected very early at top dose, they concluded that acetaminophen overdose was a direct action of its known reactive metabolite N-acetyl-*p*-benzoquinone imine, rather than a consequence of gene regulation (Ruepp et al., 2002).

Antipsychotic drugs are another kind of medication that target mitochondria. Psychotic brains present anomalies in their mitochondria, including mitochondrial dysfunction or abnormal cerebral energy metabolism, which may play an important role in the pathophysiology of schizophrenia. Together with this, mitochondrial energy metabolism might be disturbed by the antipsychotic drugs used (Modica-Napolitano et al., 2003). Various antipsychotic drugs have been available for treatment: chlorpromazine (CPZ), was in the first generation and presents serious side-effects (Freedman, 2003); clozapine (CLZ), the first atypical antipsychotic drug to present more antipsychotic effects without the adverse mobility effects of the first-generation drugs (Freedman, 2003); and quetiapine (QTP), an atypical antipsychotic drug that usually acts on both dopamine receptors and serotonin receptors (Martorell et al., 2006). Comparative proteomics of all mitochondrial proteins from the cerebral cortex and hippocampus of a rat model (Sprague-Dawley rats) in response to CPZ, CLZ and QTP antipsychotic medication demonstrated 14 differentially expressed different proteins. Six of them belong to the respiratory electron transport chain of oxidative phosphorylation, showing significant changes in protein quantity including NADH dehydrogenase 1 α subcomplex 10, NADH dehydrogenase flavoprotein 2, NADH dehydrogenase Fe-S protein 3, F1-ATPase beta subunit, ATPase, H^+ transporting, lysosomal, beta 56/58 kDa, isoform 2 and ATPase, H^+ transporting, V1 subunit A, isoform 1; demonstrating antipsychotic drug-mitochondrial interaction (Ji et al., 2009).

Dietary supplements can also act on the mitochondrial proteome. Epidemiological studies suggested that the consumption of soy-containing foods has the ability to prevent or to slow down the development of cardiovascular syndromes (Zhang. X, 2003). A systematic review suggested that a diet supplemented with soy protein isolate containing isoflavones reduces low-density lipoprotein (LDL) and cholesterol (critical risk factor in the development of cardiovascular disease), but no effects on triglycerides or high-density lipoprotein cholesterol contents were observed (Cassidy & Hooper, 2006). Proteome analysis revealed that the LDL-induced alterations of numerous proteins were reversed by the soy extracts and also by the combination of genistein/daidzein soy isoflavones. However, both treatments regulated only three proteins functionally linked to mitochondrial dysfunction and were also connected to reducing the generation of oxidized-LDL-mediated mitochondrial reactive oxygen species, which could induce damages.

Several reports demonstrate the role of specific foods in mitochondrial function (Fuchs. D et al., 2007). A nutrient-sensing target of the rapamycin pathway appears to have a conserved role in regulating life span. It has been demonstrated that the reduced nutrient-sensing target of rapamycin signaling extends yeast's chronological life-span by increasing mitochondrial oxygen consumption, in part by up-regulating mtDNA-encoded oxidative phosphorylation subunit translation (Bonawitz et al., 2007). These data demonstrate that mitochondrial dysfunction could also be related to aging. Besides, it has been demonstrated by 2D DIGE and MALDI MS/MS that the nutrient-sensing target of rapamycin signaling has a global role in regulating mitochondrial proteome dynamics and function (Pan & Shadel, 2009).

Another proteomic field that improved the understanding of drug-mitochondria interaction is in the elucidation of drug targets and the discovery of mechanisms of resistance to different pathogens. *Plasmodium falciparum* is responsible for approximately 247 million cases of malaria and one million deaths each year (WHO, 2011). The drug doxycycline is currently one of the recommended chemoprophylactic regimens for travellers visiting malaria-endemic areas in southeast Asia, Africa and South America (Gras et al., 1993). The emergence of *P. falciparum* resistance to most anti-malarial compounds has highlighted the urgency to develop novel drugs and to clarify the mechanisms of anti-malarial medications currently used. In this study, the authors analyzed protein expression changes by 2D-DIGE and iTRAQ methods in the schizont stage of the malarial parasite, following doxycycline treatment. Although some of these proteins have already been described as being deregulated by other drug treatments (Lasonder et al., 2008), numerous modifications in protein levels seem to be specific to doxycycline treatment, suggesting that apicoplasts and mitochondria are the main targets of doxycycline (Briolant et al., 2010).

Despite the progress made in these combined efforts, human mitochondrial databases have not yet been fully exploited to identify or target new candidates for drug development. In addition, the proteome of different pathologies and also the interaction between drug-pathology proteins related to pharmacological action and side effects should be further studied. On the other hand, proteomic tools can help to understand this important protein relation better, with a view to designing mitochondrial biomarkers that may be useful in drug screening, clinical diagnosis, treatment follow-up and in discovering mechanisms of drug resistance (Figure 3).

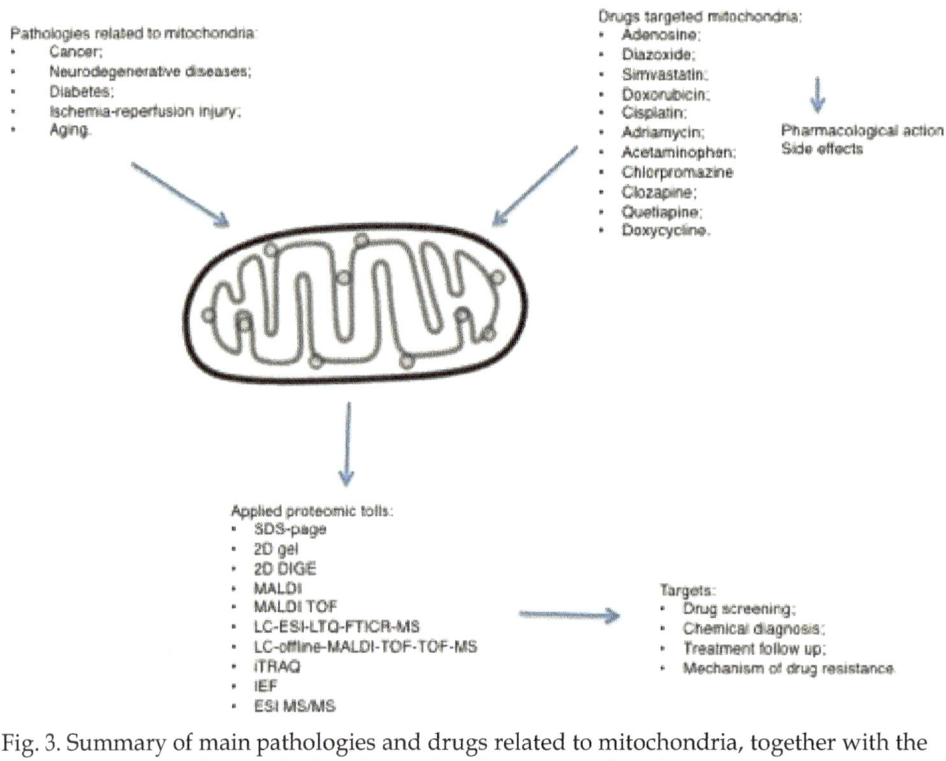

Fig. 3. Summary of main pathologies and drugs related to mitochondria, together with the main proteomic tools described in the studies above, as well as the proposed targets of this triple association.

4. Mitochondrial proteomics applied to exercise research

As reviewed by Lopez and Melov (2002), several studies have shown the characterization of complex mixtures of mitochondria proteins expressed in diseased and healthy samples, leading to a further understanding of their functions in metabolic or physiological processes. This approach has reinforced protein research, leading to important progress in the study of mitochondrial functions and cognate molecular signaling. It is well known that exercise leads to biological adaptations that are highly specific and directly dependent on duration, frequency, intensity and stimulus nature, leading this process to require intensified oxygen demand (Hawley et al., 2011). As is recognized, one of the most important contributions of mitochondria is ATP synthesis, through oxidative phosphorylation (OXPHOS). Therefore, it seems obvious that a large range of decisive phenotype modulations associated with exercise occur within mitochondria. Despite the great importance of the mitochondrial proteome in several physiologic adaptations, there are few data and many questions remaining vis-à-vis molecular signaling, interaction and activity following exercise stimulus.

In this perspective, Bo, Zhang and Ji (2010) indicated that exercise not only raises mitochondrial OXPHOS, but also exerts profound influences on mitochondrial morphology and biogenesis, being one of the most important influences on the fusion-fission process, whose action is responsible for continuous mitochondrial morphology remodeling. The mitochondrion has been seen as a dynamic networking organelle in which fusion and fission are intrinsic coupled processes. This process supports deletions of animals' damaged mitochondria according to organelle size (Kowald & Kirkwood, 2011). The complete process of mitochondrial fusion-fission has not been thoroughly elucidated, however, because there are many proteins involved in execution or modulation that remain to be described. Nevertheless, the mitochondrial dynamic appears to be specifically regulated depending on cell type or by the given function of certain tissues (Liesa et al., 2009). Mitochondrial fusion is a mechanical two-step process, where the outer and inner mitochondrial membranes are fused. This process depends on membrane potential and also the presence of GTP molecules, and is coordinated by optic atrophy gene 1 (OPA1) and mitofusins (Mfns), which promote the fusion of the lipid membrane (Liesa et al., 2009; Zorzano, 2009; Otera & Mihara, 2011). These proteins carry out various activities in promoting fusion and modulating the mitochondrial membrane (Zorzano, 2009). Moreover, according to the same author, fission is coordinated by dynamin-related protein 1 (Drp1) and Fission 1 homologue protein (Fis1) that completes these events.

Mitochondrial dynamics plays an important role in organelle functionality, contributing to an efficient bioenergy supply. The interruption of such processes leads to loss of mitochondrial activity and further diminished OXPHOS, suggesting its essentiality for mitochondrial function (Misko et al., 2010; Kowald & Kirkwood, 2011) and its contribution to the development of some neurodegenerative diseases (Westermann, 2010). Dynamic modifications in mitochondrial fusion-fission proteins during a session of extended exercise with incremental duration leads to a decrease in mitofusin Mfn1/2 expression and also an increase in Fis1 expression (Bo et al., 2010). According to the same authors, these alterations are related to exercise intensity, suggesting that fission may play a compensatory role for OXPHOS injury through improving glucoses and pyruvate uptake. This fact could maintain energy supply and prevent lactate accumulation, delaying the fatigue process associated with the enhancement of H^+ concentration. So it is possible that in severe exercise mitochondrial fission may be a powerful indicator of muscle damage (Bo et al., 2010).

The role of exercise in cardiac health promotion has been well described in literature (Ascensao et al., 2007). This cardioprotective phenotype, normally associated with endurance exercise, seems to be related to increased myocardial antioxidant capacity (Kavazis et al., 2009). Oxidative stress resulting from exercise seems to be part of physiological adaptation. Severe exercise intensities activate a cascade of intracellular sources for reactive oxygen species (ROS) and it is clear that muscle adaptation depends on this process. However, it is important to observe that excessive ROS production can negatively influence exercise performance and can also lead to long-term health consequences (Bailey et al., 2004; Sahlin et al., 2010; Sun et al., 2010). The mechanism of increased ROS production during exercise is not totally clear, but experimental evidence suggests that mitochondria are the main source of ROS production during exercise (Di Meo & Venditti, 2001; Fernstrom et al., 2007). ROS levels are also described as depending on oxygen concentrations, and an additional electron accepted during energy production is used to create superoxide, a more reactive form of oxygen, which can be converted to hydrogen peroxide (H_2O_2) (Sarsour et al., 2009). Animal cells have additional antioxidant enzymes (e.g. catalase, glutathione peroxidase), and the newly identified family of peroxidases (e.g. PRDX) to neutralize H_2O_2 (Chang et al., 2004). Peroxidases are a family with at least six isoforms in mammalian cells. One of these is the mitochondrion-specific isoform, PRDXIII, which acts in defense against oxidative stress caused by H_2O_2 produced during the mitochondrial respiratory chain process (Kavazis et al., 2009). By using the iTRAQ technique, Kavazis *et al.*, (2009) demonstrated a left ventricular remodeling after endurance exercise training in preconditioned animals. This study has shown the up-regulation of PRDXIII in subsarcolemmal mitochondrial subfraction, demonstrating a possible role of PRDXIII in heart remodeling. Exercise has also been demonstrated to reduce oxidative stress and dysfunction of mitochondria after myocardial infarction.

ATP production is well described as declining with age (Drew & Leeuwenburgh, 2003; Drew et al., 2003; Short, 2005) leading to metabolic impairment, so endurance exercise seems to be an important agent in improving and preserving mitochondrial function. Using mass spectrometry methods and the iTRAQ approach, Lanza *et al.*, (2008) demonstrated that tricarboxylic cycle enzymes and electron transport protein expression were down-regulated in older sedentary people when compared to younger subjects. On the other hand, endurance-trained elderly men exhibited an up-regulation of those proteins, suggesting that the expression level of key mitochondrial proteins may be a primary determinant for ageing. Thus, diminished oxidative capacity and regular endurance exercise appear to be beneficial in improving ATP synthesis, partially reversing some metabolic impairment caused by aging. Recently, Egan *et al.*, (2011) used the 2-D DIGE technique to demonstrate that adaptation of skeletal muscle to endurance exercise occurs within only 7 days of training with an increase in ATP generation.

Exercise is therefore recognized as an important agent in improving health, and it is also an auxiliary in numerous medical treatments and therapy. These findings about exercise have led to a better perception of the plasticity of skeletal muscle, mainly by the modulation of the mitochondrial proteome, contributing to understand muscle sensitivity to exercise stimulus. All of these results obviously indicate that phenotype changes associated with exercise are linked directly to mitochondrial proteome modulation. This fact makes mitochondrial research a promising field in sports and medical science.

5. Conclusion

In summary, data reported here clearly show the enormous importance of mitochondria in multiple processes such as drug metabolism and exercise. These processes could be better understood by the use of genomic and proteomic techniques, which are constantly improving. In this view, the use of such technologies could bring real benefits in physiological understanding and in the improvement of biotechnological research related to drug design and activity.

6. References

Aebersold, R. & Mann, M. (2003). "Mass spectrometry-based proteomics." *Nature* 422(6928): 198-207.

Akude, E., Zherebitskaya, E., Chowdhury, S.K., Smith, D.R., Dobrowsky, R.T. & Fernyhough, P. (2011). "Diminished superoxide generation is associated with respiratory chain dysfunction and changes in the mitochondrial proteome of sensory neurons from diabetic rats." *Diabetes* 60(1): 288-297.

Alberts Bruce, A.J., Julian Lewis, Martin Raff, Keith Roberts, and Peter Walter. (2002). *Molecular Biology of the Cell.* New York, Garland Science.

Arrell, D.K., Elliott, S.T., Kane, L.A., Guo, Y., Ko, Y.H., Pedersen, P.L., Robinson, J., Murata, M., Murphy, A.M., Marban, E. & Van Eyk, J.E. (2006). "Proteomic analysis of pharmacological preconditioning: novel protein targets converge to mitochondrial metabolism pathways." *Circ Res* 99(7): 706-714.

Ascensao, A., Ferreira, R. & Magalhaes, J. (2007). "Exercise-induced cardioprotection--biochemical, morphological and functional evidence in whole tissue and isolated mitochondria." *Int J Cardiol* 117(1): 16-30.

Bailey, D.M., Young, I.S., McEneny, J., Lawrenson, L., Kim, J., Barden, J. & Richardson, R.S. (2004). "Regulation of free radical outflow from an isolated muscle bed in exercising humans." *Am J Physiol Heart Circ Physiol* 287(4): H1689-1699.

Bo, H., Zhang, Y. & Ji, L.L. (2010). "Redefining the role of mitochondria in exercise: a dynamic remodeling." *Ann N Y Acad Sci* 1201: 121-128.

Bonawitz, N.D., Chatenay-Lapointe, M., Pan, Y. & Shadel, G.S. (2007). "Reduced TOR signaling extends chronological life span via increased respiration and upregulation of mitochondrial gene expression." *Cell Metab* 5(4): 265-277.

Briolant, S., Almeras, L., Belghazi, M., Boucomont-Chapeaublanc, E., Wurtz, N., Fontaine, A., Granjeaud, S., Fusai, T., Rogier, C. & Pradines, B. (2010). "Plasmodium falciparum proteome changes in response to doxycycline treatment." *Malar J* 9: 141.

Brookes, P.S., Pinner, A., Ramachandran, A., Coward, L., Barnes, S., Kim, H. & Darley-Usmar, V.M. (2002). "High throughput two-dimensional blue-native electrophoresis: a tool for functional proteomics of mitochondria and signaling complexes." *Proteomics* 2(8): 969-977.

Byrne, J.C., Downes, M.R., O'Donoghue, N., O'Keane, C., O'Neill, A., Fan, Y., Fitzpatrick, J.M., Dunn, M. & Watson, R.W. (2009). "2D-DIGE as a strategy to identify serum markers for the progression of prostate cancer." *J Proteome Res* 8(2): 942-957.

Camara, A.K., Bienengraeber, M. & Stowe, D.F. (2011). "Mitochondrial approaches to protect against cardiac ischemia and reperfusion injury." *Front Physiol* 2: 13.

Cassidy, A. & Hooper, L. (2006). "Phytoestrogens and cardiovascular disease." *J Br Menopause Soc* 12(2): 49-56.

Chan, D.C. (2006). "Mitochondria: dynamic organelles in disease, aging, and development." *Cell* 125(7): 1241-1252.

Chang, T.S., Cho, C.S., Park, S., Yu, S., Kang, S.W. & Rhee, S.G. (2004). "Peroxiredoxin III, a mitochondrion-specific peroxidase, regulates apoptotic signaling by mitochondria." *J Biol Chem* 279(40): 41975-41984.

Chipuk, J.E., Bouchier-Hayes, L. & Green, D.R. (2006). "Mitochondrial outer membrane permeabilization during apoptosis: the innocent bystander scenario." *Cell Death Differ* 13(8): 1396-1402.

Dani, D. & Dencher, N.A. (2008). "Native-DIGE: a new look at the mitochondrial membrane proteome." *Biotechnol J* 3(6): 817-822.

Davidson, D.G. & Eastham, W.N. (1966). "Acute liver necrosis following overdose of paracetamol." *Br Med J* 2(5512): 497-499.

Deluca, H.F., Engstrom, G.W. & Rasmussen, H. (1962). "The action of vitamin D and parathyroid hormone in vitro on calcium uptake and release by kidney mitochondria." *Proc Natl Acad Sci U S A* 48: 1604-1609.

Dencher, N.A., Frenzel, M., Reifschneider, N.H., Sugawa, M. & Krause, F. (2007). "Proteome alterations in rat mitochondria caused by aging." *Ann N Y Acad Sci* 1100: 291-298.

Di Marco, A., Gaetani, M. & Scarpinato, B. (1969). "Adriamycin (NSC-123,127): a new antibiotic with antitumor activity." *Cancer Chemother Rep* 53(1): 33-37.

Di Meo, S. & Venditti, P. (2001). "Mitochondria in exercise-induced oxidative stress." *Biol Signals Recept* 10(1-2): 125-140.

Doran, P., Donoghue, P., O'Connell, K., Gannon, J. & Ohlendieck, K. (2009). "Proteomics of skeletal muscle aging." *Proteomics* 9(4): 989-1003.

Drew, B. & Leeuwenburgh, C. (2003). "Method for measuring ATP production in isolated mitochondria: ATP production in brain and liver mitochondria of Fischer-344 rats with age and caloric restriction." *Am J Physiol Regul Integr Comp Physiol* 285(5): R1259-1267.

Drew, B., Phaneuf, S., Dirks, A., Selman, C., Gredilla, R., Lezza, A., Barja, G. & Leeuwenburgh, C. (2003). "Effects of aging and caloric restriction on mitochondrial energy production in gastrocnemius muscle and heart." *Am J Physiol Regul Integr Comp Physiol* 284(2): R474-480.

Egan, B., Dowling, P., O'Connor, P.L., Henry, M., Meleady, P., Zierath, J.R. & O'Gorman, D.J. (2011). "2-D DIGE analysis of the mitochondrial proteome from human skeletal muscle reveals time course-dependent remodelling in response to 14 consecutive days of endurance exercise training." *Proteomics* 11(8): 1413-1428.

Ernster, L. & Schatz, G. (1981). "Mitochondria: a historical review." *J Cell Biol* 91(3 Pt 2): 227s-255s.

Fang, X. & Lee, C.S. (2009). "Proteome characterization of mouse brain mitochondria using electrospray ionization tandem mass spectrometry." *Methods Enzymol* 457: 49-62.

Fearnley, I.M., Carroll, J. & Walker, J.E. (2007). "Proteomic analysis of the subunit composition of complex I (NADH:ubiquinone oxidoreductase) from bovine heart mitochondria." *Methods Mol Biol* 357: 103-125.

Fernstrom, M., Bakkman, L., Tonkonogi, M., Shabalina, I.G., Rozhdestvenskaya, Z., Mattsson, C.M., Enqvist, J.K., Ekblom, B. & Sahlin, K. (2007). "Reduced efficiency, but increased fat oxidation, in mitochondria from human skeletal muscle after 24-h ultraendurance exercise." *J Appl Physiol* 102(5): 1844-1849.

Ferreira, J.C., Bacurau, A.V., Bueno, C.R., Jr., Cunha, T.C., Tanaka, L.Y., Jardim, M.A., Ramires, P.R. & Brum, P.C. (2010). "Aerobic exercise training improves Ca2+

handling and redox status of skeletal muscle in mice." *Exp Biol Med (Maywood)* 235(4): 497-505.

Ferreira, R., Vitorino, R., Alves, R.M., Appell, H.J., Powers, S.K., Duarte, J.A. & Amado, F. (2010). "Subsarcolemmal and intermyofibrillar mitochondria proteome differences disclose functional specializations in skeletal muscle." *Proteomics* 10(17): 3142-3154.

Finsterer, J. & Stollberger, C. (2010). "Cardiac manifestations of mitochondrial disorders." *Eur J Heart Fail* 12(6): 637; author reply 637-638.

Forner, F., Foster, L.J., Campanaro, S., Valle, G. & Mann, M. (2006). "Quantitative proteomic comparison of rat mitochondria from muscle, heart, and liver." *Mol Cell Proteomics* 5(4): 608-619.

Forner, F., Kumar, C., Luber, C.A., Fromme, T., Klingenspor, M. & Mann, M. (2009). "Proteome differences between brown and white fat mitochondria reveal specialized metabolic functions." *Cell Metab* 10(4): 324-335.

Frederick, R.L. & Shaw, J.M. (2007). "Moving mitochondria: establishing distribution of an essential organelle." *Traffic* 8(12): 1668-1675.

Freedman, R. (2003). "Schizophrenia." *N Engl J Med* 349(18): 1738-1749.

Fuchs. D, Dirscherl. B, Schroot. J.H, Daniel. H & Wenzel. U (2007). "Proteome analysis suggests that mitochondrial dysfunction in stressed endothelial cells is reversed by a soy extract and isolated isoflavones. ." *J.Proteome.Res.* 6: 2132-2142.

Gibson, B.W. (2004). "Exploiting proteomics in the discovery of drugs that target mitochondrial oxidative damage. ." *Sci.Aging Knowledge.Environ.* 12.

Glancy, B. & Balaban, R.S. (2011). "Protein composition and function of red and white skeletal muscle mitochondria." *Am J Physiol Cell Physiol* 300(6): C1280-1290.

Gras, C., Laroche, R., Guelain, J., Martet, G., Merlin, M., Pottier, G., Guisset, M. & Touze, J.E. (1993). "[Current role of doxycycline in the chemoprophylaxis of Plasmodium falciparum malaria]." *Bull Soc Pathol Exot* 86(1): 52-55.

Gray, M.W., Burger, G. & Lang, B.F. (1999). "Mitochondrial evolution." *Science* 283(5407): 1476-1481.

Griffiths, J.R. (2001). "Causes and consequences of hypoxia and acidity in tumour microenvironments." *Bioessays* 23(3): 295-296.

Grinyer, J., McKay, M., Herbert, B. & Nevalainen, H. (2004). "Fungal proteomics: mapping the mitochondrial proteins of a Trichoderma harzianum strain applied for biological control." *Curr Genet* 45(3): 170-175.

Gygi, S.P., Rist, B., Gerber, S.A., Turecek, F., Gelb, M.H. & Aebersold, R. (1999). "Quantitative analysis of complex protein mixtures using isotope-coded affinity tags." *Nat Biotechnol* 17(10): 994-999.

Hammer, E., Bien, S., Salazar, M.G., Steil, L., Scharf, C., Hildebrandt, P., Schroeder, H.W., Kroemer, H.K., Volker, U. & Ritter, C.A. (2010). "Proteomic analysis of doxorubicin-induced changes in the proteome of HepG2cells combining 2-D DIGE and LC-MS/MS approaches." *Proteomics* 10(1): 99-114.

Harris, M.H., Vander Heiden, M.G., Kron, S.J. & Thompson, C.B. (2000). "Role of oxidative phosphorylation in Bax toxicity." *Mol Cell Biol* 20(10): 3590-3596.

Hawley, J.A., Burke, L.M., Phillips, S.M. & Spriet, L.L. (2011). "Nutritional modulation of training-induced skeletal muscle adaptations." *J Appl Physiol* 110(3): 834-845.

Herrmann, J.M. & Neupert, W. (2000). "Protein transport into mitochondria. ." *Curr Opin Microbiol* 3 (2): 210-214.

Jacoby, R.P., Millar, A.H. & Taylor, N.L. (2010). "Wheat mitochondrial proteomes provide new links between antioxidant defense and plant salinity tolerance." *J Proteome Res* 9(12): 6595-6604.

Jauslin, M.L., Meier, T., Smith, R.A. & Murphy, M.P. (2003). "Mitochondria-targeted antioxidants protect Friedreich Ataxia fibroblasts from endogenous oxidative stress more effectively than untargeted antioxidants." *FASEB J* 17(13): 1972-1974.

Ji, B., La, Y., Gao, L., Zhu, H., Tian, N., Zhang, M., Yang, Y., Zhao, X., Tang, R., Ma, G., Zhou, J., Meng, J., Ma, J., Zhang, Z., Li, H., Feng, G., Wang, Y., He, L. & Wan, C. (2009). "A comparative proteomics analysis of rat mitochondria from the cerebral cortex and hippocampus in response to antipsychotic medications." *J Proteome Res* 8(7): 3633-3641.

Jiang, X.S., Dai, J., Sheng, Q.H., Zhang, L., Xia, Q.C., Wu, J.R. & Zeng, R. (2005). "A comparative proteomic strategy for subcellular proteome research: ICAT approach coupled with bioinformatics prediction to ascertain rat liver mitochondrial proteins and indication of mitochondrial localization for catalase." *Mol Cell Proteomics* 4(1): 12-34.

Jiang, Y.J., Sun, Q., Fang, X.S. & Wang, X. (2009). "Comparative mitochondrial proteomic analysis of Rji cells exposed to adriamycin." *Mol Med* 15(5-6): 173-182.

Jin, J., Davis, J., Zhu, D., Kashima, D.T., Leroueil, M., Pan, C., Montine, K.S. & Zhang, J. (2007). "Identification of novel proteins affected by rotenone in mitochondria of dopaminergic cells." *BMC Neurosci* 8: 67.

Jones, N. (2010). "PINK1 targets dysfunctional mitochondria for autophagyin Parkinson disease." *Nat Rev Neurol* 6(4): 181.

Jullig, M., Hickey, A.J., Middleditch, M.J., Crossman, D.J., Lee, S.C. & Cooper, G.J. (2007). "Characterization of proteomic changes in cardiac mitochondria in streptozotocin-diabetic rats using iTRAQ isobaric tags." *Proteomics Clin Appl* 1(6): 565-576.

Kamp, D.W., Shacter, E. & Weitzman, S.A. (2011). "Chronic inflammation and cancer: the role of the mitochondria." *Oncology (Williston Park)* 25(5): 400-410, 413.

Kavazis, A.N., Alvarez, S., Talbert, E., Lee, Y. & Powers, S.K. (2009). "Exercise training induces a cardioprotective phenotype and alterations in cardiac subsarcolemmal and intermyofibrillar mitochondrial proteins." *Am J Physiol Heart Circ Physiol* 297(1): H144-152.

Kim, N., Lee, Y., Kim, H., Joo, H., Youm, J.B., Park, W.S., Warda, M., Cuong, D.V. & Han, J. (2006). "Potential biomarkers for ischemic heart damage identified in mitochondrial proteins by comparative proteomics." *Proteomics* 6(4): 1237-1249.

Klose, J. (1975). "Protein mapping by combined isoelectric focusing and electrophoresis of mouse tissues. A novel approach to testing for induced point mutations in mammals." *Humangenetik* 26(3): 231-243.

Koopman, W.J., Nijtmans, L.G., Dieteren, C.E., Roestenberg, P., Valsecchi, F., Smeitink, J.A. & Willems, P.H. (2010). "Mammalian mitochondrial complex I: biogenesis, regulation, and reactive oxygen species generation." *Antioxid Redox Signal* 12(12): 1431-1470.

Kowald, A. & Kirkwood, T.B. (2011). "Evolution of the mitochondrial fusion-fission cycle and its role in aging." *Proc Natl Acad Sci U S A* 108(25): 10237-10242.

Krebs, H.A. (1940). *The citric acid cycle.* , Department of Biochemistry, The University of Sheffield.

Lanza, I.R., Short, D.K., Short, K.R., Raghavakaimal, S., Basu, R., Joyner, M.J., McConnell, J.P. & Nair, K.S. (2008). "Endurance exercise as a countermeasure for aging." *Diabetes* 57(11): 2933-2942.

Lasonder, E., Janse, C.J., van Gemert, G.J., Mair, G.R., Vermunt, A.M., Douradinha, B.G., van Noort, V., Huynen, M.A., Luty, A.J., Kroeze, H., Khan, S.M., Sauerwein, R.W., Waters, A.P., Mann, M. & Stunnenberg, H.G. (2008). "Proteomic profiling of

Plasmodium sporozoite maturation identifies new proteins essential for parasite development and infectivity." *PLoS Pathog* 4(10): e1000195.

Law, M.R., Wald, N.J. & Rudnicka, A.R. (2003). "Quantifying effect of statins on low density lipoprotein cholesterol, ischaemic heart disease, and stroke: systematic review and meta-analysis." *BMJ* 326(7404): 1423.

Lee, Y.H., Boelsterli, U.A., Lin, Q. & Chung, M.C. (2008). "Proteomics profiling of hepatic mitochondria in heterozygous Sod2+/- mice, an animal model of discreet mitochondrial oxidative stress." *Proteomics* 8(3): 555-568.

Lefort, N., Yi, Z., Bowen, B., Glancy, B., De Filippis, E.A., Mapes, R., Hwang, H., Flynn, C.R., Willis, W.T., Civitarese, A., Hojlund, K. & Mandarino, L.J. (2009). "Proteome profile of functional mitochondria from human skeletal muscle using one-dimensional gel electrophoresis and HPLC-ESI-MS/MS." *J Proteomics* 72(6): 1046-1060.

Liesa, M., Palacin, M. & Zorzano, A. (2009). "Mitochondrial dynamics in mammalian health and disease." *Physiol Rev* 89(3): 799-845.

Lilley, K.S. & Friedman, D.B. (2004). "All about DIGE: quantification technology for differential-display 2D-gel proteomics." *Expert Rev Proteomics* 1(4): 401-409.

Link, A.J., Eng, J., Schieltz, D.M., Carmack, E., Mize, G.J., Morris, D.R., Garvik, B.M. & Yates, J.R., 3rd (1999). "Direct analysis of protein complexes using mass spectrometry." *Nat Biotechnol* 17(7): 676-682.

Liu, X., Kim, C.N., Yang, J., Jemmerson, R. & Wang, X. (1996). "Induction of apoptotic program in cell-free extracts: requirement for dATP and cytochrome c." *Cell* 86(1): 147-157.

Lopez, M.F. & Melov, S. (2002). "Applied proteomics: mitochondrial proteins and effect on function." *Circ Res* 90(4): 380-389.

Lovell, M.A., Xiong, S., Markesbery, W.R. & Lynn, B.C. (2005). "Quantitative proteomic analysis of mitochondria from primary neuron cultures treated with amyloid beta peptide." *Neurochem Res* 30(1): 113-122.

Lu, D., Goussev, A., Chen, J., Pannu, P., Li, Y., Mahmood, A. & Chopp, M. (2004). "Atorvastatin reduces neurological deficit and increases synaptogenesis, angiogenesis, and neuronal survival in rats subjected to traumatic brain injury." *J Neurotrauma* 21(1): 21-32.

Margulis, L. (1970). *Origin of Eukaryotic Cells.* . New Haven, Yale University Press.

Martorell, L., Segues, T., Folch, G., Valero, J., Joven, J., Labad, A. & Vilella, E. (2006). "New variants in the mitochondrial genomes of schizophrenic patients." *Eur J Hum Genet* 14(5): 520-528.

Mathy, G. & Sluse, F.E. (2008). "Mitochondrial comparative proteomics: strengths and pitfalls." *Biochim Biophys Acta* 1777(7-8): 1072-1077.

McMillin, J.B. & Dowhan, W. (2002). "Cardiolipin and apoptosis." *Biochim Biophys Acta* 1585(2-3): 97-107.

Meany, D.L., Xie, H., Thompson, L.V., Arriaga, E.A. & Griffin, T.J. (2007). "Identification of carbonylated proteins from enriched rat skeletal muscle mitochondria using affinity chromatography-stable isotope labeling and tandem mass spectrometry." *Proteomics* 7(7): 1150-1163.

Meisinger, C., Sickmann, A. & Pfanner, N. (2008). "The mitochondrial proteome: from inventory to function." *Cell* 134(1): 22-24.

Misko, A., Jiang, S., Wegorzewska, I., Milbrandt, J. & Baloh, R.H. (2010). "Mitofusin 2 is necessary for transport of axonal mitochondria and interacts with the Miro/Milton complex." *J Neurosci* 30(12): 4232-4240.

Modica-Napolitano, J.S., Lagace, C.J., Brennan, W.A. & Aprille, J.R. (2003). "Differential effects of typical and atypical neuroleptics on mitochondrial function in vitro." *Arch Pharm Res* 26(11): 951-959.

Motoyama, A. & Yates, J.R., 3rd (2008). "Multidimensional LC separations in shotgun proteomics." *Anal Chem* 80(19): 7187-7193.

Multani, P., White, C.A. & Grillo-Lopez, A. (2001). "Non-Hodgkin's lymphoma: review of conventional treatments." *Curr Pharm Biotechnol* 2(4): 279-291.

Murphy, M.P. & Smith, R.A. (2000). "Drug delivery to mitochondria: the key to mitochondrial medicine." *Adv Drug Deliv Rev* 41(2): 235-250.

O'Connell, K. & Ohlendieck, K. (2009). "Proteomic DIGE analysis of the mitochondria-enriched fraction from aged rat skeletal muscle." *Proteomics* 9(24): 5509-5524.

O'Farrell, P.H. (1975). "High resolution two-dimensional electrophoresis of proteins." *J Biol Chem* 250(10): 4007-4021.

Ong, S.B. & Hausenloy, D.J. (2010). "Mitochondrial morphology and cardiovascular disease." *Cardiovasc Res* 88(1): 16-29.

Ong, S.E., Blagoev, B., Kratchmarova, I., Kristensen, D.B., Steen, H., Pandey, A. & Mann, M. (2002). "Stable isotope labeling by amino acids in cell culture, SILAC, as a simple and accurate approach to expression proteomics." *Mol Cell Proteomics* 1(5): 376-386.

Osborne, N.N., Schwarz, M. & Pergande, G. (1996). "Protection of rabbit retina from ischemic injury by flupirtine." *Invest Ophthalmol Vis Sci* 37(2): 274-280.

Otera, H. & Mihara, K. (2011). "Molecular mechanisms and physiologic functions of mitochondrial dynamics." *J Biochem* 149(3): 241-251.

Pagliarini, D.J., Calvo, S.E., Chang, B., Sheth, S.A., Vafai, S.B., Ong, S.E., Walford, G.A., Sugiana, C., Boneh, A., Chen, W.K., Hill, D.E., Vidal, M., Evans, J.G., Thorburn, D.R., Carr, S.A. & Mootha, V.K. (2008). "A mitochondrial protein compendium elucidates complex I disease biology." *Cell* 134(1): 112-123.

Pan, Y. & Shadel, G.S. (2009). "Extension of chronological life span by reduced TOR signaling requires down-regulation of Sch9p and involves increased mitochondrial OXPHOS complex density." *Aging (Albany NY)* 1(1): 131-145.

Perovic, S., Bohm, M., Meesters, E., Meinhardt, A., Pergande, G. & Muller, W.E. (1998). "Pharmacological intervention in age-associated brain disorders by Flupirtine: Alzheimer's and prion diseases." *Mech Ageing Dev* 101(1-2): 1-19.

Petriz, B.A., Gomes, C.P., Rocha, L.A., Rezende, T.M. & Franco, O.L. (2011). "Proteomics applied to exercise physiology: a cutting-edge technology." *J Cell Physiol.*

Phillips, D., Aponte, A.M., Covian, R. & Balaban, R.S. (2011). "Intrinsic protein kinase activity in mitochondrial oxidative phosphorylation complexes." *Biochemistry* 50(13): 2515-2529.

Pienaar, I.S., Schallert, T., Hattingh, S. & Daniels, W.M. (2009). "Behavioral and quantitative mitochondrial proteome analyses of the effects of simvastatin: implications for models of neural degeneration." *J Neural Transm* 116(7): 791-806.

Rabilloud, T., Kieffer, S., Procaccio, V., Louwagie, M., Courchesne, P.L., Patterson, S.D., Martinez, P., Garin, J. & Lunardi, J. (1998). "Two-dimensional electrophoresis of human placental mitochondria and protein identification by mass spectrometry: toward a human mitochondrial proteome." *Electrophoresis* 19(6): 1006-1014.

Rajanikant, G.K., Zemke, D., Kassab, M. & Majid, A. (2007). "The therapeutic potential of statins in neurological disorders." *Curr Med Chem* 14(1): 103-112.

Reinders, J. & Sickmann, A. (2007). "Proteomics of yeast mitochondria." *Methods Mol Biol* 372: 543-557.

Ross, P.L., Huang, Y.N., Marchese, J.N., Williamson, B., Parker, K., Hattan, S., Khainovski, N., Pillai, S., Dey, S., Daniels, S., Purkayastha, S., Juhasz, P., Martin, S., Bartlet-Jones, M., He, F., Jacobson, A. & Pappin, D.J. (2004). "Multiplexed protein quantitation in Saccharomyces cerevisiae using amine-reactive isobaric tagging reagents." *Mol Cell Proteomics* 3(12): 1154-1169.

Ruepp, S.U., Tonge, R.P., Shaw, J., Wallis, N. & Pognan, F. (2002). "Genomics and proteomics analysis of acetaminophen toxicity in mouse liver." *Toxicol Sci* 65(1): 135-150.

Sahlin, K., Shabalina, I.G., Mattsson, C.M., Bakkman, L., Fernstrom, M., Rozhdestvenskaya, Z., Enqvist, J.K., Nedergaard, J., Ekblom, B. & Tonkonogi, M. (2010). "Ultraendurance exercise increases the production of reactive oxygen species in isolated mitochondria from human skeletal muscle." *J Appl Physiol* 108(4): 780-787.

Santoni, V., Molloy, M. & Rabilloud, T. (2000). "Membrane proteins and proteomics: un amour impossible?" *Electrophoresis* 21(6): 1054-1070.

Saraste, M. (1999). "Oxidative phosphorylation at the fin de siècle. ." *Science* 283: 1488-1493.

Sarsour, E.H., Kumar, M.G., Chaudhuri, L., Kalen, A.L. & Goswami, P.C. (2009). "Redox control of the cell cycle in health and disease." *Antioxid Redox Signal* 11(12): 2985-3011.

Schagger, H. & von Jagow, G. (1991). "Blue native electrophoresis for isolation of membrane protein complexes in enzymatically active form." *Anal Biochem* 199(2): 223-231.

Scheffler, I.E. (2008). *Mitochondria.* Hoboken, New Jersey, J. Wiley and Sons, Inc., .

Schirmer, T. (1998). "General and specific porins from bacterial outer membranes." *J Struct Biol* 121(2): 101-109.

Schluter, T., Struy, H. & Schonfeld, P. (2000). "Protection of mitochondrial integrity from oxidative stress by the triaminopyridine derivative flupirtine." *FEBS Lett* 481(1): 42-46.

Schwerzmann, K., Cruz-Orive, L.M., Eggman, R., Sanger, A. & Weibel, E.R. (1986). "Molecular architecture of the inner membrane of mitochondria from rat liver: a combined biochemical and stereological study." *J Cell Biol* 102(1): 97-103.

Short, K.R.B., Maureen L.; Kahl, Jane; Singh, Ravinder; Coenen-Schimke, Jill; Raghavakaimal, Sreekumar and Nair, K. Sreekumaran (2005). "Decline in skeletal muscle mitochondrial function with aging in humans." *PNAS* 102 (15): 7.

Siddik, Z.H. (2003). "Cisplatin: mode of cytotoxic action and molecular basis of resistance." *Oncogene* 22(47): 7265-7279.

Stowe, D.F. & Camara, A.K. (2009). "Mitochondrial reactive oxygen species production in excitable cells: modulators of mitochondrial and cell function." *Antioxid Redox Signal* 11(6): 1373-1414.

Sun, L., Shen, W., Liu, Z., Guan, S., Liu, J. & Ding, S. (2010). "Endurance exercise causes mitochondrial and oxidative stress in rat liver: effects of a combination of mitochondrial targeting nutrients." *Life Sci* 86(1-2): 39-44.

Tao, D., Zhu, G., Sun, L., Ma, J., Liang, Z., Zhang, W., Zhang, L. & Zhang, Y. (2009). "Serially coupled microcolumn reversed phase liquid chromatography for shotgun proteomic analysis." *Proteomics* 9(7): 2029-2036.

Taylor, N.L., Heazlewood, J.L. & Millar, A.H. (2011). "The Arabidopsis thaliana 2-D gel mitochondrial proteome: Refining the value of reference maps for assessing protein abundance, contaminants and post-translational modifications." *Proteomics* 11(9): 1720-1733.

Unlu, M., Morgan, M.E. & Minden, J.S. (1997). "Difference gel electrophoresis: a single gel method for detecting changes in protein extracts." *Electrophoresis* 18(11): 2071-2077.

van den Ecker, D., van den Brand, M.A., Bossinger, O., Mayatepek, E., Nijtmans, L.G. & Distelmaier, F. (2010). "Blue native electrophoresis to study mitochondrial complex I in C. elegans." *Anal Biochem* 407(2): 287-289.

Vega, G.L., Weiner, M.F., Lipton, A.M., Von Bergmann, K., Lutjohann, D., Moore, C. & Svetlik, D. (2003). "Reduction in levels of 24S-hydroxycholesterol by statin treatment in patients with Alzheimer disease." *Arch Neurol* 60(4): 510-515.

Wallace, D.C. (1999). "Mitochondrial diseases in man and mouse." *Science* 283(5407): 1482-1488.

Wang, D. & Lippard, S.J. (2005). "Cellular processing of platinum anticancer drugs." *Nat Rev Drug Discov* 4(4): 307-320.

Wang, J., Bai, L., Li, J., Sun, C., Zhao, J., Cui, C., Han, K., Liu, Y., Zhuo, X., Wang, T., Liu, P., Fan, F., Guan, Y. & Ma, A. (2009). "Proteomic analysis of mitochondria reveals a metabolic switch from fatty acid oxidation to glycolysis in the failing heart." *Sci China C Life Sci* 52(11): 1003-1010.

Weissig, V., Cheng, S.M. & D'Souza, G.G. (2004). "Mitochondrial pharmaceutics." *Mitochondrion* 3(4): 229-244.

Westermann, B. (2010). "Mitochondrial fusion and fission in cell life and death." *Nat Rev Mol Cell Biol* 11(12): 872-884.

WHO (2011). The world malaria reort 2008. Geneva.

Wilkins, M.R., Pasquali, C., Appel, R.D., Ou, K., Golaz, O., Sanchez, J.C., Yan, J.X., Gooley, A.A., Hughes, G., Humphery-Smith, I., Williams, K.L. & Hochstrasser, D.F. (1996). "From proteins to proteomes: large scale protein identification by two-dimensional electrophoresis and amino acid analysis." *Biotechnology (N Y)* 14(1): 61-65.

Yaffe, M.P. (1999). "The machinery of mitochondrial inheritance and behavior." *Science* 283(5407): 1493-1497.

Yoon, Y.G., Koob, M.D. & Yoo, Y.H. (2010). "Re-engineering the mitochondrial genomes in mammalian cells." *Anat Cell Biol* 43(2): 97-109.

Zhang, A., Williamson, C.D., Wong, D.S., Bullough, M.D., Brown, K.J., Hathout, Y. & Colberg-Poley, A.M. (2011). "Quantitative proteomic analyses of human cytomegalovirus-induced restructuring of endoplasmic reticulum-mitochondrial contacts at late times of infection." *Mol Cell Proteomics*.

Zhang, F., Suarez, G., Sha, J., Sierra, J.C., Peterson, J.W. & Chopra, A.K. (2009). "Phospholipase A2-activating protein (PLAA) enhances cisplatin-induced apoptosis in HeLa cells." *Cell Signal* 21(7): 1085-1099.

Zhang, J., Li, X., Mueller, M., Wang, Y., Zong, C., Deng, N., Vondriska, T.M., Liem, D.A., Yang, J.I., Korge, P., Honda, H., Weiss, J.N., Apweiler, R. & Ping, P. (2008). "Systematic characterization of the murine mitochondrial proteome using functionally validated cardiac mitochondria." *Proteomics* 8(8): 1564-1575.

Zhang, J., Liem, D.A., Mueller, M., Wang, Y., Zong, C., Deng, N., Vondriska, T.M., Korge, P., Drews, O., Maclellan, W.R., Honda, H., Weiss, J.N., Apweiler, R. & Ping, P. (2008). "Altered proteome biology of cardiac mitochondria under stress conditions." *J Proteome Res* 7(6): 2204-2214.

Zhang. X, S.X.O., Gao. Y.T, Yang. G, Li. Q, Li. H, et al., (2003). "Soy food consumption is associated with lower risk of coronary heart disease in Chinese women. ." *J.Nutr.* 133: 2874-2878.

Zorzano, A. (2009). "Regulation of mitofusin-2 expression in skeletal muscle." *Appl Physiol Nutr Metab* 34(3): 433-439.

18

Quantitative Proteomics for Investigation of Secreted Factors: Focus on Muscle Secretome

Jeanette Henningsen, Blagoy Blagoev and Irina Kratchmarova
Department of Biochemistry and Molecular Biology,
University of Southern Denmark, Odense M
Denmark

1. Introduction

The response of cells to even slight changes in the cellular microenvironment determines the reaction of the whole organism and its ability to adapt to macroenvironmental alterations. Generally, it is well recognized that the communication between cells, tissues, and organs is critical for the maintenance of the entire body homeostasis. The different cell types that build the various organs and tissues have an enormous potential to produce proteins that once secreted in the extracellular space exert their action in an auto-, para- and/or endocrine manner. It is estimated that out of the total 20.500 protein-coding genes in human, approximately 10% encode secreted proteins (Clamp et al., 2007; Skalnikova et al., 2011). The separate and combinatorial action of these ~2200 secreted proteins can influence the biology not only at adjacent sites but also have a clear effect on the whole organism (Lin et al., 2008). The secreted factors, which can range from large proteins to short peptides, are divided into different groups or classes according to their structural properties and function. The prototypical secreted proteins are represented by the group of proteins found in the blood stream and other body fluids, the components of the extracellular matrix (ECM) and enzymes released in the intestine and stomach. An intriguing group of secreted factors comprise cell surface receptor ligands, such as hormones, growth factors, and cytokines. These proteins can exert their actions either on a limited number of responsive tissues or can act on virtually all cell types dependent on the expression of their specific receptors. It is essential to decipher in depth the signaling events that are triggered by the various hormones and growth factors to understand the general mechanisms of the biological processes that occur in a strictly controlled fashion in both space and time. The processes that secreted factors influence and directly regulate range from cellular differentiation, growth and survival to apoptosis, autophagy, and ageing. In addition, a growth factor can often exert a divergent and even opposite effect depending on the cell type and cellular state. Taken in consideration the role of secreted factors in directing biological processes, malfunction of the signaling cascades orchestrated by secreted factors can have severe consequences and lead to development of a series of complicated diseases and disorders (Flier, 2001; Pedersen, 2009; Walsh, 2009). Therefore, a comprehensive characterization of secreted molecules by different cellular subtypes, tissues, and organs can contribute to the elucidation of the physiological state of a given organism and to the determination of the malfunction in diseased stages. Analyzing on a large scale and in an unbiased manner the secretome of any given cell type or tissue, which comprise a unique combination of growth factors, hormones, cytokines, inhibitory factors, and components of the extracellular environment, has become a whole distinct research field. Although still challenging, this endeavor may ultimately prove beneficial for improving human health as it can accelerate the bridging of basic research and applied medicine.

2. Proteomics

Proteomics has many sides and it is often difficult to combine the different aspects that can define or characterize this broad topic. The term proteomics was introduced in 1995, describing the entire set of proteins expressed by a given cell, tissue, or organism (Wasinger et al., 1995). At present, proteomics is defined as large scale studies of the proteomes that encompass protein expression, folding, and localization. It also includes functional analyses of large complexes within a cell, tissue, or organism as well as comparison of different proteomes. Some of the different aspects of proteomics include analysis of body fluids, defining proteomes of pathogens, investigation of tissue proteomes, characterization of signaling pathways and the effects of inhibitors and drugs. The term systems biology was also introduced to describe the incorporation of genomics, metabolomics, and proteomics data for creation of dynamic networks of interacting molecules at a system level. Typically, such studies involve following the changes in protein profiles in response to changes in the environment and determination of combined action of diverse signaling networks that lead to a differential outcome for the living organism. Obtaining and combining information for such networks is of particular importance when investigating the role of secreted factors in the regulation of major signaling events in any given cell or tissue. Functional quantitative mass spectrometry-based proteomics (QMSP) is a powerful approach for creation of maps that describe the differential expression and dynamic changes of secretomes. Correlation of these results with clinics can help resolve some of the still missing links in the development of different syndromes. In this review chapter, we focus on the latest advances in QMSP for the investigation of secreted factors and we discuss some of the issues and challenges that remain to be unveiled.

2.1 Quantitative mass spectrometry-based proteomics

The fast development of QMSP techniques added yet another dimension to the proteomic research, namely the ability to follow differences and changes of the proteomes in space and time (Aebersold and Mann, 2003; Cox and Mann, 2007; Dengjel et al., 2009). QMSP permits observation and investigation of a combination of events and interplay of pathways involving hundreds of molecules that lead to a defined outcome for the cell. It facilitates determination of even slight changes in protein expression or post-translational modifications as a result of a drug treatment, changes in the cellular environment or alterations in the total body homeostasis. Up to date, QMSP is the only available approach that can, with high confidence and in a high throughput manner, generate and combine data for the spatial and temporal order of events that take place in a cell directly at protein level in order to decipher dynamic complex processes (Dengjel et al., 2009; Rigbolt and Blagoev, 2010; Walther and Mann, 2010). There are two main QMSP strategies for relative quantitation based either on the use of stable isotopes or the label-free approach for quantitation of changes in protein abundance (Ong and Mann, 2005; Schulze and Usadel, 2010; Walther and Mann, 2010).

2.1.1 Quantitation without stable isotopes

Quantitation without stable isotopes generally encompasses a gel electrophoresis approach or a chromatography-based approach. In the gel-based approach one-dimensional or two-dimensional gel electrophoresis is used as a mean of resolving the proteins from complex mixtures. This is followed by visualization of the protein bands or spots using different types of stains or fluorescent dyes. Typically, the protein samples originating from different cellular stages are separated on a gel and then the bands or spots that show distinct changes are excised, digested with proteases and identified by mass spectrometry. A major disadvantage of two dimensional gel electrophoresis is the relatively low dynamic range and inefficient access into the gel of high or very low molecular weight proteins. This results in the identification of mainly high abundant molecules, such as cytoskeletal proteins and highly expressed metabolic enzymes (Gygi et al., 2000). Reducing the complexity of the sample can at least partially overcome such limitation. The introduction of the difference in gel electrophoresis (DIGE) approach, which allows proteins from two different samples to be separated on the same gel, led to improved quantitatively accuracy of this gel-based approach (Unlu et al., 1997).

The chromatography approach can be divided into two groups, namely peptide-based methods and protein-based methods. The peptide-based strategy relies on comparing the signal intensity of a peptide originating from one sample to the signal intensity of the same peptide originating from a different sample. The extracted ion chromatogram (XIC) for every peptide can be derived from the liquid chromatography profile of the two individual samples during the analysis by the mass spectrometer and the samples can thereby be compared quantitatively. Furthermore, a method called protein correlation profiling was established, where the total ion chromatograms of different samples are aligned and quantitative comparison of samples is then based on both retention time and accurate mass of the peptides. The relative protein quantitation is based on the fact that the peak areas obtained from liquid chromatography mass spectrometry correlate to the relative concentration of the protein in the sample (Andersen et al., 2003; Ong and Mann, 2005). It has been used to obtain semi quantitative data in complex mixtures such as human sera (Chelius and Bondarenko, 2002). A disadvantage is that it is only partially quantitative and requires highly reliable and reproducible analysis of the samples.

Another label-free mass spectrometry-based approach used to retrieve quantitative measurements is based on spectral count. The "spectral counting" method uses the numbers of peptide identification spectra obtained for each protein as representation of the protein abundance in a mixture (Liu et al., 2004). One disadvantage of the spectral count method is that it is biased toward high abundant proteins since they can mask or suppress the low-abundance ones in the sample, which is a key issue when analyzing e. g. plasma samples. The two label-free methods for quantitation, using either peptide ion intensities or spectral counts, are becoming increasingly popular, since they are simpler than the isotope-based strategy, despite being less accurate. In addition, both methods require very good reproducibility between the different liquid chromatography tandem mass spectrometry (LC-MS/MS) runs, high accuracy measurements and higher number of replica analyses. In general, the label-free approaches are widely applicable but the methods using stable isotope labels result in better accuracy of quantitation (Lundgren et al., 2010; Schulze and Usadel, 2010).

2.1.2 Quantitation using stable isotopes

The quantitative mass spectrometry-based methods utilizing stable isotopes can be achieved either by *in vivo* metabolic labeling or *in vitro* biochemical methods. The principle of the two labeling strategies is the generation of peptides labeled with stable isotopes that differ in mass from the unlabeled peptides making it possible to distinguish them within the same spectrum.

2.1.2.1 Chemical labeling strategies

The prototype of the chemical modification-based methodology for quantitation of protein is the isotope coded affinity tag (ICAT) that binds to cysteine residues (Gygi et al., 1999). It employs usage of two isotopically labeled tags - one light and one heavy, which contains eight deuterium atoms, to distinctly label the peptides originating from two separate samples. The peptides originating from one sample can thereby be distinguished from the second sample, since the heavier tag will result in a mass shift readily observable in the mass spectrum. One of the advantages of ICAT is the presence of a biotin group in the light and heavy tags allowing selective enrichment of the labeled peptides using avidin affinity chromatography, thus reducing greatly the complexity of the mixture.

ICAT has been applied to a variety of cell culture and tissue samples and has been demonstrated as a reliable and relatively easy applicable method for performing QMSP analysis. Among other applications, ICAT has been used to investigate differential expression profiles of microsomal proteins from *naive* and *in vitro*- differentiated human myeloid leukemia cells, secreted proteins during osteoclast differentiation, the dynamic changes of transcription factors during erythroid differentiation as well as comparison of livers of mice treated with different peroxisome proliferator-activated receptor agonists (Brand et al., 2004; Han et al., 2001; Kubota et al., 2003; Tian et al., 2004). Disadvantages of the ICAT strategy are that it targets only the cysteine containing peptides and the retention times of the light and heavy form during chromatographic separation are altered due to the presence of the deuterium atoms. To overcome some of those problems, a cleavable 12C- and 13C-based reagent (cICAT) has been developed, which has an improved peptide co-elution profile during the liquid chromatography separation and increased recovery after enrichment of the labeled peptides (Yi et al., 2005).

Several other chemical labeling strategies have been developed over the recent years. Probably the most popular of those being the isobaric tags for relative and absolute quantitation (iTRAQ) where the isobaric chemical groups are attached to the primary amine groups of the peptides. With iTRAQ, up to eight different conditions can be compared simultaneously since eight distinct isobaric tags for labeling are currently available. The quantitation is based on the intensities of the isotopically distinct fragments derived from the corresponding isobaric tags obtained in the peptide fragmentation spectrum. This is the main advantage of the method but it can also be a disadvantage since often a single fragment spectrum per peptide is available, thereby compromising the accuracy of quantitation (Ross et al., 2004).

2.1.2.2 Metabolic labeling

The metabolic labeling strategies rely on the incorporation of a stable isotope in proteins, while they are being *de novo* synthesized in the cell. In contrast to the standard radioactivity-based assays, the stable isotope is fully incorporated thereby encoding the whole proteome. There are two means of introducing the stable isotope using either media containing 15N labeled ammonium sulfate or media with the addition of a stable isotope labeled amino acid. The 15N labeling strategy has been used for quantitative analysis of protein phosphorylation in bacteria and a mouse melanoma cell line (Conrads et al., 2001; Oda et al., 1999). Additionally, entire organisms have been metabolically labeled using the 15N strategy, including bacteria (E. coli and Deinococcus), C. elegans, D. melanogaster, and rat (Conrads et al., 2001; Krijgsveld et al., 2003; Wu et al., 2004).

Stable Isotope Labeling by Amino Acids in Cell Culture (SILAC) is an accurate and resourceful quantitative proteomics platform, that in combination with high speed and accuracy mass spectrometry allows detailed characterization of complex biological systems (Ong et al., 2002; Ong et al., 2003). It involves usage of heavy non- radioactive stable isotope-labeled amino acids, which are incorporated directly into the newly synthesized proteins of the cell. After SILAC labeling, the entire proteome of a given cell population becomes encoded either with a light or heavier version of the same amino acid, thereby enabling direct comparison and quantitation using mass spectrometry. With SILAC, the "light" and "heavy" samples can be mixed in equal ratios at the initial stages of the workflow, which can include subsequent protein purification, interaction assay or other manipulation of the mixed sample. Combining samples prior to any further sample preparation represents a tremendous advantage, since it results in reduced quantitation errors introduced by differences in individual sample handling. Major strength of the SILAC method is the ability to discriminate true interaction partners from background, when investigating functional protein-protein interactions (Blagoev et al., 2003; Dengjel et al., 2010). Therefore, it facilitates investigation of cellular signaling cascades and creation of reliable protein interaction networks, which represents one of the biggest challenges in the field of system biology (Blagoev et al., 2004; Dengjel et al., 2009; Kratchmarova et al., 2005; Olsen et al., 2006; Osinalde et al., 2011). In addition, SILAC is invaluable for the investigation of secreted factors since it allows the distinction of specific proteins released by the cells to the extracellular environment from contaminating proteins like keratins and serum derived factors that originate from cell culture media supplements (Henningsen et al., 2010). One potential disadvantage with the SILAC protocol arises from cultures of primary cells, which usually require specific growth media with a defined formulation. Furthermore, such cells have limited division capacity in culture, whereas at least 5 population doublings are required for complete SILAC encoding of the entire proteome. Nevertheless, SILAC-based analyses have been successfully extended to include microorganisms, entire mice, and quantitation of proteins in tumor biopsies (Geiger et al., 2010; Kruger et al., 2008; Soufi et al., 2010). It was also utilized for the quantitative analyses of proteins released by omental adipose tissue explants (Alvarez-Llamas et al., 2007).

3. Application of QMSP for investigation of secreted proteins

Analysis of secreted proteins using QMSP allows in depth characterization of different cellular systems that secrete auto-, para-, and endocrine factors, which can influence the entire body homeostasis. Investigation of cellular models such as adult and embryonic stem cells, cells originating from a diseased state, immortalized cells representing various models for functional abnormalities, extends the knowledge of how changes in secretomes contribute to various types of human disorders. It also enables determination and discovery of new roads of tissue cross talk and interaction. QMSP has been applied to study secretomes of a variety of cell types and tissues including adipose cells and tissues, mouse embryonic fibroblasts, astrocytes, mesenchymal stem cells, neuronal progenitor cells, kidney, and endothelial cells (Skalnikova et al., 2011). Although, there have been several proteomics reports describing the secretory function of cells from mesenchymal origin, the role of the muscle secretome has remained elusive. A limited number of studies so far have employed mass spectrometry to elucidate the secretory function of the skeletal muscle. In a study presented by Chan and coworkers condition media (CM) was collected from differentiated C2C12 myotubes at day 5 of differentiation and analyzed by 1D-gel electrophoresis combined with matrix-assisted laser desorption/ ionization tandem mass spectrometry (MALDI-MS/MS) (Chan et al., 2007). This work led to the identification of 80 proteins released from skeletal muscle of which 27 were classified as secreted proteins based on literature searches. In another study isolated primary human skeletal muscle cells were SILAC-labeled (13C6-Lys) to make a quantitative evaluation of muscle secreted proteins between extreme obese and lean women (Hittel et al., 2009). Assessment of the identified proteins based on published literature and the Swiss-Prot database revealed 28 secreted proteins from 42 identified skeletal muscle proteins. Interestingly, the secretion of myostatin, a negative regulator of skeletal muscle growth and development but also implicated in metabolic homeostasis, was found to be markedly upregulated in extreme obesity cases. Subsequently, Yoon and colleagues presented a study investigating the effects of insulin on the secretory profile of differentiated myotubes (Yoon et al., 2009). The authors combined off-line reverse-phased HPLC fractionation with LC-MS/MS and identified 153 secreted proteins from rat L6 myotubes. Based on spectral count quantitation, 33 of these proteins were classified as differentially regulated in response to insulin. The list of secreted proteins was extracted from a total list of 254 identified proteins using three different prediction tools, Gene Ontology, SignalP, and SecretomeP. In two more recent studies, a total of 108 secreted proteins by skeletal muscle cells were identified (Chan et al., 2011; Norheim et al., 2011).

We have developed a general quantitative proteomics approach for investigation of secreted factors released by skeletal muscle cells during the course of muscle differentiation. The method utilizes a combination of SILAC labeling and advanced mass spectrometry (Fig. 1) (Henningsen et al., 2010).

Triple encoding SILAC, (Blagoev et al., 2004) was applied to investigate protein secretion at three different time points during the course of C2C12 differentiation. Initial evaluation of the differentiation protocol with SILAC-labeled cells demonstrated the formation of a high number of multinucleated myotubes and increased expression of different muscle-specific proteins. The use of three different versions of each labeled amino acid enabled the comparison of the secretome at three different time points (day 0, day 2, and day 5) during skeletal muscle differentiation. Furthermore, cells were cultured using both labeled arginine and lysine, since trypsin, which cleaves solely C-terminal to arginine and lysine, was used for in-gel digestion (Olsen et al., 2004). This "double-triple" labeling with isotopic forms of both arginine and lysine ensures that every tryptic peptide, except the C-terminal peptides of the proteins, contains at least one labeled residue and can therefore be used for quantitation (Blagoev and Mann, 2006). This increases the probability of positive protein identification and accuracy of quantitation due to the increased number of labeled peptides. It is noteworthy that under normal culture conditions cells are grown in the presence of fetal

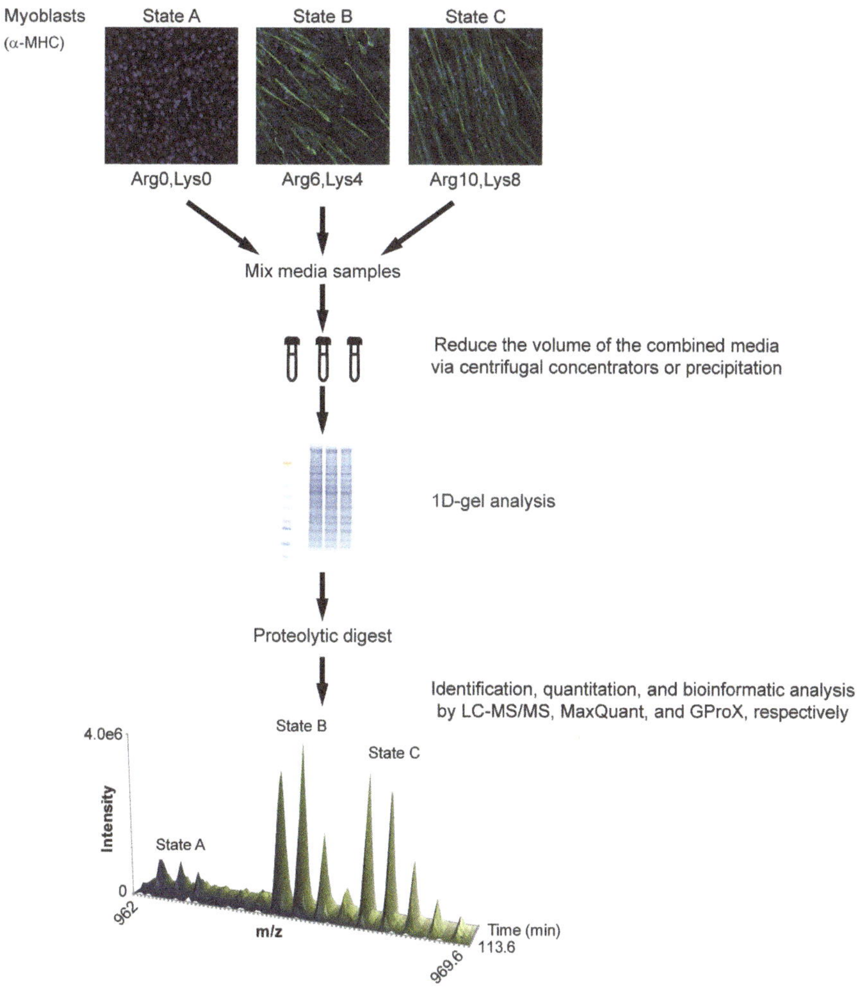

Fig. 1. General outline of QMSP for the identification and quantitation of secreted proteins.

bovine serum (FBS), but the SILAC protocol requires the use of dialyzed sera to prevent the presence of unlabeled sera-derived amino acids, which would ultimately result in inaccurate quantitation. Commercially available dFBS is dialyzed utilizing 10 kDa molecular weight cut off (MWCO) filters to remove any amino acids. Unfortunately, this also leads to the reduction of low-molecular weight proteins (<10 kDa) including certain growth factors, hormones, and cytokines, that may be needed for the growth and maintenance of certain cells. Therefore, dFBS is not compatible with all cell types and slower growth rate is observed in some cases. Ultimately, dialysis with MWCO 1,000 Da could be sufficient to remove amino acids, but it is more costly.

The myoblasts were cultured in SILAC media for at least 5 passages to ensure complete incorporation of labeled amino acids into the proteome. Before the collection of conditioned medium (CM), cells were washed and starved for 12 hours in sera-free medium to minimize the presence of sera proteins, that would interfere with the subsequent mass spectrometry (MS)-analysis. CM was collected from myoblasts on day 0 and during conversion of myoblasts into myotubes at day 2 and day 5, followed by filtration using 0.2 μm filters to remove any floating cells or cell debris, thereby reducing the risk of contaminating samples with intracellular proteins. The CM, collected from the three time points of differentiation was combined in a 1:1:1 ratio according to measured protein concentration. Subsequently, the pool of CM was concentrated by ultrafiltration using Vivaspin columns, MWCO 3,000 Da to ensure that proteins were retained in the concentrate. To reduce sample complexity, thereby effectively increasing the dynamic range of the MS-analysis, concentrated muscle-derived proteins were separated by size using 1D- gel electrophoresis. The excised gel bands were subjected to in-gel digestion and analyzed via LC-MS/MS using an linear ion trap (LTQ)-Orbitrap mass spectrometer followed by processing of the obtained data with the MaxQuant software (Box 2) (Cox and Mann, 2008; Cox et al., 2009). The described strategy resulted in the identification of 635 putatively secreted proteins by skeletal myoblasts based on the GO term "extracellular" and signal peptide prediction inbuilt in the MaxQuant and ProteinCenter. The commercially available database, ProteinCenter, (www. Proxeon.com) utilizes annotation from all major protein sequence databases including Swiss-Prot, NCBI, and Ensembl. It allows analysis of large scale proteomic studies to isolate putatively secreted factors from the total list of identified proteins. The obtained identification list of IPI numbers is filtered and extracted according to the category "extracellular" within GO term cellular component. Then, the remaining proteins are filtered using a signal peptide predictor incorporated into the ProteinCenter platform, the PrediSi algorithm. Using the SILAC strategy, 624 secreted proteins were quantitatively evaluated during the course of skeletal muscle differentiation. Proteins already known to be secreted by skeletal muscle were identified, in addition to many novel proteins not previously shown to be secreted by skeletal myoblasts. Characterization of identified secreted proteins according to GO-annotations demonstrated proteins involved in many different cellular processes including proliferation, differentiation, ECM reorganization, metabolic processes, and angiogenesis. According to the statistical analyses provided by MaxQuant, 188 secreted proteins were found to be dynamically regulated during skeletal myogenesis suggesting their regulatory involvement in skeletal muscle development, which could occur both in autocrine and paracrine manner. In a follow up study, focused on comprehensive characterization of the low abundant low molecular weight fraction of proteins secreted by muscle cells, application of triple encoding SILAC resulted in the generation of quantitative profiles of 59 growth factors and cytokines, including nine classical chemokines (Henningsen et al., 2011).

The depicted triple encoding SILAC strategy led to the characterization of the muscle secretome and creation of dynamic secretion profiles during the process of muscle differentiation. Among the identified secreted factors, we have found components of the extracellular matrix, such as collagen, fibronectin and SPARC (secreted protein acidic and rich in cysteine), growth factors, including members of the transforming growth factor and insulin-like growth factor families, members of the serpin and matrix metalloproteases classes, chemokines, and modulators. In addition, proteins such as angiopoietin-1, VEGF (Vascular endothelial growth factor), PDGF (Platelet-derived growth factor), and FGF21 (Fibroblast growth factor 21) were identified and quantitated.

Combining these results indicate that muscle is a prominent secretory organ participating actively in the general regulation of body homeostasis. The muscle specific secreted factors exert their effects in local and/or systemic manner. In Henningsen et. al., 2010 we have identified and characterized the semaphorins as a new family of muscle secreted proteins. Semaphorins constitute a large family of secreted, GPI-anchored, and transmembrane proteins defined by a conserved semaphorin (sema) domain in their amino terminus (Gherardi et al., 2004; Neufeld and Kessler, 2008; Roth et al., 2009; Serini et al., 2009; Suzuki et al., 2008; Zhou et al., 2008). Initially, semaphorins were described as important regulators of axon guidance during neuronal development. However, an increasing number of studies have recognized the semaphorins as pleiotropic signaling molecules influencing a wide array of biological processes, such as angiogenesis, immune responses, and organ morphogenesis. In addition, semaphorins have also been linked to various pathologies including cancer and different diseases of the nervous system (Neufeld and Kessler, 2008; Roth et al., 2009). Currently, the mammalian semaphorin gene family consists of 20 members and although expression of individual semaphorins has been best described in the nervous system, semaphorins appear to be expressed by most if not all tissues (Yazdani and Terman, 2006). We have identified several members of the semaphorin family belonging to different subfamilies to be secreted from skeletal myoblasts including the soluble Sema3A, Sema3B, Sema3D, Sema3E, the transmembrane Sema4B, Sema4C, and Sema6A, and finally the GPI-linked Sema7A. Examination of the dynamic secretion profiles of the identified semaphorins demonstrated differential secretion of Sema3A, Sema3D, Sema3E, Sema6A, and Sema7A during the course of C2C12 myoblast differentiation. Interestingly, secretion of Sema3A, Sema3E, Sema3D, and Sema6A was markedly enhanced at the early stage of the differentiation, indicating that they may serve a role during the initial phase of the conversion process. In contrast, a gradually increased secretion of Sema7A was observed during differentiation, suggesting that Sema7A plays a role both during early and terminal differentiation. Identification of both the transmembrane and GPI-anchor semaphorins in the media would suggest that they are released from the plasma membrane in a soluble form either by proteolytic shedding, in the case of Sema4 and Sema6, or proteolytic cleavage catalyzed by a phospholipase, in the case of Sema7A. Earlier studies have shown that the enzymatic activity of metalloproteases can generate and modulate the activity of a soluble form of Sema4D (Basile et al., 2007; Elhabazi et al., 2001). Indeed, we did observe an increased secretion of various proteases including MMP-2. Western blot analysis of sema6A in conditioned media collected from C2C12 myoblasts during differentiation supported the idea of Sema6A shedding, as the secreted protein migrated at an apparent molecular weight corresponding to the size of the extracellular domain (approx. 71 kDa) and not to the size of the full-length Sema6A (approx. 113 kDa). Different members of the semaphorin family have been shown to orchestrate the development of different organs including bone, lung, kidney, and the cardiovascular system (Roth et al., 2009; Tamagnone and Giordano, 2006). The number of studies investigating the function of semaphorins in skeletal muscle development and regeneration are more limited. So far, studies have demonstrated an enhanced expression of Sema4C but no alterations of Sema4B expression during C2C12 myogenesis were detected (Ko et al., 2005; Wu et al., 2007). In addition, enhanced expression of Sema4C was also observed *in vivo* in injury-induced skeletal muscle regeneration. Targeted knockdown of Sema4C expression by siRNA caused inhibition of C2C12 myotube formation, demonstrating that semaphorins could exert an active autocrine/paracrine function in myogenesis. Interestingly, animal models have suggested that semaphorins could be important paracrine factors regulating neurogenesis during skeletal muscle growth, development, and regeneration. A delayed transient increase of Sema3A expression was observed in response to muscle-induced injury (Tatsumi et al., 2009). In addition, a similar delay of Sema3A expression and secretion was seen in isolated skeletal muscle cells in response to HGF, which is an essential factor in muscle growth and regeneration. In our study, we have identified both Sema3A and Sema4C to be released by C2C12 myoblasts during differentiation.

We have analyzed the mRNA and protein expression of selected regulated members of the semaphorin family (Sema3A, Sema3E, Sema6A, and Sema7A) to investigate if their dynamic secretion pattern was regulated by post-transcriptional and post-translational mechanisms. Only minor changes were observed in the mRNA expression of Sema3A, Sema3E, Sema6A, and Sema7A. The mRNA expression of Sema3A and Sema7A remained constant during differentiation, whereas there was a slight decrease and increase in the level of Sema3E and Sema6A, respectively. We found that the high levels of secreted Sema3A and Sema3E at early stage of myotube formation did not reflect the intracellular protein levels of these semaphorins. Expression of Sema3A protein remained constant, whereas a slight decrease was observed of Sema3E protein expression in accordance with the corresponding RNA profile of Sema3A and Sema3E. Moreover, although the intracellular level of Sema7A protein was increased at day 5 of differentiation, it did not correlate with the gradually enhanced level of secreted protein. These finding shows that the level of secreted semaphorin proteins can be regulated both by post-transcriptional and post-translational mechanisms. This is in agreement with previous findings in which imperfect correlation between RNA and protein expression was observed (Bonaldi et al., 2008; de Godoy et al., 2008; Kratchmarova et al., 2002). It also emphasizes the necessity to quantitatively investigate protein abundance to understand the functional role exhibited by individual genes and their corresponding proteins. These results clearly illustrate, that when studying the complex nature of the secreted factors it is important to observe both the intracellular level of proteins and their secretion profiles since they might differ due to post-translational modification or modulation of their release via the secretory pathway, turnover rate, and/or processing.

4. Pitfalls of the studies on secreted proteins

One of the major challenges in secretome studies is the identification and classification of secreted proteins from the total number of identified proteins from the proteomics experiment. Secreted proteins are released in the extracellular space via two routes: the classical and non-classical secretory pathways (Box 1).

4.1 Secretory pathway, classical

Majority of eukaryotic proteins are secreted by the classical endoplasmic reticulum (ER)-Golgi secretory pathway consisting of a number of distinct membrane-bound compartments interconnected by vesicular traffic (Baines and Zhang, 2007; De Matteis and Luini; Nickel and Rabouille, 2009; Nickel and Wieland, 1998; Park and Loh, 2008; Pelham, 1996; Strating and Martens, 2009). Many basic cellular functions take place in the ER including folding of newly synthesized transmembrane and secretory proteins, lipid synthesis, and the storage

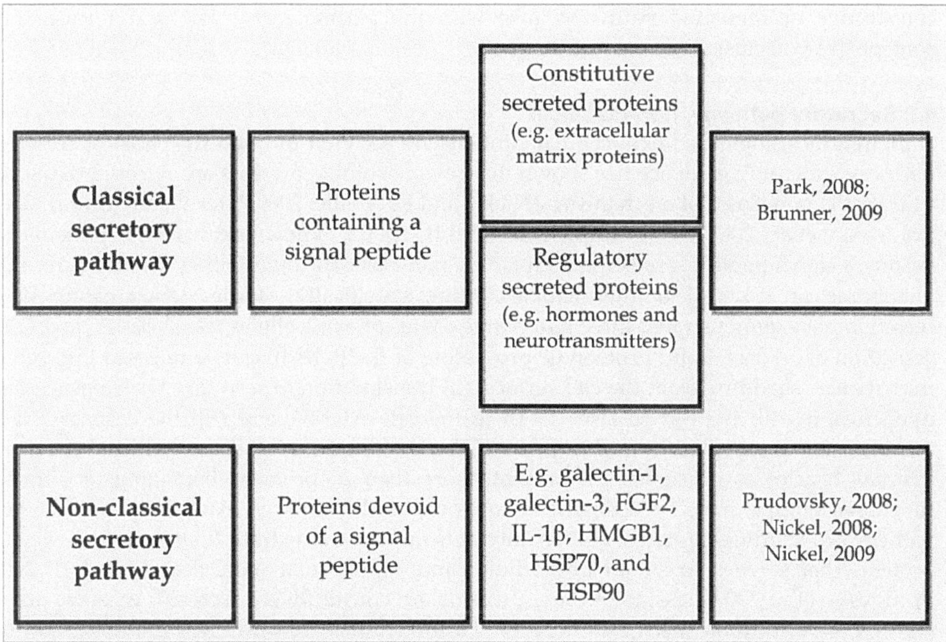

Box 1. Classification of secretory pathways

of high concentrations of calcium ions (Marie et al., 2008; Mayor and Riezman, 2004; Sallese et al., 2009; Strating and Martens, 2009). In addition, post-translational modifications of soluble and membrane proteins occur in the ER lumen including oxidation of proline, N-linked glycosylation, proteolytic processing, formation of disulfide bonds, oligomerization, and attachment of a GPI-anchor. Whereas the main functions of the Golgi apparatus include carbohydrate synthesis, O-linked glycosylation, processing, post-translational modification, and sorting both proteins and lipids (De Matteis and Luini, 2008; Marie et al., 2008; Marsh and Howell, 2002). Regardless of their subsequent fate, most proteins containing a N-terminal or internal signal sequence peptide can be targeted to the ER membrane. These include transmembrane proteins destined to reside in the ER, plasma membrane or other organellar membranes as well as soluble proteins destined to the lumen of an organelle or for secretion. With the exception of mitochondria, nuclei, and peroxisomes, all other organelles receive their proteins via the ER. Signal peptides show extreme variations in their length and amino acid composition, but do contain three distinct domains: a positively charged N-terminal region, a hydrophobic core region, typically consisting of at least 6 hydrophobic residues, and C-terminal region of polar uncharged residues (Hiller et al., 2004). Soluble proteins are transported from the Golgi to the cell exterior via the constitutive secretory pathway transporting proteins directly to the cell surface or the regulated secretory pathway in which soluble proteins and other substances are initially stored in secretory vesicles, which release proteins to the extracellular space upon extracellular signals (Brunner et al., 2009; De Matteis and Luini, 2008; Strating and Martens, 2009). The latter pathway only exists in specialized secretory cells including pancreatic β-cell releasing insulin from secretory vesicles, nerve cells, and endocrine cells. The secretory vesicles of the constitutive or regulated pathways fuse with the plasma membrane and release their contents by exocytosis.

4.2 Secretory pathway, non-classical

Although most identified extracellular proteins are secreted through the classical secretory pathway, emerging evidence has shown that several soluble proteins are released to the cell exterior via non-classical mechanisms (Nickel and Rabouille, 2009; Nickel and Seedorf, 2008; Prudovsky et al., 2008). For example FGF2 and IL-1β, well known extracellular proteins but lacking a signal peptide, are being secreted by non-classical routes either directly across the membrane or via vesicle intermediates. More specifically, studies investigating IL-1β secretion have demonstrated three alternative routes of extracellular translocation involving activation of caspase 1 and proteolytic processing of IL-1β. IL-1β can be released through (i) microvesicle shedding from the cell surface, (ii) translocation to secretory lysosomes, which upon fusion with the PM releases IL-1β to the cell exterior, and (iii) the caspase 1-Il-1β complex can be captured by endosomal vesicles creating multivesicular bodies that release internal vesicles as exosomes. At present, more than 20 proteins, belonging to different functional groups, have been described to be released to the cell exterior by non-classical pathways, including proteins that mainly function in the extracellular space as well as proteins that serve a role both intracellular and extracellular (Nickel and Seedorf, 2008; Prudovsky et al., 2008). Some of these proteins are constitutively secreted, whereas others are first released upon specific stimulation. Future studies are warranted to understand the biological function and regulation of the many different secretory pathways as well as the number and function of proteins devoid of a signal peptide but released to the extracellular space. Secretion of proteins by alternative pathways, which require interaction with other proteins and/or proteolytic activation, could impose additional levels of regulation to protein secretion (Nickel and Rabouille, 2009; Prudovsky et al., 2008). In addition, alternative secretion of signal peptide containing proteins that bypass the Golgi apparatus, could cause alterations in the structures of post-transcriptional modifications, such as glycosylation, or prevent proper proteolytic processing. This could be a way to modulate the biological activity of secreted proteins under certain physiological conditions.

In addition to the two general pathways of secretion, proteins are also being released to the cell exterior due to apoptosis or cell leakage, thereby contaminating the pool of true secreted proteins. In this regard, the increased performance of MS-instrumentation not only improves the dynamic range for the identification of secreted proteins but also increases the number of identified proteins originating from the intracellular space. One example was presented in the study by Henningsen et al., 2011 focusing on the low molecular weight proteins. The quantitative mass spectrometry analysis resulted in the identification of more than 2000 proteins however, less than 25% of these proteins were predicted to be secreted according to conventional database analyses based on the GO term extracellular and signal peptide prediction. Among the predicted secreted proteins, there were also tubulins, a number of ribosomal proteins, and membrane proteins that are not encountered as being truly secreted. Nevertheless, some of the cytoskeletal and ribosomal proteins have been demonstrated to be part of the exosomes and as such are being released in the extracellular environment. Major part of the exosomes consists of tubulins and Tsg101, which is a well-known exosome marker, was also identified as a secreted protein (Henningsen et al., 2011; Thery et al., 2002). Different tools are being used to classify the extracellular compartment in various secretome studies, most commonly being assessment based on literature searches, GO-annotations and/or algorithms predicting secretion by classical (SignalP) or non-classical (SecretomeP) mechanisms (Box 2). Extraction of secreted proteins based on previous reported studies is extremely time-consuming considering the large number of identified proteins by today's advanced MS. In addition, this will only result in the identification of proteins already shown by experimental data to be secreted. Isolation of secreted proteins from a large list of identified proteins can be done combining GO classification as extracellular and/or prediction of a signal peptide. However, all these tools do come with certain restrictions that could lead to either false positive or false negative identifications of secretion status. The presence of a signal peptide is not restricted to extracellular proteins. Proteins destined for other intracellular compartments, such as the ER or Golgi, also contains a signal peptide. In addition, GO terms are assigned according to different parameters, including computational analyses of sequences in addition to experimental data. Again, predictions based on sequence information could result in false positive identification of secreted proteins as well. Prediction tools always have their own limitations and therefore bona fide secreted proteins could also be lost by these tools. Most affected in this regard are the proteins released from cells by non-conventional mechanisms whose number is still low but steadily increasing (Nickel and Rabouille, 2009; Prudovsky et al., 2008).

Open source software and databases

MaxQuant (http://maxquant.org): Advanced software program used as a tool for both protein identification and quantitation (Cox and Mann, 2008; Cox et al., 2009).

SignalP (http://www.cbs.dtu.dk/services/SignalP): Predicting the presence of a signal peptide, suggesting proteins could be secreted through the classical pathway (Bendtsen et al., 2004b; Emanuelsson et al., 2007).

SecretomeP (http://www.cbs.dtu.dk/services/SecretomeP): Prediction of proteins to be secreted by non-classical mechanisms (Bendtsen et al., 2004a).

QuickGO provided by the Gene Ontology Annotation (GOA) group (http://www.ebi.ac.uk/GOA): Bioinformatics resource integrating various databases to assign subcellular localization and functional annotation according to GO terms (Barrell et al., 2009; Binns et al., 2009).

GProX (http://gprox.sourceforge.net): Bioinformatics platform, which support the analysis and visualization of large-scale proteomics data (Rigbolt et al., 2011).

Commercially available database

ProteinCenter (http://www.proxeon.com): Software tool combining several data bases to analyze the biological context of complex proteomics experiments.

Box 2. Software and databases commonly used in quantitative mass spectrometry-based proteomics research of secreted proteins

The high number of identified proteins in the QMSP experiments, which are not classified as secreted could be present in the extracellular space (conditioned medium) due to cell leakage or release of intracellular proteins from necrotic or apoptotic cells. The apoptotic process is a normal process that all cells grown in culture undergo at a given time point. However, the number of dead cells is limited since the protocol for collection of media is optimized such as to reduce the number of dying cells. In addition, the collected CM is typically filtrated using a 0.2 μm filter to ensure removal of any dead cells and thereby to reduce contamination from intracellular proteins. The presence of intracellular proteins might be explained by other structures present in the extracellular space such as exosomes and their cargo. Another point is that prediction of a signal peptide by itself does not exclude the possibility that these proteins are in fact located in other intracellular compartments of the cells, such as the ER and Golgi. On the other hand, an increasing number of proteins are being recognized as extracellular despite lacking a signal peptide and thought to be released through non-classical pathways (Nickel and Rabouille, 2009; Prudovsky et al., 2008). In the literature, more than 20 proteins devoid of any signal peptide have been shown to reside in the extracellular space and being released by non-conventional mechanisms. SecretomeP (Box 2) has been designed to predict non-classical secreted proteins (Bendtsen et al., 2004a). For that purpose 13 known human non-classical secreted proteins were analyzed, but no specific sequence motif was identified to characterize non-classical secretion. Instead, the non-classical software for prediction was developed using the multiple sequence features of the 13 non-classical secreted proteins combined with sequence information obtained from more than 3,000 classical secreted proteins. Due to the limited number of identified non-classical proteins, the value of this prediction approach is difficult to assess. Submitting either the murine or human sequence of galectin-1 to SecretomeP resulted in probability score of < 0.5, thereby exemplifying a false negative identification. Galectin-1 is a well-known extracellular protein lacking a signal peptide but released by non-conventional ways (Hughes, 1999; Sango et al., 2004). On the other hand HMGB1, also not containing a signal peptide and mainly known for its role as a chromatin modifying protein, is also serving an extracellular function suggesting that proteins with typically intracellular functions could also be released to the cell exterior (Bonaldi et al., 2003 2002; Gardella et al., 2002). Future studies will help to elucidate how many proteins deficient in a signal peptide are being released to the extracellular space. Classifying proteins as extracellular based on GO annotation can also lead to false negative or false positive classifications. GO annotation are based both on experimental data but also on computational analysis of sequence information. With the increasing number of biomarker directed studies analyzing biofluids by mass spectrometry, the number of classified secreted proteins is steadily increasing. The increased number of identified secreted proteins could be due to improvements of mass spectrometry technology, which increased the overall sensitivity of protein identification, but could also be artifacts derived from dead cells floating around in the circulation.

In summary, combination of different tools and manually curated data might be beneficial when validating the large lists obtained from QMSP experiments focusing on secreted factors. Nevertheless, release of cellular components can occur via microvesicles and/or exosomes adding to the complexity of secretome studies, thus some of the factors commonly counted as contaminants might be truly secreted ones.

4.3 Serum contaminants

Mammalian cell culture models are broadly used in proteomics experiments and often contamination with bovine serum proteins, originating from the serum supplement used for the culturing of cells, is observed in the results from the mass spectrometric analyses. Naturally, when studying the proteins released by specific types of cells, one of the biggest challenges remains the presence of serum proteins that could interfere with the identification of proteins secreted by the cells. Presence of serum proteins in the sample can disrupt the concentration of the CM as well as interfere with the MS analysis, masking the presence of other proteins. It has been estimated that a 10% FBS serum complement, which is commonly added to the culture media, adds 5-6 mg/ml protein to the media and even extensive washing of the cells might not be sufficient to remove the bovine proteins to levels below the detection limit of the mass spectrometer (Bunkenborg et al., 2010). The sera-derived proteins could be falsely identified as proteins being secreted by the cells due to sequence homology between species. One suggested solution to exclude bovine contaminants was based on expanding the database to include both the human and the bovine proteome. Another alternative is to extend the database to include known bovine contaminants as a common contaminant list, which is already incorporated in the data analysis by programs such as MaxQuant (Bunkenborg et al., 2010; Henningsen et al., 2011; Henningsen et al., 2010). In this way, it is possible to exclude the proteins recognized as contaminants from the initial list of identifications and thereby to minimize the number of identifications originating from sera proteins. Nevertheless, the SILAC strategy is so far the best known applicable method to investigate secreted factors by a given type of cells since the metabolic labeling makes it possible to distinguish cell-derived secreted proteins, as these are SILAC labeled, from residual sera proteins. Only proteins that are synthesized in the cells in the presence of the heavy SILAC amino acid will be labeled, thereby these are easily distinguished from sera contaminants, which remain unlabeled. In addition, the accuracy of protein quantitation could also be compromised by the presence of sera proteins in the samples. It is therefore advisable to perform a replica experiment with reverse SILAC labeling strategy (Schulze and Mann, 2004), which is an easy solution to overcome this possible drawback as well as to ensure high quality quantitation of bona fide secreted proteins.

4.4 Post-translational modifications of secreted proteins

Glycosylation of secreted proteins is one of the most abundant post-translational modifications (PTM), which affects the proteins folding, stability, and activity. The oligosaccharides are linked to the proteins via asparagine (N-linked) or serine/threonine (O-linked) residues. Enrichment of secreted proteins through their glycan structures is an alternative experimental strategy for the identification of secreted proteins. Various types of enrichment methods have been utilized to capture glycosylated proteins, one of the common approaches being lectin affinity chromatography. In an elegant study by Zielinska et al., the combinatorial use of optimized lectin-based enrichment step, subcellular fractionation, deglycosylation assays, SILAC labeling, advanced mass spectrometry followed by integrative bioinformatic analyses resulted in the identification of 6367 N-glycosylation sites on 2352 proteins in four mouse tissues and blood plasma. N-glycosylation was found to occur exclusively on secreted proteins, on the extracellular face of membrane proteins, and on the lumenal side of ER, Golgi apparatus, and lysosomes

(Zielinska et al., 2010). In a complementary study using formalin-fixed paraffin-embedded tissue samples, 1500 N-glycosylation sites were found underlying the increased sensitivity and accuracy of the mass spectrometry-based proteomics for identification of post-translationally modified proteins, even in fixed samples. The comparison of fresh tissue using SILAC-labeled mouse (Kruger et al., 2008) with the paraffin embedded tissue showed no significant qualitative or quantitative differences between these samples, either at protein or peptide level, thereby permitting the use of this methodology in clinical studies (Ostasiewicz et al., 2010).
Hydroxyproline is another type of PTM that is identified predominantly on components of the extracellular matrix and especially on different types of collagens. We have recently reported the identification of 299 unique high-confidence hydroxyproline sites from 48 distinct secreted proteins in muscle cells, representing the largest data set so far on this proline modification. 231 of the modified prolines were located on various collagen types with a large variation of the number of modified sites per individual protein. The number ranged from 1 site on collagen alpha-3 type VI to more than 70 on collagen alpha-1 type I, highlighting the importance of the proline modification in maintaining the structure of the collagens. Motif sequence analysis revealed the canonical motif previously reported for collagen proteins as well as a novel hydroxyproline motif. Modified peptides containing hydroxyproline sites extend over more than 40 proteins including fatty acid binding protein (FABP), several components of the ECM such as SPARC, fibronectin, Lama2, perlecan, and different inhibitors of proteolytic enzymes such as serine protease inhibitors (serpinf1 and serphinh1) and the metalloproteinase inhibitor 2 (Timp2). These results indicate that hydroxyproline could serve as an important secondary modification to confer protein stability and interaction with other secreted proteins.

5. Conclusion

The rapid development of MS-instrumentation combined with the advances of quantitative proteomics strategies, such as SILAC, has had a tremendous impact in the analysis of complex biological systems. QMSP is increasingly becoming an essential approach, especially for the characterization of entire secretomes and generation of dynamic quantitative profiles of secreted factors during the course of cellular differentiation or in response to drugs, inhibitors, and modulators. Although there have been a marked improvement of the proteomics strategies to characterize secretomes, many challenges still remain: minimizing the suppressive effect of growth supplements present in the sample during MS analyses, identification of whole tissue secretomes, collection of samples under specific conditions to avoid induction of cell death, identification of low abundant low molecular weight proteins. However, the most critical point presented by secretome studies today is to isolate the bona fide secreted proteins and to validate the obtained results. Integrative approaches that combine highly advanced proteomics methodology followed by biological functional analyses can lead to the creation of secretome maps that underline tissue crosstalk and communication.

6. Acknowledgment

This work was supported by a grant from the Novo Nordisk Foundation, the Lundbeck Foundation and the Augustinus Foundation. IK is supported by grants from the Danish

Natural Science Research Council and the Danish Medical Research Council. BB is supported by grant from the Lundbeck Foundation and the Danish Natural Science Research Council.

7. References

Aebersold, R., and M. Mann. 2003. Mass spectrometry-based proteomics. *Nature*. 422:198-207.

Alvarez-Llamas, G., E. Szalowska, M.P. de Vries, D. Weening, K. Landman, A. Hoek, B.H. Wolffenbuttel, H. Roelofsen, and R.J. Vonk. 2007. Characterization of the human visceral adipose tissue secretome. *Mol. Cell. Proteomics*. 6:589-600.

Andersen, J.S., C.J. Wilkinson, T. Mayor, P. Mortensen, E.A. Nigg, and M. Mann. 2003. Proteomic characterization of the human centrosome by protein correlation profiling. *Nature*. 426:570-574.

Baines, A.C., and B. Zhang. 2007. Receptor-mediated protein transport in the early secretory pathway. *Trends Biochem. Sci.* 32:381-388.

Barrell, D., E. Dimmer, R.P. Huntley, D. Binns, C. O'Donovan, and R. Apweiler. 2009. The GOA database in 2009--an integrated Gene Ontology Annotation resource. *Nucleic acids research*. 37:D396-403.

Basile, J.R., K. Holmbeck, T.H. Bugge, and J.S. Gutkind. 2007. MT1-MMP controls tumor-induced angiogenesis through the release of semaphorin 4D. *J. Biol. Chem.* 282:6899-6905.

Bendtsen, J.D., L.J. Jensen, N. Blom, G. Von Heijne, and S. Brunak. 2004a. Feature-based prediction of non-classical and leaderless protein secretion. *Protein Eng. Des. Sel.* 17:349-356.

Bendtsen, J.D., H. Nielsen, G. von Heijne, and S. Brunak. 2004b. Improved prediction of signal peptides: SignalP 3.0. *Journal of molecular biology*. 340:783-795.

Binns, D., E. Dimmer, R. Huntley, D. Barrell, C. O'Donovan, and R. Apweiler. 2009. QuickGO: a web-based tool for Gene Ontology searching. *Bioinformatics*. 25:3045-3046.

Blagoev, B., I. Kratchmarova, S.E. Ong, M. Nielsen, L.J. Foster, and M. Mann. 2003. A proteomics strategy to elucidate functional protein-protein interactions applied to EGF signaling. *Nat. Biotechnol.* 21:315-318.

Blagoev, B., and M. Mann. 2006. Quantitative proteomics to study mitogen-activated protein kinases. *Methods*. 40:243-250.

Blagoev, B., S.E. Ong, I. Kratchmarova, and M. Mann. 2004. Temporal analysis of phosphotyrosine-dependent signaling networks by quantitative proteomics. *Nat. Biotechnol.* 22:1139-1145.

Bonaldi, T., T. Straub, J. Cox, C. Kumar, P.B. Becker, and M. Mann. 2008. Combined use of RNAi and quantitative proteomics to study gene function in Drosophila. *Mol. Cell.* 31:762-772.

Bonaldi, T., F. Talamo, P. Scaffidi, D. Ferrera, A. Porto, A. Bachi, A. Rubartelli, A. Agresti, and M.E. Bianchi. 2003. Monocytic cells hyperacetylate chromatin protein HMGB1 to redirect it towards secretion. *EMBO J.* 22:5551-5560.

Brand, M., J.A. Ranish, N.T. Kummer, J. Hamilton, K. Igarashi, C. Francastel, T.H. Chi, G.R. Crabtree, R. Aebersold, and M. Groudine. 2004. Dynamic changes in transcription factor complexes during erythroid differentiation revealed by quantitative proteomics. *Nat Struct Mol Biol*. 11:73-80.

Brunner, Y., D. Schvartz, Y. Coute, and J.C. Sanchez. 2009. Proteomics of regulated secretory organelles. *Mass Spectrom. Rev.* 28:844-867.

Bunkenborg, J., G.E. Garcia, M.I. Paz, J.S. Andersen, and H. Molina. 2010. The minotaur proteome: avoiding cross-species identifications deriving from bovine serum in cell culture models. *Proteomics*. 10:3040-3044.

Chan, C.Y., O. Masui, O. Krakovska, V.E. Belozerov, S. Voisin, S. Ghanny, J. Chen, D. Moyez, P. Zhu, K.R. Evans, J.C. McDermott, and K.W. Siu. 2011. Identification of differentially regulated secretome components during skeletal myogenesis. *Molecular & cellular proteomics : MCP*. 10:M110 004804.

Chan, X.C., J.C. McDermott, and K.W. Siu. 2007. Identification of secreted proteins during skeletal muscle development. *J. Proteome Res.* 6:698-710.

Chelius, D., and P.V. Bondarenko. 2002. Quantitative profiling of proteins in complex mixtures using liquid chromatography and mass spectrometry. *J Proteome Res.* 1:317-323.

Clamp, M., B. Fry, M. Kamal, X. Xie, J. Cuff, M.F. Lin, M. Kellis, K. Lindblad-Toh, and E.S. Lander. 2007. Distinguishing protein-coding and noncoding genes in the human genome. *Proceedings of the National Academy of Sciences of the United States of America*. 104:19428-19433.

Conrads, T.P., K. Alving, T.D. Veenstra, M.E. Belov, G.A. Anderson, D.J. Anderson, M.S. Lipton, L. Pasa-Tolic, H.R. Udseth, W.B. Chrisler, B.D. Thrall, and R.D. Smith. 2001. Quantitative analysis of bacterial and mammalian proteomes using a combination of cysteine affinity tags and 15N-metabolic labeling. *Anal Chem*. 73:2132-2139.

Cox, J., and M. Mann. 2007. Is proteomics the new genomics? *Cell*. 130:395-398.

Cox, J., and M. Mann. 2008. MaxQuant enables high peptide identification rates, individualized p.p.b.-range mass accuracies and proteome-wide protein quantification. *Nat. Biotechnol.* 26:1367-1372.

Cox, J., I. Matic, M. Hilger, N. Nagaraj, M. Selbach, J.V. Olsen, and M. Mann. 2009. A practical guide to the MaxQuant computational platform for SILAC-based quantitative proteomics. *Nat. Protoc.* 4:698-705.

de Godoy, L.M., J.V. Olsen, J. Cox, M.L. Nielsen, N.C. Hubner, F. Frohlich, T.C. Walther, and M. Mann. 2008. Comprehensive mass-spectrometry-based proteome quantification of haploid versus diploid yeast. *Nature*. 455:1251-1254.

De Matteis, M.A., and A. Luini. 2008. Exiting the Golgi complex. *Nat. Rev. Mol. Cell Biol.* 9:273-284.

Dengjel, J., I. Kratchmarova, and B. Blagoev. 2009. Receptor tyrosine kinase signaling: a view from quantitative proteomics. *Mol. Biosyst.* 5:1112-1121.

Dengjel, J., I. Kratchmarova, and B. Blagoev. 2010. Mapping protein-protein interactions by quantitative proteomics. *Methods Mol Biol*. 658:267-278.

Elhabazi, A., S. Delaire, A. Bensussan, L. Boumsell, and G. Bismuth. 2001. Biological activity of soluble CD100. I. The extracellular region of CD100 is released from the surface of T lymphocytes by regulated proteolysis. *J. Immunol.* 166:4341-4347.

Emanuelsson, O., S. Brunak, G. von Heijne, and H. Nielsen. 2007. Locating proteins in the cell using TargetP, SignalP and related tools. *Nature protocols*. 2:953-971.

Flier, J.S. 2001. Diabetes. The missing link with obesity? *Nature*. 409:292-293.

Gardella, S., C. Andrei, D. Ferrera, L.V. Lotti, M.R. Torrisi, M.E. Bianchi, and A. Rubartelli. 2002. The nuclear protein HMGB1 is secreted by monocytes via a non-classical, vesicle-mediated secretory pathway. *EMBO Rep.* 3:995-1001.
Geiger, T., J. Cox, P. Ostasiewicz, J.R. Wisniewski, and M. Mann. 2010. Super-SILAC mix for quantitative proteomics of human tumor tissue. *Nature methods.* 7:383-385.
Gherardi, E., C.A. Love, R.M. Esnouf, and E.Y. Jones. 2004. The sema domain. *Curr. Opin. Struct. Biol.* 14:669-678.
Gygi, S.P., G.L. Corthals, Y. Zhang, Y. Rochon, and R. Aebersold. 2000. Evaluation of two-dimensional gel electrophoresis-based proteome analysis technology. *Proc Natl Acad Sci U S A.* 97:9390-9395.
Gygi, S.P., B. Rist, S.A. Gerber, F. Turecek, M.H. Gelb, and R. Aebersold. 1999. Quantitative analysis of complex protein mixtures using isotope-coded affinity tags. *Nat. Biotechnol.* 17:994-999.
Han, D.K., J. Eng, H. Zhou, and R. Aebersold. 2001. Quantitative profiling of differentiation-induced microsomal proteins using isotope-coded affinity tags and mass spectrometry. *Nat Biotechnol.* 19:946-951.
Henningsen, J., B.K. Pedersen, and I. Kratchmarova. 2011. Quantitative analysis of the secretion of the MCP family of chemokines by muscle cells. *Mol Biosyst.* 7:311-321.
Henningsen, J., K.T. Rigbolt, B. Blagoev, B.K. Pedersen, and I. Kratchmarova. 2010. Dynamics of the Skeletal Muscle Secretome during Myoblast Differentiation. *Mol. Cell. Proteomics.* 9:2482-2496.
Hiller, K., A. Grote, M. Scheer, R. Munch, and D. Jahn. 2004. PrediSi: prediction of signal peptides and their cleavage positions. *Nucleic Acids Res.* 32:W375-379.
Hittel, D.S., J.R. Berggren, J. Shearer, K. Boyle, and J.A. Houmard. 2009. Increased secretion and expression of myostatin in skeletal muscle from extremely obese women. *Diabetes.* 58:30-38.
Hughes, R.C. 1999. Secretion of the galectin family of mammalian carbohydrate-binding proteins. *Biochim. Biophys. Acta.* 1473:172-185.
Ko, J.A., T. Gondo, S. Inagaki, and M. Inui. 2005. Requirement of the transmembrane semaphorin Sema4C for myogenic differentiation. *FEBS Lett.* 579:2236-2242.
Kratchmarova, I., B. Blagoev, M. Haack-Sorensen, M. Kassem, and M. Mann. 2005. Mechanism of divergent growth factor effects in mesenchymal stem cell differentiation. *Science.* 308:1472-1477.
Kratchmarova, I., D.E. Kalume, B. Blagoev, P.E. Scherer, A.V. Podtelejnikov, H. Molina, P.E. Bickel, J.S. Andersen, M.M. Fernandez, J. Bunkenborg, P. Roepstorff, K. Kristiansen, H.F. Lodish, M. Mann, and A. Pandey. 2002. A proteomic approach for identification of secreted proteins during the differentiation of 3T3-L1 preadipocytes to adipocytes. *Mol. Cell. Proteomics.* 1:213-222.
Krijgsveld, J., R.F. Ketting, T. Mahmoudi, J. Johansen, M. Artal-Sanz, C.P. Verrijzer, R.H. Plasterk, and A.J. Heck. 2003. Metabolic labeling of C. elegans and D. melanogaster for quantitative proteomics. *Nat Biotechnol.* 21:927-931.
Kruger, M., M. Moser, S. Ussar, I. Thievessen, C.A. Luber, F. Forner, S. Schmidt, S. Zanivan, R. Fassler, and M. Mann. 2008. SILAC mouse for quantitative proteomics uncovers kindlin-3 as an essential factor for red blood cell function. *Cell.* 134:353-364.
Kubota, K., K. Wakabayashi, and T. Matsuoka. 2003. Proteome analysis of secreted proteins during osteoclast differentiation using two different methods: two-dimensional

electrophoresis and isotope-coded affinity tags analysis with two-dimensional chromatography. *Proteomics*. 3:616-626.

Lin, H., E. Lee, K. Hestir, C. Leo, M. Huang, E. Bosch, R. Halenbeck, G. Wu, A. Zhou, D. Behrens, D. Hollenbaugh, T. Linnemann, M. Qin, J. Wong, K. Chu, S.K. Doberstein, and L.T. Williams. 2008. Discovery of a cytokine and its receptor by functional screening of the extracellular proteome. *Science*. 320:807-811.

Lundgren, D.H., S.I. Hwang, L. Wu, and D.K. Han. 2010. Role of spectral counting in quantitative proteomics. *Expert review of proteomics*. 7:39-53.

Marie, M., R. Sannerud, H. Avsnes Dale, and J. Saraste. 2008. Take the 'A' train: on fast tracks to the cell surface. *Cell. Mol. Life Sci.* 65:2859-2874.

Marsh, B.J., and K.E. Howell. 2002. The mammalian Golgi--complex debates. *Nat. Rev. Mol. Cell Biol.* 3:789-795.

Mayor, S., and H. Riezman. 2004. Sorting GPI-anchored proteins. *Nat. Rev. Mol. Cell Biol.* 5:110-120.

Neufeld, G., and O. Kessler. 2008. The semaphorins: versatile regulators of tumour progression and tumour angiogenesis. *Nat. Rev. Cancer*. 8:632-645.

Nickel, W., and C. Rabouille. 2009. Mechanisms of regulated unconventional protein secretion. *Nat. Rev. Mol. Cell Biol.* 10:148-155.

Nickel, W., and M. Seedorf. 2008. Unconventional mechanisms of protein transport to the cell surface of eukaryotic cells. *Annu. Rev. Cell Dev. Biol.* 24:287-308.

Nickel, W., and F.T. Wieland. 1998. Biosynthetic protein transport through the early secretory pathway. *Histochem. Cell Biol.* 109:477-486.

Norheim, F., T. Raastad, B. Thiede, A.C. Rustan, C.A. Drevon, and F. Haugen. 2011. Proteomic identification of secreted proteins from human skeletal muscle cells and expression in response to strength training. *American journal of physiology. Endocrinology and metabolism.*

Oda, Y., K. Huang, F.R. Cross, D. Cowburn, and B.T. Chait. 1999. Accurate quantitation of protein expression and site-specific phosphorylation. *Proc. Natl. Acad. Sci. U. S. A.* 96:6591-6596.

Olsen, J.V., B. Blagoev, F. Gnad, B. Macek, C. Kumar, P. Mortensen, and M. Mann. 2006. Global, in vivo, and site-specific phosphorylation dynamics in signaling networks. *Cell*. 127:635-648.

Olsen, J.V., S.E. Ong, and M. Mann. 2004. Trypsin cleaves exclusively C-terminal to arginine and lysine residues. *Mol. Cell. Proteomics*. 3:608-614.

Ong, S.E., B. Blagoev, I. Kratchmarova, D.B. Kristensen, H. Steen, A. Pandey, and M. Mann. 2002. Stable isotope labeling by amino acids in cell culture, SILAC, as a simple and accurate approach to expression proteomics. *Mol. Cell. Proteomics*. 1:376-386.

Ong, S.E., I. Kratchmarova, and M. Mann. 2003. Properties of 13C-substituted arginine in stable isotope labeling by amino acids in cell culture (SILAC). *J. Proteome Res.* 2:173-181.

Ong, S.E., and M. Mann. 2005. Mass spectrometry-based proteomics turns quantitative. *Nat. Chem. Biol.* 1:252-262.

Osinalde, N., H. Moss, O. Arrizabalaga, M.J. Omaetxebarria, B. Blagoev, A.M. Zubiaga, A. Fullaondo, J.M. Arizmendi, and I. Kratchmarova. 2011. Interleukin-2 signaling pathway analysis by quantitative phosphoproteomics. *Journal of proteomics*.

Ostasiewicz, P., D.F. Zielinska, M. Mann, and J.R. Wisniewski. 2010. Proteome, phosphoproteome, and N-glycoproteome are quantitatively preserved in formalin-fixed paraffin-embedded tissue and analyzable by high-resolution mass spectrometry. *Journal of proteome research*. 9:3688-3700.

Park, J.J., and Y.P. Loh. 2008. How peptide hormone vesicles are transported to the secretion site for exocytosis. *Mol. Endocrinol.* 22:2583-2595.

Pedersen, B.K. 2009. The diseasome of physical inactivity--and the role of myokines in muscle--fat cross talk. *J. Physiol.* 587:5559-5568.

Pelham, H.R. 1996. The dynamic organisation of the secretory pathway. *Cell Struct. Funct.* 21:413-419.

Prudovsky, I., F. Tarantini, M. Landriscina, D. Neivandt, R. Soldi, A. Kirov, D. Small, K.M. Kathir, D. Rajalingam, and T.K. Kumar. 2008. Secretion without Golgi. *J. Cell. Biochem.* 103:1327-1343.

Rigbolt, K.T., and B. Blagoev. 2010. Proteome-wide quantitation by SILAC. *Methods Mol Biol.* 658:187-204.

Rigbolt, K.T., J.T. Vanselow, and B. Blagoev. 2011. GProX, a User-Friendly Platform for Bioinformatics Analysis and Visualization of Quantitative Proteomics Data. *Molecular & cellular proteomics : MCP*. 10:O110 007450.

Ross, P.L., Y.N. Huang, J.N. Marchese, B. Williamson, K. Parker, S. Hattan, N. Khainovski, S. Pillai, S. Dey, S. Daniels, S. Purkayastha, P. Juhasz, S. Martin, M. Bartlet-Jones, F. He, A. Jacobson, and D.J. Pappin. 2004. Multiplexed protein quantitation in Saccharomyces cerevisiae using amine-reactive isobaric tagging reagents. *Molecular & cellular proteomics : MCP*. 3:1154-1169.

Roth, L., E. Koncina, S. Satkauskas, G. Cremel, D. Aunis, and D. Bagnard. 2009. The many faces of semaphorins: from development to pathology. *Cell. Mol. Life Sci.* 66:649-666.

Sallese, M., M. Giannotta, and A. Luini. 2009. Coordination of the secretory compartments via inter-organelle signalling. *Semin. Cell Dev. Biol.* 20:801-809.

Sango, K., A. Tokashiki, K. Ajiki, M. Horie, H. Kawano, K. Watabe, H. Horie, and T. Kadoya. 2004. Synthesis, localization and externalization of galectin-1 in mature dorsal root ganglion neurons and Schwann cells. *Eur. J. Neurosci.* 19:55-64.

Schulze, W.X., and M. Mann. 2004. A novel proteomic screen for peptide-protein interactions. *The Journal of biological chemistry*. 279:10756-10764.

Schulze, W.X., and B. Usadel. 2010. Quantitation in mass-spectrometry-based proteomics. *Annual review of plant biology*. 61:491-516.

Serini, G., F. Maione, E. Giraudo, and F. Bussolino. 2009. Semaphorins and tumor angiogenesis. *Angiogenesis*. 12:187-193.

Skalnikova, H., J. Motlik, S.J. Gadher, and H. Kovarova. 2011. Mapping of the secretome of primary isolates of mammalian cells, stem cells and derived cell lines. *Proteomics*. 11:691-708.

Soufi, B., C. Kumar, F. Gnad, M. Mann, I. Mijakovic, and B. Macek. 2010. Stable isotope labeling by amino acids in cell culture (SILAC) applied to quantitative proteomics of Bacillus subtilis. *Journal of proteome research*. 9:3638-3646.

Strating, J.R., and G.J. Martens. 2009. The p24 family and selective transport processes at the ER-Golgi interface. *Biol. Cell.* 101:495-509.

Suzuki, K., A. Kumanogoh, and H. Kikutani. 2008. Semaphorins and their receptors in immune cell interactions. *Nat. Immunol.* 9:17-23.

Tamagnone, L., and S. Giordano. 2006. Semaphorin pathways orchestrate osteogenesis. *Nat. Cell Biol.* 8:545-547.

Tatsumi, R., Y. Sankoda, J.E. Anderson, Y. Sato, W. Mizunoya, N. Shimizu, T. Suzuki, M. Yamada, R.P. Rhoads, Jr., Y. Ikeuchi, and R.E. Allen. 2009. Possible implication of satellite cells in regenerative motoneuritogenesis: HGF upregulates neural chemorepellent Sema3A during myogenic differentiation. *Am J Physiol Cell Physiol.* 297:C238-252.

Thery, C., L. Zitvogel, and S. Amigorena. 2002. Exosomes: composition, biogenesis and function. *Nature reviews. Immunology.* 2:569-579.

Tian, Q., S.B. Stepaniants, M. Mao, L. Weng, M.C. Feetham, M.J. Doyle, E.C. Yi, H. Dai, V. Thorsson, J. Eng, D. Goodlett, J.P. Berger, B. Gunter, P.S. Linseley, R.B. Stoughton, R. Aebersold, S.J. Collins, W.A. Hanlon, and L.E. Hood. 2004. Integrated genomic and proteomic analyses of gene expression in Mammalian cells. *Mol Cell Proteomics.* 3:960-969.

Unlu, M., M.E. Morgan, and J.S. Minden. 1997. Difference gel electrophoresis: a single gel method for detecting changes in protein extracts. *Electrophoresis.* 18:2071-2077.

Walsh, K. 2009. Adipokines, myokines and cardiovascular disease. *Circ. J.* 73:13-18.

Walther, T.C., and M. Mann. 2010. Mass spectrometry-based proteomics in cell biology. *The Journal of cell biology.* 190:491-500.

Wasinger, V.C., S.J. Cordwell, A. Cerpa-Poljak, J.X. Yan, A.A. Gooley, M.R. Wilkins, M.W. Duncan, R. Harris, K.L. Williams, and I. Humphery-Smith. 1995. Progress with gene-product mapping of the Mollicutes: Mycoplasma genitalium. *Electrophoresis.* 16:1090-1094.

Wu, C.C., M.J. MacCoss, K.E. Howell, D.E. Matthews, and J.R. Yates, 3rd. 2004. Metabolic labeling of mammalian organisms with stable isotopes for quantitative proteomic analysis. *Anal Chem.* 76:4951-4959.

Wu, H., X. Wang, S. Liu, Y. Wu, T. Zhao, X. Chen, L. Zhu, Y. Wu, X. Ding, X. Peng, J. Yuan, X. Wang, W. Fan, and M. Fan. 2007. Sema4C participates in myogenic differentiation in vivo and in vitro through the p38 MAPK pathway. *Eur. J. Cell Biol.* 86:331-344.

Yazdani, U., and J.R. Terman. 2006. The semaphorins. *Genome Biol.* 7:211.

Yi, E.C., X.J. Li, K. Cooke, H. Lee, B. Raught, A. Page, V. Aneliunas, P. Hieter, D.R. Goodlett, and R. Aebersold. 2005. Increased quantitative proteome coverage with (13)C/(12)C-based, acid-cleavable isotope-coded affinity tag reagent and modified data acquisition scheme. *Proteomics.* 5:380-387.

Yoon, J.H., K. Yea, J. Kim, Y.S. Choi, S. Park, H. Lee, C.S. Lee, P.G. Suh, and S.H. Ryu. 2009. Comparative proteomic analysis of the insulin-induced L6 myotube secretome. *Proteomics.* 9:51-60.

Zhou, Y., R.A. Gunput, and R.J. Pasterkamp. 2008. Semaphorin signaling: progress made and promises ahead. *Trends Biochem. Sci.* 33:161-170.

Zielinska, D.F., F. Gnad, J.R. Wisniewski, and M. Mann. 2010. Precision mapping of an in vivo N-glycoproteome reveals rigid topological and sequence constraints. *Cell.* 141:897-907.

19

Proteomic Analysis of Plasma Membrane Proteins in an *In Vitro* Blood-Brain Barrier Model

Sophie Duban-Deweer, Johan Hachani, Barbara Deracinois, Roméo Cecchelli, Christophe Flahaut and Yannis Karamanos
Laboratoire de Physiopathologie de la Barrière Hémato-Encéphalique, Université d'Artois, Lens
France

1. Introduction

Although several cell types have important regulatory roles in the induction and maintenance of a properly functioning blood-brain barrier (BBB) [Abbott et al., 2006; Armulik et al., 2010], it is clear that brain capillary endothelial cells (BCECs) constitute the barrier *per se* in histological terms. In the central nervous system's blood vessels, BCECs are closely interconnected by tight junctions and form a continuous, circular tube lining the basal membrane in which pericytes are embedded. The basal membrane surface is itself covered by a continuous sleeve of astrocyte endfeet (Fig. 1). The BBB is one of the most important physiological structures in the maintenance of brain homeostasis.

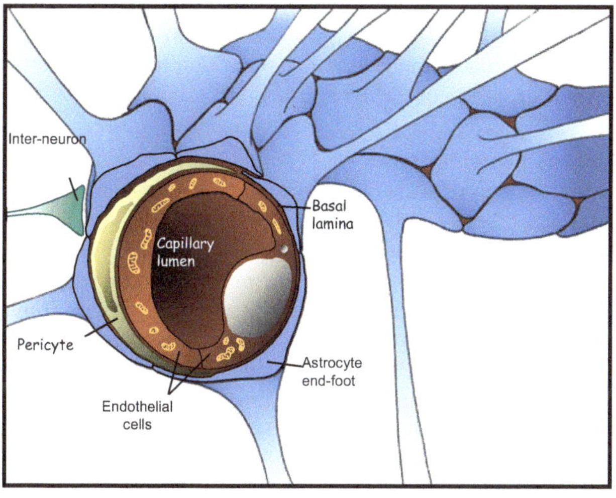

Fig. 1. Brain capillary endothelial cells constitute the core of the BBB. The endothelial cells are surrounded by a tubular sheath of astrocyte end-feet. Pericytes are embedded in the basal lamina (between the endothelium and the astrocyte end-feet). Reprinted from [Pottiez et al., 2009a], with permission from Elsevier).

The BBB is a dynamic, regulatory interface that controls the molecular and cellular exchanges between the bloodstream and the brain compartment [Abbott et al., 2010]. The BCECs' barrier function depends on the acquisition and maintenance of characteristic features (referred to as the "BBB phenotype"), such as the absence of endothelial fenestrae, decrease in the number of endocytosis vesicles, the reinforcement of tight junctions and changes in the expression pattern of certain proteins. Overall, these physiological characteristics condition cell polarisation and permeation, transendothelial electrical resistance and a number of metabolic, receptor-based and transport functions. The latter mainly rely on the properties of the BCECs' plasma membrane (PM). Relevant information regarding the lipid composition of the whole cell and of the apical and basolateral PMs has been reported [Tewes & Galla, 2001]. The latter authors demonstrated that each PM shows a unique lipid composition; the apical PM is enriched in phosphatidylcholine, whereas the basolateral PM is enriched in sphingomyelin and glucosylceramide. It has also been observed that co-culture with glioma C6 cells is able to induce a more *in vivo*-like fatty acid pattern in BCEC-based BBB models, although the intensity of these changes did not reach *in vivo* levels [Kramer et al., 2002]. Given the vital physiological functions performed by membrane lipids this aspect merits further investigation. In contrast, the PM's protein moieties have been extensively studied. The protein composition of the PM is determined by the balance between membrane protein sorting, internalization and recycling. Briefly, biosynthesized PM proteins are translocated from the endoplasmic reticulum to the Golgi apparatus, where they undergo posttranslational modifications. Proteins are then sorted to the apical or basal membrane of polarized cells. Some PM proteins are subsequently internalised and sequestrated in lysosomes and then degraded or recycled to the cell surface; endocytic adaptor proteins may have a pivotal role in this process [Howes et al., 2010; Kelly & Owen, 2011; O'Bryan, 2010; Reider & Wendland, 2011]. Plasma membrane proteins are involved in many BBB functions, including (i) cell-extracellular matrix interactions, (ii) the cell-cell junctions (especially tight junctions) that impede paracellular transport and polarise the cells, (iii) the molecular transport systems that regulate the exchange of nutrients and enable the passage of signalling molecules across the BBB and (iv) cell signalling via the expression of PM receptors [Leth-Larsen et al., 2010].

1.1 Plasma membrane proteins

Integral PM proteins are polypeptides whose particular physicochemical properties enable insertion into the lipid bilayer and interaction with both the extracellular environment and/or the intracellular compartment. In all transmembrane polypeptides examined to date, the membrane-spanning domains are α-helices or multiple β-strands. Most integral proteins span the entire phospholipid bilayer with one or more membrane domains. The domains may have as few as four amino acid residues or as many as several hundred. The integral insertion of proteins into the PM means that the side chains of buried amino acids have Van der Waals interactions with the fatty acyl chains and shield the peptide bond's polar carbonyl and imino groups. Indeed, integral proteins containing membrane-spanning α-helical domains are composed mainly of uncharged hydrophobic amino acids. These properties probably make spanning regions more resistant to proteolysis by the trypsin enzyme used in most proteomics protocols. However, hydrophobic helices are often flanked by positively charged amino acids (i.e. lysine and arginine) thought to stabilize the helix by neutralizing the helix's dipole moment and interacting with negatively charged phospholipid head groups. The second class of transmembrane proteins displays a radically different structure in which several β strands form a barrel-shaped structure with a central pore. These strands contain predominantly polar amino acids and no long hydrophobic segments. Nevertheless, the outward-facing side groups on each of the β-strands are hydrophobic and interact with the membrane lipids' fatty acyl groups, whereas the side chains facing the inside are mainly hydrophilic [Lodish et al., 2000]. Interestingly, several posttranslational modifications that do not occur in the cytosol (such as disulphide bond formation and glycosylation) enhance the stability of PM or secreted proteins prior to their exposure to the extracellular milieu. Overall, these particularities can dramatically decrease the PM proteins' sensitivity to trypsin digestion. Newly synthesized proteins can also be targeted to the PM via the covalent attachment of a lipid anchor. Indeed, some proteins bind to the PM's cytosolic surface via a covalently attached fatty acid (e.g. palmitate or myristate) or isoprene group (e.g. a farnesyl or geranyl group, whereas proteins from the PM's outer leaflet are tethered some distance out from the surface by a glycosylphosphatidylinositol (GPI) anchor [Paulick & Bertozzi, 2008].

1.2 Proteomics of the plasma membrane

Traditionally, mass spectrometry (MS)-based identification methods, chromatography and common cell biology techniques can be combined to form powerful tools for the proteomic mapping of PM proteins. Although major technical progress in MS continues to be made [Savas et al., 2011], the extraction, purification, separation and analysis of PM proteins remains problematic due to the latter's low abundance, poor solubility in aqueous solution and micro-heterogeneity [Santoni et al., 2000]. It is now clear that the development of complementary approaches is a prerequisite for the comprehensive analysis of PM proteins, including protein isolation and enrichment strategies that best preserve certain functional states and minimize the loss of transient and/or peripherally associated non-transmembrane proteins [Helbig et al., 2010], (Fig. 2). Polarized cells are present in many different organs and so their PMs have heterogeneous morphological and functional domains. Conventionally, PM proteomics can be performed with either cells cultured in suspension or adherent cells. Fig. 2 illustrates the importance of choosing the right method for the isolation of PMs and membrane sub- and microdomains and summarizes the different methods used in PM proteome analysis. The analysis can be divided into three experimental steps, all of which are challenging: (i) PM protein enrichment, (ii) separation and quantification and (iii) identification [Sprenger & Jensen, 2010].

1.3 Plasma membrane protein enrichment

Plasma membrane protein enrichment can be achieved either directly by extraction of membrane proteins or indirectly by pre-purification of the PM itself (or part of the PM) prior to proteome analysis. In view of the PM proteins' physicochemical properties, it is tempting to use of amphoteric agents (such as detergents) for enrichment. However, aqueous phase proteins will also be more soluble and may not necessarily be separated from the PM proteins. In contrast, the enrichment of membrane proteins based on two-phase partitioning (i.e. an aqueous phase and an organic phase) has been widely used and has proved its utility. The PM proteins can then be separated from aqueous proteins, due to the difference in hydrophobicity. Another way of directly studying the PM protein content involves its evaluation through its peptide fingerprinting. To this end, cell surface proteins undergo a "proteolytic shaving" procedure. The resulting peptides are purified, separated and then identified by liquid chromatography - tandem MS (LC-MS/MS). Although the proteolytic

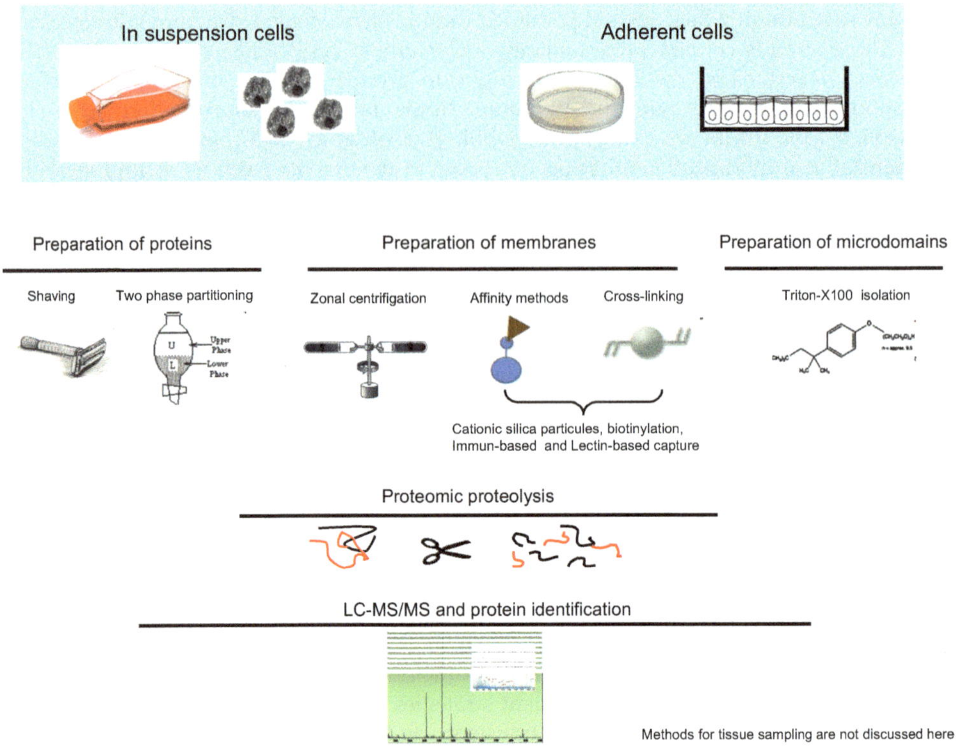

Fig. 2. A schematic drawing of complementary strategies for the comprehensive proteomic analysis of PM proteins. Approaches which best preserve certain functional states and minimize the loss of transient and/or peripherally associated non-transmembrane proteins are preferable [Helbig et al., 2010].

shaving offers many advantages in theory (because surface-exposed peptides are more water-soluble than their intrabilayer counterparts), the main drawback of this approach relates to its tendency to trigger cell lysis and thus the significant contamination of surface-exposed membrane peptides with cytosol-derived peptides. The glycosylation of PM proteins also prevents proteases from accessing the polypeptide moiety [Cordwell & Thingholm, 2010].

In view of the PM's lipid composition, membrane pre-purification and separation from soluble proteins is conventionally performed by zone centrifugation with a density gradient. Most of the PM-associated (peripheral) proteins are recovered with the integral PM protein fraction - which can constitute a drawback or an advantage. To overcome this problem, additional high-salt, high-pH washing steps can be used to form easily separable membrane sheets that lack peripheral proteins. Furthermore, plasma, mitochondrial and endoplasmic reticulum membranes all have similar densities and so membrane fractions prepared by ultracentrifugation often contain a mixture of the three [Chen et al., 2006].

In fact, the most frequently used methods for the enrichment of PMs are those based on affinity chromatography, cationic colloidal silica particles, cell biotinylation or a tissue-specific polyclonal antiserum [Agarwal & Shusta, 2009; Shusta et al., 2002]. The cell surface membrane proteins may be covalently labelled (e.g. in biotinylation) or not (e.g. with cationic silica and antibodies). The label serves as an anchor for silica bead- or magnetic bead-based separation. Loosely PM-associated proteins can always be removed by high-salt/high-pH washing [Josic & Clifton, 2007]. Similarly, the generally glycosylated PM proteins can be affinity-purified with lectin-based chromatography media [Cordwell & Thingholm, 2010].

At a higher organizational level, the topological mapping of plasma protein complexes requires the use of chemical or photo- crosslinking prior to unavoidable cell lysis, to keep them in a close-to-native state. Crosslinkers are often homo- or hetero-bifunctional agents absorbed on the cell surface [Back et al., 2003]; after chemical or photonic triggering, polymerization leads to the formation of a network that entraps PM proteins [Cordwell & Thingholm, 2010]. The proteomic needs in this field are increasing. A recent review described a new strategy and recent progress in the field of chemical cross-linking coupled to MS [Tang & Bruce, 2010].

Last but not least, membrane enrichment can be achieved by purifying microdomain components (e.g. caveolae, rafts and tetraspannin domains) enriched in the cholesterol and sphingolipids that give these cell surface structures their concave shape. This method exploits the poor solubility of membrane microstructure lipids vis-à-vis certain detergents [Zheng & Foster, 2009] (hence the term "detergent-resistant membranes"). Indeed, cholesterol- and sphingolipid-enriched membranes are insoluble in cold, non-ionic detergents (Triton X-family, NP-40, Tween, etc.) and their low buoyancy makes them amenable to purification by density gradient centrifugation. However, the main drawback of this method relates to the detergents' ability to break up protein-protein interactions. It is important to note that membrane surface labelling and affinity purification can also be used to isolate this particular protein population.

1.4 The state of the art in BBB PM proteomics

Proteomics studies of the PM in human umbilical vein endothelial cells (HUVECs) [Karsan et al., 2005; Sprenger et al., 2004] and aortic endothelial cells [Dauly et al., 2006] have been initiated in the last decade. However, the phenotypic characteristics of these types of endothelial cell (EC) differ from those of BCECs. Hence, the use of non-brain ECs in *in vitro* BBB models is subject to debate [Cecchelli et al., 2007; Prieto et al., 2004].

To date, the very few studies to have focused on BBB EC proteomics can be divided into two distinct categories. The first category is outside the scope of the present review but is mentioned here for the sake of completeness. It concerns mid- to high-throughput proteomics initiated with *in vivo* or *in vitro* cells and that seek to answer a well-defined question (e.g. to identify the broadest possible protein expression profile in the brain microvascular endothelium [Haseloff et al., 2003; Lu Q. et al., 2008; Pottiez et al., 2010]; investigate cerebral ischemia [Haqqani et al., 2007; Haqqani et al., 2005; Haseloff et al., 2006] or evaluate a differential solubility approach for the characterization of EC proteins [Lu L. et al., 2007; Murugesan et al., 2011; Pottiez et al., 2009b]. Nevertheless, some PM proteins have been identified in the course of these high-throughput studies. The second category of truly BBB-focused PM proteomic studies arose in 2008 with the work by Terasaki et al.. These researchers used the elegant principle of isotopic dilution (see [Brun et al., 2009] for a review) to achieve the absolute quantification of 34 proteins known to be of significant interest. This list of membrane transporter and receptor proteins has recently been expanded to 114, following a human brain microvessel study [Uchida et al., 2011]. In addition to studies focusing on known BBB PM proteins, an indirect method based on a multiplex expression cloning strategy after fluorescence activated cell sorting with a tissue-specific polyclonal antiserum has been developed [Agarwal & Shusta, 2009; Shusta et al., 2002]. The latter researchers identified a total of 30 BBB membrane proteins at the transcript level. Even though the expression of the corresponding gene products remains to be confirmed, these results constitute a considerable advance. Given that most PM proteins are glycosylated, the leverage of this post-translational modification for addressing PM proteins is tempting. However, large-scale glycoproteomics studies have only recently been reported. Indeed, a methodology based on hydrazine capture of membrane and secreted glycoproteins [Haqqani et al., 2011] revealed an enrichment in glycoprotein content (over 90%) and led to the identification of 23 new glycoproteins (i.e. not referenced as such in the Uniprot database). The full study results will doubtless be published soon.

1.5 Cell surface biotinylation

Chemical labelling of cell surface proteins is a novel methodology for the isolation of new target proteins. One of the major advantages of this approach is that the labelling reagent's chemical properties can be chosen to suit the biological structures that are being targeted. Cell surface biotinylation is a selective technology for the capture of PM proteins. This technology comprises several steps: (i) the selective labelling of proteins with a biotinylating reagent, (ii) the capture of biotinylated proteins with avidin-coated magnetic beads, resins etc. and (iii) elution and digestion (or, for increased specificity, digestion and elution) of the biotinylated proteins [Scheurer et al., 2005].

Using our *in vitro* BBB co-culture model [Dehouck et al., 1990], we have initiated a differential PM proteome approach that selects, separates and identifies BCEC cell surface proteins that are expressed differently in bovine BCECs with limited BBB functions versus those with re-induced BBB functions. This method is based on biotinylation of bovine BCECs' cell surface proteins with the reagent sulfosuccinimidyl-2-[biotinamido]ethyl-1,3-dithiopropionate (sulfo-NHS-SS-biotin), in which biotin is coupled to a reactive ester group. The NHS group undergoes a nucleophilic substitution reaction with the primary amines of protein amino acids (mainly lysine residues, depending on the local pH). Due to the low dissociation constant for biotin and streptavidin, the use of a cleavable spacer arm containing a disulphide bond facilitates the release of biotinylated proteins after capture on immobilized streptavidin [Elia, 2008]. Moreover, the sulfo-NHS-ester derivatives of biotin are preferable for use in PM labelling because they are more soluble in water than NHS-esters alone. This enables reactions to be performed in the absence of polar aprotic solvents and membrane permeabilizing reagents like dimethylsulfoxyde and dimethylformamide. Furthermore, the sulfo-NHS-esters are membrane-impermeable reagents, which reduces interference from cytosolic components [Daniels & Amara, 1998; Elia, 2008]. After biotinylation and hypotonic cell lysis, biotin-labelled proteins can be captured on streptavidin-coated magnetic beads and on-bead digested by trypsin. The eluted peptides are separated with nano-liquid chromatography (nano-LC) coupled to a MALDI-TOF/TOF mass spectrometer. Proteins are then identified on the basis of the MS-fragmented peptide spectra via a protein-database search with Mascot software (Matrix Science Ltd, London, UK).

2. Materials and methods

2.1 Cell culture

Bovine BCECs were isolated and characterized as described previously [Meresse et al., 1989]. Petri dishes (diameter: 100 mm) were coated with an in-house preparation of rat tail collagen (2 mg/mL) in ten-fold concentrated Dulbecco's Modified Eagle's Medium (DMEM) from GIBCO (Invitrogen Corporation, Carlsbad, CA, USA) and 0.4 M NaOH. The BCECs (4 x 10^5 cells/mL) were seeded and cultured in DMEM supplemented with 10% (v/v) heat-inactivated foetal calf serum, 10% (v/v) heat-inactivated horse serum (Hyclone Laboratories, Logan, UT, USA), 2 mM glutamine, 50 mg/mL gentamicin (Biochrome Ltd, Cambridge, UK) and 1 ng/mL basic fibroblast growth factor (GIBCO). The culture medium was refreshed every 2 days until confluence (after around 6 days, typically). Co-cultures were set in Transwell™ cell culture inserts (diameter: 100 mm; pore size: 0.4 mm; Corning Inc., New York, NY, USA) coated on the upper side with rat tail collagen. Endothelial cells were then seeded onto the inserts and transferred to a 100 mm Petri dish containing glial cells prepared according to Booher and Sensenbrenner [Booher & Sensenbrenner, 1972]. After 12 days of co-culture (in the same medium as mentioned above), the re-induction of BBB properties in the BCECs was checked by measuring the paracellular permeability coefficient of Lucifer Yellow carbohydrazide (Pe^{LY}) and by immunostaining the main tight junction proteins (occludin and claudin-5) and the associated intracellular scaffolding protein zona occludens 1 (ZO-1). Endothelial cell biotinylation and harvesting were performed after 12 days of co-culture.

2.2 Cell surface biotinylation and cell harvesting

Bovine BCEC biotinylation was performed by slightly modifying the previously reported method [Zhao et al., 2004]. Endothelial cells were washed three times with prewarmed (37°C) calcium- and magnesium-free PBS (CMF-PBS, pH 7.4) and gently shaken for 15 min at 37°C in CMF-PBS supplemented with 3 mg EZ-link sulfo-NHS-SS-biotin (Thermo Scientific, Cergy Pontoise, France) per Petri dish. The labelling reaction was quenched by adding 1 mL of 40 mM glycine in CMF-PBS, pH 8.0. Excess quenching buffer was removed by washing the cells twice in CMF-PBS.

The cells were harvested by adding collagenase type XI (*Clostridium histolyticum*, Sigma, Lyon, France) as described previously [Pottiez et al., 2009b]. Briefly, bovine BCECs were incubated for 15 min with 1.5 mL of a 0.1% w/v collagenase solution. The cell suspension was harvested, washed three times in PBS and pelleted at 500 x *g* for 5 min at 4°C. The cell pellets were stored at -80°C until protein extraction.

2.3 Preparation of biotinylated cell surface proteins

Bovine BCEC pellets were lysed with 800 µL of ice-cold hypotonic buffer [10 Mm HEPES, pH 7.5, 1.5 mM $MgCl_2$, 10 mM KCl, protease inhibitor cocktail) [Zhao et al., 2004] and incubated on ice for 30 min. The cells were lysed by dounce homogenization (50 passes) and then sonicated two times (30 W, 20 s). Unbroken cells and nuclei were pelleted from the cell homogenate by centrifugation at 1,000 x *g* for 10 min at 4 °C. Aliquots of supernatants and entire pellets were stored at -20°C prior to dot blot biotinylation control.

The KCl concentration in the supernatants was adjusted to 150 mM. An aliquot (300 µL) of streptavidin magnetic beads (10 mg beads/mL, prewashed four times with hypotonic buffer) was added to supernatants. The supernatant/bead suspensions were rotated at room temperature (RT) for 90 min and then pelleted using a magnetic plate. To obtain the biotinylated protein fraction, the resulting preparations were washed three times with 500 µL of ice-cold 1 M KCl for 15 min, three times again with 500 µL of ice-cold 0.1 M Na_2CO_3, pH 11.5 and lastly once with ice-cold hypotonic buffer for 10 min. The trypsin digestion was performed directly on the beads.

2.4 On-bead proteolysis and isolation of tryptic peptides

The on-bead proteolysis of biotinylated protein fractions was carried out overnight at 37°C in 400 µL of a proteolysis buffer containing 40 mM NH_4CO_3 (pH 8.0), 0.5 mM $CaCl_2$ and 12.5 ng/µL trypsin (Promega, Charbonnières-les-Bains, France). The enzyme reaction was stopped by heat denaturation at 100°C for 5 min. The magnetic beads were pelleted using a magnetic plate and the tryptic digest peptides were transferred into a clean microtube.

The peptides attached to the streptavidin-coupled beads were eluted from beads by means of a reduction reaction for 15 min at 60°C with 100 µL of 40 mM NH_4CO_3 (pH 8.0) containing 200 mM dithiothreitol (to disrupt the disulphide bond in the sulfo-NHS-SS-biotin). The eluate was pooled and tryptic peptides were concentrated under vacuum and immediately resolubilized in 30 µL of 0.1% TFA/10% acetonitrile/water prior to nano-LC separation.

2.5 Nano-LC-MALDI-TOF-MS/MS experiments

Separations were performed on an U3000 nano-LC system (Dionex-LC-Packings, Sunnyvale, CA, USA). After a pre-concentration step (C18 cartridge, 300 µm, 1 mm), the peptide samples were separated on a Pepmap C18 column (75 µm, 15 cm) using an acetonitrile gradient from 5% to 15% over 10 min, from 15% to 65% over 38 min and from 65% to 100% over 15 min and, lastly, 15 min in 100% acetonitrile. The flow was set to 300 nl/min and 115 fractions were automatically collected (one per 30 s) on an AnchorChip™ MALDI target using a Proteineer™ fraction collector (Bruker Daltonics, Bremen, Germany). Next, 2 µl of MALDI matrix (0.3 mg/ml α-cyano-4-hydroxycinnamic acid in acetone:ethanol:0.1% TFA-acidified water, 3:6:1 v/v/v) were added during the collection process. The MS and MS/MS measurements were performed off-line using an Ultraflex™ II TOF/TOF mass spectrometer (Bruker Daltonics) in automatic mode (using FlexControl™ 2.4 software), reflectron mode (for MALDI-TOF PMF) or LIFT mode (for MALDI-TOF/TOF peptide fragmentation fingerprint (PFF)). External calibration over the 1000-3500 mass range was performed with the $[M+H]^+$ mono-isotopic ions of bradykinins 1-7, angiotensin I, angiotensin II, substance P, bombesin and adrenocorticotropic hormone (clips 1-17 and clips 18-39) from a peptide calibration standard kit (Bruker Daltonics). Briefly, a 25 kV accelerating voltage, a 26.3 kV reflector voltage and a 160 ns pulsed ion extraction were used to obtain the MS spectrum. Each spectrum was produced by accumulating data from 500 laser shots. Peptide fragmentation was driven by Warp-LC software 1.0 (Bruker Daltonics) with the following parameters: signal-to-noise ratio > 15, more than 3 MS/MS by fraction if the MS signal was available, 0.15 Da of MS tolerance for peak merge and the elimination of peaks which appears in more than 35% of fractions. Precursor ions were accelerated to 8 kV and selected in a timed ion gate. Metastable ions generated by laser-induced decomposition were further accelerated by 19 kV in the LIFT cell and their masses were measured in reflectron mode. Peak lists were generated from MS and MS/MS spectra using Flexanalysis™ 2.4 software (Bruker Daltonics). Database searches with Mascot 2.2 (Matrix Science Ltd) using combined PMF and PFF datasets were performed in the UniProt 56.0 and 56.6 databases via ProteinScape 1.3 (Bruker Daltonics). A mass tolerance of 75 ppm and 1 missing cleavage site were allowed for PMF, with an MS/MS tolerance of 0.5 Da and 1 missing cleavage site allowed for MS/MS searching. The relevance of protein identities was judged according to the probability-based Mowse score [Perkins et al., 1999], calculated with $p < 0.05$.

2.6 Bioinformatics resources and sorting protein lists

Two FASTA sequence protein datasets were extracted from UniProt using the sequence retrieval system at the European Bioinformatics Institute [Zdobnov et al., 2002]. The first FASTA sequence dataset corresponds to the list (with 18,187 entries) of all mammalian proteins having at least one transmembrane domain (the SRS-coding criteria are as follows: [uniprot-Taxonomy:mammalia*] & [uniprot-FtKey:transmem*]). The second FASTA sequence dataset corresponds to the list (424,819 entries) of all mammalian proteins lacking transmembrane domains (the SRS-coding criteria are as follows: [uniprot-Taxonomy:mammalia*] ! [uniprot-FtKey:transmem*]). The FASTA sequence datasets were subjected to *in silico* trypsin proteolysis using Proteogest [Cagney et al., 2003] and the following command line: >perl proteogest.pl –i *filename* –c trypsin –d –a –g1.

The protein lists were compared using nwCompare software [Pont & Fournie, 2010] and classified according to the Protein Analysis Through Evolutionary Relationships (PANTHER) system [Mi et al., 2007; Thomas et al., 2003] (www.pantherdb.org). PANTHER is a resource in which genes have been functionally classified by expert biologists on the basis of published scientific experimental evidence and evolutionary relationships. Proteins are classified into families and subfamilies of shared function, which are then categorized by molecular function and biological process ontology terms.

2.7 Fluorescence microscopy

For fluorescence microscopy observations, the BCECs were biotinylated according to the above-described method, except that a non-cleavable biotinylation reagent (sulfosuccinimidyl-6-[biotinamido]-6-hexanamido hexanoate; EZ-link sulfo-NHS-LC-biotin (Thermo Scientific, Cergy Pontoise, France)) was used. Filters with BCECs were fixed for 10 min in 2% w/v paraformaldehyde at RT and washed in PBS. Biotinylated proteins were revealed by incubation with a Streptavidin-Cy3 conjugate (1:50 v/v) for 30 min. After washing with PBS, cells were incubated for 2 min with the nuclear stain Hoechst 33258 (1 µg/mL) and the filter sections were mounted in Mowiol (Merck, France). Fluorescence was visualized with a Leica DMR fluorescence microscope (Leica Microsystems, Wetzlar, Germany).

2.8 Dot blots for estimating the biotinylation efficiency

Briefly, 15 µg of proteins from pellets and supernatants were dot-blotted on a nitrocellulose membrane. The membrane was incubated in blocking buffer [5% bovine serum albumin (BSA) in 20 mM Tris-HCl, 150 mM NaCl; pH 7.5, and 0.05% Tween-20 (TBS-T)] for one hour at RT and then immersed for 30 min at RT in a solution of alkaline phosphatase-conjugated avidin (1:1000 v/v in BSA/TBS-T). After three 15-min washes with TBS-T and one 10-minute wash with TBS (20 mM Tris-HCl, 150 mM NaCl; pH 7.5), the membrane was incubated with 5-bromo-4-chloro-3-indoyl phosphate p-toluidine salt/p-nitro blue tetrazolium chloride substrate solution. The reaction was stopped by rinsing with deionised water during gentle shaking. The membrane image was acquired at 300 dpi with a Umax Scanner (Amersham Biosciences, Orsay, France) and stored in a Tagged Image File format.

3. Results and discussion

3.1 Confirmation of BBB-like properties

Once primary capillary ECs are isolated *in vitro*, they rapidly lose some of their BBB functions. The cells' barrier properties were restored by a 12-day co-culture in which bovine

BCECs were seeded on the upper side of a filter placed in a Petri box and glial cells were seeded on the underside (see the Materials and Methods for details). Re-induction of BBB properties was confirmed by the fact that Pe^{LY} for bovine BCECs with re-induced BBB functions (0.6×10^{-3} cm/min) was just over half that for cells with limited BBB functions (1.0×10^{-3} cm/min). Immunostaining also confirmed the presence and localization of the main tight junction proteins occludin and claudin-5 and the associated protein ZO-1, as described elsewhere by our group [Gosselet et al., 2009; Pottiez et al., 2009b].

3.2 Assessment of the susceptibility of BCEC membrane proteins to trypsin cleavage

Prior to MS identification, membrane proteins are usually cleaved by proteolytic enzymes. Whatever the protein studied, trypsin is often considered as the enzyme of choice for proteomics, because it (i) has a specific cleavage site (on the C-terminal side of Arg- Xaa and Lys-Xaa, except when Xaa is a Pro), (ii) generates peptides of the right length for MS (in terms of sensitivity and accuracy) because the relatively high abundance of Arg and Lys (around 6%, compared with 10% for Leu, the most life abundant amino acid) and (iii) yields peptides with positive trapped charges. Due to the hydrophobic nature of PM proteins, several improvements of trypsin-based digestion methods have been especially developed to improve trypsin accessibility to proteins of interest. Most use buffers containing organic solvents (methanol, acetone, acetonitrile, etc.) or detergents (SDS, CYMAL-5, n-octylglucoside, etc.) ([Lu X. & Zhu, 2005]; see [Josic & Clifton, 2007] for a review).
Other enzymes can also be used in this essential step in proteomics [Wu et al., 2003]. Other methods involve enzyme-free, hydrolytic cleavage using various combinations of acidic conditions, cyanogen bromide and microwave irradiation [Josic & Clifton, 2007; Zhong et al., 2005]. These enzyme-free methods cleave either specifically at methionine (with an average abundance of around 2.5%) or non-specifically at any peptide bond [Zhong et al., 2005]. Clearly, it is important to choose the right cleavage method when seeking to reduce bias and erroneous conclusions in the proteomic identification of membrane proteins.
The susceptibility of mammalian PM proteins to trypsin cleavage was assessed *in silico*. The two Uniprot FASTA sequence datasets (corresponding to all known mammalian transmembrane proteins and non-transmembrane proteins, respectively) were analysed with Proteogest software. This Perl-written software performs the *in silico* trypsin digestion of all listed proteins and lists the generated peptides according to length or isotopic mass. Expression of the results as histograms (Fig. 3) shows that the overall distribution of tryptic peptides (in terms of length or isotopic mass) is essentially the same for both datasets and suggests that the susceptibility of mammalian transmembrane proteins does not differ from that of non-transmembrane proteins.
As expected, the length-based distribution of peptides matches the isotopic mass distribution. Additionally, more than 75% of the potential trypsin-generated peptides in each dataset have fewer than 30 amino acids or an isotopic mass below 3000 atomic mass units, meaning that mass measurement or mass fragmentation will give unambiguous results. Even though between 10 and 17% of the *in silico* peptides have an isotopic mass below 500 atomic mass units, more than 50% of the potentially generated peptides are located in the optimal mass range for standard mass spectrometers.

3.3 Assessment of *in vitro* biotinylation

The efficiency of *in vitro* biotinylation with the non-cleavable reagent (EZ-link sulfo-NHS-LC-biotin) was assessed by florescence microscopy. The fluorescence pattern and intensity

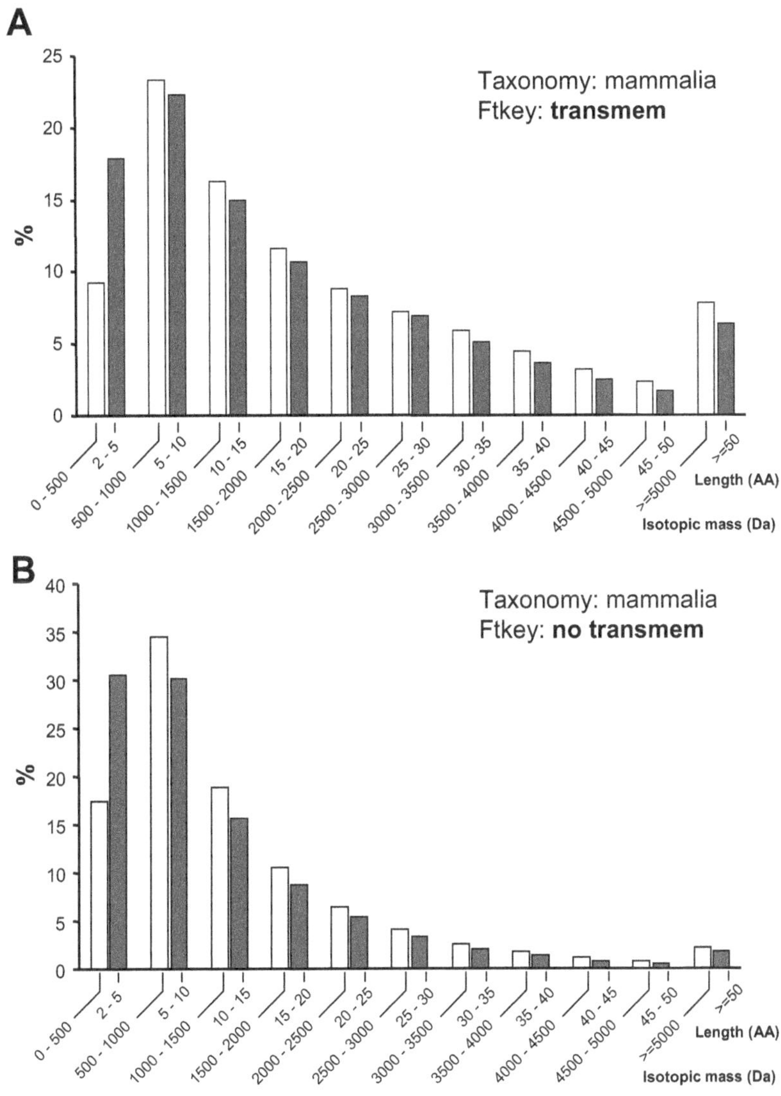

Fig. 3. Histograms of peptide counts according to the number of amino acid residues (AA) or the isotopic mass after *in silico* trypsin digestion with Proteogest [Cagney et al., 2003] of FASTA sequence datasets for (A) all mammalian proteins displaying at least one transmembrane domain (18,187 entries) and (B) all mammalian proteins lacking transmembrane domains (424,819 entries). The command line was >perl proteogest.pl –i *filename* –c trypsin –d –a –g1. The histograms show that the overall distribution of tryptic peptides (in terms of length or isotopic mass) is essentially the same in the two datasets and suggest that the trypsin susceptibility of mammalian transmembrane proteins does not significantly differ from that of non-transmembrane proteins.

did not differ significantly from one condition to another (Fig. 4) and the signal was principally located at the cell boundaries (red colour). Likewise, the EC permeabilities (deduced from the Pe^{LY} values) evolved similarly in treated and untreated cells.. Taken as a whole, these findings demonstrated that biotinylation did not affect the integrity of the BBB and did not introduce experimental bias.

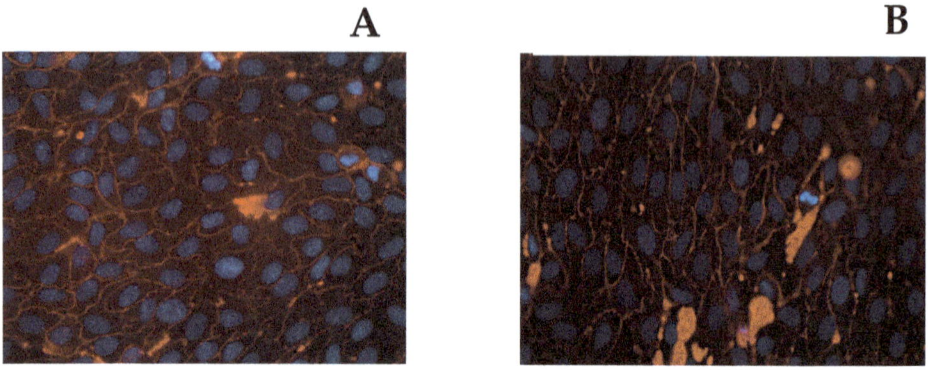

Fig. 4. Fluorescence microscopy of a bovine BCEC monolayer with limited BBB functions ("Lim. BBB", panel A) or re-induced BBB functions (Re-ind. BBB, panel B). The monolayers were biotinylated with a non-cleavable reagent (EZ-link sulfo-NHS-LC-biotin). Biotinylated proteins were revealed by incubation with a Streptavidin-Cy3 conjugate (in red), whereas nuclei were stained with Hoechst 33258 (in blue).

3.4 Nano-LC-MALDI-TOF-MS/MS maps

After *in vitro* biotinylation, adherent bovine BCECs with limited or re-induced BBB functions were detached from the extracellular matrix by collagenase treatment, in order to avoid proteolytic damage to the PM proteins. The collected cells were lysed in ice-cold hypotonic buffer and pelleted at 1,000 x *g* for 10 min at 4 °C. Biotinylated proteins in the supernatant were trapped using streptavidin-coupled magnetic beads. Elution of non-bound proteins was monitored with dot blots. Biotinylated proteins immobilised on the streptavidin-coated magnetic beads were then on-bead digested with trypsin. The resulting peptides were collected, released by reduction and concentrated prior to nano-LC-MALDI-TOF/TOF mass spectrometry analysis.
Typical chromatograms for each of the two conditions are shown in Fig. 5. As with two-dimensional gel electrophoresis, these peptide maps provide an overall, graphic representation of a sample's peptide diversity and abundance. The fact that the chromatograms for limited or re-induced BBB sample differ significantly underlines the quality of the sample preparation. Indeed, chromatograms that are too similar and/or too dense reflect inefficient labelling and purification, leading to the identification of a large set of cytosolic proteins.

3.5 Protein identification

Proteins were identified according to published guidelines [Wilkins et al., 2006] on the basis of PFF data. Briefly, the MS/MS data of all fragmented peptides were processed with the Mascot search algorithm, which compares the experimental MS/MS data to the theoretical

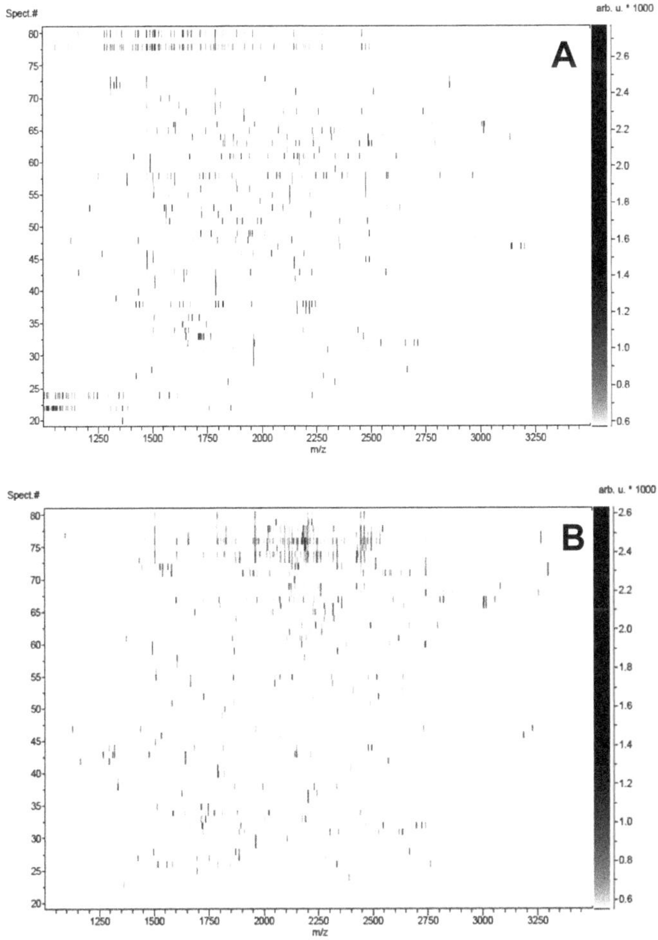

Fig. 5. Nano-LC-MALDI-TOF/TOF mass spectrometry analysis. The figure shows typical chromatograms of tryptic digests of *in vitro* biotinylated bovine BCECs monolayers with limited BBB functions (panel A) and re-induced BBB functions (panel B). The Y axis corresponds to the chromatographic retention time (expressed as a spectrum number, Spect. #), whereas the X axis displays the mass/charge (m/z) ratio of the detected peptide ions. Each peptide is characterized by its retention time (Spect. #) and molecular mass (more exactly, its isotopic distribution). Peptide abundance is grey-scale coded; the darker the signal, the more abundant the peptide.

data from the *in silico* digestion of all database-referenced proteins (or subsets of the latter). The concordance between experimental and theoretical data is then expressed as a Mascot score (-10 x log10 (p), where p is the likelihood (with 95% confidence) than the match is not due to chance). In other words, if the Mascot score for a given peptide is above the predefine threshold, the matching is not probably due to chance (and vice versa). Ultimately, the scores for each peptide matching the same protein are summed.

An illustration of the rigorousness of protein identification is shown in Fig. 6 for the sodium/potassium-transporting ATPase subunit alpha-1 precursor (AT1A1_BOVIN), a protein with 10 transmembrane domains. This catalytic subunit is located at the PM and enables creation of the electrochemical gradient required for the active transport of various nutrients. The mature form of bovine AT1A1 is composed of 1016 amino acids and has an average molecular weight of around 112 kDa. The individual identification scores of the three peptides belonging to this protein are presented in the summary box in Fig. 6. All the scores are over the chance-related threshold, demonstrating that the identification is relevant. Hence, the cumulative Mascot score of 168.6 for AT1A1 denotes unambiguous identification.

The location of the matching peptides (in bold red type) within the protein amino acid sequence shows that they are clustered in the large cytosolic region (described as "potential" in Uniprot database (aa #337 to #770)) of the Na^+/K^+-transporting ATPase subunit. Accordingly, no transmembrane domain-containing peptides served as the basis for protein identification, suggesting that the hydrophilic (i.e. cytoplasmic) regions of a given, non-denatured protein are more accessible to trypsin than their hydrophobic counterparts. Lastly, a typical MS/MS spectrum is shown in Fig. 6. The precursor ions displaying an m/z ratio of 2834.3838 atomic mass units are in-source fragmented and all the generated daughter ions had an m/z ratio below that of the parent ions. The mass differences between daughter ions allow deducing the amino acid sequence.

A typical nano-LC MS/MS analysis reported 761 fragmented peptides from samples of BCECs with limited BBB functions, whereas 957 fragmented peptides were reported for samples of BCECs with re-induced BBB functions. The efficient MS fragmentation led to the identification of 145 and 124 proteins in BCEC samples with limited and re-induced BBB functions, respectively. Sixty-three proteins were common to both conditions (Figure 7A). Following duplicate experiments on fraction-specific proteins, only 51 and 32 proteins were identified twice in BCECs with limited BBB functions and re-induced BBB functions, respectively. In all, this approach identified 211 distinct genes, of which 58 are referenced in Uniprot as coding for membrane-related proteins. Five of the 63 common proteins were PM or membrane-associated proteins, whereas 2 and 3 membrane-related proteins were identified in fraction-specific protein sets from BCECs with limited and re-induced BBB functions, respectively. Of the 15 membrane-related proteins (Figure 7B), 5 had more than one transmembrane domain (range: 2 to 17), 4 had a single transmembrane domain and 6 were lipid-anchored. Hence, the majority of membrane-related proteins were anchored to the membrane by a single domain or a lipid moiety.

3.6 Sorting protein lists

After conversion of identified proteins into their corresponding gene names via web-available bioinformatics resources, protein lists were sorted with PANTHER. The cellular locations of identified proteins (Fig. 8) were similar in the two kinds of BCEC. The protein sorting results showed that about two thirds of the identified proteins came from the cytoplasm or the PM, whereas a quarter were related to the endoplasmic reticulum, the mitochondrion, the nucleus and secreted proteins. Very few of the identified proteins belonged to the cell junction, endosome or Golgi apparatus. This ranking shows that very few proteins belonging to cytoplasm or secreted proteins (or proteins added to the cell culture medium) were recovered, despite their cellular abundance. Our findings demonstrate the efficiency of the enrichment approach used in the present study, even though only about 30 proteins came from the BCEC PM.

AT1A1_BOVIN

Sodium/potassium-transporting ATPase subunit alpha-1 precursor (EC 3.6.3.9)

Score: 168 Sequence Coverage [%]: 5.4 No. of unique Peptides: 3

MW [kDa]: 112 pI: 5. 36

m/z meas.	Δ m/z [ppm]	Score	Range	Sequence
2834.3838	-0.17	76.9	525-549	K.EQPLDEELKDAFQNAYLELGGLGER.V
1236.6960	-8.00	34.7	646-656	R.LNIPVSQVNPR.D
2464.1980	-1.80	57.0	742-764	K.QAADMILLDDNFASIVTGVEEGR.L

Matched peptides shown in **Bold Red**

451 ESALLKCIEV CCGSVKEMRE RYTKIVEIPF NSTNKYQLSI HKNANAGEPR
501 HLLVMKGAPE RILDRCSSIL IHGK**EQPLDE ELKDAFQNAY LELGGLGER**V
551 LGFCHLLLPD EQFPEGFQFD TDDVNFPVDN LCFVGLISMI DPPRAAVPDA
601 VGKCRSAGIK VIMVTGDHPI TAKAIAKGVG IISEGNETVE DIAAR**LNIPV**
651 **SQVNPR**DARA CVVHGSDLKD MTPEQLDDIL KYHTEIVFAR TSPQQKLIIV
701 EGCQRQGAIV AVTGDGVNDS PALKKADIGV AMGIAGSDVS K**QAADMILLD**
751 **DNFASIVTGV EEGR**LIFDNL KKSIAYTLTS NIPEITPFLI FIANIPLPL
801 GTVTILCIDL GTDMVPAISL AYEQAESDIM KRQPRNPQTD KLVNERLISM

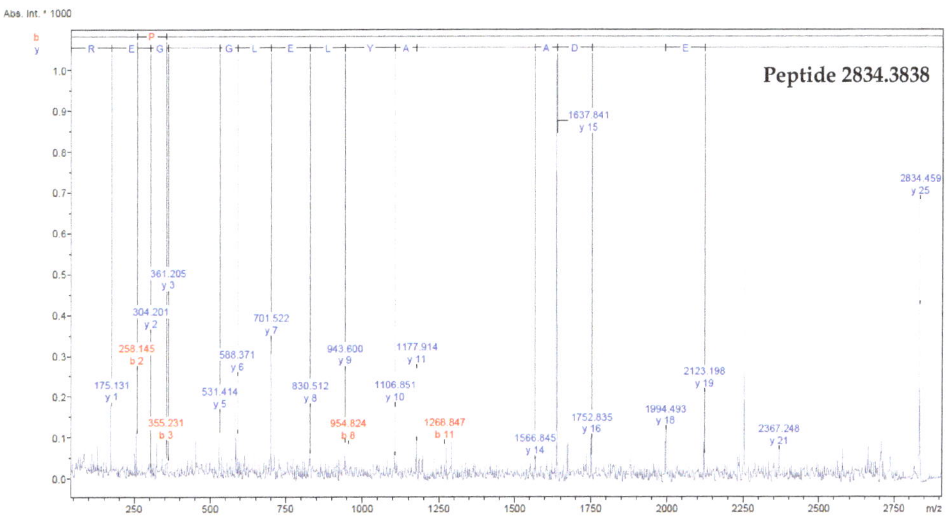

Fig. 6. Identification of AT1A1_BOVIN (sodium/potassium-transporting ATPase subunit alpha-1 precursor). The summary report describes some of the structural characteristics of the three matching peptides. The high Mascot scores correspond to an unambiguous identification. The sequences of the matching peptides are highlighted in bold red type within the AT1A1 amino acid sequence. For the sake of clarity, the amino acid sequence displayed here is truncated (ranging from amino acids #451 to #850). Lastly, the MS/MS spectrum of ionized peptides of 2834.3838 atomic mass units illustrates the amino acid sequence deduction.

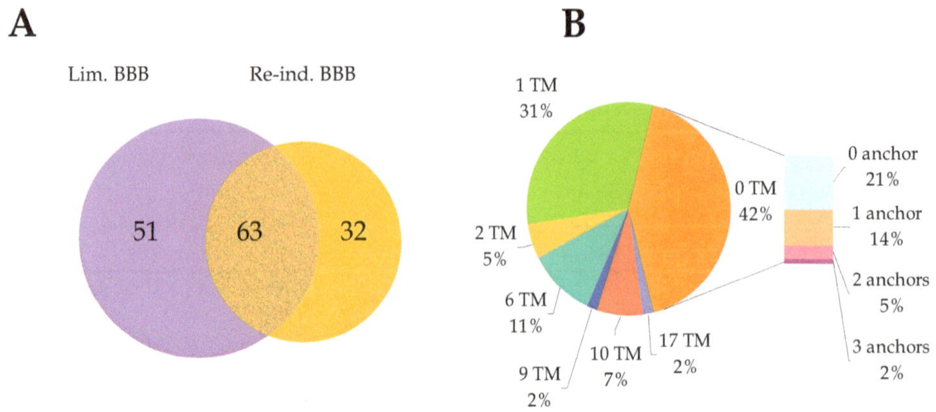

Fig. 7. Overall distribution of proteins identified using this approach. Panel A: A Venn diagram of proteins identified in BCECs with limited BBB functions and re-induced BBB functions, respectively, showing the distribution of proteins identified in both conditions and in only one condition. Panel B: The distribution of membrane-related proteins according to the number of transmembrane domains and the presence of a lipid anchor.

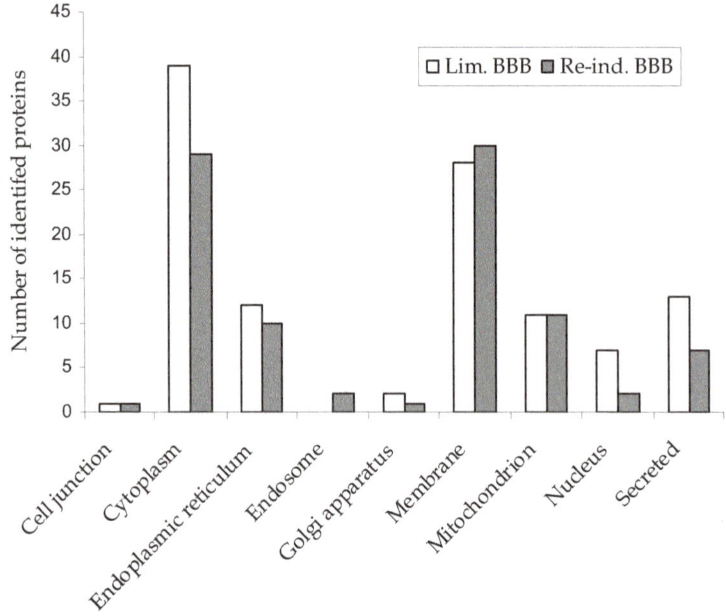

Fig. 8. Cellular location-based sorting of identified proteins. The white histogram shows the sorting results for proteins in samples of BCECs with limited BBB functions (Lim. BBB) and the grey histogram depicts the result for BCECs with re-induced BBB (Re-ind. BBB) functions. Clearly, the grey and white histograms are very similar. More than 50% of the identified proteins were related to the cytoplasm and membrane. The remaining proteins were related to the mitochondrion, the nucleus and secretory pathways.

The sorting of protein lists by molecular function is presented in Fig. 9. Proteins identified from the bovine BCECs with limited (Fig. 9A) or re-induced (Fig. 9B) BBB functions could be divided into 8 and 9 activity classes, respectively, of which 7 were common (binding, catalytic activity, enzyme regulation activity, ion channel activity, receptor activity, transporter activity and structural molecule activity). Briefly, there were twice as many proteins with catalytic or receptor activity for BCECs with re-induced BBB functions than for BCECs with limited BBB functions. In contrast, the proteins involved in binding, enzyme regulation activity and structural molecule activity were less represented (at least two fold) in BCECs with re-induced BBB functions. Interestingly, proteins displaying transcription regulation activity were only identified in BCECs with limited BBB functions; whereas lists from BCECs with re-induced BBB functions also included proteins with motor activity and antioxidant activity.

As expected for our experimental model, 59% of the 211 identified proteins were identified as bovine proteins. Indeed, certain proteins not yet reported in bovine samples were identified on the basis of inter-species sequence homologies. Given their location, this subset of proteins complements the results of our previous work, in which we used a large-scale electrophoresis- and chromatography-based approach to identify more than 430 cytoplasmic proteins [Pottiez et al., 2010]. Proteins found in both BCECs with limited and re-induced BBB functions will not be discussed further here.

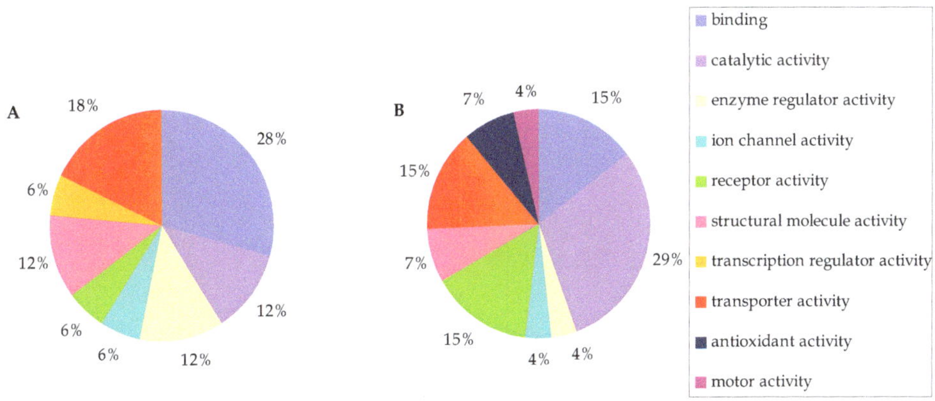

Fig. 9. Distribution of the proteins specifically identified in each condition according to their molecular function. The lists were generated under the PANTHER classification system. Proteins only identified in samples of BCECs with limited BBB function were distributed across 8 categories (Panel A), whereas those only identified in samples from BCECs with re-induced BBB functions were distributed over 9 categories (panel B).

The literature-based sorting of proteins identified in one condition only generated a lot of valuable information. A selected subset of these proteins is presented in Table 1. All of the listed proteins are found in the inner mitochondria membrane, the endoplasmic reticulum, the Golgi membrane and the vesicle membrane as well as the PM; this shows that the biotinylation reaction takes also place inside the cell, despite the experimental precautions taken. However, for the first time, we report a few PM proteins that had not previously been

Table 1.

Lim. BBB							
Protein name	Gene name [a]	Accession number [a]	pI [b]	MW (kDa) [b]	Seq. Cov. (%) [c]	Matched peptides	Biological Process
Class I histocompatibility antigen	*1b04*	P30382	5.4	40.4	7.2	2	Histocompatibility antigen
ATP-binding cassette sub-family C member 8	*Abcc8*	Q09427	9.1	177.0	1.2	2	Transport
Very long-chain specific acyl-CoA dehydrogenase	*Acadvl*	P48818	9.5	70.6	2.6	1	Lipid metabolism
Cell division control protein 42 homolog	*Cdc42*	Q2KJ93	6.2	21.2	8.9	1	Small GTPase mediated signal transduction
Cytoskeleton-associated protein 4	*Ckap4*	Q07065	5.6	66.0	2.5	1	Membrane fraction
Integrin alpha-D	*Itgad*	Q13349	5.4	126.7	2.4	2	Cell adhesion
Myosin-Ic	*Myo1c*	Q27966	9.9	121.9	4.6	3	Protein transport
Nitric oxide synthase, endothelial	*Nos3*	P29473	6.5	133.2	2.4	1	Blood vessel remodeling
Platelet endothelial cell adhesion molecule	*Pecam1*	P51866	7.0	82.5	4.7	2	Cell adhesion
Spectrin beta chain, brain	*Sptbn1*	Q01082	5.3	274.4	1.0	2	Actin filament capping

Re-ind. BBB							
Protein name	Gene name [a]	Accession number [a]	pI [b]	MW (kDa) [b]	Seq Cov (%) [c]	Matched peptides	Biological Process
Neutral cholesterol ester hydrolase 1	*Nceh1*	Q1JQE6	6.2	46.0	3.4	1	Lipid catabolic process
Dysferlin	*Dysf*	A6QQP7	5.3	237.1	0.9	1	Vesicle fusion
EH domain-containing protein	*Ehd2*	Q9NZN4	6.0	61.1	5.0	2	Endocytic recycling
Guanine nucleotide-binding protein subunit beta-2-like	*Gnb2l1*	P63243	8.9	35.1	5.0	1	Apoptosis
Moesin	*Msn*	Q2HJ49	5.8	67.9	3.6	1	Membrane to membrane docking
Myoferlin	*Myof*	Q69ZN7	5.8	233.2	0.7	1	Plasma membrane repair
Membrane-associated progesterone receptor component 1	*Pgrmc1*	Q17QC0	4.4	21.6	4.6	1	Receptor activity
1-acyl-sn-glycerol-3-phosphate acyltransferase alpha	*Agpat1*	Q95JH2	10.3	32.0	7.3	1	Phospholipid biosynthesis
Ras-related protein Rab-35	*Rab35*	Q15286	9.4	23.0	9.0	1	Protein transport
Transforming protein RhoA	*Rhoa*	P61585	5.8	21.8	8.8	1	Small GTPase mediated signal transduction
Signal peptidase complex subunit 2	*Spcs2*	Q28250	9.5	24.9	8.4	1	Signal peptide processing
Translocon-associated protein subunit delta	*Ssr4*	Q2TBX5	5.4	18.8	11.0	1	Intracellular protein transport
Transmembrane 9 superfamily member 4	*Tm9sf4*	A5D7E2	6.2	74.3	3.0	1	Cytoplasmic vesicule
Zinc transporter 1	*Slc30a1*	Q9Y6M5	6.0	55.3	3.9	1	Ion transport

a Gene name and accession number according to Uniprot. b Isoelectric point (pI) and molecular weight (MW). c Sequence coverage.

Table 1. List of identified plasma membrane proteins that were present only in solo-cultured (Lim. BBB)or in co-culured (re-ind. BBB) BCECs.

identified as such in BCECs (notably integrin alpha-D, nitric oxide synthase 3, dysferlin, myoferlin, transmembrane 9 superfamily member 4) and confirmed the presence of previously reported PM proteins (notably ATP-binding cassette sub-family C member 8, platelet endothelial cell adhesion molecule and Na^+/K^+ ATPase) [Uchida et al., 2011]. Although moesin is not a PM protein, it appears to be associated with the PM in BCECs with re-induced BBB functions (as previously reported [Pottiez et al., 2009b]).

In vivo BCECs displaying a BBB phenotype display specific endocytic trafficking that regulates (at least in part) the molecular exchanges between the blood and the brain [Abbott et al., 2010]. Interestingly, our samples from BCECs with re-induced BBB functions contained several proteins involved in cellular endocytosis, endocytic recycling, membrane trafficking and receptor internalization, such as EH domain-containing protein 2, myoferlin, dysferlin and certain cellular partners. Ferlin proteins are calcium-sensing proteins involved in vesicle trafficking and PM repair [Glover & Brown, 2007] and regulate the fusion of lipid vesicles at the PM. Myoferlin is reportedly strongly expressed in ECs and vascular tissues and was identified in a proteomics study of caveolae/lipid raft microdomains [Bernatchez et al., 2007]. Repression of myoferlin expression reduces not only lipid vesicle fusion in ECs but also protein expression levels of the vascular endothelial growth factor receptor-2 (VEGFR-2). In contrast to dysferlin, myoferlin regulates the membrane stability and function of VEGFR-2, [Sharma et al., 2010]. Dysferlin has been reported as a new marker for leaky brain blood vessels [Hochmeister et al., 2006].

Furthermore, *in vitro* myoferlin gene silencing not only decreases both clathrin- and caveolin-/raft-dependent endocytosis [Bernatchez et al., 2009] but also attenuates the expression of the angiogenic second tyrosine kinase receptor (Tie-2) [Yu et al., 2011]. In general, myoferlin appears to be critical for endocytosis events in ECs and could be a potential candidate for drug-mediated enhancement of transcytosis pathway and/or angiogenic targets. Accordingly, it has been shown that caveolin's main effect is to retain dysferlin at the cell surface [Hernandez-Deviez et al., 2008]; this inhibits the endocytosis of dysferlin through clathrin-independent pathway and therefore reinforces its PM-resealing activity. Recently, Doherty et al. have described a third interaction partner, EH domain-containing protein 2 (EHD2) [Doherty et al., 2008]. Although its role was demonstrated in myoblasts, EHD2 is an endocytic recycling protein that interacts with myoferlin to regulate lipid vesicle fusion. EHD2 binds to lipid membranes and deforms them into tubules. The protein regulates trafficking from the PM by controlling Rac1 activity [Benjamin et al., 2011] and is important for internalization of the glucose-transporter 4 (GLUT-4) [Park et al., 2004] Lastly, EHD2 is required for the translocation of a newly identified ferlin-like protein (Fer1L5) to the PM [Posey et al., 2011].

4. Conclusions

The aim of our study was to determine the distribution and the nature of PM proteins in BCECs displaying the BBB phenotype. Based in our BBB *in vitro* model, we developed a strategy for labelling these proteins (with biotin), isolating them (with streptavidin affinity chromatography) and identify them (with nano-LC MS/MS). The most frequently used methods for the enrichment of PMs are based on affinity chromatography, cationic colloidal silica particles, cell biotinylation or a tissue-specific polyclonal antiserum. We decided to use a biotinylation approach because it avoids many of the drawbacks of the other methods. For example, proteolytic shaving offers many advantages in theory (since surface-exposed peptides are more water-soluble than their intrabilayer counterparts) but is handicapped by its tendency to trigger cell lysis and thus significantly contaminate surface-exposed membrane peptides with cytosol-derived peptides.

By using the biotinylation approach, we showed that very few cytoplasmic proteins, secreted proteins or proteins added to the cell culture medium were recovered - despite their relatively high cellular abundance. We reported on the novel identification of transmembrane and membrane-associated proteins in bovine BCECs displaying the BBB phenotype. Our findings demonstrated the efficiency of the enrichment approach used, even though only about 30 proteins came from the BCEC PM. The proteins are variously involved in cellular endocytosis, membrane trafficking and receptor internalization and may thus have significant roles in BBB function. The fact that transmembrane and membrane-associated proteins accounted for less than half the identified proteins shows how difficult it still is to isolate, solubilise and digest hydrophobic proteins of low cellular abundance. Our results suggest that the specific properties of PM proteins must be taken into account when seeking to improve biotinylation, purification and identification methods. Moreover, the glycocalyx can also impede biotinylation [Ueno, 2009]. The biotinylation targeting could probably be improved by the use of new biotin derivatives that are less likely to cross the PM.

Furthermore, the present study reports the identification of several proteins involved in cellular endocytosis, membrane trafficking and receptor internalization (such as EHD2 and myoferlin), together with their cellular partners. These proteins and the pathways of which they are a part may become new targets for increasing drug transport across the BBB.

5. Acknowledgments

This research was funded by the Ministère de la Recherche et de l'Enseignement Supérieur and Oseo-Anvar. The mass spectrometry facilities used for this study were funded by the European Regional Development Fund, the Fonds d'Industrialisation des Bassins Miniers (FIBM), the Ministère de l'Education Nationale, de l'Enseignement Supérieur et de la Recherche and the Université d'Artois. We thank Dr F. Pont (INSERM, Toulouse) for his help with use of nwCompare software.

6. References

Abbott, N. J., Patabendige, A. A., Dolman, D. E., Yusof, S. R. & Begley, D. J. (2010). Structure and function of the blood-brain barrier. *Neurobiol Dis*, Vol. 37, No. 1, (Jan 2010), pp. 13-25.

Abbott, N. J., Ronnback, L. & Hansson, E. (2006). Astrocyte-endothelial interactions at the blood-brain barrier. *Nat Rev Neurosci*, Vol. 7, No. 1, (Jan 2006), pp. 41-53.

Agarwal, N.Shusta, E. V. (2009). Multiplex expression cloning of blood-brain barrier membrane proteins. *Proteomics*, Vol. 9, No. 4, (Feb 2009), pp. 1099-108, ISSN 1615-9861.

Armulik, A., Genove, G., Mae, M., Nisancioglu, M. H., Wallgard, E., Niaudet, C., He, L., Norlin, J., Lindblom, P., Strittmatter, K., Johansson, B. R. & Betsholtz, C. (2010).

Pericytes regulate the blood-brain barrier. *Nature*, Vol. 468, No. 7323, (Nov 25 2010), pp. 557-61.

Back, J. W., de Jong, L., Muijsers, A. O. & de Koster, C. G. (2003). Chemical cross-linking and mass spectrometry for protein structural modeling. *J Mol Biol*, Vol. 331, No. 2, (Aug 8 2003), pp. 303-13.

Benjamin, S., Weidberg, H., Rapaport, D., Pekar, O., Nudelman, M., Segal, D., Hirschberg, K., Katzav, S., Ehrlich, M. & Horowitz, M. (2011). EHD2 mediates trafficking from the plasma membrane by modulating Rac1 activity. *Biochem J*, Vol. No. (Jul 15 2011), pp.

Bernatchez, P. N., Acevedo, L., Fernandez-Hernando, C., Murata, T., Chalouni, C., Kim, J., Erdjument-Bromage, H., Shah, V., Gratton, J. P., McNally, E. M., Tempst, P. & Sessa, W. C. (2007). Myoferlin regulates vascular endothelial growth factor receptor-2 stability and function. *J Biol Chem*, Vol. 282, No. 42, (Oct 19 2007), pp. 30745-53.

Bernatchez, P. N., Sharma, A., Kodaman, P. & Sessa, W. C. (2009). Myoferlin is critical for endocytosis in endothelial cells. *Am J Physiol Cell Physiol*, Vol. 297, No. 3, (Sep 2009), pp. C484-92.

Booher, J.Sensenbrenner, M. (1972). Growth and cultivation of dissociated neurons and glial cells from embryonic chick, rat and human brain in flask cultures. *Neurobiology*, Vol. 2, No. 3, (n.d. 1972), pp. 97-105.

Brun, V., Masselon, C., Garin, J. & Dupuis, A. (2009). Isotope dilution strategies for absolute quantitative proteomics. *Journal of proteomics*, Vol. 72, No. 5, (Jul 21 2009), pp. 740-9, ISSN 1876-7737.

Cagney, G., Amiri, S., Premawaradena, T., Lindo, M. & Emili, A. (2003). In silico proteome analysis to facilitate proteomics experiments using mass spectrometry. *Proteome Sci*, Vol. 1, No. 1, (Aug 13 2003), pp. 5.

Cecchelli, R., Berezowski, V., Lundquist, S., Culot, M., Renftel, M., Dehouck, M. P. & Fenart, L. (2007). Modelling of the blood-brain barrier in drug discovery and development. *Nat Rev Drug Discov*, Vol. 6, No. 8, (Aug 2007), pp. 650-61.

Chen, P., Li, X., Sun, Y., Liu, Z., Cao, R., He, Q., Wang, M., Xiong, J., Xie, J., Wang, X. & Liang, S. (2006). Proteomic analysis of rat hippocampal plasma membrane: characterization of potential neuronal-specific plasma membrane proteins. *J Neurochem*, Vol. 98, No. 4, (Aug 2006), pp. 1126-40.

Cordwell, S. J.Thingholm, T. E. (2010). Technologies for plasma membrane proteomics. *Proteomics*, Vol. 10, No. 4, (Feb 2010), pp. 611-27.

Daniels, G. M.Amara, S. G. (1998). Selective labeling of neurotransmitter transporters at the cell surface. *Methods Enzymol*, Vol. 296, No. 1998), pp. 307-18.

Dauly, C., Perlman, D. H., Costello, C. E. & McComb, M. E. (2006). Protein separation and characterization by np-RP-HPLC followed by intact MALDI-TOF mass spectrometry and peptide mass mapping analyses. *J Proteome Res*, Vol. 5, No. 7, (Jul 2006), pp. 1688-700.

Dehouck, M. P., Meresse, S., Delorme, P., Fruchart, J. C. & Cecchelli, R. (1990). An easier, reproducible, and mass-production method to study the blood-brain barrier in vitro. *J Neurochem*, Vol. 54, No. 5, (May 1990), pp. 1798-1801.

Doherty, K. R., Demonbreun, A. R., Wallace, G. Q., Cave, A., Posey, A. D., Heretis, K., Pytel, P. & McNally, E. M. (2008). The endocytic recycling protein EHD2 interacts with myoferlin to regulate myoblast fusion. *J Biol Chem*, Vol. 283, No. 29, (Jul 18 2008), pp. 20252-60.

Elia, G. (2008). Biotinylation reagents for the study of cell surface proteins. *Proteomics*, Vol. 8, No. 19, (Oct 2008), pp. 4012-24.

Glover, L.Brown, R. H., Jr. (2007). Dysferlin in membrane trafficking and patch repair. *Traffic*, Vol. 8, No. 7, (Jul 2007), pp. 785-94.

Gosselet, F., Candela, P., Sevin, E., Berezowski, V., Cecchelli, R. & Fenart, L. (2009). Transcriptional profiles of receptors and transporters involved in brain cholesterol homeostasis at the blood-brain barrier: use of an in vitro model. *Brain Res*, Vol. 1249, No. (Jan 16 2009), pp. 34-42.

Haqqani, A. S., Hill, J. J., Mullen, J. & Stanimirovic, D. B. (2011). Methods to study glycoproteins at the blood-brain barrier using mass spectrometry. *Methods in molecular biology*, Vol. 686, No. (Nov 2011), pp. 337-53, ISSN 1940-6029.

Haqqani, A. S., Kelly, J., Baumann, E., Haseloff, R. F., Blasig, I. E. & Stanimirovic, D. B. (2007). Protein markers of ischemic insult in brain endothelial cells identified using 2D gel electrophoresis and ICAT-based quantitative proteomics. *Journal of proteome research*, Vol. 6, No. 1, (Jan 2007), pp. 226-39, ISSN 1535-3893.

Haqqani, A. S., Nesic, M., Preston, E., Baumann, E., Kelly, J. & Stanimirovic, D. (2005). Characterization of vascular protein expression patterns in cerebral ischemia/reperfusion using laser capture microdissection and ICAT-nanoLC-MS/MS. *The FASEB journal: official publication of the Federation of American Societies for Experimental Biology*, Vol. 19, No. 13, (Nov 2005), pp. 1809-21, ISSN 1530-6860.

Haseloff, R. F., Krause, E., Bigl, M., Mikoteit, K., Stanimirovic, D. & Blasig, I. E. (2006). Differential protein expression in brain capillary endothelial cells induced by hypoxia and posthypoxic reoxygenation. *Proteomics*, Vol. 6, No. 6, (Mar 2006), pp. 1803-9.

Haseloff, R. F., Krause, E. & Blasig, I. E. (2003). Proteomics of brain endothelium. Separation of proteins by two-dimensional gel electrophoresis and identification by mass spectrometry. *Methods Mol Med*, Vol. 89, No. (Sep 2003), pp. 465-77.

Helbig, A. O., Heck, A. J. & Slijper, M. (2010). Exploring the membrane proteome-challenges and analytical strategies. *J Proteomics*, Vol. 73, No. 5, (Mar 10 2010), pp. 868-78.

Hernandez-Deviez, D. J., Howes, M. T., Laval, S. H., Bushby, K., Hancock, J. F. & Parton, R. G. (2008). Caveolin regulates endocytosis of the muscle repair protein, dysferlin. *J Biol Chem*, Vol. 283, No. 10, (Mar 7 2008), pp. 6476-88.

Hochmeister, S., Grundtner, R., Bauer, J., Engelhardt, B., Lyck, R., Gordon, G., Korosec, T., Kutzelnigg, A., Berger, J. J., Bradl, M., Bittner, R. E. & Lassmann, H. (2006). Dysferlin is a new marker for leaky brain blood vessels in multiple sclerosis. *J Neuropathol Exp Neurol*, Vol. 65, No. 9, (Sep 2006), pp. 855-65.

Howes, M. T., Mayor, S. & Parton, R. G. (2010). Molecules, mechanisms, and cellular roles of clathrin-independent endocytosis. *Curr Opin Cell Biol*, Vol. 22, No. 4, (Aug 2010), pp. 519-27.

Josic, D.Clifton, J. G. (2007). Mammalian plasma membrane proteomics. *Proteomics*, Vol. 7, No. 16, (Aug 2007), pp. 3010-29.

Karsan, A., Blonder, J., Law, J., Yaquian, E., Lucas, D. A., Conrads, T. P. & Veenstra, T. (2005). Proteomic analysis of lipid microdomains from lipopolysaccharide-activated human endothelial cells. *J Proteome Res*, Vol. 4, No. 2, (Mar-Apr 2005), pp. 349-57.

Kelly, B. T.Owen, D. J. (2011). Endocytic sorting of transmembrane protein cargo. *Curr Opin Cell Biol*, Vol. No. (Mar 28 2011), pp.

Kramer, S. D., Schutz, Y. B., Wunderli-Allenspach, H., Abbott, N. J. & Begley, D. J. (2002). Lipids in blood-brain barrier models in vitro II: Influence of glial cells on lipid classes and lipid fatty acids. *In Vitro Cell Dev Biol Anim*, Vol. 38, No. 10, (Nov-Dec 2002), pp. 566-71.

Leth-Larsen, R., Lund, R. R. & Ditzel, H. J. (2010). Plasma membrane proteomics and its application in clinical cancer biomarker discovery. *Mol Cell Proteomics*, Vol. 9, No. 7, (Jul 2010), pp. 1369-82,

Lodish, H., Berk, A., Zipursky, S., Matsudaira, P., Baltimore, D. & Darnell, J. (2000). W. H. Freeman, New York.

Lu, L., Yang, P. Y., Rui, Y., Kang, H., Zhang, J., Zhang, J. P. & Feng, W. H. (2007). Comparative proteome analysis of rat brain and coronary microvascular endothelial cells. *Physiol Res*, Vol. 56, No. 2, (Mar 2007), pp. 159-68.

Lu, Q., Murugesan, N., Macdonald, J. A., Wu, S. L., Pachter, J. S. & Hancock, W. S. (2008). Analysis of mouse brain microvascular endothelium using immuno-laser capture microdissection coupled to a hybrid linear ion trap with Fourier transform-mass spectrometry proteomics platform. *Electrophoresis*, Vol. 29, No. 12, (Jun 2008), pp. 2689-95.

Lu, X.Zhu, H. (2005). Tube-gel digestion: a novel proteomic approach for high throughput analysis of membrane proteins. *Mol Cell Proteomics*, Vol. 4, No. 12, (Dec 2005), pp. 1948-58,

Meresse, S., Dehouck, M. P., Delorme, P., Bensaid, M., Tauber, J. P., Delbart, C., Fruchart, J. C. & Cecchelli, R. (1989). Bovine brain endothelial cells express tight junctions and monoamine oxidase activity in long-term culture. *J Neurochem*, Vol. 53, No. 5, (Nov 1989), pp. 1363-71.

Mi, H., Dong, Q., Muruganujan, A., Gaudet, P., Lewis, S. & Thomas, P. D. (2007). PANTHER version 7: improved phylogenetic trees, orthologs and collaboration with the Gene Ontology Consortium. *Nucleic Acids Res*, Vol. 38, No. Database issue, (Jan 2007), pp. D204-10.

Murugesan, N., Macdonald, J. A., Lu, Q., Wu, S. L., Hancock, W. S. & Pachter, J. S. (2011). Analysis of mouse brain microvascular endothelium using laser capture microdissection coupled with proteomics. *Methods in molecular biology*, Vol. 686, No. (Nov 2011), pp. 297-311, ISSN 1940-6029.

O'Bryan, J. P. (2010). Intersecting pathways in cell biology. *Sci Signal*, Vol. 3, No. 152, (Dec 2010), pp. re10.

Park, S. Y., Ha, B. G., Choi, G. H., Ryu, J., Kim, B., Jung, C. Y. & Lee, W. (2004). EHD2 interacts with the insulin-responsive glucose transporter (GLUT4) in rat adipocytes and may participate in insulin-induced GLUT4 recruitment. *Biochemistry*, Vol. 43, No. 23, (Jun 15 2004), pp. 7552-62.

Paulick, M. G.Bertozzi, C. R. (2008). The glycosylphosphatidylinositol anchor: a complex membrane-anchoring structure for proteins. *Biochemistry*, Vol. 47, No. 27, (Jul 8 2008), pp. 6991-7000.

Perkins, D. N., Pappin, D. J., Creasy, D. M. & Cottrell, J. S. (1999). Probability-based protein identification by searching sequence databases using mass spectrometry data. *Electrophoresis*, Vol. 20, No. 18, (Dec 1999), pp. 3551-67.

Pont, F.Fournie, J. J. (2010). Sorting protein lists with nwCompare: a simple and fast algorithm for n-way comparison of proteomic data files. *Proteomics*, Vol. 10, No. 5, (Mar 2010), pp. 1091-4.

Posey, A. D., Jr., Pytel, P., Gardikiotes, K., Demonbreun, A. R., Rainey, M., George, M., Band, H. & McNally, E. M. (2011). Endocytic recycling proteins EHD1 and EHD2 interact with fer-1-like-5 (Fer1L5) and mediate myoblast fusion. *J Biol Chem*, Vol. 286, No. 9, (Mar 4 2011), pp. 7379-88.

Pottiez, G., Deracinois, B., Duban-Deweer, S., Cecchelli, R., Fenart, L., Karamanos, Y. & Flahaut, C. (2010). A large-scale electrophoresis- and chromatography-based determination of gene expression profiles in bovine brain capillary endothelial cells after the re-induction of blood-brain barrier properties. *Proteome Sci*, Vol. 8, No. (Nov 2010), pp. 57.

Pottiez, G., Flahaut, C., Cecchelli, R. & Karamanos, Y. (2009a). Understanding the blood-brain barrier using gene and protein expression profiling technologies. *Brain Res Rev*, Vol. 62, No. 1, (Dec 11 2009a), pp. 83-98.

Pottiez, G., Sevin, E., Cecchelli, R., Karamanos, Y. & Flahaut, C. (2009b). Actin, gelsolin and filamin-A are dynamic actors in the cytoskeleton remodelling contributing to the blood brain barrier phenotype. *Proteomics*, Vol. 9, No. 5, (Mar 2009b), pp. 1207-19.

Prieto, P., Blaauboer, B. J., de Boer, A. G., Boveri, M., Cecchelli, R., Clemedson, C., Coecke, S., Forsby, A., Galla, H. J., Garberg, P., Greenwood, J., Price, A. & Tahti, H. (2004). Blood-brain barrier in vitro models and their application in toxicology. The report and recommendations of ECVAM Workshop 49. *Altern Lab Anim*, Vol. 32, No. 1, (Mar 2004), pp. 37-50.

Reider, A.Wendland, B. (2011). Endocytic adaptors - social networking at the plasma membrane. *J Cell Sci*, Vol. 124, No. Pt 10, (May 15 2011), pp. 1613-22.

Santoni, V., Molloy, M. & Rabilloud, T. (2000). Membrane proteins and proteomics: un amour impossible? *Electrophoresis*, Vol. 21, No. 6, (Apr 2000), pp. 1054-70.

Savas, J. N., Stein, B. D., Wu, C. C. & Yates, J. R., 3rd. (2011). Mass spectrometry accelerates membrane protein analysis. *Trends Biochem Sci*, Vol. No. (May 25 2011), pp.

Scheurer, S. B., Roesli, C., Neri, D. & Elia, G. (2005). A comparison of different biotinylation reagents, tryptic digestion procedures, and mass spectrometric techniques for 2-D peptide mapping of membrane proteins. *Proteomics*, Vol. 5, No. 12, (Aug 2005), pp. 3035-9.

Sharma, A., Yu, C., Leung, C., Trane, A., Lau, M., Utokaparch, S., Shaheen, F., Sheibani, N. & Bernatchez, P. (2010). A new role for the muscle repair protein dysferlin in endothelial cell adhesion and angiogenesis. *Arterioscler Thromb Vasc Biol*, Vol. 30, No. 11, (Nov 2010), pp. 2196-204.

Shusta, E. V., Boado, R. J. & Pardridge, W. M. (2002). Vascular proteomics and subtractive antibody expression cloning. *Molecular & cellular proteomics: MCP*, Vol. 1, No. 1, (Jan 2002), pp. 75-82, ISSN 1535-9476.

Sprenger, R. R.Jensen, O. N. (2010). Proteomics and the dynamic plasma membrane: Quo Vadis? *Proteomics*, Vol. 10, No. 22, (Nov 2010), pp. 3997-4011.

Sprenger, R. R., Speijer, D., Back, J. W., De Koster, C. G., Pannekoek, H. & Horrevoets, A. J. (2004). Comparative proteomics of human endothelial cell caveolae and rafts using two-dimensional gel electrophoresis and mass spectrometry. *Electrophoresis*, Vol. 25, No. 1, (Jan 2004), pp. 156-72.

Tang, X.Bruce, J. E. (2010). A new cross-linking strategy: protein interaction reporter (PIR) technology for protein-protein interaction studies. *Mol Biosyst*, Vol. 6, No. 6, (Jun 2010), pp. 939-47.

Tewes, B. J.Galla, H. J. (2001). Lipid polarity in brain capillary endothelial cells. *Endothelium*, Vol. 8, No. 3, (Feb 2001), pp. 207-20.

Thomas, P. D., Campbell, M. J., Kejariwal, A., Mi, H., Karlak, B., Daverman, R., Diemer, K., Muruganujan, A. & Narechania, A. (2003). PANTHER: a library of protein families and subfamilies indexed by function. *Genome Res*, Vol. 13, No. 9, (Sep 2003), pp. 2129-41.

Uchida, Y., Ohtsuki, S., Katsukura, Y., Ikeda, C., Suzuki, T., Kamiie, J. & Terasaki, T. (2011). Quantitative targeted absolute proteomics of human blood-brain barrier transporters and receptors. *Journal of neurochemistry*, Vol. 117, No. 2, (Apr 2011), pp. 333-45, ISSN 1471-4159.

Ueno, M. (2009). Mechanisms of the penetration of blood-borne substances into the brain. *Curr Neuropharmacol*, Vol. 7, No. 2, (Jun 2009), pp. 142-9.

Wilkins, M. R., Appel, R. D., Van Eyk, J. E., Chung, M. C., Gorg, A., Hecker, M., Huber, L. A., Langen, H., Link, A. J., Paik, Y. K., Patterson, S. D., Pennington, S. R., Rabilloud, T., Simpson, R. J., Weiss, W. & Dunn, M. J. (2006). Guidelines for the next 10 years of proteomics. *Proteomics*, Vol. 6, No. 1, (Jan 2006), pp. 4-8.

Wu, C. C., MacCoss, M. J., Howell, K. E. & Yates, J. R., 3rd. (2003). A method for the comprehensive proteomic analysis of membrane proteins. *Nat Biotechnol*, Vol. 21, No. 5, (May 2003), pp. 532-8.

Yu, C., Sharma, A., Trane, A., Utokaparch, S., Leung, C. & Bernatchez, P. (2011). Myoferlin gene silencing decreases Tie-2 expression in vitro and angiogenesis in vivo. *Vascul Pharmacol*, Vol. No. (May 6 2011), pp.

Zdobnov, E. M., Lopez, R., Apweiler, R. & Etzold, T. (2002). The EBI SRS server-new features. *Bioinformatics*, Vol. 18, No. 8, (Aug 2002), pp. 1149-50.

Zhao, Y., Zhang, W., Kho, Y. & Zhao, Y. (2004). Proteomic analysis of integral plasma membrane proteins. *Anal Chem*, Vol. 76, No. 7, (Apr 1 2004), pp. 1817-23.

Zheng, Y. Z.Foster, L. J. (2009). Biochemical and proteomic approaches for the study of membrane microdomains. *J Proteomics*, Vol. 72, No. 1, (Feb 15 2009), pp. 12-22.

Zhong, H., Marcus, S. L. & Li, L. (2005). Microwave-assisted acid hydrolysis of proteins combined with liquid chromatography MALDI MS/MS for protein identification. *J Am Soc Mass Spectrom*, Vol. 16, No. 4, (Apr 2005), pp. 471-81.

Permissions

The contributors of this book come from diverse backgrounds, making this book a truly international effort. This book will bring forth new frontiers with its revolutionizing research information and detailed analysis of the nascent developments around the world.

We would like to thank Tsz-Kwong Man, PhD and Ricardo J. Flores, MD, for lending their expertise to make the book truly unique. They have played a crucial role in the development of this book. Without their invaluable contribution this book wouldn't have been possible. They have made vital efforts to compile up to date information on the varied aspects of this subject to make this book a valuable addition to the collection of many professionals and students.

This book was conceptualized with the vision of imparting up-to-date information and advanced data in this field. To ensure the same, a matchless editorial board was set up. Every individual on the board went through rigorous rounds of assessment to prove their worth. After which they invested a large part of their time researching and compiling the most relevant data for our readers. Conferences and sessions were held from time to time between the editorial board and the contributing authors to present the data in the most comprehensible form. The editorial team has worked tirelessly to provide valuable and valid information to help people across the globe.

Every chapter published in this book has been scrutinized by our experts. Their significance has been extensively debated. The topics covered herein carry significant findings which will fuel the growth of the discipline. They may even be implemented as practical applications or may be referred to as a beginning point for another development. Chapters in this book were first published by InTech; hereby published with permission under the Creative Commons Attribution License or equivalent.

The editorial board has been involved in producing this book since its inception. They have spent rigorous hours researching and exploring the diverse topics which have resulted in the successful publishing of this book. They have passed on their knowledge of decades through this book. To expedite this challenging task, the publisher supported the team at every step. A small team of assistant editors was also appointed to further simplify the editing procedure and attain best results for the readers.

Our editorial team has been hand-picked from every corner of the world. Their multi-ethnicity adds dynamic inputs to the discussions which result in innovative outcomes. These outcomes are then further discussed with the researchers and contributors who give their valuable feedback and opinion regarding the same. The feedback is then collaborated with the researches and they are edited in a comprehensive manner to aid the understanding of the subject.

Apart from the editorial board, the designing team has also invested a significant amount of their time in understanding the subject and creating the most relevant covers. They scrutinized every image to scout for the most suitable representation of the subject and create an appropriate cover for the book.

The publishing team has been involved in this book since its early stages. They were actively engaged in every process, be it collecting the data, connecting with the contributors or procuring relevant information. The team has been an ardent support to the editorial, designing and production team. Their endless efforts to recruit the best for this project, has resulted in the accomplishment of this book. They are a veteran in the field of academics and their pool of knowledge is as vast as their experience in printing. Their expertise and guidance has proved useful at every step. Their uncompromising quality standards have made this book an exceptional effort. Their encouragement from time to time has been an inspiration for everyone.

The publisher and the editorial board hope that this book will prove to be a valuable piece of knowledge for researchers, students, practitioners and scholars across the globe.

List of Contributors

Lepedda Antonio Junior, Zinellu Elisabetta and Formato Marilena
University of Sassari/Dipartimento di Scienze Fisiologiche, Biochimiche e Cellulari, Italy

Delfin Albert Amal Raj
Mass Spectrometry and Proteomics, Institute of Protein Biochemistry - CNR, Naples, Italy
Department of Internal Medicine, Chair of Nephrology, Faculty of Medicine, Second University of Naples, Naples, Italy

Giovambattista Capasso
Department of Internal Medicine, Chair of Nephrology, Faculty of Medicine, Second University of Naples, Naples, Italy

Immacolata Fiume and Gabriella Pocsfalvi
Mass Spectrometry and Proteomics, Institute of Protein Biochemistry - CNR, Naples, Italy

Linda Papa
Graduate Medical Education, Orlando Health, Department of Emergency Medicine
University of Florida, College of Medicine, Florida State University, College of Medicine, University of Central Florida, College of Medicine, Orlando Regional Medical Center, Orlando, Florida, USA

Peter S. Podobed, Gordon M. Kirby and Tami A. Martino
Cardiovascular Research Group, Biomedical Sciences, University of Guelph, Ontario, Canada

Mei-Ling Tsai, Shu-Hui Chen, Chih-Ching Chang and Ming-Ho Wu
National Cheng Kung University, Taiwan, Republic of China

Jone Mitxelena, Asier Fullaondo and Ana M. Zubiaga
Dept. Genetics, Physical Anthropology and Animal Physiology, University of the Basque Country, UPV/EHU, Bilbao, Spain

Nerea Osinalde and Jesus M. Arizmendi
Dept. Biochemistry and Molecular Biology, University of the Basque Country, UPV/EHU, Bilbao, Spain

Federica Dabbeni-Sala and Amit Kumar Rai
Department of Pharmacology, University of Padova, Padova

Giovanna Lippe
Department of Food Science, University of Udine, Udine, Italy

Kenneth Ka Ho Lee
Stem Cell and Regeneration Thematic Research Programme, School of Biomedical Sciences, Chinese University of Hong Kong, Shatin, N.T., Hong Kong
Joint JUN-CUHK Key Laboratories for Regenerative Medicine, Ministry of Education, JiNan University, Guangzhou, China

Mei KuenTang, Elve Chen, Yao Yao and Henry Siu Sum Lee
Stem Cell and Regeneration Thematic Research Programme, School of Biomedical Sciences, Chinese University of Hong Kong, Shatin, N.T., Hong Kong

John Yeuk-Hon Chan
Joint JUN-CUHK Key Laboratories for Regenerative Medicine, Ministry of Education, JiNan University, Guangzhou, China

Yiu Loon Chui
Department of Chemical Pathology, Sir Y.K. Pao Centre for Cancer, Prince of Wales Hospital, Chinese University of Hong Kong, Shatin, N.T., Hong Kong

Olivia Miu Yung Ngan
Department of Biology, University of Michigan, Ann Arbor, USA

Lindsey A. Miles, Nagyung Baik, Shahrzad Lighvani, William B. Kiosses and John R. Yates III
The Scripps Research Institute, USA

Nicholas M. Andronicos
CSIRO Livestock Industries, Armidale, NSW, Australia

Emily I. Chen
Stony Brook University, USA

Hongdong Bai
Veterans Administration San Diego Healthcare System, USA

Caitlin M. Parmer
Yale University, USA

Mark P. Kamps
University of California, San Diego, USA

Samir Nangia and Robert J. Parmer
Veterans Administration San Diego Healthcare System, USA
University of California, San Diego, USA

Noriko Yokoyama
State University of New York at Stony Brook, Stony Brook, New York, USA

Virgilio J. J. Cadete and Grzegorz Sawicki
University of Saskatchewan, College of Medicine, Department of Pharmacology, Canada

Yi-Jun Qi
College of Medicine, Henan University, P.R. China

Jen-Fu Chiu
College of Medicine, Shantou University and University of Hong Kong, P.R. China

Francisco José Fernández-Gómez, Susanna Schraen-Maschke and Luc Buée
Inserm UMR837 - Alzheimer & Tauopathies - Jean-Pierre Aubert Reserch Center, Université de Lille Droit & Santé, Lille, France

Isabelle Sirois, Alexey V. Pshezhetsky and Marie-Josée Hébert
Université de Montréal, Canada

Alexandra Chicheportiche, Mathieu Daynac, François D. Boussin and Marc-André Mouthon
CEA DSV iRCM SCSR, Laboratoire de Radiopathologie, F-92265 Fontenay-aux-Roses, France
INSERM, U967, F-92265 Fontenay-aux-Roses, France
Université Paris Diderot, Sorbonne Paris Cité, UMR 967, F-92265 Fontenay-aux-Roses, France
Université Paris Sud, UMR 967, F-92265 Fontenay-aux-Roses, Institut de Radiobiologie Cellulaire et Moléculaire, Fontenay-aux-Roses, France

François Chevalier, Jordane Depagne and Pascale Bertrand
CEA DSV iRCM, Plateforme de Protéomique, F-92265 Fontenay-aux-Roses, France

Florian Fröhlich, Tobias C. Walther and Romain Christiano
Yale University School of Medicine, Department of Cell Biology, USA

Bernardo A. Petriz, Jeeser A. Almeida, Mirna S. Freire, Luiz A. O. Rocha, Taia M. B. Rezende and Octavio L. Franco
Center of Proteomic and Biochemical Analyses, Postgraduate, Program in Genomic Sciences and Biotechnology, Catholic University of Brasília, Brasília-DF, Brazil

Jeanette Henningsen, Blagoy Blagoev and Irina Kratchmarova
Department of Biochemistry and Molecular Biology, University of Southern Denmark, Odense M, Denmark

Sophie Duban-Deweer, Johan Hachani, Barbara Deracinois, Roméo Cecchelli, Christophe Flahaut and Yannis Karamanos
Laboratoire de Physiopathologie de la Barrière Hémato-Encéphalique, Université d'Artois, Lens, France